Orthopaedic and Trauma Nursing

For Churchill Livingstone:

Senior Commissioning Editor: Ninette Premdas
Project Development Manager: Dinah Thom
Project Manager: Jane Dingwall
Designer: Judith Wright
Illustration Manager: Bruce Hogarth

Orthopaedic and Trauma Nursing

Edited by

Julia D Kneale BSc(Hons) RN RNT

Senior Lecturer, Department of Nursing, Faculty of Health, University of Central Lancashire, Preston, UK

Peter S Davis MBE BEd(Hons) MA CertEd DN(Lond) RGN ONC

Senior Health Lecturer, University of Nottingham, UK

Foreword by

Mary Powell OBE SRN MCSO ONC

Formerly Matron, Robert Jones and Agnes Hunt Orthopaedic Hospital, Oswestry, Shropshire, UK

SECOND EDITION

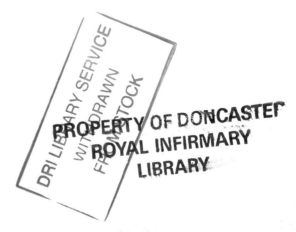

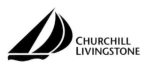

CHURCHILL LIVINGSTONE

EDINBURGH LONDON NEW YORK OXFORD PHILADELPHIA ST LOUIS SYDNEY TORONTO 2005

First edition 1994
Second edition 2005

ISBN 0 443 06182 3

British Library Cataloguing in Publication Data
A catalogue record for this book is available from the British Library

Library of Congress Cataloging in Publication Data
A catalog record for this book is available from the Library of Congress

Note
Knowledge and best practice in this field are constantly changing. As new
research and experience broaden our knowledge, changes in practice, treatment
and drug therapy may become necessary or appropriate. Readers are advised to
check the most current information provided (i) on procedures featured or (ii) by
the manufacturer of each product to be administered, to verify the recommended
dose or formula, the method and duration of administration, and contraindications.
It is the responsibility of the practitioner, relying on their own experience and
knowledge of the patient, to make diagnoses, to determine dosages and the best
treatment for each individual patient, and to take all appropriate safety
precautions. To the fullest extent of the law, neither the publisher nor the
editors assumes any liability for any injury and/or damage.

The Publisher

your source for books,
journals and multimedia
in the health sciences
www.elsevierhealth.com

The
Publisher's
policy is to use
**paper manufactured
from sustainable forests**

Printed in China

Contents

Contributors

Ann Allsworth DipHE PGC
*Clinical Nurse Specialist, Royal National Orthopaedic
Hospital, Stanmore, Middlesex, UK*

John Burden BSc RGN ONC RNT (*retired*)
*Freelance Lecturer in Orthopaedic Nursing,
Borehamwood, Herts, UK*

Michelle Cage RGN N78 ENB 997/998
*Clinical Nurse Specialist in Rheumatology, Harold
Wood Hospital, Romford, Essex, UK*

Sharon Church RGN ONC DIPN
PGDipAdvancedClinRheum
*Clinical Nurse Specialist in Rheumatology, Outpatient
Department, Harold Wood Hospital, Romford,
Essex, UK*

Jennifer Cody MSc RGN
*General Manager, Accident and Emergency
Department, Basildon Hospital, Basildon,
Essex, UK*

Peter S Davis MBE BEd(Hons) MA CertEd DN(Lond)
RGN ONC
Senior Health Lecturer, University of Nottingham, UK

Naomi Flasher RGN PGDipClinRheumNursing
*Clinical Nurse Specialist, Oldchurch Hospital,
Romford, Essex, UK*

Dinah Gould BSc MPhil PhD RGN RNT
*Professor of Applied Biology, School of Nursing, City
University, London, UK*

Julie Gregory BA(Hons) MSc RGN ONC
*Acute Pain Nurse Specialist, Royal Bolton Hospital,
Bolton, UK*

Chris Henry MSc RGN ONC FETC ENB 237
*CLIC Specialist Nurse (Cancer and Leukaemia in
Childhood) in Orthopaedic Oncology, London Bone
Tumour Service, Royal National Orthopaedic
Hospital/UCLH, Stanmore, Middlesex, UK*

Rebecca Jester BSc(Hons) PhD RN ONC DPSN RNT
*Reader in Clinical Nursing, University of West of
England, Bristol, UK*

Julia Judd RGN RSCN ENB 219/970/MSc Student
*Paediatric Orthopaedic Nurse Practitioner,
Southampton General Hospital, Southampton, UK*

Julia D Kneale BSc(Hons) RN RNT WN219
*Senior Lecturer, Department of Nursing,
Faculty of Health, University of Central Lancashire,
Preston, UK*

Christine Knight MSc SRN ONC RCNT RNT CertHealthEd
DipNurs
*Health Lecturer, Nottingham University School of
Nursing, Queen's Medical Centre, Nottingham, UK*

Christine Love RGN ONC DNCert MSc BEd(Hons)
DipN(Lon) CertEd
*Formerly Senior Lecturer in Orthopaedic Nursing,
Faculty of Health Care Sciences, St George's Hospital
Medical School, London, UK*

Brian Lucas BA(Hons) MSc PGDipHE RN ENB 219
*Orthopaedic Advanced Practice Nurse, Whipps Cross
Hospital, London, UK*

Seamus O'Brien BSc(Hons) DipN(Lond) RGN
*Outcome Assessment Manager, Outcome Assessment
Unit, Musgrave Park Hospital, Belfast, UK*

Julie Santy BSc(Hons) MSc RGN ENB 219 RNT
Lecturer, University of Hull, Hull, UK

Mike Smith MSc PGDipEd RN
Co-ordinator Masters in Clinical Nursing (Orthopaedic Stream), Lecturer, Edwin Cowan University, Perth, Australia
Staff Development Educator Centre of Nursing Evidence Based Practice, Education and Research, Royal Perth Hospital, Perth, Australia

Beverley Wellington BSc(Hons) RGN ONC DipC/N CertCNEL CertManagement (open) CertCounsellingSkills
Clinical Nurse Specialist, Victoria Infirmary, Glasgow, UK
Lecturer in Orthopaedics, University of Paisley, UK

Liz Wright RGN RSCN ENB 219/970/MSc Student
Paediatric Orthopaedic Nurse Practitioner, Southampton General Hospital, Southampton, UK

Foreword

Orthopaedic and trauma nurses can learn about their patients' conditions from the same sources as their medical colleagues, but the nursing care required by these patients is a different discipline which is admirably and ably described in the pages of this book.

There is a helpful Preface, which describes the scope of the book, stating that 'the principle focus is on the nursing care and management of the patient rather than his condition'. This approach is carried forward in the earliest chapters, which are particularly impressive and which cover a huge tapestry of nursing care.

There is a brief historical review, which leads to discussion of the changes that have influenced this specialty and the modern methods of delivering nursing care. At the same time, orthopaedic nursing theory and concepts are highlighted. The process of rehabilitation is described as returning the patient as far as possible to his normal lifestyle, and throughout the book it is rewarding to note that stress is laid on the nurse's role in prevention of complications which hinder or prevent this happy outcome.

It is perhaps invidious to mention individual chapters since each is written by an expert in his or her field and has its own message, so I shall highlight just a few. I found it rewarding to read in Chapter 5 the word 'constipation'. Patients with orthopaedic conditions who have problems with immobility are especially likely to develop this disagreeable condition. It is noticeable that many patients discharged from hospital, who because of their condition were unable to use normal toilet facilities, have no complaints regarding their treatment and care, except the discomfort due to lack of attention to this problem. It seems that patients in hospital worry more about their bowels than about their wounds.

Since the title of the book is 'Orthopaedic and Trauma Nursing' it is interesting to note the inclusion and extensive coverage of rheumatic diseases. There was a time when 'rheumatology' was regarded as part and parcel of orthopaedics, but the multidisciplinary approach to this condition caused it to be 'hived-off', and indeed the specialty has its own Forum under the aegis of the Royal College of Nursing.

Another chapter worthy of comment is Chapter 17, Osteoarthritis and Total Joint Replacements. I mention it because it could be postulated that the operations described here have done more to improve the lifestyle of more people than those of any other specialty.

Another chapter, which makes gripping reading, describes one of the most demanding of nursing activities. It is that relating to spinal cord injuries. Indeed, it should be required reading for all nurses because it recognises the fact that patients who have suffered this devastating injury are often initially received in an 'ordinary' casualty department. Early transfer to a specialist centre is strongly recommended, and suggests that, should this be delayed, advice should be sought from the staff of a specialist centre. The matter-of-fact tone of this chapter carries its own emphasis on the nursing responsibilities inherent in the care and rehabilitation of these patients.

Later chapters follow on each other until the whole gamut of nursing care of patients with neuro-muscular-skeletal conditions is described.

In conclusion, Julia Kneale and Peter Davis have done a wonderful job, not only in their own presentations but also in recruiting contributors and in collating this book. It presents orthopaedic and trauma nursing care to a depth never reached before. I am confident of its value and success.

Mary Powell OBE

Preface to the Second Edition

Musculoskeletal nursing has changed dramatically over the last 100 years. It will continue to do so in the 21st century. This book reflects current practice issues at national and local levels, as well as individual patient care.

Orthopaedic and trauma nursing are distinct in terms of the reason for admission but many of the underpinning concepts and rationales for care are the same. This book brings together the pertinent issues related to both arenas, exploring the implications for practice in a wide variety of healthcare settings and the evidence basis for clinical decisions. The arena of care is varied, resulting in more orthopaedic practitioners working across clinical areas such as acute wards, clinics, community hospitals, nursing homes and in patients' homes. These changes are reflected within the text.

This edition of *Orthopaedic and Trauma Nursing* has an accessible style and format. It is primarily aimed at qualified nurses working in a range of clinical orthopaedic and trauma-related areas. By addressing paediatric and adult nursing issues, the book will appeal to practitioners involved in the care of patients across the age spectrum. Those studying the specialty at both diploma and degree level will find it invaluable, while pre-registration students will find it a useful reference source.

The initial 12 chapters focus on nursing and practice principles that underpin orthopaedic patient care, whatever the cause of the musculoskeletal condition or injury. Chapters 1–3 set the current scene for practice in the 21st century, reviewing a variety of influences on practice, including how practice is developed and supported, changes in the setting of orthopaedic nursing care and how that care is organised. Chapter 4 explains the anatomical and physiological basis of skeletal growth, development and repair; this chapter underpins the discussions in later chapters. Chapters 5 and 6 address the principles of why patients must be encouraged to move and why and how movement should be restricted.

Fundamental issues relating to all patients are addressed throughout the book and are expanded on in specifically focused chapters. The principles of pain management, including assessment and the analgesic drugs used in musculoskeletal practice, are discussed in Chapter 7. The nutritional implications of skeletal development, injury and healing are described in Chapter 8. Chapter 9 introduces the concept of epidemiology. Recognition of the incidence and prevalence of illness and trauma is not often discussed in detail, yet recognising epidemiological influences allows environmental causes to be identified and can support the planning of healthcare provision. Chapters 10 and 11 review the causes of infection, prevention of infection and the more common skeletal infections. Chapter 12 introduces the admission process for patients through preadmission clinics and for those admitted following a trauma incident.

The principal focus of the book is on the nursing care and management of the patient rather than his or her condition. The preceding chapters set the scene for the discussion of care related to specific conditions and injuries. For ease of discussion, the second half of the book is divided into chapters focusing on specific conditions and injuries commonly seen in practice. Clinical experts involved in specific practice fields have written or been referred to in the writing of these chapters. The care of children and adolescents is a vast area of practice; the principal paediatric orthopaedic and trauma issues are addressed in

Chapter 13. Bone tumours and the nursing implications for patients with bone cancer and metastases are discussed in Chapter 14. The field of rheumatology care is addressed in Chapters 15 and 16, identifying the special needs of patients with long-term health problems. Chapter 17 covers osteoarthritis and the developments in joint replacement surgery. Spinal conditions and trauma are divided into three chapters: Chapter 18 addresses skeletal spinal conditions and injuries including disc trauma, Chapter 19 reviews osteoporosis care and Chapter 20 the nursing care of patients with an acute spinal cord injury. Chapter 21 discusses the nursing care of patients with upper limb problems and Chapter 22 the implications of nerve injuries. Pelvic and lower limb conditions and injuries are reviewed in Chapters 23 and 24 respectively. The significance of sports injuries and overuse injuries are addressed in the final two chapters.

This text provides a foundation for clinical decision making based on current knowledge and understanding. The theoretical concepts and practice applications will guide practitioners in their nursing decisions about patient care. Each chapter is supported by a comprehensive reference list, and many include additional relevant reading titles, making a valuable resource for those wanting to explore the evidence basis for practice further.

Lancashire, 2005   *Julia D Kneale*

Acknowledgements

Many friends and colleagues have contributed directly and indirectly to the production of this book. The first acknowledgement is to Peter Davis, who initiated the writing and development of this text, based on his original book *Nursing the Orthopaedic Patient*; his advice and encouragement have been invaluable.

Special thanks are owed to the contributors of the original text, whose work has been read and referred to by countless orthopaedic nurses in the last 10 years. My thanks also to all the contributors to this text – thank you for your time and efforts without which this text would not be as comprehensive. In addition our thanks go to all the orthopaedic nurses I have worked with, been inspired by and learnt from, and especially the orthopaedic students I had in mind when writing.

I particularly thank Julie Santy and Jenny Booth for their unstinting support and enthusiasm that carried me through. The encouragement of various colleagues at the University of Central Lancashire and those in practice has been tremendous, in particular Liz Walker, Sam Pollitt, Barbara Condliffe and Hilary Wallbank; thank you for your forbearance, listening and mugs of tea.

My thanks to Dinah Thom, Associate Editor with Elsevier Ltd, who has cajoled, supported and encouraged me to persevere throughout.

Finally, my thanks go to family and friends, particularly my father, Richard, and Gemma, Alistair, Linda and Peter, with whom I have not spent as much time as I would have liked.

Julia D Kneale

Chapter 1

Orthopaedic and trauma nursing

Julia D Kneale

Orthopaedic and trauma nursing is a dynamic specialty with a history of changing, often dramatically, in reaction to developments in society, healthcare provision, disease patterns technology, medical and nursing developments and, of course, patient needs. This ability to react and adapt will continue to shape the specialty in the future.

Many of the changes seen in the last 20 years have related to increased life expectancy, increased emphasis on the prevention of ill health and accidents, shorter periods of hospital care, increased community-based healthcare and changes in the multidisciplinary team in terms of roles and increased collaboration. Nursing has and will continue to adapt to these challenges.

The demographic changes have led to an increased elderly population, more of whom are fit, active and independent in their eighth and ninth decades. There are also fewer children affected by severe long-term physical disability because health problems are being identified earlier and improvements have been made in surgical and therapy techniques to correct musculoskeletal problems.

The demands, costs and provision of resources for healthcare in the public and private sectors constantly change, increasing the complexity of providing care at the appropriate time and place. This has led to the constant need to review and develop new healthcare practices. Technology such as telemedicine and digital radiographic techniques now allow patients to be treated and monitored without having to travel for several hours to a specialist centre or clinic. Future improvements in health technology will lead to more developments in these areas of health provision.

While the focus of this book is predominantly on the physical causes of ill health, readers must remember that the psychological, spiritual, cultural and social aspects of an illness are of equal and sometimes greater importance for the patient and their family. The experience and severity of a condition such as rheumatoid arthritis, or a symptom such as pain, will vary over time, in different situations and with other events occurring in the patient's life. They need to be supported when adapting to any changes caused by ill health, surgery or trauma. The orthopaedic nurse must recognise these needs and act accordingly.

The role of the family in healthcare has also changed. There are fewer extended families with homes large enough for three generations to live together. The greater movement of people nationally and internationally has led to fewer families being close enough to support each other when ill. Yet within healthcare, the family and carers are relied on and involved in patient care, especially with the increase in community-based care, although many are elderly or in full-time employment, restricting their ability to be full-time carers. Not all patients and family members are able or willing to be involved in healthcare nor are they equipped to do so and this must be respected (Footner 1997).

The speed and impact of changes in nursing can be exciting and exhilarating as the boundaries of practice are challenged. The development of evidence-based healthcare and the increased involvement of nurses in research will ensure practice remains current and relevant. All practitioners have a responsibility to keep up to date with the latest best practice evidence, research, publications and to accept being challenged by their peers, patients and others. This brings with it new challenges about how to keep up to date, the role of continuing education and lifelong learning in orthopaedic and nursing practice, which requires a questioning and enquiring approach to practice to be developed with appropriate support.

Orthopaedic and trauma nurses are involved in a wide range of specialist roles, nursing developments and collaborative working approaches. They need to understand how changes and challenges affect themselves, their peers, patients, carers and others. Specialist orthopaedic nurses are often in a prime position to lead nursing practice. The development of leadership skills must therefore be supported to ensure an appropriate approach is taken, that inspires, innovates, supports and empowers the nursing team and patients.

It is this diversity of interest, challenges and experiences which makes orthopaedic and trauma care a dynamic specialty.

HISTORICAL VIEW

The most significant and obvious change in orthopaedic nursing is seen in the derivation of the term from the Greek language, in which *orthos* means straight and *paedios* means child, the implication being that the specialty developed from the needs of children affected by crippling musculoskeletal problems. Indeed, when the first orthopaedic nurse was appointed in 1841, the majority of patients were children with congenital and developmental conditions including spinal curvatures and foot deformities (Davis 1994). The majority of orthopaedic patients are now adults with traumatic injuries and conditions related to old age.

The history of orthopaedic nursing in Britain covers the developments of nursing and medicine over the 19th and 20th centuries. The first orthopaedic hospital, now the Royal Orthopaedic Hospital, Birmingham, opened in 1871. This was well before the first preliminary training school for nurses opened in 1890. Dame Agnes Hunt (1867–1948) opened her home for crippled children in Baschurch, near Oswestry, which, with the help of Sir Robert Jones, became an orthopaedic hospital in 1900. Other hospitals continued to open across the country, leading in the 1920s to concerns about the recruitment and training of orthopaedic nurses.

Following the support of the British Orthopaedic Association and the General Nursing Council, a nationally recognised and standardised 2-year training for nurses in orthopaedic hospitals was established in 1937. This course offered a good grounding in nursing skills prior to commencing nursing or physiotherapy training. Approval was also given for a 1-year course for qualified nurses (Davis 2002) and from this point all orthopaedic courses have developed. The more recent changes in nursing education, especially the integration of nurse education into universities, have led to orthopaedic courses now being available at diploma, degree and postgraduate level in Britain.

The science and art of nursing have also evolved. The art of nursing is exemplified in the interaction between the nurse and patient. Good relationships are based on interpersonal and communication skills, and knowing when to remain quiet, sit and listen to a patient. Intuitive nursing actions develop from knowledge, skills, values and beliefs, with expert nurses developing intuitive feelings, awareness and confidence through experience (Benner 1982). These attributes enable the nurse to judge when to act and when to empower patients to take control of their own health and care (Artless & Richmond 2000). The science of nursing involves the application of knowledge and skills to specific patients' needs. Nurses need to keep pace with changes in nursing and medical knowledge and adapt to the technology involved in care. In addition, they need expert knowledge of the patient's orthopaedic condition, to understand how their needs can be met and how complications are prevented (Powell 1986).

Many aspects of the content and delivery of orthopaedic courses and the principles of care can be traced back to the vision, energy and determination of the pioneers of orthopaedic nursing (Davis 1994). These changes have paved the way for orthopaedic and trauma nursing to move from (Davis 1994):

- a medical to a nursing model of care
- an illness-focused to a health-focused approach
- viewing the patient as a disease or condition to a holistic patient-centred view of care.

Orthopaedic care will continue to evolve and develop to meet the challenges and needs of society, healthcare and patients. Orthopaedic nurses need to adapt, meet these challenges and continue to lead healthcare developments in the future. Several current influences on orthopaedic nursing are broadly discussed here: taking a health and health promotion approach, changes in the setting of orthopaedic care, the development of an evidence-based healthcare approach and leading developments in healthcare. Other influences are mentioned briefly, as they are expanded on in later chapters.

HEALTH

Health is a very individual, subjective concept; we each have our own perception of what being healthy is. This dynamic changeable state requires an ability to adapt to circumstances, including changes in quality of life and the interplay of attitudes, emotions, thoughts and feelings. Kiger (1995) discusses four dimensions of health: physical, social, mental and spiritual. These need to be in a state of balance; if one

is upset, it can lead to an imbalance in one or more of the others. For example, a rugby player with a knee injury (physical health imbalance) is unable to play as part of a team (social imbalance); the resultant lack of social interaction can cause withdrawal or depression (mental imbalance) and if immobility affects his ability to take part in all the rites and practices of his religion, a spiritual imbalance may occur.

Being healthy reflects a person's definition of health, their personal goals, expectations, age, circumstances, environment and ability to live healthily in their own terms. Other factors affecting health include lifestyle, genetics, the available health services, political and economic factors and personal health beliefs (Bright 1997).

Kiger (1995) views health as a continuum ranging from ill health due to disease to optimal health as evident in a sense of well-being. We move along this continuum in either direction at different times. The health professional's role is to enable patients to move along the continuum within the confines of their particular health expectations and potential, to achieve an optimal health state. Hence a client who is mentally well adjusted, independent, physically and socially active but who happens to have had a below-knee amputation can still achieve their optimal health despite the physical disability. Having an insight into how patients view their health is essential for understanding healing and health promotion and maximising the benefits of health education.

HEALTH TRENDS

Social, cultural and demographic changes over the last 100 years have had a dramatic impact on the provision of healthcare. The impacts on orthopaedic and trauma nursing can be seen in:

- increased life expectancy with more people living into older age, leading to more patients presenting with degenerative conditions such as osteoarthritis and osteoporosis
- changes in the workplace, causing musculo-skeletal stress injuries
- increased leisure time, resulting in sports injuries
- changes in infectious diseases with the emergence of multiresistant pathogens, the resurgence in tuberculosis and the eradication of polio in many countries

- reduction in amputations, permanent disability and death rates from traumatic injuries as a result of surgical and technological advances.

These changes will continue, requiring orthopaedic services to adjust accordingly. Understanding the influences of these trends on health enables resources to be allocated accordingly.

ILL HEALTH PREVENTION

Cohen (1997) identifies the important role orthopaedic nurses play in using their knowledge, experience and practice skills to interrupt a patient's cycle of ill health and poor health behaviours. Using a health-orientated approach to nursing practice can enable the promotion of health and prevention of ill health.

There are three accepted approaches to preventing ill health.

1 **Primary prevention**: actions taken before a disease or disability occur; this includes accident prevention, immunisation and advice on preventing sports injuries.

2 **Secondary prevention**: the early detection and treatment of health problems; for example, a nurse-led clinic for hip screening (Haugh et al 1997), bone densitometry scans and nutritional screening.

3 **Tertiary prevention**: aims to avoid the progression of ill health and potential complications, for instance by limiting further rheumatoid joint damage. Harada et al's (1995) study employed this approach when using balance and walking assessments prior to tailored exercise programmes for elderly participants. The results showed that programmes based on preventing, delaying or reversing mobility deterioration benefit the elderly by promoting independence and mobility.

HEALTH PROMOTION

Health professionals have a moral and professional responsibility to be involved in maintaining and improving the health of patients and the community. Health promotion and education based on the prevention of disease and a good quality of life is an essential aspect of orthopaedic and trauma nursing. To be effective health promoters, nurses require a broad understanding of factors influencing disease and illness, such as genetic predisposition, age, gender, economic, social and psychological

conditions, individual response and the immune system (Davis 1994).

Models of health promotion

Health promotion involves a variety of activities within and outside the hospital environment (Latter 1996, Simnett 1995). Collins (1997) proposes a model of health that relates to both an individual and a community, reflecting the personal nature of health and the broader health of a religious, geographical, cultural or societal community. The model seeks to explain a complex activity by identifying the level of health promotion activity to use in different situations. At an individual level, the model identifies five issues that interrelate and affect the health of the patient (Table 1.1), while the health needs of the community encompass four components within the model. These will differ between each person and change over time.

Whitehead (1999a) raises the debate about who is best placed to provide effective health promotion. He challenges nurses to look at health promotion from new and radical approaches rather than traditional viewpoints as these can have limited scope for long-term effectiveness. Whitehead (1999b) further suggests that most nurses adopt a medical or prevention-focused strategy rather than an empowerment-based model. This fits with the nurse being seen as an expert and places the responsibility for changing behaviours with the client but this can lead to a 'blame culture' when the patient is unable to change.

In all aspects of health promotion and education, care must be exercised to prevent value judgements, implications of criticism or removing the patient's right to choose their lifestyle. There are never any guarantees that a patient will change their health behaviours, either in the short term or permanently, although additional unexpected benefits can be found. Edwards' (1998) study of teenage girls aimed to discover their diet and exercise habits. From the results, a campaign was developed using a multiprofessional approach involving a dietician, general practice surgeries, school nurses, teachers and practice nurses. This multi-strategy approach was evaluated through a follow-up questionnaire. Overall, the girls' behaviours were not significantly improved but the campaign raised awareness of the importance of maximising peak bone mass among the wider community, including the teachers who were in a position to continue

Table 1.1   Health promotion model (Collins 1997)

Health promotion activities	Influences on orthopaedic nursing
Individual	
Psychosocial influences	• Development of the nurse–patient relationship • Provision of information and advice to reduce the stress of procedures and surgery
Microphysical environment	• Involves the patient's care environment, ward and home layout • Health and safety advice when teaching a patient to use a walking aid
Patient's background	• Relates to social class, gender, culture and education • Includes education and information on nutrition that benefits skeletal health
Patient's behaviours	• Encompasses smoking habits and participation in rehabilitation programmes • Promoting and supporting smoking cessation programmes and advice on reducing the risk of injury during exercise and leisure activities
Work situation	• Relates to health and safety practices, including ergonomics • Occupational health issues relating to moving and handling patients safely
Community	
Political and economic environment	• Involves housing policies and local health provision • Bone density screening for those at high risk of osteoporosis and hip fracture
Macrophysical environment	• Relates to food sources, air quality, road safety • Accident prevention including multiprofessional approaches to falls prevention programmes
Social justice and equity	• Would include promoting work-based health insurance, disability and social benefits • Access for all to community facilities
Community control and cohesiveness	• Involvement of the community and healthcare staff in identifying, planning and implementing community health strategies • Patient support groups, involvement in community networks, school and youth group activities

influencing health behaviours through the school curriculum.

Any health education activity needs to be complementary to the nursing and multidisciplinary team approach to care. For orthopaedic patients this usually means enabling the client to move towards self-care and empowerment in taking health decisions that lead to establishing and maintaining an optimum healthy lifestyle. It includes the prevention of ill health or further injury, enabling identification of illness as well as preventing its progression and complications.

Kiger (1995) identifies five approaches to health education, each offering positive aspects and drawbacks when planning and implementing health education for orthopaedic and trauma clients, each being appropriate for use at different times and in particular circumstances.

1 The **political action model** accepts that everyone has rights, including the right to health. People cannot always act alone to achieve this; they need support to challenge political powers or to change their environment. Examples of activities include highlighting inequalities in care, lobbying for accident prevention schemes and ensuring appropriate equipment is provided to reduce occupational injuries, including back injuries from moving patients.

2 A **media or propaganda model** aims to persuade, motivate and make people change their behaviours. It assumes the media know what is right and good for society but the media also play on the public's emotions and assumes that health is marketable. Consequently, the messages can be misleading and often have only short-lived effects because they require people to change their preferred

behaviour. This is typically seen in the need to repeat road safety and drink driving campaigns.

3 **Community models** accept that professional and lay people can work together to create change through involvement in decision making and actions. It enables and empowers people towards self and communal help through community safety and health screening programmes, for example tuberculosis screening.

4 An **information-giving or medical model** provides information based on the professional's expertise. It assumes the patient understands the information and is in a position to carry out decisions based on the facts but ignores their financial and social resources, internal motivation and ability to change behaviours permanently. This approach is authoritarian and dictatorial, so has limited permanent impact, as seen when patients are advised to exercise, stop smoking or lose weight but fail to do so.

5 The **educational model** accepts that beliefs, values and feelings influence behaviours. The aim is to lead the client towards discovery, taking opportunities as they arise to motivate, help and enable them to make decisions for themselves. The educational approach involves both emotional (affective) and intellectual (cognitive) learning, using an androgogical approach. It will not change the community resources available and may bring the client into conflict with different value systems; for example, educating a patient about exercise can engender different values and create problems about access to sports resources.

Nurses need to understand the context in which health choices are made and to take a leading role in health promotion and education. No single health promotion or health education approach, including those briefly explored here, will be ideal. These models offer an insight only into how practitioners can influence the health decisions of others and why they may or may not be effective.

CARE SETTINGS

Although musculoskeletal care mainly takes place within the acute hospital environment, orthopaedic and trauma nurses are working in a variety of healthcare settings. This has led to an increased diversity in orthopaedic nursing roles.

TRAUMA CARE

Several developments within trauma care have reduced the impact of injuries, enabling patients to reach hospital in a more stable condition (McEwan 2002) including:

- injury prevention at national, local and personal levels
- prehospital care and the training of paramedic teams
- triage both at the scene of an accident and in the accident and emergency (A & E) department
- the implementation of rapid assessment processes
- the improved management of trauma patients in hospital.

Trauma assessment courses have enabled a systematic approach to emergency care. They have also led to nurses developing their skills in identifying injuries, assessing patients and managing their emergency care within a skilled multidisciplinary team approach. Although these activities relate to the care of patients prior to their arrival on a trauma ward, they have had a great impact on the health of the trauma patient, their treatment and recovery from injury.

The trauma nurse coordinator role has facilitated the admission of patients, allowing a smoother transfer of care from one unit to another. The remit of these roles varies widely but specific advantages are seen in:

- improved communication between the A & E department and trauma wards
- reduced time spent in the A & E department, especially for elderly patients
- improved care of trauma patients admitted to non-trauma wards if the coordinator has a role in supporting the care of patients admitted to other wards
- improved communication between the operating department and trauma wards, with smoother running of trauma theatre lists, particularly when the coordinator has a role in planning theatre lists.

For trauma ward nurses, developments in medical management, especially the increased use of limb-salvaging techniques and external fixation, have led to a dramatic reduction in the use of traction. However, these have brought new nursing challenges, for example in identifying best practice in pin-site care and psychological problems relating to body image. Nursing care has changed to meet these demands.

At the other end of the patient's journey, the involvement of trauma nurses in rehabilitation is changing. More patients are referred within days of their injury or surgery to intermediate care. This has led to more patients receiving their rehabilitation care in less acute settings. Equally, trauma nurses have developed new roles that facilitate the transfer of patients into intermediate care, long-term rehabilitation or the community. Schemes linked to local nursing homes and hospital-at-home are increasing in number.

MUSCULOSKELETAL CARE

Within other areas of musculoskeletal care, other new roles are continuing to develop. More osteoporosis and rheumatology nurse specialist roles are available to support patients and practitioners. These are often both hospital and community based, some with research and specific education remits linked to local academic centres.

A prime example of practice development, now seen in most centres for orthopaedic surgery, is the use of preadmission clinics. These have facilitated the reduction in patient length of hospital stay and reduced the number of patients who have their surgery cancelled on the day of admission. Many are multidisciplinary, involving nursing, anaesthetic, physiotherapy and occupational therapy assessments of the patients. These clinics have enabled nurses to develop their skills in patient assessment, diagnostic processes and interpretation of medical investigations. In some areas, a home assessment is also completed prior to admission for surgery. These developments have ensured that patients are fitter, better prepared for their surgery, more informed about their care and, where possible, their active cooperation in treatment regimes and rehabilitation is promoted.

REHABILITATION

Rehabilitation is moving away from the traditional medical model to one that crosses professional, health, hospital, community and agency boundaries (McEwan 2002). When good rehabilitation services are provided, the patient's length of hospital stay is reduced, ensuring they spend no longer than necessary in the acute care setting.

The aim of rehabilitation is to maximise the patient's independence, physically and socially, allowing them to return to their normal place of living wherever possible. Plans for rehabilitation care begin in the preadmission clinic or on admission for a trauma patient, with many patients being transferred to intermediate care or long-term rehabilitation once recovered from the immediate effects of their trauma and surgery.

Rehabilitation care must include the cognitive and emotional aspects of recovery. Trauma patients are particularly vulnerable to psychological changes, especially an altered body image or stress from the trauma event, medical interventions, loss and bereavement. These reactions are also seen in patients following planned surgery but can be preempted; for example, patients having an external fixator for a leg-lengthening procedure are offered information, education and support through the preadmission clinic or outpatient services.

The rehabilitation environment is also changing with more patients being transferred to intermediate care in a rehabilitation unit, community hospital, elderly care unit or hospital-at-home facility. The rehabilitation setting must have an appropriate mix of nurses and therapists. The orthopaedic nurse is ideally placed to act as the coordinator of rehabilitation care (McEwan 2002) and to be the lead practitioner of the service. This change from medically led services reflects the development of practice and practitioners to meet the needs of patients and the service in the 21st century. The increase in generic healthcare worker roles has enhanced this area of care and increased the flexibility of the rehabilitation team.

COMMUNITY ROLES

The development of hospital-at-home schemes is just one of many community-based orthopaedic nursing roles. In paediatric care, the orthopaedic nurse may be involved in providing home nursing care for a child and support for parents caring for their child on traction, with an external fixator or in a hip spica. In adult care, the nurse may be involved in falls assessment, home assessments and acting as a support link between the acute care and intermediate care environments.

When at home, more patients are integrating traditional medical care with complementary therapies to alleviate their pain, increase mobility, reduce swelling, relax or provide the motivation to continue their level of activity. For some patients, these therapies are part of their lifestyle and they may forget or not realise that occasionally interactions and contraindications exist between, for instance, homeopathic remedies and medical drugs that can affect the potency and effectiveness of both forms of treatment. Orthopaedic nurses need to develop an awareness of the role these therapies may play in patient care, especially for those with long-term musculoskeletal problems.

The community aspects of orthopaedic and trauma roles are likely to develop further in the future. In particular, there is likely to be increased integration and collaboration between primary and secondary care services that will provide new avenues for orthopaedic nurses and nursing developments.

EVIDENCE-BASED HEALTHCARE

Traditionally nurses learnt their skills and nursing practices from more senior and experienced practitioners. This led to practice being primarily built on tradition and ritual. The current approach to nurse education is to foster and sustain an environment of enquiry that encourages innovation and proactive learning in both the academic and practice settings. This has led to the questioning of traditional or ritualistic practices and encouraged enquiry into the best approaches to healthcare. Consequently, more nurses are developing their awareness of how evidence relates to practice and are reviewing the evidence for decision-making and practice skills.

The types of evidence sought and identified will vary (Kneale 2000), each having its own role in influencing practice. Examples include:

- audit results: to identify urinary tract infection rates
- colleagues: to enquire how another unit manages its preadmission clinic
- literature: to review guidelines on pin-site care
- conferences and study days: to extend knowledge and share experiences
- local and national networks: to gain support and information from colleagues
- research: to review an area of practice such as wound care
- systematic reviews: to identify best practice based on research

- guidelines: to implement best practice as identified through benchmarking.

Orthopaedic nurses need to develop their skills to evaluate evidence. Included in this range of skills are literature searching, identifying and reviewing evidence, critical reading and evaluative skills. From these develop the ability to identify the value, quality, validity and reliability of different forms of evidence. The development of these skills needs to be fostered and encouraged.

Evidence of good practice is of little relevance if not applied at a strategic, local or individual level. This evidence-based approach to practice involves the integration of the evidence with clinical experience and patient choice (Sackett et al 1996). The evidence is critically reviewed in the context of current practice and if found to be relevant, is then integrated into clinical decisions. The evidence therefore does not dictate actions but informs them, ensuring individual patient needs, variations in practice and patient preferences are incorporated into the decision-making process.

As the evidence will change over time, practice must be reevaluated regularly. Being able to keep up to date is just one of the barriers to evidence-based practice that need to be addressed by strong leadership and support (Adams 2001).

DEVELOPING A RESEARCH CULTURE

Although the volume of nursing research is increasing, only a small number of orthopaedic nursing research papers are published each year. Many of these are studies carried out as part of higher degrees. Not all orthopaedic nurses want to be actively involved in developing and participating in research studies. However, every nurse has a responsibility to be aware of the results of research and other evidence that relates to their practice and to implement those findings where appropriate.

Encouraging nurses to take an active role as part of a research team allows the development and understanding of research implications (O'Brien & Davis 1997) and strategies (Box 1.1). Many of these are short-term opportunities to be involved in medically orientated research studies. They provide a positive opportunity for understanding the value and influence of research and its application to practice and allow the nurse time to decide if research is a career path they want to follow. Even if the nurse does not remain within a research role,

Box 1.1 Issues and strategies learned from involvement in research teams (from O'Brien & Davis 1997)

- Liaison with the research and development departments, audit department, research coordinator and others
- Study development:
  - Research design
  - Ethical implications
  - Ethics committee applications, role of local and multicentre research ethic committees
  - Applications for funding
  - Communication with others in the team including full-time researchers, academic support, managers, medical colleagues, general practitioners, physiotherapists, engineers, statisticians
- Study implementation:
  - Providing information on the study for practitioners, patients and others affected by the study
  - Coordinating the recruitment and randomisation of participants
  - Informed consent process
  - Data collection
  - Data analysis
  - Problem solving
- On completion:
  - Report writing
  - Dissemination and publication of findings through presentations, posters, conferences and articles

the skills learned are transferable to other areas of practice.

Developing a research culture within orthopaedic nursing is essential for the future of the specialty. Encouraging everyone with an interest in research to become active is ideal but not straightforward. All nurses need to develop their awareness of research implications; they need support and encouragement to achieve this. Managers need to view this as a normal part of staff development and education that supports practice now and in the future. Building capacity and capability in research is essential for the nursing profession (DoH 2003) but there are few orthopaedic nurses developing research-orientated careers. To encourage more research activities, there needs to be an increase in the number of orthopaedic research posts and other roles requiring the post holder to carry out primary orthopaedic nursing research.

LEADERSHIP IN PRACTICE

Effective leadership in clinical practice is one of the cornerstones of enabling healthcare to grow (DoH 2000) and is a key factor in enabling staff to face the challenges of practice (Simons 2003). However, leadership is a complex phenomenon.

Leadership must not be confused with management. Although effective managers are likely to be good leaders, not all leaders are managers. Effective leaders develop a variety of attributes, including self-awareness, recognition of their own values, beliefs and confidence, recognition of how they contribute to the workplace, their communication styles and ability to listen to and inspire others. They learn from experience, are willing to challenge, be challenged and move forwards.

Orthopaedic and trauma nurses need to lead practice, by being proactive and empowered to instigate and develop innovations (Simons 2003). Developing these attributes requires self-examination, personal development and increasing awareness of how the organisation functions. Having an understanding of the local and national political issues that impact on practice allows an effective leader to put practice developments into an organisational context; consequently they often become involved in the wider organisation rather than just their specific area of work (Simons 2003).

Networking with others is essential to develop support both within and outside the organisation; this includes identifying role models, mentors or clinical supervisors. Such networks include national and local orthopaedic associations as well as internal organisational networks of peers leading practice developments. Attending, presenting and sharing innovations in practice through study days, conferences and publications bring leaders into contact with other like-minded practitioners who can provide valuable support and be a resource in the future. Such networks are likely to include university researchers and lecturers who are involved directly or indirectly in practice developments.

An effective leader will build a successful, patient-focused team that utilises the team members' skills through support and facilitation rather than day-to-day supervision and control. They will have a vision that identifies future directions, inspires and motivates others, creating order rather than chaos, fostering and setting criteria that measure success, for example, by benchmarking progress and evaluating outcomes (Allen 1995).

Having a vision is important at both individual and organisational levels as many innovations in practice, large and small, have evolved from a vision of how practice could be. To be successful, the vision must be shared and owned by those involved who agree that it is the right way to move. Allen (1995, p41) offers some guidelines for organisations developing effective visions which are also applicable at a ward, team or individual level.

- Visions should be timeless: the vision is established with the idea that it will not be changed again, although this is unlikely as practice is constantly evolving.
- The means of achieving the vision, the goals and objectives, must be flexible to ensure the vision is accomplished.
- The vision and the means to achieve it should be based on agreed principles.
- The vision should involve all the organisation's members because it will depend on their participation if it is to be implemented successfully.

Nicholls (1994) identifies the effect of the leader on others, both collectively and individually, in relation to the environment and events. Taking an inspirational leadership approach engages others in a vision that inspires them to give their best response. A transformational leadership style engages others (Kouzes & Posner 1995), enabling them to develop beyond their current capability. Other characteristics of transformational leaders include:

- knowing each member of the team and treating them individually
- communicating with all involved at an appropriate level
- putting important issues into simple, easily understood terms
- instilling a sense of pride, respect and trust
- being careful problem solvers.

The components of this style (Box 1.2) are used within leadership courses (Simons 2003) to enable participants to identify and develop their own leadership qualities (Sheridan & Corney 2003a, b).

As transformational leaders inspire others, they also pay attention to their own concerns and developmental needs, helping them to look at new ways of thinking and learning. When their goal is achieved

---

Box 1.2 Key areas of clinical leadership (Sheridan & Corney 2003a, b)

- **Encouraging the heart:** includes recognising contributions, celebrating success, focusing on what can be achieved, being positive
- **Inspiring a shared vision:** listening to team members, stating the team's values, respecting opinions, motivating others, valuing others' ability, diversity and capability
- **Challenging the process:** developing new ways of thinking, seeking opportunities, taking risks, being proactive
- **Modelling the way:** setting an example, requires consistent value and belief systems, respect for others, welcoming criticisms, aiming for small achievements that lead to bigger successes
- **Enabling others to act:** involves enabling others, encouraging team members' contributions, feedback through performance reviews and mentorship

---

successfully, the leader may leave but their vision is still valid as the team has a sense of ownership of the project (Cacioppe 1997).

By empowering the team to excel, enabling others to change and cope with change, the leader is demonstrating leadership from inside, drawing out people's strengths and engendering trust (Kerfoot 2001). The potential leaders of the future need encouragement to develop their leadership skills as well as their practice abilities. This approach is to be applauded and encouraged within orthopaedic and trauma nursing now and in the future.

CONCLUSION

The dynamic nature of nursing, nursing education and medical care is evident in orthopaedic nursing which has a long-established history of practice challenges, innovations and developments. The challenges of meeting patients' health needs, changes in the setting of orthopaedic care and the development of an evidence-based approach to practice illustrate some of the ways in which the specialty has evolved. The pioneering orthopaedic nurses, particularly Dame Agnes Hunt and Mary Powell, have proven an inspiration to many. Current practitioners are developing similarly inspirational roles, acting as leaders of practice and encouraging others to find innovative ways of developing practice that meets patients' needs.

Experienced practitioners are able to use their knowledge of the principles of orthopaedic and trauma nursing, combined with knowledge from nursing, medical and other therapies, to ensure the delivery of clinically effective nursing, that is appropriate for the individual patient and of the highest quality. This ensures a holistic approach to care, that integrates theory, evidence and research with nursing expertise and practice.

Further reading

Audit Commission 2000 The way to go home: rehabilitation and remedial services for older people. Audit Commission, London

Evans D, Head MJ, Speller V 1994 Assuring quality in health promotion. Health Authority, London

Gillespie LD, Gillespie WJ, Robertson MC et al 2004 Interventions for preventing falls in elderly people (Cochrane review).The Cochrane Library, Issue 1. John Wiley & Sons, Chichester, UK

Heiber K 1998 Mobility health assessment. Orthopaedic Nursing 17(4): 30–35

Long AF, Kneafsey R, Ryan J, Berry J 2002 The role of the nurse within the multidisciplinary rehabilitation team. Journal of Advanced Nursing 37(1): 70–78

MacMahon D 2001 Intermediate care: a challenge to specialty of geriatric medicine or its renaissance? Age and Ageing 30 (Suppl 3): 19–23

Martin F, Oyewole A, Moloney A 1991 A randomised controlled trial of a high support hospital discharge team for elderly people. Age and Ageing 23: 228–234

Mills D, Muscari M 1998 Adolescent health: preventing sports injuries. American Journal of Nursing 98(7): 58, 60

Nazarko L 2001 Quality outcomes in rehabilitation. Nursing Management 8(2): 22–26

Rosenstock IM, Stretcher VJ, Becker MH 1988 Social learning theory and the health belief model. Health Education Quarterly 15(2): 175–183

Scriven A, Orme J 1996 Health promotion: professional perspectives. Macmillan, Basingstoke

Sheppard S, Iliffe S 2004 Hospital-at-home versus in-patient hospital care (Cochrane review). The Cochrane Library, Issue 1. John Wiley & Sons, Chichester, UK

Sidell M, Jones L, Katz J et al 1997 Debates and dilemmas in promoting health: a reader. Macmillan, Basingstoke

Steiner A 1997 Intermediate care: a conceptual framework and review of the literature. King's Fund, London

Steiner A 2001 Intermediate care: a good thing. Age and Ageing 30 (Suppl 3): 33–39

Swift CG 2001 Falls in later life and their consequences – implementing effective services. British Medical Journal 322: 855–857

Vaughan B, Lathlean J 1999 Intermediate care: model in practice. King's Fund, London

Young J 2000 Rehabilitation and older people. British Medical Journal 313: 677

References

Adams D 2001 Breaking down the barriers: perceptions of factors that influence the use of evidence in practice. Journal of Orthopaedic Nursing 5(4): 170–175

Allen R 1995 On a clear day you can have a vision: visioning model for everyone. Leadership and Organisational Development Journal 16(4): 39–44

Artless E, Richmond C 2000 The art and science of orthopaedic nursing. Journal of Orthopaedic Nursing 4(1): 4–9

Benner P 1982 From novice to expert. American Journal of Nursing 83(3): 402–407

Bright JS 1997 Health promotion in nursing practice. In: Bright JS (ed) Health promotion in clinical practice. Baillière Tindall, London

Cacioppe R 1997 Leadership moment by moment. Leadership and Organization Development Journal 18(7): 335–345

Cohen S 1997 Using a health belief model to promote increased well-being in obese patients with chronic low back pain. Journal of Orthopaedic Nursing 1(2): 89–93

Collins T 1997 Models of health: pervasive, persuasive and politically charged. In: Sidell M, Jones L, Katz J, Peberdy A (eds) Debates and dilemmas in promoting health: a reader. Macmillan, Basingstoke

Davis PS 1994 Changing orthopaedic nursing. In: Davis PS (ed) Nursing the orthopaedic patient. Churchill Livingstone, Edinburgh

Davis PS 2002 The perpetual fight for education. Journal of Orthopaedic Nursing 6(2): 62–63

Department of Health 2000 The NHS plan: a plan for invest-ment, a plan for reform. Stationery Office, London

Department of Health 2003 Towards a strategy for nursing research and development. Stationery Office, London

Edwards M 1998 Health promotion: maximising bone mass in young women. Community Practitioner 71(7/8): 256–259

Footner A 1997 It's all a question of nursing. Journal of Orthopaedic Nursing 1(4): 171–172

Harada N, Chiu V, Fowler E et al 1995 Physical therapy to improve functioning of older people in residential care facilities. Physical Therapy 75(9): 830–838

Haugh P, Trainor B, Kernohan G 1997 Nurses detecting infant hip abnormalities. Journal of Orthopaedic Nursing 1(1): 11–16

Keerfoot K 2001 Leading from the inside. Dermatology Nursing 13(1): 42, 74

Kiger AM 1995 Teaching for health, 2nd edn. Churchill Livingstone, Edinburgh

Kneale JD 2000 Evidence-based practice and orthopaedic nursing. Journal of Orthopaedic Nursing 4(1): 16–21

Kouzes J, Posner B 1995 The leadership challenge: how to get extraordinary things done in organisations. Jossey-Bass, San Francisco

Latter S 1996 The potential for health promotion in hospital nursing practice. In: Scriven A, Orme J (eds) Health promotion: professional perspectives. Macmillan, Basingstoke

McEwan Y 2002 Trauma and rehabilitation: the way forward. Journal of Orthopaedic Nursing 6(1): 2–4

Nicholls J 1994 The 'heart, head and hands' of transforming leadership. Leadership and Organisational Development Journal 15(6): 8–15

O'Brien S, Davis PS 1997 Should orthopaedic nurses only be involved in nursing research? Journal of Orthopaedic Nursing 1(1): 2–3

Powell M 1986 Orthopaedic nursing and rehabilitation, 9th edn. Churchill Livingstone, Edinburgh

Sackett DL, Rosenberg WM, Gray JA et al 1996 Evidence-based medicine: what it is and what it isn't. British Medical Journal 312(7023): 71–72

Sheridan M, Corney B 2003a Clinical leadership. Part 2 transforming leadership. Professional Nurse 18(12): 716–717

Sheridan M, Corney B 2003b Clinical leadership. Part 3 how to foster a leading role for everyone. Professional Nurse 19(1): 56–57

Simons F 2003 Clinical leadership. Part 1 key components of the programme. Professional Nurse 18(11): 656–657

Simnett I 1995 Managing health promotion: developing healthy organisations and communities. John Wiley, Chichester

Whitehead D 1999a Health promotion within an orthopaedic setting: a differing perspective. Journal of Orthopaedic Nursing 3(1): 2–4

Whitehead D 1999b The application of health promoting practice within the orthopaedic setting. Journal of Orthopaedic Nursing 3(2): 101–107

Chapter 2

The scope of care

Rebecca Jester

INTRODUCTION

As we begin the 21st century, nursing in general and orthopaedic nursing in particular continue to face the issue of constant change, not only within the profession itself but also in relation to the environments in which care takes place. This chapter seeks to set out the issues that orthopaedic nurses encounter in providing quality care for patients in a variety of primary, community and tertiary settings.

The changes in healthcare over the last decades and developments in nursing generally have led to a proliferation of specialist and advancing roles within orthopaedic and trauma nursing, including the role of nurse consultant. This chapter explores the potential impact of these changes on the environment of care, the development of new nursing roles on service provision, the implications of nurse prescribing and the requirement for nurses to develop challenging new skills in evaluating patient outcomes through patient satisfaction surveys, measures of functional outcomes and economic evaluations of new services.

CHANGES IN THE ENVIRONMENT OF CARE

Traditionally orthopaedic care has been delivered mainly within inpatient settings. In recent years, there has been a move towards the provision of orthopaedic care within community, primary and outpatient settings. This shift in emphasis aims to minimise the institutional separation of primary and secondary care, promoting seamless integrated services for patients and their families while maximising the efficient use of available resources. The major developments exemplifying the transference of responsibility from secondary to primary care are:

- early screening and preoperative assessment in primary care for elective surgery patients
- more minor surgery in general practice
- more hospital-at-home schemes
- more community hospitals offering rehabilitation and step-down services
- fewer follow-up appointments in the outpatient department
- the provision of health maintenance and health promotion services in primary care.

These developments present orthopaedic nurses and other members of the multidisciplinary team with specific challenges. Practitioners need to adapt their expertise and skills in orthopaedic care to a variety of settings, to facilitate liaison between primary and secondary care and ensure orthopaedic patients receive high-quality, evidence-based care and treatment. This chapter discusses these developments in the context of orthopaedic nursing, focusing predominantly on hospital-at-home schemes.

PREOPERATIVE ASSESSMENT IN PRIMARY CARE

Traditionally orthopaedic patients booked for elective surgery have been assessed in hospital-based preoperative assessment units. These services are often nurse led, providing an opportunity for a comprehensive assessment of the patient to ensure they are suitable for orthopaedic surgery and anaesthesia. The nurse can use the opportunity to provide detailed information for the patient and carer about the surgery and postoperative care.

The preoperative assessment normally takes place 2–4 weeks before the date of surgery (see Chapter 12 for a detailed discussion of preoperative assessment care). The timing of the preoperative assessment can mean that if significant health problems such as uncontrolled hypertension or fungal infections of the feet are found, it is too late to treat the problem effectively before the planned date of admission, leading to either postponement or cancellation of the surgery. This frequent scenario leads to bitter disappointment for the patient concerned who has often been waiting months for surgery to alleviate their severe pain and disability. In addition, it requires a 'fit' patient to be admitted at

relatively short notice in order to avoid wastage of surgery time.

To address these difficulties, as soon as a decision is made for the patient to have planned orthopaedic surgery, they need to have an early health screening to detect any significant health problems. There is then time for these problems to be treated effectively before the date of surgery, avoiding cancellation or postponement. Such early screening can be conducted in the primary care setting. Orthopaedic nurses have a significant role to play in ensuring the effectiveness of health screening and the provision of appropriate preoperative patient information at this time.

Orthopaedic liaison nurse

A specialist liaison orthopaedic nurse can lead and coordinate the assessment process and liaise between the primary and secondary care environments. The nurse is responsible for conducting an early screening assessment and identifying any deleterious health or social problems that could adversely affect the planned surgery, anaesthesia, recovery, rehabilitation or discharge plans.

The liaison nurse would communicate with the primary care team and hospital staff, to ensure the patient receives any required investigations and treatment to optimise their health status prior to surgery. If the liaison nurse continues to monitor and communicate with the patient whilst they are waiting for their surgery, the nurse would be in a position to detect any subsequent changes in the patient's health or social status and manage these appropriately.

This process will then ensure that when the patient attends the preoperative assessment clinic, there is a minimal chance of any significant factor being discovered that adversely affects the forthcoming surgery.

The Pathway model

An alternative model is a community-based 'Pathway' team comprising community nurses and social workers, with occupational therapy input. As soon as the patient is placed on the waiting list, a referral is made to the appropriate Pathway team who then contacts the patient to arrange an initial home visit and assessment. The Pathway's nurse then conducts preoperative investigations such as blood pressure recording, full blood count and Doppler assessment of vascular competence, in the patient's home. If health or social problems are detected the necessary referral and treatments are instigated.

The Pathway team liaises closely with the hospital-based preoperative assessment unit to pass on information about the progress of the patient in terms of their fitness and suitability for surgery and anaesthesia. This model supports the use of patient-held records, so when the patient attends the preoperative assessment unit, the assessing nurse has access to all previous assessment and investigation data.

A potential advantage of the Pathway model is that a member of the team can visit the patient whilst they are in hospital following their surgery and in their own home following discharge. This provides continuity of care and affords the opportunity for the patient and their family to build up a strong therapeutic relationship with the Pathway team.

Clearly, the knowledge and skills of the team must include orthopaedic, preoperative assessment, community and primary care expertise. This provides an ideal environment for sharing of skills and knowledge for orthopaedic, primary and community nurses, providing an opportunity for rotation of roles between Pathway and preoperative assessment units.

MINOR SURGERY IN GENERAL PRACTICE

The shift in emphasis toward a primary care-led health service has resulted in more minor orthopaedic surgery being carried out in general practice. Minor procedures, such as removal of ganglions or removal of wires, can be effectively managed within the primary care setting, providing a more convenient option for patients and more effective use of orthopaedic day surgery beds. Clearly, orthopaedic nurses have a role to play in helping staff in primary care to develop and implement this type of service, specifically in relation to patient information and proactive evidence-based complication prevention.

HOSPITAL-AT-HOME

In recent years there has been a proliferation of hospital-at-home (HaH) type schemes, which aim to facilitate early discharge of patients from hospital, prevent admission or provide palliative care in patients' homes. HaH may be defined as 'providing treatment that otherwise would require inpatient care, in the patient's home, always for a time limited period' (Shepperd & Illiffe 1998, p344).

A HaH can facilitate discharge for elective or trauma patients as early as 3–4 days following total joint replacement or open reduction and internal fixation of a femoral neck fracture. Clearly, this early discharge of patients has major implications for the dependency of remaining inpatients, making it necessary to review the skill mix and establishment of inpatient orthopaedic and trauma units to reflect the change in caseloads.

Such schemes provide intensive levels of care for rehabilitation of acutely ill patients in their own home, which is distinctly different from the broad range of social and nursing care provided by existing community services (Marks 1991). Unnecessary admissions to hospital are prevented by supporting patients requiring intravenous therapy such as antibiotics for late sepsis of surgical wounds or steroid therapy for exacerbation of rheumatoid arthritis in their own home.

The genesis of HaH schemes in the UK has been in part a response to:

- the dramatic reduction in the number of acute hospital beds (Vaughan 1995)
- a shift in emphasis away from tertiary to community-based healthcare (DoH 1989)
- the realisation that prolonged hospitalisation, particularly for the elderly, is not therapeutically beneficial (Pitts & Phillips 1998)
- the increasing demographic proportion and number of elderly people requiring healthcare (Carr-Hill & Dalley 1999).

These factors, in addition to the need to control burgeoning healthcare costs, have led providers of healthcare services to rethink the modes of delivery for specific patient groups, including elective orthopaedic and trauma patients across all age groups.

Effectiveness of HaH

To date there is a deficit of empirical evidence to support the widespread adoption of HaH schemes. This is exemplified in Shepperd & Illiffe's (1998) systematic review of HaH schemes, which concluded that there were only five studies, all from the 1970s and 1980s, of sufficient power and quality to be included in the review. A small number of studies have compared early discharge to HaH and traditional inpatient care for orthopaedic patients in terms of cost and effectiveness.

A study by Jester & Hicks (2003a, b) of primary total hip and knee replacement patients reported that

HaH was preferable to inpatient care in relation to increased patient satisfaction and reduced joint stiffness and that it is less costly due to the reduction in the length of stay and cost per treatment day. Shepperd et al (1998) affirmed significantly greater improvements in quality of life for total hip replacement patients discharged early to HaH compared to inpatient rehabilitation. However, the same study reported that HaH was not suitable for knee replacement patients as 30% of the sample were unable to access the scheme due to postoperative complications.

One of the issues raised by Jester (2003) is giving patients and informal carers the choice about whether to be involved in an early discharge scheme. HaH will not be desirable or feasible for all patients; it is here that orthopaedic nurses have an important role in assessing patients' and carers' ability to cope with early discharge. The patient's ability to cope is dependent on many factors including the appropriateness of the home situation in terms of access, having a telephone and the availability of a suitable co-resident adult to take on the informal carer role.

Consideration of the patient's general health status is needed. Entry criteria and appropriate assessments are needed to assess current and past health status, including factors such as any history of deep vein thrombosis, pulmonary embolism, uncontrolled diabetes, unstable hypertension or a significant history of mental health problems. The presence of these may increase potential patient risks if they are discharged early to HaH. Psychological factors such as a patient's locus of control, stress and coping strategies need to be included in the assessment process (Jester 2003).

The ability and willingness of a family member or significant other to take on the role of informal carer is essential. It is advisable to assess patient and carer suitability separately to avoid either party feeling pressurised to make a decision. Tables 2.1 and 2.2 provide simple screening tools to assess the suitability of patients and informal carers, providing a useful adjunct to the patient's past medical and social history.

Models of HaH

There are two organisational models of the HaH scheme (Haggard 1996, Hughes & Gordon 1995).

Type one. The first model is the creation of a specialised team, usually hospital based, and often

Table 2.1   Assessment tool to assess the suitability of patients for early discharge to HaH (Jester 2003)

	Yes	No
1 It is very important to me to be able to return home as soon as possible after my operation	☐	☐
2 I believe that the progress I make after my operation is largely within my own control	☐	☐
3 Being in hospital makes me feel out of control of what is happening to me	☐	☐
4 I would feel very anxious to be discharged home 3–4 days after my operation, even if visited frequently by the HaH team	☐	☐
5 It is very important to me to be surrounded by other patients who have undergone similar types of operation	☐	☐
6 It is very important to me to see a doctor at least daily for the first week following my operation	☐	☐
7 I would recuperate much better after my operation in my own home being visited regularly by nurses and physiotherapists rather than remaining in hospital	☐	☐
8 If I went home early after my operation I would be tempted to let my family do everything for me rather than trying myself	☐	☐
9 I would be well supported by my family if I were discharged home 3–4 days following my operation	☐	☐
10 Being in hospital makes me feel very anxious	☐	☐

Scoring of the index:
Items 1, 2, 3, 7, 9 and 10   score   Yes = 1   and   No = 0
Items 4, 5, 6 and 8   score   Yes = 0   and   No = 1
The higher the score, the more suitable the patient is for early discharge to HaH.

linked to a surgical specialty (Hughes & Gordon 1995), often known as hospital outreach or early discharge schemes. Examples of this model in the UK include COPE (Community Orthopaedic Project in Essex) (Bosanquet & Zajaler 1992) and ROCS (Royal Orthopaedic Community Scheme) in the West Midlands (Jester & Hicks 2003a, b).

These models are coordinated by practitioners from the acute sector, recruited to the scheme for their specialist skills, knowledge and training in orthopaedic and trauma care. The medical responsibility for the patient remains with the relevant orthopaedic consultant.

The advantage of this model is that the practitioners are experts in the high-technology interventions some patients require. The hospital-based orthopaedic consultants generally feel confident to discharge their patients early to the scheme if they know the HaH team have the relevant specialist skills and training. Marks (1991) affirms this, stating that:

Just as hospital care is highly specialised, so high technology care at home requires specialist skills and

sophisticated equipment. Certain kinds of paediatric, orthopaedic, respiratory, stoma and cancer care may involve training over and above that for district nursing. (p29)

In addition, if a problem develops with the patient at home, the outreach team have relatively easy access to readmit the patient to the orthopaedic unit or to arrange for them to be seen by the orthopaedic consultant in the outpatient clinic.

The specialist team model has potential disadvantages such as difficulty in defining the boundaries between the existing community nursing services and the HaH schemes. Detailed admission and discharge criteria to HaH must be agreed and if necessary, following discharge from HaH, patients can be referred to the community nursing services.

Type two. The second type of organisational model suggested by Hughes & Gordon (1995) is 'a community-based, generic HaH service for a geographically defined population which admits patients with all types of illnesses' (p27). These schemes are an extension of the existing community

Table 2.2 Assessment tool to assess the suitability of informal carers to take on the care-giving role (Jester 2003)

	Yes	No
1 It is very important to me that my relative returns home as soon as possible after their operation	☐	☐
2 I would enjoy actively participating in my relative's care	☐	☐
3 Being discharged early would put my relative at risk of developing complications	☐	☐
4 I would feel very anxious to leave my relative at home while I went out for short periods of time, e.g. to visit local shops	☐	☐
5 My relative would receive better care if they were discharged early to HaH rather than remaining in hospital	☐	☐
6 I would not be able to cope with helping my relative with activities such as washing, dressing and transferring	☐	☐
7 Providing help for my relative if they were discharged early to HaH would be very disruptive for me	☐	☐
8 I feel I would have to stay awake during the night in case my relative needed help	☐	☐
9 I would receive a great deal of support from family and friends if I took on the care-giving role	☐	☐
10 Reducing the amount of travelling to and from the hospital for visiting would be a real benefit to me	☐	☐

Scoring of the index:
Items 1, 2, 5, 9 and 10   score   yes = 1 and No = 0
Items 3, 4, 6, 7 and 8   score   yes = 0 and No = 1
The higher the score, the more suitable the relative is to take on the informal carer role.

nursing services, using the community nurses to provide care.

Haggard (1996) supports the idea of community nurses taking on the acute interventions for HaH patients, stating that 'It was learned that GPs are confident in their attached district nursing staff and willing to delegate the care of HaH patients to them; and that the staff enjoyed using their acute level skills' (p37). This does not mean that hospital-based consultants would be so willing to refer their patients for early discharge to a scheme that is staffed only by community nurses. They may consider that the community nurses do not have recent up-to-date orthopaedic specialist and acute care skills and knowledge. The concept of 'enjoying' carrying out acute-level care is not synonymous with having the skills and knowledge to cope with the rapidly changing technology, especially if they have not received additional training and updating.

Transference of skills and knowledge

Billingham & Boyd (1997) suggest that despite sharing a basic training with other nurses, there are salient divergences between community nursing and hospital nursing. Community nurses work within the patient's own home where the nurse is a guest. This has legal and ethical implications when entry to a patient's home is refused despite the need for care being known. Community nurses work in relative isolation compared to hospital nurses and have relatively little medical direction. Working in semi-isolation has implications for personal safety, sharing good practice, autonomy and clinical reasoning.

Orthopaedic nurses working on a HaH scheme must be prepared to take on increased levels of professional autonomy and enhanced decision making. This necessitates educational preparation and an ongoing system of peer support facilitated by clinical supervision, action learning sets and other similar modes of ongoing professional development and support.

Working in HaH teams requires a degree of multiskilling between nurses and therapists because it is not cost effective to replicate patient visits. Nurses undertake skills traditionally deemed the domain of therapists, such as measuring the range of movement, gait assessment, measuring for and fitting aids to daily living. Therapists in turn undertake nursing skills such as wound assessment and dressings, pain assessment and administration of medication. Multiskilling can provide a rewarding expansion to the normal scope of practice for nurses and therapists, maximising opportunities for interdisciplinary care.

It would seem that both organisational models have advantages and disadvantages; consequently, it would be prudent to develop an eclectic model encompassing the advantages of both. This may be achieved in several ways. First, the development of a specialist educational pathway could prepare nurses employed on HaH schemes. Alternatively, specialist hospital and community nurses could rotate settings on a regular basis as midwives currently do in the UK. Rotation between community and hospital settings would help to break down professional rivalry, enhancing cooperation and sharing of good practice.

A third option would encourage existing schemes to endeavour to employ a combination of acute hospital nurses and community nurses so that the skill mix would facilitate the care needed by patients on HaH. This third model would be the most feasible and relatively easy to organise as it addresses issues such as multiskilling and professional autonomy that are vital to consider as such schemes generally reduce the medical input compared to inpatient care.

Clearly educational preparation of nurses working within the specialty of orthopaedics must include preparation to transfer orthopaedic skills and knowledge to the community setting. The orthopaedic nursing curriculum must therefore reflect the shift in patient management toward primary and community-based care.

FEWER FOLLOW-UP APPOINTMENTS IN OUTPATIENT DEPARTMENT

Follow-up appointments in hospital outpatient departments often provide unsatisfactory experiences. Areas of dissatisfaction include arduous journeys to and from the hospital, long waiting times, lack of privacy and little time for patients to ask questions and develop therapeutic relationships with healthcare professionals.

Specialist orthopaedic nurses are in an ideal position to provide follow-up services for many patient groups; for example, the 6-week and 6-month reviews after joint replacement surgery, falls prevention follow-up services and the monitoring of casts and external fixators. Transferring these services to a primary care setting involves a collaborative project between general practitioners, practice nurses and specialist orthopaedic nurses to minimise some of the difficulties with traditional outpatient follow-up reported earlier.

HEALTH MAINTENANCE AND HEALTH PROMOTION SERVICES IN PRIMARY CARE

There are many instances within primary care where orthopaedic nurses could use their expertise to promote health and well-being for orthopaedic patients of all age groups.

Elective surgery adult patients can benefit from health maintenance clinics, which aim to manage their symptoms and promote optimum health prior to their surgery. Symptom relief in terms of pain assessment along with a review and the modification of analgesia can significantly improve patients' physical and psychological well-being. Gait assessment, provision of appropriate walking aids and weight reduction may also provide interim relief from joint pain and disability. In addition, aids to daily living such as handrails, raised toilet seats and helping hands may optimise patients' independence whilst waiting for elective surgery such as total joint replacement.

Health promotion and maintenance services can serve an important function in the prevention of falls and preventing and detecting osteoporosis. There is a huge potential for orthopaedic nurses to work in liaison with their primary care partners to develop and implement these services.

REHABILITATION AND STEP-DOWN SERVICES

The need to maximise the number of patients being admitted to both trauma and elective orthopaedic hospital beds has resulted in a proliferation of initiatives to transfer patients needing rehabilitation or convalescence to community hospitals or designated step-down beds within nursing homes. This type of initiative clearly has the potential to reduce waiting lists and release beds for acute orthopaedic interventions. It is important to view these services as part of the continuum of care and treatment, preventing disjointed or fragmented care.

A number of orthopaedic liaison posts have developed with the specific remit of identifying

suitable patients for transfer to such services, ensuring they continue to receive appropriate evidence-based orthopaedic care and rehabilitation in the step-down facility. It is essential that the patient and their family are involved in any decisions about transfer to rehabilitation or step-down care.

THE SCOPE OF ORTHOPAEDIC NURSING PRACTICE

Over the past 20–30 years in America, there has been a proliferation of advanced nurse practitioner (ANP) roles. The impetus for the development of the ANP role was a national shortage of medical practitioners, particularly within isolated rural communities. Advanced nurse practitioners are educated to Master's degree level and register with the state in which they practise. They have gained a high degree of professional autonomy including, in many cases, full prescribing rights. In orthopaedics and trauma, the ANP role has evolved to meet patient and practice needs. Although aspects of the role vary between states, it generally involves advanced holistic health assessment skills, enhanced clinical decision making and prescription of medication and other treatment options.

As in America, the impetus for the development of specialist and advanced roles in UK nursing was an anticipated shortage of junior medical staff resulting from the reduction in junior doctors' hours.

In Britain, *The scope of professional practice* (UKCC 1992) gave practitioners, for the first time, the opportunity to examine and develop their practice according to patients' needs and move away from the concepts of extended and expanded roles. Following this, the UKCC (1994) set out criteria and definitions for four spheres of professional practice: novice, primary, specialist and advanced.

The professional body subsequently opened a register for specialist practitioners, stipulating that entry to the register required completion of a validated educational programme to at least first degree level or Master's level, plus a minimum of 3 years postregistration experience within the specific field of practice. The educational preparation for a specialist nurse practitioner (SNP) must comprise equal proportions of practice and theory. Jester (1997) explains how a Master's degree orthopaedic pathway can be facilitated by the use of negotiated clinical learning contracts, ensuring a strong partnership between the educational institution, the student, the consultant preceptor and the relevant manager to develop the student's skills and knowledge and to develop orthopaedic practice in line with the sponsoring organisation's strategic plans. As the professional bodies have failed to agree on the differentiation between specialist and advanced practice, advanced nurse practitioners have not gained registration status in Britain.

SPECIALIST NURSE PRACTITIONERS AND CLINICAL NURSE SPECIALISTS

The emergence of the SNP register created a degree of uncertainty for the traditional role of clinical nurse specialist (CNS) that had developed over the previous 20 years in Britain. No statutory regulation for the title of clinical nurse specialist exists, leading to a wide variation in their educational preparation, experience, clinical role and level of competence. Hameric (1988) defined the four subroles of a CNS as:

- expert practitioner
- researcher
- educator
- consultant.

These subroles appear to be almost identical to the UKCC (1994) definition of a registered SNP.

There appears to be very little difference between the CNS and SNP roles, except that the latter is protected by specified educational preparation, a minimum amount of clinical experience within the specialty and by professional registration. Registration is clearly important to maintain standards of practice, protecting the public and enhancing the professional standing of nurses taking on additional responsibilities.

By the very nature of their work with a specific group of patients, all nurses holding an orthopaedic qualification could be designated as specialists. This is affirmed by the work of Santy (2001) who identified a number of specialist roles and responsibilities specific to orthopaedic nurses. However, we must be cautious in our differentiation between nurses working within a specialty and registered specialist nurse practitioners. The latter are educated and prepared to work at a higher level in terms of patient assessment, diagnostic and clinical reasoning skills and pushing the boundaries of practice forward.

Specialist nurse practitioners frequently work autonomously, undertaking responsibilities formerly considered the domain of medical or therapy professionals. Examples of this include nurse practitioner follow-up clinics for total joint replacement patients (Jackson 2003) and knee triage clinics. There are many potential advantages of these roles including:

- the reduction of waiting lists
- freeing senior medical staff to see more complex cases
- offering patients a more holistic consultation
- maximising interprofessional working
- providing continuity of care and treatment for patients.

Generally, CNSs and SNPs have no managerial authority over others. Their influence over the quality of patient care comes from clinical leadership, role modelling and ability to act as a change agent. Through the research element of their role, they can influence improvements in practice by investigating clinical problems and using research-based literature to underpin practice and policy.

It is important, though, for those advancing practice through specialist roles to remain firmly rooted in the ethos of nursing, striving to be maxi nurses as opposed to mini doctors (Castledine 1995). In the context of informed consent and user involvement in service provision, it is imperative that orthopaedic specialist nurses explain to patients their role and professional background, especially when carrying out procedures normally performed by a medical practitioner.

NURSE CONSULTANTS

In 1999, the Department of Health (DoH) published 'making a difference: strengthening the nursing, midwifery and health visiting contribution to health and healthcare'. This sets out four levels of practice as illustrated in Table 2.3. Of particular relevance to this chapter are levels 3 and 4, which define the level of competence, experience and educational preparation required for nurses working at specialist and nurse consultant level.

The development of nurse consultant posts was in response to the reduction in junior doctors' hours, while keeping experienced clinical nurses within practice by offering commensurate salaries and opportunities to develop nursing practice to a higher level. To date, the DoH and professional bodies have

Table 2.3   A new career framework for nurses, midwives and health visitors (DoH 1999)

	Typically people will, at a minimum, be competent ...	Typically posts will include ...	Typically people here will have been educated and trained to ...
1	To provide basic and routine personal care and a limited range of clinical interventions routine to the care setting under the supervision of a registered nurse	Cadets, healthcare assistants and other clinical support workers	NVQ levels 1, 2, or 3
2	To do the above and exercise clinical judgement and assume professional responsibility and accountability for the assessment of health needs, planning, delivery and evaluation of routine and direct care. Direct and supervise the work of support workers and mentor students	Both newly registered nurses and established registered practitioners in a variety of jobs and specialties in both hospital and community and primary care settings	Higher education diploma or first degree level, hold professional registration and in some cases additional specialist-specific professional qualifications
3	To do the above and assume significant clinical or public health leadership of registered practitioners and others, and/or clinical management and/or specialist care	Experienced senior registered practitioners in a diverse range of posts including ward sisters, community nurses and **clinical nurse specialists**	First or Master's degree level, hold professional registration and in many cases additional specialist-specific professional qualifications
4	To do the above and provide expert care, to provide clinical or public health leadership and consultancy to senior registered practitioners and others and initiate and lead significant practice, education and service development	Experienced and expert practitioners holding **nurse consultant posts**	Master's or doctorate level, hold professional registration and additional specialist-specific professional qualifications commensurate with standards for recognition of a higher level of practice

not stipulated regulation of the nurse consultant title through registration. This may lead to mirroring the earlier situation encountered by CNS posts, resulting in regional and national variations in terms of experience, qualifications, role and salary. The DoH (1999) specifies that nurse consultants must spend at least 50% of their available time in expert clinical practice in contact with patients and clients and that their responsibilities are within four main areas:

- expert practice
- professional leadership and consultancy
- education and development
- service development linked to research and evaluation.

To date the majority of nurse consultant posts have developed in areas such as critical care, oncology and mental health. However, a small but significant number have been appointed in orthopaedics and trauma. The precise nature and scope of the role depend on local negotiation between the individual, relevant medical consultants and managers, based on patient and service need. Being a consultant in all areas of orthopaedic and trauma care would be an impossible goal. It is likely that nurse consultants will inevitably subspecialise to achieve the level of expertise required, possibly continuing the current trend that reflects medical consultant subspecialties. Examples to date include posts in orthopaedic oncology, trauma and spinal care. From a legal perspective, statute does not stipulate the boundaries between nursing and medical practice except in terms of nurse prescribing.

NURSE PRESCRIBING

Since the late 1990s, a number of DoH directives have aimed to provide nurses with limited prescribing rights. In the first instance, district nurses and health visitors were, after educational preparation, able to prescribe from the formulary for district nurses and health visitors. The formulary initially was mainly composed of a variety of wound dressings, wound cleaning agents and urinary catheters.

An extension of independent prescribing was sanctioned by the DoH in 2001 with the development of the nurse prescribers' extended formulary covering four main areas of clinical practice: minor ailments, minor injuries, palliative care and health promotion. The extended formulary includes all general sales list pharmacy medicines and a limited list of prescription-only medicines. The items comprising the extended formulary are only for use in treating patients within the four specified areas of practice. Within the minor injuries category, there are only four conditions related to the musculoskeletal system: back and neck pain of acute and uncomplicated origin, soft tissue injury and sprains.

To be eligible as an independent prescriber using the extended formulary, a nurse must successfully complete educational preparation comprising 25 days of theory and 12 days of supervised practice with a medical practitioner.

The extended formulary in its present format does not appear to meet the prescribing needs of nurses in advanced roles within orthopaedics and trauma. The current alternative is to carry out supplementary prescribing under patient group directives. This allows individual nurses working within advanced roles to administer prescription-only medications without having to obtain a medically signed prescription for each individual patient. Examples could include intraarticular local anaesthetics and steroids, local anaesthesia prior to fine needle biopsy and titration of first-line drugs used in the treatment of rheumatoid arthritis. Patient directives need to be agreed by the individual healthcare organisation and the medical team responsible for patients treated under the directive.

To support nurses in advanced practice roles, it is important for them to have full prescribing rights after completion of appropriate educational preparation and supervised practice. The current restrictions on independent prescribing rights may hinder the potential for the development of autonomous practitioners and the provision of a high-quality seamless service.

PROFESSIONAL AUTONOMY AND DECISION MAKING

Clearly advanced nursing roles in orthopaedics and trauma require practitioners to exercise higher levels of professional autonomy and decision making. *The NHS plan* (DoH 2000) sets out a clear agenda to challenge hierarchical ways of working in the NHS with an emphasis on greater flexibility and autonomy for healthcare professionals such as nurses and therapists. The plan states that nurses and therapists should be afforded greater opportunities for decision making specifically in relation to the admission and discharge of patients.

SETTING UP AND EVALUATING NURSE-LED SERVICES

Many of those taking on advanced roles are developing their own nurse-led services, which need careful planning and organisation. The first stage is to develop a proposal for the service, which addresses the following issues:

- the rationale for the development of the service
- whether it is replacing an existing service or is a new provision
- who will be delivering the service, their experience and education requirements
- the additional resources required to set up the service
- the anticipated benefits of the development
- the protocols, guidelines or directives required
- how the service will be evaluated
- issues around vicarious liability
- who will be involved in the planning of the service. The planning team may include: user involvement, the orthopaedic medical team, other members of the multidisciplinary team, managers, primary care team involved, administrators and significant others.

This list is not exhaustive but a guide to the main issues for consideration. As with any change, it is important for those affected to be kept informed of the developments and actively involved in the decision-making process. Resistance to new nurse-led services can come from clinicians and patients, particularly if they replace services previously provided by medical staff. This is minimised by involving the stakeholders in the change process and by providing empirical evidence of why the nurse-led service will improve efficiency and the quality of healthcare provision.

Once the proposal for the development is accepted, it is important that patients understand that a nurse rather than a doctor will see them and manage their care. This can be explained in a letter asking them to attend a relevant clinic or prior to admission to hospital. When patients access the service, the nurse practitioner must reinforce their role to ensure the validity of any consent to carry out a procedure.

EVALUATING NURSE-LED SERVICES

The evaluation of any nurse-led service is essential to establish its effectiveness. It may be appropriate to compare service provision between, for instance, nurse-led and medically led rehabilitation care, in terms of both cost and effectiveness, especially if a new intervention has been approved on a time-limited pilot basis.

The precise details of what to include in a comprehensive evaluation will vary depending on the nature of the service provided. However, it is reasonable to expect an evaluation to include the following:

- ascertaining patient satisfaction with practitioners' involvement in their care
- measuring patient outcomes such as the degree of knee flexion or walking gait
- auditing the nature and number of complications; for example, thrombosis and plaster sore rates or delayed discharges
- reviewing the nature and number of complaints
- determining the cost of the service including the costs incurred or saved by other departments
- auditing clinic waiting times and the number of patients who fail to attend appointments
- establishing the views of other members of the multidisciplinary team about the nurse-led service.

Patient satisfaction, patient outcomes and economic evaluation are discussed here to provide a background to the theoretical, evidence-based approach for evaluating nurse-led interventions.

PATIENT SATISFACTION

Providers of healthcare are increasingly expected to supply information relating to patient outcomes and clinical effectiveness (DoH 1998) following various treatment interventions. In addition to quantitative health outcome measures such as rates of mortality and morbidity, incidence of complications, readmission rates, length of hospital stay and functional improvements, patient satisfaction is considered to be a valid outcome measure (Walsh & Walsh 1999).

Patient satisfaction is more than a customer relations exercise. Patients' participation in their care and satisfaction with care delivery directly influence treatment compliance and patient well-being (Bowling 1992, Ley 1990). Hardy et al (1996) suggest three important reasons for ascertaining patient satisfaction, which are:

- patient satisfaction is known to be associated with better health outcome
- dissatisfied patients are often unable to take their custom elsewhere
- the need to develop a consumer-based service model of healthcare.

Ley (1990) focuses on communication, satisfaction and compliance in relation to their impact upon each other, suggesting that poor communication between patients and healthcare practitioners results in patient dissatisfaction, which in turn results in poor or non-compliance with medical advice and treatment. Hence, poor or non-compliance with treatment can have a severe negative impact on patient progress and recovery.

The positive impact of satisfaction on health is discussed by Hall et al (1990), who suggest two possible reasons: firstly 'that satisfied patients are more likely to adhere to medical advice and secondly that satisfaction has a placebo type effect on psychological well being, which in turn has a positive effect on physical health' (p24). Consequently dissatisfied patients experience stress and anxiety, which has a subsequent negative impact on their physical well-being. The negative impact of the psychological distress specifically relates to effects on the patient's immune and cardiovascular systems (Atkinson et al 1990).

Despite the wealth of evidence to support the importance of patient satisfaction, Walsh & Walsh (1999) suggest that satisfaction is an elusive and subjective quality, which means different things to different people.

Patient satisfaction must be viewed as a valuable measure of the quality of care provided, making it an important aspect for evaluating and comparing nurse-led services in orthopaedics. For examples of patient satisfaction measures, see Table 2.4.

Measuring patient satisfaction

In reality, patients cannot vote with their feet as the NHS has a monopoly over healthcare provision

Table 2.4 Examples of patient satisfaction measures

Measure	Issues addressed
Medical Interview Satisfaction Scale (Wolf et al 1978)	Three aspects of satisfaction with physician intervention: Cognitive aspects: the quality and amount of information provided by the doctor Affective aspects: the amount that the patient feels that the doctor listens, understands and is interested in them. Behavioural aspect: the patient's evaluation of the doctor's competence
Newcastle Satisfaction with Nursing Scale (NSNS) (Walsh & Walsh 1999)	NSNS examines patients' satisfaction with a variety of dimensions of nursing activity and attitude, such as nurses' empathy toward patients and level of competence
Hall & Dornan (1988)	Recognises 11 aspects of patient satisfaction: humaneness, informativeness, overall quality, competence, access, cost, facilities, health outcome, continuity, attention to psychosocial problems and bureaucracy
Rubin (1990)	Suggests 3 domains of patient satisfaction: health improvement, affective state such as anxiety or depression, and sense of safety and security
Hospital Patient Satisfaction Index (HPSI) (Hardy & West 1994)	Embraces theories of organisational participation and socialisation

except for those able to afford private healthcare. Therefore, it is essential to ensure that interventions are evaluated in terms of patient satisfaction in addition to professionals' views of the outcome.

Ley (1990) states that investigators concentrate on specific aspects of patient satisfaction, such as communication between patient and healthcare professionals, as predictors of patient satisfaction. This can be viewed as a reductionist model which focuses on a single indicator rather than taking a holistic approach that examines satisfaction with the total care experience, as with the Hall & Dornan (1988) model.

Additional factors that impact on patients' perceptions of satisfaction include their gender, age, social status, education level, cultural background, previous experiences with healthcare (Forbes & Brown 1995) and social class (Bowling 1992). Patient satisfaction is therefore a multidimensional concept involving physical, social and psychological components (Hall & Dornan 1988, Rubin 1990).

Many patient satisfaction tools lack validity and reliability; consequently, the results lack sensitivity or are unable to identify accurately the components of satisfaction (Walsh & Walsh 1999). Measures that focus on physical amenities, hotel aspects of care and process indicators such as waiting times are within the remit of NHS management. These fail to address the fundamental psychological components of satisfaction or the process and outcome of clinical aspects of care, so may not reflect the issues considered important by patients.

Ley (1975) reports a curvilinear relationship between the percentage of patients reporting satisfaction and the time since discharge from hospital or since their consultation. Ley suggests that levels of satisfaction are higher within 1 week of discharge from hospital than measures taken between 2 and 4 weeks after discharge but that levels of satisfaction rose again 8 weeks following discharge. This refutes the earlier work by Spelman et al (1966) who reported that satisfaction increased with increasing time since discharge. The stress experienced by inpatients from their ill health and separation from their family, home and normal routine may be influencing the correlation between time and the levels of satisfaction, as patients' stress diminishes on return to home.

It is imperative for those collecting and collating patient satisfaction data to remain neutral and assure patients that their confidentiality and anonymity will be respected (Fitzpatrick & Hopkins 1993). To ensure neutrality, practitioners must ensure that an independent individual administers and collects data pertaining to patient satisfaction with their own service.

PATIENT OUTCOMES

Clinical governance (DoH 1998) has necessitated the systematic collection of patient outcome data to demonstrate clinical effectiveness. Prior to this, ad hoc data collection resulted in problems of comparing the efficiency and quality of many health-care interventions such as joint replacement surgery. Clinical governance has led to systematic data collection using valid and reliable methods. The outcome data are then available for the National Institute of Clinical Excellence (NICE), which monitors and compares provider units and is then able to highlight centres of excellence and enforce recommendations to improve practice.

Measuring changes to healthcare delivery methods ensures that patients receive appropriate, safe and high-quality care. Nurse-led services are no exception; they must demonstrate the provision of a viable alternative to the traditional medically led service, while ensuring that patient safety and quality of care are not compromised.

MEASURING FUNCTIONAL OUTCOMES

Historically, outcome measures can be traced back to Florence Nightingale, who devised a system for comparing death rates by diagnostic category during the Crimean war (Pynsent et al 1993).

An outcome is described by Bulstrode (1993) as a measure of change, the endpoint being compared to the situation prior to the intervention. Additionally Bulstrode (1993) describes an outcome as having relative value rather than being an absolute.

There are several methods of measuring outcomes as used, for example, following joint replacement surgery (Bowling 1997).

• Physical tests of function, such as assessment of the range of movement, stability of the joint or radiological evidence. However, these do not measure the impact of a disease such as osteoarthritis or an intervention such as surgery, on the individual patient.
• Direct observation of patient behaviours is useful but can be intrusive for patients and very time consuming for the clinician.
• Interviewing patients enables practitioners to ascertain the patients' perceptions of the outcomes following an intervention. This approach is affirmed by Garland (1988) who suggests that quality of life measures focus on health as perceived by the patient,

rather than on the status of the prosthesis or other technical concerns that are not directly related or relevant to patients. For instance, attainment of 90° or more knee flexion following a knee replacement is of little importance to a patient if they are pain free and can function within their lives as they wish to. The problems of patients self-reporting outcomes include individual reactions to apparently similar levels of physical impairment, which in turn is dependent on their expectations, priorities and prior experiences (Bowling 1997). Changes in patients' perceptions of their functional ability will also vary with time so a one-off snapshot will not give an accurate picture. Additionally patients' memories can be poor, especially when comparing pain prior to a procedure to that afterwards (Pynsent et al 1993).

Generic versus disease-specific measures

Self-reported measures of health are subclassified into two main groups: generic and disease specific (Table 2.5). These are often used together to give a more comprehensive measure of patient outcome (Kantz et al 1992).

Generic measures of health aim to measure the multifaceted nature of health and well-being, so they should be comprehensive and include items relating to social and psychological health as well as physical health (Newell 1996). They are useful for assessing health in large diverse populations or when a comparison between several conditions is required (Bowling 1997), for example to compare patients having a hip replacement following osteoarthritis with those with rheumatoid arthritis. The main disadvantage of these measures is their lack of specificity and sensitivity in identifying condition-specific aspects (Hutchinson & Fowler 1992).

Disease-specific measures are designed specifically to encapsulate the impact of a specific disease process on an individual (Newell 1996) and maximise the chance of detecting small but significant changes in health status and levels of disease severity, which are essential aspects of clinical research on the disease concerned (Bowling 1997, McKenna 1993).

The disadvantage of disease-specific measures is that their specificity renders them unsuitable for comparing health across diverse patient groups.

There are a plethora of disease-specific measures used within the field of orthopaedics to assess outcomes (Table 2.5). However, it is important to consider validity, reliability, specificity, sensitivity, ease of completion, scoring and the process of analysis

Table 2.5 Examples of generic and disease-specific measures

Generic measures	Disease-specific measures
• Sickness Impact Profile (Deyo et al 1982)	• Oxford hip and knee scores
• Nottingham Health Profile (Hunt 1986)	• Western Ontario and McMaster Arthritis Index (WOMAC) (Bellamy et al 1988)
• Short Form 36 Health Survey Questionnaire (Ware & Sherbourne 1993)	• Harris Hip Score (Harris 1969)
• Dartmouth COOP Function Charts (Nelson et al 1993)	• Arthritis Impact Measurement Scale (AIMS) (Meenan et al 1980)

before deciding upon which measure to use (Bowling 1997, Newell 1996).

ECONOMIC EVALUATION

No government or authority is likely to favour health innovations that are potentially more costly than existing healthcare provisions. This includes the introduction of prevention measures such as screening everyone for osteoporosis, as the financial outcomes from the reduction in fractures will be seen in future decades, while the cost of screening and fracture prevention therapy occurs immediately.

Investigating the cost-effectiveness of a service is an essential component of evaluating the suitability and acceptability of nurse-led interventions. The type of economic evaluation used (Table 2.6) will depend on the results of previously carried out clinical effectiveness outcomes.

Table 2.6 Methods of evaluating cost effectiveness

Cost minimisation analysis (CMA)	CMA calculates the difference in monetary terms between two interventions, for example HaH versus inpatient rehabilitation. It assumes that both interventions are equally effective in terms of outcome. The intervention that costs less is considered to be more cost effective (Gold et al 1996)
Cost–benefit analysis (CBA)	CBA measures in monetary terms the benefits and the costs of an intervention and offers the bottom line of a benefit–cost ratio in monetary figures (Beauchamp & Childress 1989). The monetary value is apportioned to health consequences by calculating willingness to pay via surveying opinions on the trade-offs between health and money, and human capital calculated on the basis of the produce value of people in the economy (Gold et al 1996). It involves apportioning a monetary figure to improvements in outcome, such as a reduction in joint stiffness, by calculating how reduced stiffness would equate to reduced consumption of analgesic and antiinflammatory medication or how patients would claim less mobility allowance.
	Alternatively, CBA can lay out the information on costs and benefits to aid a decision about whether any gains provided by the experimental treatment are worth the extra costs involved (Donaldson et al 1996).
	The CBA model endorses ethical principles of balancing benefits, such as improvement in health, against monetary cost
Cost-effectiveness analysis (CEA)	This compares the relative value of two or more interventions in achieving better health or outcomes with the results presented as a cost-effectiveness ratio (Fig. 2.1), where the denominator reflects the gain in health effects achieved and the numerator reflects the cost of obtaining the health gain (Gold et al 1996). If one of the interventions is both more effective and less costly than the alternative, there is no need to calculate a cost-effectiveness ratio.
	CEA is a tool for improving social welfare by maximising the aggregate health effect achievable at the lowest possible cost (Gold et al 1996). The foundations of CEA encompass welfare economics. CEA provides a method of comparing interventions so that decision makers can maximise health benefit with finite resources and supports the rationale that any alteration in the mode of healthcare delivery has economic and social consequences, for example the development of community-based services

Doubilet et al (1986) provide a comprehensive definition of the term cost effective, suggesting it should be used for cases where one strategy is more cost effective than another, where it is:

- less costly and at least as effective

- more effective and more costly but the additional benefits are worth the additional cost, or
- less effective and less costly but the benefit of the rival strategy is not worth its extra cost.

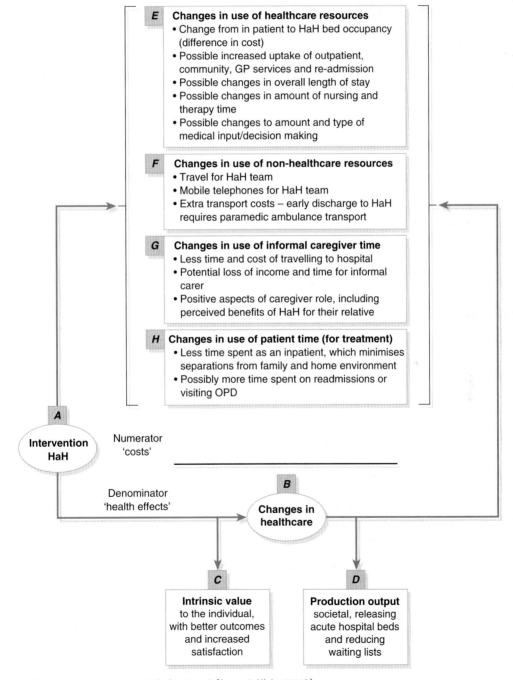

E Changes in use of healthcare resources
- Change from in patient to HaH bed occupancy (difference in cost)
- Possible increased uptake of outpatient, community, GP services and re-admission
- Possible changes in overall length of stay
- Possible changes in amount of nursing and therapy time
- Possible changes to amount and type of medical input/decision making

F Changes in use of non-healthcare resources
- Travel for HaH team
- Mobile telephones for HaH team
- Extra transport costs – early discharge to HaH requires paramedic ambulance transport

G Changes in use of informal caregiver time
- Less time and cost of travelling to hospital
- Potential loss of income and time for informal carer
- Positive aspects of caregiver role, including perceived benefits of HaH for their relative

H Changes in use of patient time (for treatment)
- Less time spent as an inpatient, which minimises separations from family and home environment
- Possibly more time spent on readmissions or visiting OPD

A Intervention HaH

Numerator 'costs'

Denominator 'health effects'

B Changes in healthcare

C Intrinsic value to the individual, with better outcomes and increased satisfaction

D Production output societal, releasing acute hospital beds and reducing waiting lists

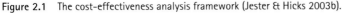

Figure 2.1 The cost-effectiveness analysis framework (Jester & Hicks 2003b).

Donaldson et al (1996) suggest economic evaluation techniques cannot be predetermined until the results of parallel investigation into the effectiveness of the intervention are known.

Calculating and comparing costs for nurse-led services is complex and must encompass the costs incurred by patients and families, as well as any shift in cost from hospital to community and outpatient services.

Literature relating to economic analysis suggests that there are several types of data that should be collected which include both direct and indirect costs (Donaldson et al 1996). Direct costs apply to items such as clinical investigations, medications, nursing and therapy interventions and patient transport such as ambulance journeys. Indirect costs relate to items such as the overhead costs of running a hospital or clinic, including the utility costs, maintenance of the building and administration. However, it is important not just to examine the direct and indirect costs but also to monitor any shift in the costs incurred. For example, if following consultation at a nurse-led orthopaedic clinic, patients have to visit their general practitioner for a different analgesia prescription, this increases the primary care costs in comparison to patients attending a medically led clinic where costs of the issued prescription and dispensing of the analgesia are covered by the hospital. This emphasises the importance of nurse practitioners involved in such services having the relevant prescribing rights.

The complexity of ensuring that all relevant costs are included within an economic evaluation necessitates the use of a structured framework underpinned by theoretical relevance, rather than an ad hoc approach. Figure 2.1 show the complexity of an actual economic comparison of HaH versus inpatient interventions, using a cost-effectiveness framework (Jester & Hicks 2003b).

CONCLUSION

This chapter has critically explored the complex nature of the significant shift in the focus of orthopaedic care from a hospital to a community and primary care based model. Orthopaedic nurses need to continue to develop professionally to facilitate the transaction of orthopaedic nursing skills, knowledge and experience into new settings.

The proliferation of advanced practice roles and nurse-led services has benefits and drawbacks for patients, practitioners and healthcare provision which need to be accounted for when evaluating the potential of, or provision of, a new service. Opportunities to develop advanced practice roles in orthopaedics provide the potential to improve patient services and allow practitioners to optimise their experience and knowledge in providing evidence-based care. This has resulted in nurses being required to understand how their services can be evaluated using outcome measures and economic evaluations. These areas are new challenges for orthopaedic practitioners and the specialism as a whole.

Further reading

Abramowitz A, Cote A, Berry E 1987 Analysing patient satisfaction: a multi-analytical approach. Quality Review Bulletin 13(4): 122–130

Doering E 1983 Factors influencing inpatient satisfaction with care. Quality Review Bulletin 9(10): 291–299

Greenfield S, Kaplan S, Ware J 1985 Expanding patient involvement in care. Annals of Internal Medicine 102: 520–528

Humphris D (ed) 1994 The clinical nurse specialist: issues in practice. Macmillan, Basingstoke

McDaniel C, Nash J 1990 Compendium of instruments measuring patient satisfaction with nursing care. Quality Review Bulletin May: 182–188

References

Atkinson R, Atkinson R, Smith E et al 1990 Introduction to psychology, 10th edn. Harcourt Brace Jovanovich Publishing, London

Beauchamp T, Childress J 1989 Principles of biomedical ethics, 3rd edn. Oxford University Press, Oxford

Bellamy N, Buchanan W, Goldsmith C et al 1988 Validation study of WOMAC: a health status instrument for measuring clinically important patient-relevant outcomes

following total hip or knee arthroplasty in osteoarthritis. Journal of Orthopaedics and Rheumatology 1: 95–108

Billingham K, Boyd M 1997 Developing clinical expertise in community nursing. In: Gastrell P, Edwards J (eds) Community health nursing: frameworks for practice. Baillière Tindall, London

Bosanquet N, Zajaler A 1992 Community Orthopaedic Project in Essex (COPE): an evaluation. RHBNC/

St Mary's University of London Health Policy Unit, London

Bowling A 1992 Assessing health needs and measuring patient satisfaction. Nursing Times 88(31): 31–34

Bowling A 1997 Measuring health: a review of quality of life measurement scales, 2nd edn. Open University Press, Buckingham

Bulstrode C 1993 Outcome measures and their analysis. In: Pynsent P, Fairbank J, Carr A (eds) Outcome measures in orthopaedics. Butterworth-Heinemann, Oxford

Carr-Hill R, Dalley G 1999 Estimating demand pressures arising from need for social services for older people. University of York, Centre for Health Economics, York

Castledine G 1995 Defining specialist nursing. British Journal of Nursing 4(5): 264–265

Department of Health (DoH) 1989 Caring for people: community care in the next decade and beyond. HMSO, London

Department of Health (DoH) 1998 The new NHS: modern, dependable. NHSE, London

Department of Health (DoH) 1999 Making a difference: strengthening the nursing, midwifery and health visiting contribution. NHSE, London

Department of Health (DoH) 2000 The NHS plan: a plan for investment, a plan for reform. NHSE, London

Department of Health (DoH) 2001 Nurse prescribing. www.doh.gov.uk/nurseprescribing

Deyo R, Inui T, Leninger J 1982 Physical and psychological functioning in rheumatoid arthritis. Clinical use of a self-administered instrument. Archives of Internal Medicine 142: 878–882

Donaldson C, Hundley V, McIntosh E 1996 Using economics alongside clinical trials: why we cannot choose the evaluation technique in advance. Health Economics 5: 267–269

Doubilet P, Weinstein M, McNeil B 1986 Use and misuse of the term 'cost effective' in medicine. New England Journal of Medicine 314: 253–256

Fitzpatrick R, Hopkins A 1993 Measurement of patients' satisfaction with their care. Royal College of Physicians, London

Forbes M, Brown H 1995 Developing an instrument for measuring patient satisfaction. AORN Journal 61(4): 737–743

Garland J 1988 A shift in focus for orthopaedic clinical outcome studies. AAOS Bulletin 30/31: 4

Gold M, Siegel J, Russell L et al 1996 Cost-effectiveness in health and medicine. Oxford University Press, Oxford

Haggard L 1996 Hospitals at home. In: Gordon P, Hadley J (eds) Extending primary care: polyclinics, resource centres, hospitals at home. Radcliffe Medical Press, Oxford

Hall J, Dornan M 1988 What patients think about their medical care and how often they are asked: a meta-analysis of the satisfaction literature. Social Science and Medicine 27: 935–939

Hall J, Feldstein M, Fretwell M 1990 Older patients' health status and satisfaction with medical care in an HMO population. Medical Care 28: 261–270

Hameric AB 1988 Executive practice. Clinical Nurse Specialist 2(3): 118

Hardy G, West M 1994 Happy talk. Health Service Journal 7: 24–26

Hardy G, West M, Hill F 1996 Components and predictors of patient satisfaction. British Journal of Health Psychology 1: 65–85

Harris W 1969 Traumatic arthritis of the hip after dislocation in acetabular fractures: treatment by mould arthroplasty. Journal of Bone and Joint Surgery 51A: 737–755

Hughes J, Gordon P 1995 Hospital and primary care: breaking the boundaries. King's Fund Centre, London

Hunt S 1986 Measuring health status. Croom Helm, Beckenham

Hutchinson A, Fowler P 1992 Outcome measures for primary health care: what are the research priorities? British Journal of General Practice 4(2): 227–231

Jackson R 2003 Advancing nursing practice for orthopaedic outpatients. Journal of Orthopaedic Nursing 7(1): 10–14

Jester R 1997 The development and implementation of an orthopaedic pathway leading to specialist/advanced practitioner status. Journal of Orthopaedic Nursing 1(2): 85–88

Jester R 2003 Early discharge to hospital at home: should it be a matter of choice? Journal of Orthopaedic Nursing 7(2): 64–69

Jester R, Hicks C 2003a Using cost-effectiveness analysis to compare hospital at home and in-patient interventions Part 1. Journal of Clinical Nursing 12: 13–19

Jester R, Hicks C 2003b Using cost-effectiveness analysis to compare hospital at home and in-patient interventions Part 2. Journal of Clinical Nursing 12: 20–27

Kantz E, Harris W, Levitsky K et al 1992 Methods for assessing condition-specific and generic functional status after total knee replacement. Medical Care 30 (Suppl): 5

Ley P 1975 Complaints by hospital staff and patients: a review of the literature. Bulletin of the British Psychology Society 25: 115–120

Ley P 1990 Communicating with patients: improving communication, satisfaction and compliance. Chapman and Hall, London

Marks L 1991 Home and hospital care: redrawing the boundaries. Research report 9. King's Fund Institute, London

McKenna S 1993 The Nottingham Health Profile. In: Bowling A (ed) Measuring disease. Open University Press, Buckingham

Meenan R, Gertman P, Mason J 1980 Measuring health status in arthritis. Arthritis/Rheumatology 23: 146–152

Nelson E, Landgraf J, Hay D 1993 The COOP function charts: a system to measure patients' function in physicians' offices. In: Bowling A (ed) Measuring disease. Open University Press, Buckingham

Newell R 1996 Measuring health. Open University Press, Buckingham

Pitts M, Phillips K 1998 The psychology of health: an introduction, 2nd edn. Routledge, London

Pynsent P, Fairbank J, Carr A 1993 Outcome measures in orthopaedics. Butterworth-Heinemann, Oxford

Rubin H 1990 Patient evaluation of hospital care: a review of the literature. Medical Care 28 (Suppl): 3–9

Santy J 2001 An investigation of the reality of nursing work with orthopaedic patients. Journal of Orthopaedic Nursing 5(1): 22–29

Shepperd S, Illiffe S 1998 The effectiveness of hospital at home compared with in-patient hospital care: a systematic review. Journal of Public Health Medicine 20(3): 344–350

Shepperd S, Harwood D, Jenkinson C et al 1998 Randomised controlled trial comparing hospital at home care with inpatient care: 3 month follow up of health outcomes. British Medical Journal 316: 1786–1891

Spelman M, Ley P, Jones C 1966 How do we improve doctor–patient communications in our hospitals? World Hospitals 2: 126–134

United Kingdom Central Council (UKCC) 1992 The scope of professional practice. United Kingdom Central Council, London

United Kingdom Central Council (UKCC) 1994 The future of professional practice: the Council's standards for education and practice following registration. United Kingdom Central Council, London

Vaughan B 1995 Who cares? Hospital, home or somewhere in between: the case for intermediate services. Journal of Clinical Nursing 4: 341–342

Walsh M, Walsh A 1999 Measuring patient satisfaction with nursing care: experience of using the Newcastle Satisfaction with Nursing Scale. Journal of Advanced Nursing 29(2): 307–315

Ware JE, Sherbourne CD 1993 The MOS 36-item short-form health survey (SF36) 1: conceptual framework and item selection. Medical Care 30: 473–483

Wolf M, Putnam S, James S et al 1978 The Medical Interview Satisfaction Scale: Development of a scale to measure patient perception of physician behaviour. Journal of Behavioural Medicine 1: 391–401

Chapter 3

Orthopaedic nursing theory and concepts

Julie Santy

INTRODUCTION

In recent years the definition and shaping of orthopaedic nursing practice have been built on a foundation of increasing knowledge and theory development. This knowledge and theory, which has gathered pace considerably in the last two decades, has enabled orthopaedic nursing to make great strides forward in professionalisation of the specialty and in the development of theory and practice. This chapter aims to capture some of the philosophy, theory and concepts pertinent to orthopaedic nursing and to enable the reader to integrate them into practice.

Theory in nursing provides us with an approach to thinking about practice. It allows us to think critically about the actions of nurses and to debate the issues that matter to nurses and those they provide care for. It provides a way of identifying, exploring and expressing key ideas about practice (Walker & Avant 1995).

Theory provides nurses with a perspective from which to view situations, a means of organising the many aspects of patient care and in particular to interpret and analyse the findings of assessment processes. This allows nurses to practise purposefully and systematically, with control over client outcomes. If, however, nursing theory is to guide nursing practice, the critical issue in choosing a specific theory for a nursing specialism such as orthopaedic nursing is its 'fit' between the philosophical assumptions the theory makes and the reality of nursing practice (Raudonis & Acton 1997).

Nursing is a combination of an art and a science, with nursing theory attempting to take knowledge about nursing and integrate it with practice. Nursing is dependent on scientific knowledge, aesthetic perception, personal understanding and moral choices in order to provide effective care (Artless & Richmond 2000). These practical as well as theoretical matters affect everyday clinical situations for orthopaedic nurses.

Most nursing theories are underpinned by philosophy, which allows us to scrutinise the underpinning values and beliefs of orthopaedic nursing. Nursing theory is also underpinned by descriptions and explanations of specific concepts. A grasp of these concepts allows us to understand, with greater clarity, a number of important and instrumental aspects of practice. Without an understanding of these underpinning issues, no orthopaedic nurse is able to consider their own practice and that of others in sufficient detail to allow it to develop in ways beneficial to clinical care. It is the intention of this chapter to present some of the theory relevant to orthopaedic nursing in a way that offers the reader the opportunity to consider whether and how such theory can be applied to their orthopaedic nursing practice.

THE NATURE OF NURSING

Orthopaedic nursing, like all other disciplines in nursing, is visualised as both an art and a science which, together with knowledge, are essential for providing high-quality care. The art of nursing involves consideration of the values, beliefs, and cognitive elements of nursing practice. The science involves reasoning and decision making based on scientific knowledge as well as that which comes from nursing art (Artless & Richmond 2000).

Fawcett (1995) proposes that a theory of nursing is based around four concepts or ideas that are central to the understanding of what it is that directs nursing and what nurses do. These concepts are: the person, health, the environment and nursing itself. This explanation is dominant within many publications on nursing theory (McGee 1998) and is used here as a framework for elucidating orthopaedic nursing theory.

THE PERSON

Orthopaedic nursing is focused on:

- the care of an individual, family or other group
- where a musculoskeletal disorder, trauma or their consequences are present

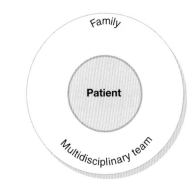

Figure 3.1 The patient as the pivot of care.

- involving people of all age groups from birth to old age and
- involving people from across all socio-economic, cultural and ethnic groups.

Each person is viewed as an individual with a diverse and complex set of problems and needs. Consequently, they are viewed as a whole, including physical, psychosocial and environmental factors affecting their health. In orthopaedic nursing, the patient is seen very clearly as the central pivot of care, with their family and the multidisciplinary team around them (Fig. 3.1).

HEALTH

Musculoskeletal problems can be acute or chronic with the effects potentially being wide reaching. Most obvious are the presence of pain and the impact on mobility that can be visualised as a continuum of the patient's desired health status and degree of altered health status. The role of the nurse is to assist the patient in moving towards or achieving their desired health status or to adapt to an altered health status (Balcombe 1994). Many musculoskeletal disorders and traumatic injuries lead to a permanent and long-term disability so rehabilitation has to be the central focus of recovery once the acute stage is over.

Consideration of health status is important for providing holistic, patient-centred care. This involves attention to psychological and social well-being as well as the physical aspects of health. It is equally important to consider the psychological aspect of, for example, joint replacement surgery or major trauma as it is to consider the physical issues. As these events affect all aspects of patients' lives they must also be considered in a sociocultural context.

THE ENVIRONMENT

The patient's contact with orthopaedic nursing can take place in all healthcare settings and healthcare environments. The trauma patient's care journey will be different to that of the patient with a more chronic condition and to the experiences of a patient having elective orthopaedic surgery.

Orthopaedic nursing skills are required in all settings including the accident and emergency department, acute hospital ward, operating department, rehabilitation unit, outpatients department and nursing home, as well as other distinct settings within the community. The challenge for nurses working in these settings is to ensure that a seamless and high-quality service is provided, no matter what part of the journey the patient is on (Lucas 2002).

It is important for orthopaedic nurses to consider the patient's environment in a global context. Healthcare is provided across all frontiers with specific issues surrounding migration. Nursing theory is no longer confined to national boundaries but must be considered within environments as diverse as a large multicultural metropolis, to rural areas in developing countries. The patterns of orthopaedic problems vary from one environment to the next but the nursing skills required are similar in each environment and are transferable to different settings once the cultural context is taken into account.

NURSING

The role of the orthopaedic nurse has been described as 'the harmonist' (Santy 2001). Orthopaedic nurses act as harmonists within the disruption caused to patients by orthopaedic disorders, surgery or trauma, providing a link between the many environments on the patient's journey. This is in keeping with McMahon's (1998) therapeutic activities in nursing, which range through developing the nurse–patient relationship, caring and comforting, to using evidence-based physical interventions, teaching, manipulation of the environment and adopting complementary health practices. The harmonist role therefore fosters a holistic approach to patient care.

CORE ACTIVITIES OF ORTHOPAEDIC NURSING

Six core activities (Fig. 3.2) have been identified for orthopaedic nursing (Santy 2001). These fit in with

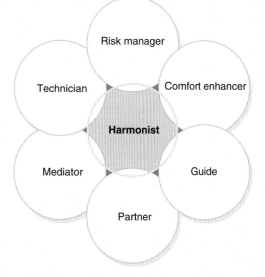

Figure 3.2   A concentric model of orthopaedic nursing (Santy 2001).

the work of Love (1995) who takes a different approach to identifying the activities of the orthopaedic nurse although the activities can be mapped against the harmonist model.

These activities require varying degrees of knowledge, experience and skill from those practising the art and science of orthopaedic nursing. It is often specialised knowledge of the musculoskeletal system and the factors involved in the related disorders and trauma that make the orthopaedic nurse instrumental in patients' recovery and rehabilitation. Experienced orthopaedic nurses develop a special sense of how musculoskeletal problems affect an individual's posture and movement, and identify nursing needs from these. This is often called the 'orthopaedic eye' (Powell 1986). This view of orthopaedic nursing is still developing and its use as a framework for understanding practice and as a tool for developing competencies for orthopaedic nursing is a role for the future.

PARTNER

The partner role in orthopaedic nursing is a complex phenomenon, discussed in the nursing literature in a variety of different ways. McMahon (1998) describes the therapeutic partnership in nursing and refers to Muetzel's (1988) three concepts of partnership, intimacy and reciprocity. Patients who receive supportive interaction in their treatment and nursing do better than those who are isolated or feel alone. When the nurse, as provider of care, becomes a partner with the patient, the results can be synergistic (Scherwitz et al 1997) and lead to positive outcomes. This nursing function involves building a relationship with the client, similar to that of a friend. Some writers in nursing have termed this a therapeutic relationship (McMahon 1998); it is built on trust and rapport and usually involves a degree of advocacy.

One of the important aspects for the nurse is being someone who can be trusted, who feels like a friend but also has inside knowledge of the 'system', of what is happening and what is likely to happen to the patient during and after their journey through care. This being a friend 'in the know' is very important in the engendering of trust, reducing the patient's anxiety, and is best fulfilled when the nurse promotes trust by making an effort to get to know and spend time with the patient. Trust is also earned by the demonstration of skill and knowledge (Fosbinder 1994) in dealing with the patient and others. As the patient's trustee, the nurse has a particular role to play as a mediator between the medical world and the patient, acting as translator for the patient, ensuring they understand what is happening and what the implications might be. In particular, this role fulfils the client's need for information about their condition, surgery and management; for example, the patient admitted for elective surgery will be less anxious when the nurse has explained what will happen to them and what the potential results can be. Most importantly, the patient feels there is someone with whom they can share fears and in whom they can place trust.

GUIDE

Orthopaedic patients in particular have a discrepancy between their mobility, ambulation needs and capabilities (Ouellet & Rush 1998), and their ability to self-care. The nurse has a vital role to play in helping the patient to overcome this deficit through rehabilitation. The nurse first has to motivate the patient to put effort into their rehabilitation and use all the skills of a good trainer or mentor to enable the patient's progression towards their goal achievement (Geelen & Soons 1996). This aspect of care often involves being with the patient whilst they mobilise, providing psychological and physical

support along with constructive feedback and encouragement.

There is considerable debate about the role of the nurse in rehabilitation, particularly in the field of elderly care. Many question whether the nurse has an active role to play and what the nursing rehabilitation interventions are (Ellul et al 1993, Johnson 1995, Myco 1984). There is a distinct nursing role arising from the trustee and translator aspects fostered in the working relationship.

The word 'encouragement' is often used to describe the motivating role in rehabilitation. This is closely linked to the friend-trustee role because of the need for the patient to have confidence and trust in the nurse who takes responsibility for their motivation and guidance in rehabilitation, a position that other health professionals cannot fulfil in the short amounts of time they spend with patients in comparison to nurses. Some of this involves acting as a coach to the patient during the early phase of remobilisation and rehabilitation. The role of the orthopaedic nurse in rehabilitation will be considered in further detail later in this chapter.

COMFORT ENHANCER

There is a wealth of literature discussing the role of comfort in well-being, linking the achievement of patient comfort to the concept of caring (Fagerstrom et al 1998, Morse et al 1994).

There are two aspects of comfort in the orthopaedic setting. The first is the maintenance of a suitable fluid and dietary intake, fulfilment of elimination needs, the need for privacy and dignity as well as the maintenance of personal standards of hygiene and dress. A great deal of comfort enhancement involves positioning plus moving and handling techniques, requiring considerable specialist skills, especially for the patient confined to bed (Bjork 1995, Morse & Procter 1998). Moving and handling is closely related to risk management in terms of musculoskeletal safety and the prevention of the complications of immobility such as pressure damage development.

The second area of importance in comfort enhancement is the assessment and management of pain related to the orthopaedic condition and its management. Orthopaedic nurses use a variety of ways of assessing and managing pain to ensure comfort can be gained without the need for unnecessary analgesic administration.

MEDIATOR

The orthopaedic nurse acts as mediator, coordinator and gatekeeper. This nursing role, in all phases of care, sees the nurse acting as a link between the patient, the interdisciplinary and interagency teams, family and friends. As a result of the 24-hour nature of nurses' contact with the patient, they are best placed to hold detailed information and understanding of the patient's problems and needs.

The nurse holds the final key to discharge, making decisions about the patient's fitness to leave the relative safety of the hospital or other healthcare facility and coordinating the activities that facilitate this. This involves communication with other health professionals and agencies as well as the patient's family, ensuring that all are working effectively towards the common goal of recovery, rehabilitation and adaptation.

RISK MANAGER

The orthopaedic nurse acts as the main manager of risk for the patient. Following trauma and orthopaedic surgery, complications are a major concern, making prevention and early recognition essential for avoiding any short- or long-term effects. The risks of potential and actual complications tend to fall into four major categories related to:

1 immobility
2 the peri- and postoperative period
3 the injury
4 those due to management and treatment.

The most common complications are pressure ulcers, wound infections and osteomyelitis, post fall syndrome, chest infection, deep vein thrombosis, pulmonary embolus, fat embolus and compartment syndrome. In many instances interventions to prevent their development fall within the scope of nursing practice, with orthopaedic nurses developing expertise in their recognition and management.

These risks and their management are a highly specialised area of orthopaedic nursing practice, related to the specialist management of orthopaedic problems. Knowledge of these and the ability to assess and record the risks, signs, monitoring parameters and appropriate nursing interventions are essential in providing effective nursing care (Slye 1991). Once a risk has become a reality, the nursing activity tends to move into the technical domain.

TECHNICIAN

Increasingly the orthopaedic nurse has a technical role to play in many aspects of patient management and care, generally in support of the medical and surgical treatment and management of orthopaedic and traumatic conditions.

In the trauma setting this is often related to the strategies used to stabilise fractures, including the application and care of casts and appliances, the application and management of traction, the care of external fixators and skeletal pins and the use and management of electronic apparatus in the care of the patient such as infusion pumps and monitoring equipment.

As nursing practice moves forward and extends its scope, these technical activities will increase. Orthopaedic nurses are now commonly working in situations requiring technical skills related to diagnosis and care management.

A PHILOSOPHY OF CARING

Caring is increasingly seen as a concept central in the theory and practice of all areas of nursing. It is, however, a nebulous concept, probably one of the hardest to define and identify in practice (Payle 2001), yet when asked what nurses do, many people would answer that they 'care'.

The term 'caring' is used in descriptions of nursing practice, with many theorists debating the importance and meaning of the concept of caring. At its simplest, caring can be described as the performance of acts or omissions towards another person that lead to a beneficial result. It is a natural human trait and an important part of how we behave morally towards others in society (Cortis & Kendrick 2003). As such, it is not necessarily a trait exclusive to nursing but is often attached to nursing ideals.

The altruistic goal of nursing is to care for the health of individuals, families and communities, with many authors agreeing that the care provided by nurses has the potential to restore health (Jackson & Borbasi 2002) because of its therapeutic nature. The concept of caring encompasses the ethical themes of holism, compassion, empathy and communication which are essential to the healing aspect of nursing care (Greenwood 2002) and central to clinical and technical competence (Fosbinder 1994).

Watson's theory (1994) of caring identifies 10 factors involved in caring (Box 3.1) that begin to offer

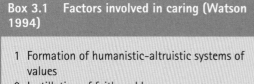

Box 3.1   Factors involved in caring (Watson 1994)

1   Formation of humanistic–altruistic systems of values
2   Instillation of faith and hope
3   Cultivation of sensitivity to one's self and to others
4   Development of a helping, trusting, human caring relationship
5   Promotion and acceptance of the expression of positive and negative feelings
6   Systematic use of a creative problem-solving caring process
7   Promotion of transpersonal teaching and learning
8   Provision for a supportive, protective and/or corrective mental, physical, societal and spiritual environment
9   Assistance with gratification of human needs
10 Allowance for existential, phenomenological and spiritual forces

some ideas on how caring may manifest itself in orthopaedic nursing practice and offers important pointers for how practice should be conducted. As yet there is no specific definition of caring within orthopaedic nursing; this would seem to be a good area for future development of nursing theory for the specialty.

HOLISM

Holism is a philosophical ideal that suggests human beings require wholeness and integrity to make life worth living (Owen & Holmes 1993); this links in many ways to the concepts of caring. Seeing human beings as whole people rather than just specific aspects of their personhood is a basic moral issue in modern society. The development of the concept of holism reflects the fact that a historical approach to healthcare did not always recognise the importance of considering every aspect of a person. Medicine in particular tended to focus on the illness rather than the whole person affected by that illness. Holism encourages us to focus on the physical aspects of care along with the psychological, spiritual, cultural, social and economic aspects of an individual's experience of life.

The focus on holism in nursing is therefore central to its humanistic practice (Kolcaba 1997) and an important moral aspect of care. Without it, patients become objects of care rather than partners with care providers. Many nursing models and theories include holism within their central ideals as an important aspect of the goal of nursing. In orthopaedic nursing practice, holistic approaches to care encourage the individual to be viewed as a human being with many physical and psychological issues contributing to their nursing needs rather than viewing the individual as, for example, an isolated limb injury or condition.

MOBILITY

The nature of musculoskeletal disorders and injury suggests that the notion of mobility is central to orthopaedic nursing and the nature of the orthopaedic patient (Balcombe 1994). Mobility is an important concept that appears frequently in discussions about nursing care, in care plans and in the orthopaedic nursing literature.

Mobility is central to maintenance of independence but is often severely impaired by orthopaedic conditions, surgery and trauma. Orthopaedic nurses need to understand its features in detail as their main role is in improving the mobility of patients and clients. Underpinning this knowledge must be an understanding of how the musculoskeletal and neurological systems affect mobility and how psychosocial issues can affect it. For example, an older person with arthritis may have considerable difficulty in mobilising but in addition, depression associated with pain or isolation can add to their mobility problems.

Ouellet & Rush (1998) offer orthopaedic nurses a conceptual model of mobility that allows understanding in more detail than was previously possible. This model, based on research work with nurses and patients, offers an understanding on several levels.

● **Mobility capacity**: this component suggests there is a finite capacity in each human being for movement and mobility. The natural mobility of joints, for example, varies from one individual to another, as does the shape of limbs; these make a difference to the smoothness and ease of movement. The mobility capacity emphasises that not all aspects of mobility are physical as there are additional social and cognitive factors influencing, for example, the ability to move around in the world and conceive movement. However, for the majority of orthopaedic patients there is some degree of mobility restriction due to their condition, surgery or trauma.

- **Forces**: this component considers the forces that either facilitate or impede mobility. For the orthopaedic patient, these can be many and far reaching, including issues such as personal characteristics, motivation, human presence, environmental elements, personality factors, mobility resources, perceptions and well-being.
- **Actuation**: this refers to the act of putting into motion an individual's mobility capacity. People who are able to move freely, effortlessly and independently are perceived to have a high level of mobility. In contrast, when impediment and restrictions to mobility are evident, people are perceived to have a low level of mobility.
- **Pattern**: this refers to the idea that mobility patterns can shift and change constantly; for example, an individual's mobility pattern will vary greatly during a phase of healthcare and even during different parts of a day. This is important when considering the best time of day and best approach to rehabilitation activities. Patients with rheumatoid arthritis often experience more stiffness in the morning; consequently many rheumatology units deliberately schedule hydrotherapy sessions or a warm bath in the morning to help reduce this effect before other patient activities can take place.
- **Consequences**: this refers to the outcomes of mobility. When client mobility improves there is a perceived increase in the quality of life with enhanced physical health, positive feelings about self, a greater sense of control and a brighter outlook on life.

Ouellet & Rush's (1998) work is central to an understanding of mobility and must be pivotal to all orthopaedic nursing theory, with any future theory development including consideration of the concept of mobility. This work has set the scene for future research in this area.

NURSING MODELS

Nursing models provide a framework on which to base nursing practice and are overtly seen in the documentation of care used. A number of well-known nursing models can be linked to orthopaedic nursing for a variety of reasons. The following section considers examples of how models can be applied to this specialised area of practice.

It is not within the scope of this chapter to discuss in detail all the major nursing models that might apply to orthopaedic nursing. However, it is important to consider the role that some of these might play. The models presented briefly here are linked to their particular relevance to orthopaedic nursing. There are many texts that elucidate the applicability of these and other nursing models to nursing practice that allow the orthopaedic nurse to consider them in more detail. Relevant texts are included in the Further Reading and Reference lists at the end of this chapter.

A MODEL FOR ORTHOPAEDIC NURSING

The only model to date specifically devised for orthopaedic nursing is Balcombe's Model of Orthopaedic Nursing (1994). This is built on the assumption that assisting the individual to regain mobility and resume their previous function or to adapt to changes in their life is central to a definition of orthopaedic nursing. The patient's desired health status is central to the goals of nursing as well as other medical and paramedical interventions. There are many factors acting on the patient's desired health status such as the physical, psychological, cultural, social, religious and personal relationships (Fig. 3.3). The model suggests that nurses achieve this through acting as a counsellor, teacher, agent for change, negotiator and manager.

There are a number of considerations for patient assessment with a central focus on mobility (Fig. 3.4). We can see elements of these in the harmonist model (Santy 2001) and in Ouellet & Rush's (1998) work on mobility.

Although this model places orthopaedic nursing in context, one of its drawbacks is that it does not specifically identify the nature of orthopaedic nursing as a distinct specialism, different from other nursing specialisms. Like many models, it presents ideas about the nature of nursing and its sphere of influence but it gives very little detail about the role of the nurse.

Balcombe (1994) links this model to practice by identifying how it can be used, but very few orthopaedic nurses can articulate its use in practice and more work is required to define its practical manifestations.

This is one of the real issues underpinning the problems with the use of nursing models. Nurses

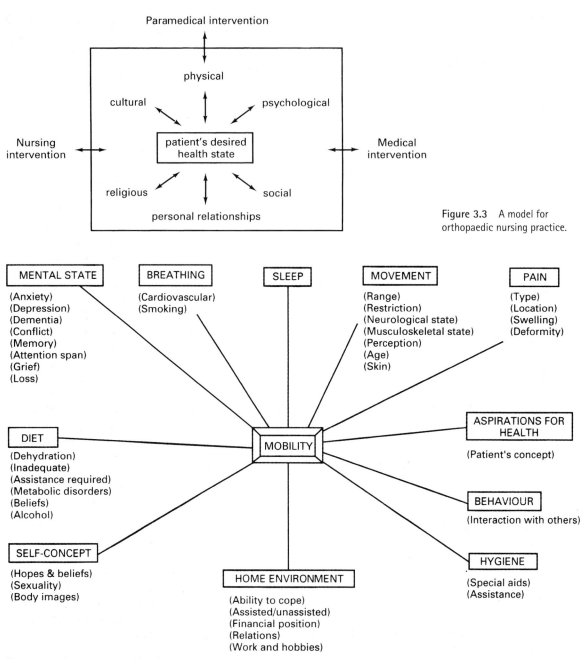

Figure 3.3 A model for orthopaedic nursing practice.

Figure 3.4 Assessment considerations.

often cannot clearly see ways in which the theories presented can be translated into practice in the form of interventions. In reality, most nursing models are used as frameworks for assessment. This is certainly true of the Roper, Logan and Tierney Activities of Living model, which is the model most commonly used in orthopaedic nursing practice in the UK.

ACTIVITIES OF LIVING

First published in *The elements of nursing* (1980), the Roper, Logan and Tierney model was an attempt to present nursing students with a conceptual framework identifying the theoretical base that underpins nursing practice (Roper et al 2000). Created

Box 3.2   Activities of living

- Maintaining a safe environment
- Communicating
- Breathing
- Eating and drinking
- Eliminating
- Personal cleansing and dressing
- Controlling body temperature
- Mobilising
- Working and playing
- Expressing sexuality
- Sleeping
- Dying

Box 3.3   An example of the Roper, Logan and Tierney ALs model in practice

Heather has rheumatoid arthritis. The joints of her hands and feet are severely affected which causes a considerable degree of disability. She has been admitted to hospital for a right total hip replacement with a view to resolving the pain in this extremely arthritic joint and allowing her to be more independent at home.

In the immediate period before surgery, Heather's assessment using the activities of living identified needs centred on maintaining a safe environment and communication in preparation for surgery. Heather's needs for information and psychological preparation are paramount at this stage. Her dependence/independence continuum focuses highly on independence and Heather requires little other care in the preoperative period.

In the immediate period following surgery, assessment continues and identifies that Heather's dependence/independence continuum highlights dependence in many areas. Nursing interventions focus on ensuring that all Heather's needs are met while the impact of her recent surgery prevents her from being independent. Her independence returns in a variety of areas over time. Once Heather is independently caring for herself in most respects, including mobilising sufficiently well to manage other activities of living in her home and community, she is ready for discharge with primary care support. Her need for knowledge and information at each stage is continuous.

originally for education purposes, it was adopted in the UK as a model to support clinical nursing practice and is widely used in many orthopaedic settings to this day.

Four central concepts underpin this model: activities of living (ALs) (Box 3.2), lifespan, the dependence to independence continuum and factors influencing ALs. As the central component of the module, the activities of living provide a way of describing what living means, enabling nurses to focus on those ALs that affect a patient at a given time.

This model is pertinent to orthopaedic nursing since musculoskeletal disorders and injury can severely affect an individual's dependence to independence continuum and their ability to maintain their ALs. Importantly, mobility is considered one of the activities of living along with recognition that other factors influence these activities, namely: biological, psychological, sociocultural, environmental and politicoeconomic factors. These areas also affect the orthopaedic patient's recovery from illness and injury. There is recognition of the influence of lifespan, taking into account the development of human beings from birth to death and their differing needs and influences at each stage in life. This reflects the 'cradle to grave' nature of orthopaedic nursing. Equally, the dependence to independence continuum recognises that at various stages, both in life and in the course of illness, disease or injury, a variety of factors affect an individual's ability to live life independently.

Often nurses use the 12 activities as aids to assessment. The model tends to work best when the patient's underlying needs are physical but it is important that the nurse uses a knowledge of these physical needs to gain a deeper understanding of the person's needs outside the physical domain, such as psychological and sociocultural needs (Aggleton & Chalmers 2000). Box 3.3 gives an example of how this model might be used in practice.

SELF-CARE

The work of Dorothea Orem (Orem 2001) presents a model of nursing that has been in development since the 1970s and has moved forwards during the intervening time. Orem sees human beings as self-determined individuals who act deliberately in pursuit of their own goals. The central concept within the model is the self-care capabilities human beings possess, which allow the individual to control and regulate their own functioning and development. Self-care is the maintenance of the equilibrium between self-care needs and the capacity an individual possesses to meet those needs. In ill health, the balance between the power to self-care and the demand for self-care can lead to a 'self-care deficit', resulting in the need for nursing care (Aggleton & Chalmers 2000).

There are eight universal self-care requisites.

1   Sufficient intake of air.
2   Sufficient intake of water.
3   Sufficient intake of food.
4   Satisfactory eliminative functions.
5   Activity balanced with rest.
6   Balance between solitude and social interaction.
7   Prevention of hazards to human life, human functioning and human well-being.
8   Promotion of human function and development within social groups in accordance with human potential, known human limitations and the desire for normalcy.

The model suggests that a person's ability to undertake self-care is affected by a number of factors including age, gender, sociocultural issues, patterns of living, environment, the availability of appropriate resources for self-care, along with ill health and injury. A healthy person is likely to have appropriate care abilities to meet their needs. An individual who is disabled, ill or injured will have additional demands known as 'health deviation self-care' needs. These link to changes in a person's physical structure, physical function or behaviour. It is easy to see how changes to physical form and function can apply to the orthopaedic patient.

In terms of nursing care, Orem identifies the need for the nurse and patient to undertake activities to help meet self-care deficits (Aggleton & Chalmers 2000). Some broad ways for the nurse to help patients are identified as:

- doing for or acting for another
- guiding or directing another
- providing physical support
- providing an environment supportive of development
- teaching another.

This model is well suited to orthopaedic nursing because of the need to focus on the individual's ability to self-care resulting from their disorder, illness or injury and their future ability to self-care

---

Box 3.4   An example of the Orem self-care model in practice

Mrs Wright is 79 years old. She lives alone in a house she shared with her husband all their married life until he died 5 years ago. Mrs Wright is very independent and has always looked after herself very well with minimal help from her daughter who lives 2 miles away.

Mrs Wright fell whilst rushing to answer the telephone, sustaining an intertrochanteric fracture of the right proximal femur for which she has undergone surgery to insert a dynamic hip screw.

The nurses caring for Mrs Wright after her surgery use Orem's model of self-care to inform the care they give. Mrs Wright is learning to walk again after her surgery. During this time there are clear changes within her physical structure and function following the fracture and surgery that have led to self-care deficits in the following areas:

- sufficient intake of food and water
- satisfactory eliminative functions
- activity balanced with rest
- prevention of hazards
- promotion of human function.

A care plan is carefully negotiated with Mrs Wright who is very keen to return to her own home but recognises her current self-care deficits; she is willing to work with the nurses who will guide and direct her in her mobilisation. Mrs Wright and the nurse agree that in order for her needs to be fulfilled the nurses will initially need to do things for her. This phase of 'acting for' her will gradually change over time, reducing the amount of 'doing for' that is provided and increasing the guiding and directing along with the provision of psychological support.

Although it takes 14 days for Mrs Wright to be discharged from hospital, she gradually increases her mobility, resulting in a reduction in her self-care deficits sufficient to allow her to return home. Mrs Wright's discharge plan includes:

- her daughter helping her to bed at night as she is still finding the stairs difficult (prevention of hazards, activity balanced with rest)
- a commode has been placed downstairs for during the day (satisfactory eliminative functions) and
- Mrs Wright's daughter will shop and cook for her mother in the evenings until her mobility has improved enough to allow her to make more than a sandwich (sufficient intake of food).

once recovery and rehabilitation have taken place. The eight self-care requisites help identify nursing needs and the five ways of helping enable the nurse to consider which interventions are appropriate when planning care. Box 3.4 gives an example of how this model might be used in practice.

THE ROY ADAPTATION MODEL

Roy's model of nursing sees human beings as unified entities made up of three main systems: biological, psychological and social. These constantly interact both within the individual and within the environment. As they can affect each other, each system is constantly striving for stability within itself and in its relationship with the others. When an individual becomes disabled, ill or injured, there may be some imbalance within these systems and in their relationship with each other, leading to the need for nursing care (Aggleton & Chalmers 2000).

Roy presents human beings as individuals who are constantly reacting and adapting to changes in the three systems and their environment. These changes are referred to as stimuli. Individuals can react to these stimuli with either adaptive responses or ineffective responses. Nursing aims to promote adaptive responses through physical, psychological and social nursing interventions.

Roy's theory of nursing is about the science and practice that expand adaptive abilities and enhance person and environment transformation. It utilises nursing goals to promote adaptation for individuals and groups through the adaptive responses, thus contributing to health, quality of life and dying with dignity. This is achieved by assessing behaviour and the factors that influence adaptive abilities, by intervening to expand those abilities and by enhancing environmental interactions (Aggleton & Chalmers 2000). Box 3.5 gives an example of how this model might be used in practice.

USING NURSING MODELS AND THEORIES

The models described above are not an exhaustive reference to models relevant to orthopaedic nursing practice. Nursing teams may find elements of these and other models useful in guiding their practice. Indeed, the development of a specific model that fits orthopaedic nursing is likely to result from a combination of these ideas.

Box 3.5   An example of the Roy adaptation model in practice

Mike is a 26 year old who sustained a compound fracture of the right tibia in a motorcycle accident. He was admitted to the orthopaedic trauma ward from the operating theatre following application of an external fixator device to his right lower leg. The initial nursing assessment identifies needs in all four adaptive modes. The following are examples.

- **Physiological adaptive mode:** the nurse identifies maladaptation related to Mike's fracture, tissue damage and enforced immobility. Homoeostasis is not maintained. Swelling and an open wound are assessed as having the potential to lead to further maladaptation and possible compromise of the tissue, blood and nerve supply. Nursing interventions focus on the need to increase the physiological adaptation to tissue damage by elevating the limb and undertaking regularly observations designed to recognise alterations in sensation, warmth and movement.
- **Self-concept adaptive mode:** the nurse recognises the potential for Mike's maladaptation to the presence of the external fixator, recognising the need to consider the psychological consequences of this. The nursing interventions focus on helping Mike to decrease the stimuli causing distress by helping him understand the purpose and management of the external fixator.
- **Role function adaptive mode:** the nurse identifies Mike's concerns about his personal life and his current and future work. Nursing interventions centre on maintaining Mike's contact with his normal world and allowing him to discuss and work through his fears about the future.
- **Interdependency adaptive mode:** later assessments indicated maladaptation due to Mike feeling isolated from his friends and family as a result of hospitalisation and restricted mobility. Nursing interventions centre on preventing the isolation by involving family and friends in Mike's care and discharge plans.

There is a tendency in the 21st century to move away from the development of nursing models, which were a feature of nursing in the 1980s and 1990s, to a more integrated approach in the delivery and documentation of nursing care. Nursing models and their documentation are often seen as being unwieldy, difficult and time consuming to use. Developments such as critical pathways are more likely to be a part of the future in this area of practice. However, it is important only to move in this direction whilst remembering the underpinning theory of nursing practice.

One of the problems with some nursing models is the need for them to move forward in time along with developments in nursing practice. This has not always been the case. Orthopaedic nurses and nurse theorists need to consider how these ideas can be developed for nursing in the 21st century.

THE NURSING PROCESS

In all nursing models, the nursing process is central to articulating the essence of the model of practice (McGee 1998). The introduction of the nursing process in the UK in the late 1970s and early 1980s provided a means of translating nursing models into a usable form. The process provides a logical way of thinking about patients and their needs through assessing, planning, implementing and evaluating care. It gives a structure to thinking about and planning nursing care and is central to the structure of most nursing documentation.

INTEGRATED CARE PATHWAYS

An integrated care pathway (ICP) is both a tool and a concept that embeds guidelines, protocols, locally agreed evidence-based and patient-centred best practice into everyday individual patient care. In addition, and uniquely to ICPs, they record deviations from planned care in the form of variances.

An ICP aims to have (National Electronic Library for Health 2003):

- the right people
- doing the right things
- in the right order
- at the right time
- in the right place
- with the right outcome
- all with attention to the patient experience and
- comparing planned care with the care actually given.

ICPs are now a common alternative approach to care planning. The idea brings together all the

professional groups involved in patient care, arriving at a consensus about standards of care and expected outcomes for selected patient groups (Walsh 1998). This idea works particularly well in orthopaedic care where a patient's pathway of care is expected to follow a set pattern. ICPs are often used in areas where patients can be grouped according to their injury, disorder, surgery or investigations; for example, patients who have sustained a proximal femoral fracture (hip fracture), have chronic back pain from a disc prolapse or are undergoing total joint arthroplasty surgery.

The pathway concept acknowledges that each individual's care is largely similar, with variations that do not greatly affect the main focus of care. When patient care deviates from the usual pathway, the reasons for this are identified, documented and used to monitor the quality of care provided. This idea suggests that individualised care has gone too far, resulting in nurses treating each patient as an exception to the norm.

The additional benefits of critical pathways are the reduction in the amount of documentation health professionals need to complete, the fostering of multidisciplinary working and the ability to free practitioners' time so they can deal with specific problems as they occur rather than worrying about the potential problems.

The use of ICPs has allowed different healthcare institutions to make comparisons between the care provided in each area and to share innovations and improvements through a collaborative approach.

Other names sometimes used to describe ICPs are listed in Box 3.6. These variations developed in different settings but share many of the central concepts

---

Box 3.6   Variations of terms used for integrated care pathways

- Anticipated recovery pathways (ARPs)
- Multidisciplinary pathways of care (MPCs)
- Care protocols
- Critical care pathways
- Pathways of care
- Care packages
- Collaborative care pathways
- CareMaps®
- Care profiles

of ICPs. A genuine ICP is characterised by (National Electronic Library for Health 2003):

- systematic actions for consistent best practice and continuous improvements in patient care, all with attention to the patient experience
- patient-centred approaches built into packages of care for identified patient grouping
- providing continuous feedback via variance tracking and analysis
- multidisciplinary approaches based on roles, competence and responsibility
- mapping and modelling of clinical and non-clinical care processes
- incorporating order and priorities, including guidelines and protocols
- including standards and outcomes.

The use of ICPs is increasing in trauma and elective orthopaedic surgery and this trend is likely to continue in the future. The current health service agenda values mutidisciplinarity, collaboration and clinical effectiveness and ICPs are seen as one tool able to foster these ideas. However, full integration of all members of the multidisciplinary team within a care pathway that covers the full duration of the patient's journey is still rare. Orthopaedic nurses need to embrace these ideas within their practice, whilst ensuring that the underpinning theory and philosophy of nursing are not lost.

CONTINUITY OF CARE

The way in which nursing is organised to ensure that each patient has received the care they require has been a major discussion point in the profession for many decades. Central to the current argument is the idea that care is most effective and acceptable to patients when provided by the smallest number of team members possible.

In the 1970s and 1980s, nursing began to move away from the allocation of tasks to patient allocation. Small groups of nurses became responsible for the care of a group of patients during a shift rather than undertaking specific tasks for all patients. This enables the patient to build up a valuable and important trusting relationship between themselves and those caring for them. Ideally, a patient in hospital or in the community should have their care provided regularly by as few healthcare workers as possible. This seems to be particularly important in orthopaedic

settings where the patient's contact with the health system is likely to be more prolonged than in many other settings. This principle is the basis of the provision of continuity of care.

To support the approach, the concept of the named nurse developed in the UK in the early 1990s. This was originally intended to enhance nursing practice through allocating a specific nurse to the care of an individual patient. The standard set was that each patient should have a nurse who is well known to them and takes responsibility for their care plan and implementation of that care. This idea stresses the importance of the nurse–patient relationship and the idea of individual and collective responsibility for care. Consequently, the named nurse approach is often seen as both a mode of care delivery and a philosophy of nursing (Pontin 1999).

The idea of named nursing was based on the concept of primary nursing, a mode of care delivery developed in the USA in the 1980s that took this idea a number of steps further. Primary nursing was developed to ensure patient-centred care delivery within limited resources, increasing the involvement of nurses in shaping the care of their patients whilst increasing their job satisfaction (Botishwarelo 2003). The primary nurse was the professional who took direct 24-hour responsibility for the patient's plan of care and, whenever possible, led and delivered that care with a team of nurses. The idea allows for continuity of care during the entire 24-hour period and has been instrumental in a number of nursing developments and increased nursing autonomy. This mode of care delivery has also been seen as a philosophy for nursing (Pontin 1999).

Many of the benefits of the primary nursing system have yet to be proven through empirical inquiry but it has been embraced in orthopaedic nursing to a degree and it remains a feature of care in a number of orthopaedic units in the UK. The notion of primary nursing has led to a number of further sideways developments such as team nursing. Team nursing works on a similar principle to primary nursing but is less focused on the role of the primary nurse, focusing instead on nurses working in small teams to provide care for small groups of patients within a ward, unit or community.

A further development of this is key working and case management where the central professional who makes decisions about the patient's plan of care can be a nurse or another health professional such as a physiotherapist, occupational therapist or social worker, depending on the patient's central needs.

This idea has yet to take off in the orthopaedic setting in the UK.

THE PHILOSOPHY OF REHABILITATION

Rehabilitation is often seen as central to orthopaedic nursing (Powell 1986) as the means of restoring a person to their normal life (Hawkey & Williams 2001). One of the major problems for patients who have an orthopaedic condition, surgery or sustained trauma is the physical disability that can lead to dependency.

The nurse is the health professional who has most contact with the client, largely due to the unique 24-hour nature of nursing and its focus on the client's physical needs. This offers often unrealised opportunities for the nurse to develop strategies to enhance the patient's rehabilitation potential. There has been considerable debate over the last two decades regarding the role of the nurse in rehabilitation, particularly whether there is a therapeutic role for the nurse. Nursing practice in this area has been slow to focus attention on the patient's desires and psychological needs that impact on successful rehabilitation. The literature that considers these issues recognises that nurses have not yet defined a role in rehabilitation other than that focusing on physical needs (Nolan et al 1997, Waters & Luker 1996) and orthopaedic nursing is no exception.

Hawkey & Williams (2001) identify eight categories that are central to evolving rehabilitation nursing and these need to be considered within any orthopaedic rehabilitation context.

- Essential nursing skills
- Therapeutic practice
- Coordination
- Education
- Advocacy
- Political awareness
- Advice and counselling
- Clinical governance.

MOTIVATION

Motivation is a concept often seen as central to successful rehabilitation. Rehabilitation professionals have long suspected that a client's motivation plays an important role in determining the outcome of therapy. It is commensurate with many factors such as self-efficacy, contextual support, emotions, needs, incentives, rewards (Geelen & Soons 1996, Rensick 1996, Thomas 1999), courage and encouragement (Beck 1994).

This complex phenomenon may influence the successful rehabilitation of orthopaedic patients. Many factors are likely to influence rehabilitation motivation, including goals, humour, caring and kindness, belief in the staff and rehabilitation, encouragement, basic personality, power within relationships, domination in rehabilitation, responses to domination and beliefs (Rensick 1996). In particular, involvement of the client in decision making appears to be vital.

ENCOURAGEMENT

Basic concepts are often taken for granted, ignored or dismissed as simplistic. Encouragement is one such concept. The word is in daily use in nursing practice yet there is to date no nursing literature that has examined it as either a concept or an intervention.

The nature of disease, ill health and injury causes individuals to frequently suffer from fear, helplessness, frustration, lack of motivation and discouragement. A potentially important and untapped aspect of the caring role in nursing may be to use encouragement practices to dissipate fear, demotivation and discouragement and thereby facilitate recovery and health. The literature indicates that to encourage is to promote and activate social interest and a sense of belonging, value, worthwhileness and welcome in the human community (Dinkmeyer & Eckstein 1995).

In Adlerian psychology, the loss of courage or discouragement is understood to be the basis of mistaken and dysfunctional behaviour, seen for example in a patient's reluctance to take an active part in their rehabilitation.

Encouragement is mainly discussed in the literature of educational psychology, the field in which the most evaluative research has taken place in an attempt to identify the benefits of encouragement. Carns & Carns (1998) offer the following elements of encouragement seen in educational psychology which lend themselves well to an elucidation of encouragement in rehabilitation nursing practice.

- Value individuals as they are.
- Use words that build the individual's self-esteem.
- Plan for experiences that create success.
- Demonstrate genuineness to individuals.
- Demonstrate non-verbal acceptance through touch.

- Use humour.
- Spend regular time with individuals.
- Recognise effort.
- Avoid emphasis on disabilities.
- Show appreciation for the individual's cooperation.
- Avoid comparing individuals.

Such strategies are likely to be useful to nurses when encouraging orthopaedic patients during rehabilitation. Put simply, verbal encouragement while completing a difficult mobility task can make all the difference to patients' rehabilitation outcomes.

CONCLUSION

Theory is now integral to orthopaedic nursing and is likely to become an increasing feature of practice as the 21st century progresses. Systems are now in place that will allow such theory to develop and further work on the part of practitioners, theorists and researchers will reap rewards in the future. This chapter has highlighted only some of the many theories and concepts that interface with orthopaedic nursing. It is not exhaustive and the enquiring orthopaedic nurse needs to keep constantly up to date with the literature that helps to apply theory to practice.

Further reading

Holland K, Jenkins J, Soloman J, Whittam S 2003 Applying the Roper, Logan and Tierney model in practice. Churchill Livingstone, Edinburgh

References

Aggleton P, Chalmers H 2000 Nursing models and nursing practice, 2nd edn. Macmillan, Basingstoke

Artless E, Richmond C 2000 The art and science of orthopaedic nursing. Journal of Orthopaedic Nursing 4(1): 4–9

Balcombe K 1994 Using a nursing model: a model for orthopaedic nursing. In: Davis P (ed) Nursing the orthopaedic patient. Churchill Livingstone, Edinburgh

Beck RJ 1994 Encouragement as a vehicle to empowerment in counselling: an existential perspective. Journal of Rehabilitation 60(3): 6–11

Bjork IT 1995 Neglected conflicts in the discipline of nursing: perceptions of the importance and value of practical skill. Journal of Advanced Nursing 22(1): 6–12

Botishwarelo T 2003 The phenomenon of primary nursing: beyond the ordinary. Creative Nursing 1(1): 12–13

Carns MR, Carns AW 1998 A review of the professional literature concerning the consistency of the definition and application of Adlerian encouragement. Journal of Individual Psychology 54(1): 72–89

Cortis JD, Kendrick K 2003 Nursing ethics, caring and culture. Nursing Ethics 10(1): 77–88

Dinkmeyer D, Eckstein D 1995 Leadership by encouragement. St Lucie Press, USA

Ellul J, Watkins C, Ferguson N, Barer D 1993 Increasing patient engagement in rehabilitation activities. Clinical Rehabilitation 7: 297–302

Fagerstrom L, Eriksson K, Enberg IB 1998 The patient's perceived caring needs as a message of suffering. Journal of Advanced Nursing 28(5): 978–987

Fawcett J 1995 Analysis and evaluation of conceptual models of nursing, 3rd edn. Davis, Philadelphia

Fosbinder D 1994 Patient perceptions of nursing care: an emerging theory of interpersonal competence. Journal of Advanced Nursing 20(6): 1085–1093

Geelen R, Soons P 1996 Rehabilitation: an 'everyday' motivation model. Patient Education and Counselling 28(1): 69–77

Greenwood J 2002 The caring conundrum. In: Daly J, Speedy S, Jackson D, Darbyshire P (eds) Contexts of nursing: an introduction. Blackwell, Oxford

Hawkey B, Williams J 2001 Rehabilitation: the nurses' role. Journal of Orthopaedic Nursing 5(2): 81–88

Jackson D, Borbasi S 2002 The caring conundrum: should caring be the basis of nursing practice and scholarship? In: Daly J, Speedy S, Jackson D, Darbyshire P (eds) Contexts of nursing: an introduction. Blackwell, Oxford

Johnson J 1995 Achieving effective rehabilitation outcome: does the nurse have a role? British Journal of Therapy and Rehabilitation 2(3): 113–118

Kolcaba R 1997 The primary holisms in nursing. Journal of Advanced Nursing 25: 290–296

Love C 1995 Orthopaedic nursing: study of its specialty status. Nursing Standard 9(44): 36–40

Lucas B 2002 Orthopaedic patient journeys: a UK perspective. Journal of Orthopaedic Nursing 6(2): 86–89

McGee P 1998 Models for nursing practice: a pattern for practical care. Stanley Thornes, Cheltenham

McMahon R 1998 Therapeutic nursing: theory, issues and practice. In: McMahon R, Pearson S (eds) Nursing as therapy, 2nd edn. Stanley Thornes, Cheltenham

Morse JM, Procter A 1998 Maintaining patient endurance … the comfort work of trauma nurses. Clinical Nursing Research 7(3): 250–274

Morse JM, Bortoff JL, Hutchinson S 1994 The phenomenology of comfort. Journal of Advanced Nursing 20(1): 189–195

Muetzel P-A 1988 Therapeutic nursing. In: Pearson A (ed) Primary nursing. Chapman and Hall, London

Myco F 1984 Stroke and its rehabilitation: the perceived role of the nurse in medical and nursing literature. Journal of Advanced Nursing 9: 429–439

National Electronic Library for Health (2003) Integrated care pathways. Available online at: www.nelh.nhs.uk/carepathways/intro

Nolan M, Booth S, Nolan J 1997 New directions in rehabilitation: exploring the nursing contribution. English National Board, London

Orem DE 2001 Nursing: concepts and practice, 6th edn. Mosby, St Louis

Ouellet LL, Rush KL 1998 Conceptual model of client mobility. Journal of Orthopaedic Nursing 2(3): 132–135

Owen MJ, Holmes CA 1993 Holism in the discourse of nursing. Journal of Advanced Nursing 18: 1688–1695

Payle J 2001 An archaeology of caring knowledge. Journal of Advanced Nursing 36(2): 188–198

Pontin D 1999 Primary nursing: a mode of care or a philosophy of nursing? Journal of Advanced Nursing 29(3): 584–592

Powell M 1986 Orthopaedic nursing and rehabilitation. Churchill Livingstone, Edinburgh

Raudonis BM, Acton GJ 1997 Theory-based nursing practice. Journal of Advanced Nursing 26(1): 138–145

Rensick B 1996 Motivation in geriatric rehabilitation. Image. Journal of Nursing Scholarship 28(1): 41–45

Roper N, Logan W, Tierney AJ 1980 The elements of nursing. Churchill Livingstone, Edinburgh

Roper N, Logan W, Tierney AJ 2000 The Roper, Logan and Tierney model of nursing: based on activities of living. Churchill Livingstone, Edinburgh

Santy J 2001 An investigation of the reality of nursing work with orthopaedic patients. Journal of Orthopaedic Nursing 5(1): 22–29

Scherwitz LW, Rountree R, Delvitt P 1997 Wound caring is more than wound care: the provider as a partner. Ostomy Wound Management 43(9): 42–44, 46, 48

Slye DA 1991 Orthopaedic complications: compartment syndrome, fat embolism syndrome and venous thromboembolism. Nursing Clinics of North America 26(1): 113–132

Thomas D 1999 The nurse as psychological support in rehabilitation. In: Smith M (ed) Rehabilitation in adult nursing practice. Churchill Livingstone, Edinburgh

Walker LO, Avant LC 1995 Strategies for theory construction in nursing, 3rd edn. Prentice Hall, New Jersey

Walsh M 1998 Models and critical pathways in clinical nursing. Baillière Tindall, London

Waters K, Luker L 1996 Staff perspectives on the role of the nurse in rehabilitation wards for elderly people. Journal of Clinical Nursing 5(2): 103–114

Watson J 1994 Applying the art and science of human caring. National League for Nursing, New York

Chapter 4

The locomotor system

Christine Knight, Amanda Mathew, Judith K Muir

INTRODUCTION

An understanding of the locomotor system is central to orthopaedic nursing and caring for people with mobility problems. Movement involves biomechanics, the musculoskeletal system, joints and levers, the neural system and biochemistry. These elements combine and influence the way in which people maintain their body posture, form and function. This chapter provides a quick reference to the anatomy and physiology of the locomotor system. In view of the increasing proportion of elderly people in the population, it also discusses some of the current theories of ageing in relation to the locomotor system.

THE SKELETAL SYSTEM

The skeletal system is the framework of the body. It consists of bone and associated connective tissue such as cartilage and dense fibrous tissue. Bone is a specialised form of connective tissue and is important for its mechanical properties and the maintenance of mineral homoeostasis.

FUNCTIONS OF THE SKELETON

The functions of the skeleton are as follows:

- **Support**: the skeleton provides a framework for the body, with surface markings for the attachment and insertion of muscles.
- **Protection**: the skeleton maintains body shape, protecting from injury many of the internal organs such as the brain, heart, lungs and spinal cord.

- **Movement**: bones and muscles act as levers, producing body movements through joints.
- **Mineral storage**: bones store minerals such as calcium and phosphorus.
- **Blood cell formation**: red bone marrow produces red blood cells, white blood cells and platelets. This process is called haematopoiesis.

NORMAL BONE STRUCTURE

Bone tissue is highly vascular, combining organic and inorganic material. A system of collagenous fibres forms the organic component, providing resilience and flexibility. The inorganic material consists mainly of mineral salts which form a matrix providing strength and weight-bearing capabilities. Bone is three times stronger than wood and as tensile as cast iron. It is the strength and rigidity of this matrix that give bone its characteristics.

Bone is composed of two types of specialised cells, arising from different stem cells (Fig. 4.1).

1 Osteogenic cells are unspecialised cells derived from the mesenchyme. These are to be found in the periosteum, endosteum, Haversian and Volkmann's canals.
   - Osteoblasts do not have mitotic potential. They are involved in bone formation by secreting organic components and mineral salts. They are found on the surface of bones.

- Osteocytes are osteoblasts that become trapped within bone and do not have mitotic potential. They maintain the structure of the bone tissue.

2 Osteoclasts develop from the macrophage–monocyte system. Their function involves the resorption of bone; as a result they have the key role in the continuous modelling of bone.

Chemical composition

Bone is normally made up of organic (30–35%) and inorganic (65–70%) material. The organic component consists of protein fibres which are mainly collagen. These collagen fibres make up 90–95% of the organic matrix.

Mineral salts, such as those of calcium and phosphorus, predominate in the inorganic component. These complex crystals combine to produce rod-shaped hydroxyapatite crystals (Fig. 4.2) that are uniform in shape. The ratio of calcium content to phosphorus content varies depending on the nutritional state of the individual. The levels are controlled by the parathyroid hormone and calcitonin produced in the parathyroid and thyroid glands.

Other substances are present, attached in the form of ions:

- magnesium
- sodium

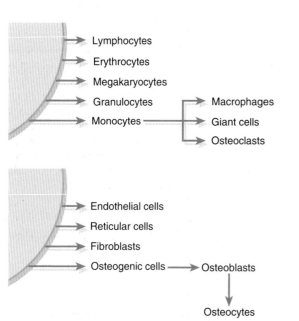

Figure 4.1 Origin of bone cells.

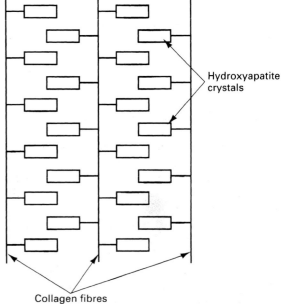

Figure 4.2 Hydroxyapatite crystals.

- potassium
- carbonate.

The chemical composition of bone makes it susceptible to damage. For example, radioactive chemicals attach strongly to the hydroxyapatite crystals. This includes emissions from nuclear power stations such as uranium, plutonium and strontium. These destructive chemicals are ionically similar to calcium and phosphorus; these do not pass out of the body but accumulate and irradiate bone marrow.

TYPES OF BONE

The density of bone varies. There are two major types of bone with differences in weight, strength and function:

- compact (dense) bone
- cancellous (spongy) bone.

Compact bone is denser bone tissue with few spaces, whereas cancellous bone has larger spaces filled with red bone marrow. The distribution of compact and cancellous bone is illustrated in Figure 4.3.

Compact bone

A layer of compact bone surrounds cancellous bone. This layer is thicker in the diaphysis than the epiphysis. In addition to providing support and protection, it resists any weight directed through the long bone.

Compact bone is dense with a concentric ring structure. Blood vessels and nerves enter the bone substance from its outer covering, the periosteum, through the Volkmann's canals. Central (Haversian) canals run longitudinally and contain blood vessels and nerves which have merged with vessels from the Volkmann's canals and the medullary cavity.

The Haversian canals are surrounded by rings of a hard calcified bone, known as concentric lamellae. In between the lamellae are spaces called lacunae which contain osteocytes. Small canals called canaliculi radiate from these osteocytes. Circumferential lamellae form flat plates and surround the outer surface of the compact bone. In cross-section (Fig. 4.4) a Haversian system (osteon) consists of a single Haversian canal, associated concentric lamellae and osteocytes.

Compact bone is made up of an intricate network allowing the passage of nutrients from the periosteum and endosteum to the osteocytes, with the removal of waste products passing in the opposite direction.

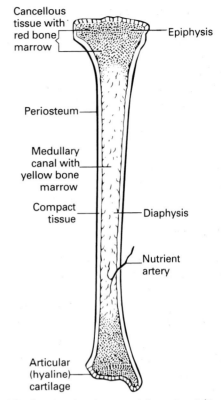

Figure 4.3   A mature long bone, partially sectioned. (From Waugh & Grant 2001.)

Cancellous bone

Cancellous bone consists of a latticework of thin plates of compact bone called trabeculae which are laid down along lines of stress. Each trabecula comprises several lamellae containing layers of lacunae filled with osteocytes. The osteocytes are linked with other osteocytes through the canaliculi, from where they obtain their nutrients via the circulating blood.

Although cancellous bone is lighter and less strong than compact bone, its irregular, spongy nature provides a large internal surface for blood-forming cells. Red bone marrow, contained in the axial skeleton, remains active in blood cell formation even in adult life. Yellow bone marrow, which replaces red marrow in the appendicular skeleton of adult life, retains the ability to produce blood cells if stimulated by deficiency.

STRUCTURE OF A LONG BONE

A typical long bone (Fig. 4.5) consists of the following components.

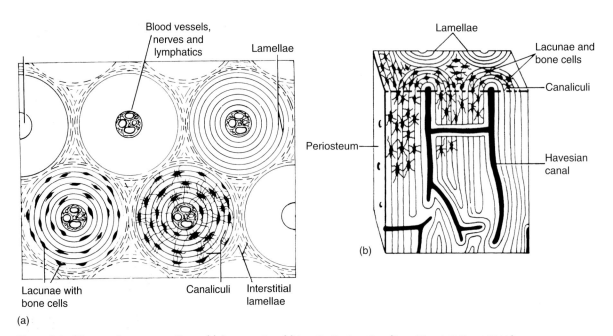

Figure 4.4   Microscopic structure of bone. (a) Cross-section. (b) Longitudinal section. (From Waugh & Grant 2001.)

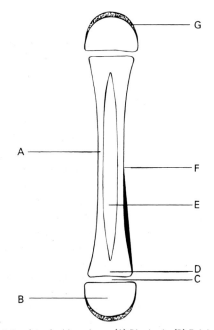

Figure 4.5   A typical long bone. (A) Diaphysis. (B) Epiphysis. (C) Epiphyseal plate. (D) Metaphysis. (E) Medullary cavity. (F) Periosteum. (G) Articular hyaline cartilage. (From Gunn 1996.)

- **Diaphysis**: the shaft of a long bone.
- **Epiphysis**: these are at the ends of a long bone.
- **Epiphyseal plate**: this consists of cartilage and joins the diaphysis to the epiphysis in mature bone.

This is the area where most growth in length takes place. Growth stops when all of the epiphyseal plate is fully ossified, usually in the late teens to early 20s. The area where the diaphysis joins the epiphyseal plate may be referred to as the metaphysis.

- **Periosteum**: this is essential for bone growth, repair and nutrition. It covers the outer surface of the bone. The periosteum has a dense outer fibrous layer composed of connective tissue, containing blood vessels, nerves and lymphatic vessels. The inner layer contains elastic fibres, a few osteoclasts, a single layer of osteoblasts, osteoprogenitor cells and blood vessels. Where ligaments and tendons attach, the periosteal fibres become continuous with the fibres of the tendon or ligament. Perforating fibres called Sharpey's fibres allow the attachment of ligaments and fibres to the bone by penetrating the periosteum.
- **Endosteum**: the lining of the medullary cavity of the bone. It consists of a single layer of osteoprogenitor cells, osteoblasts and some osteoclasts.
- **Medullary cavity**: this is found within the diaphysis of long bones and in smaller cavities in the epiphysis. The medullary cavity contains yellow marrow or red marrow.

BONE FORMATION

The embryonic development of bone involves the migration of mesenchymal tissue into the area where bone formation is to begin. The mesenchymal cells increase in size and number and differentiate into osteogenic cells. Then the osteogenic cells differentiate into osteoblasts or chondroblasts. In the embryo, fibrous membranes and cartilage are shaped like bone. Ossification begins around the 6th or 7th week of embryonic life.

Embryonic (fetal) bone

The fetal bones are outlined as fibrous or cartilagenous tissue. As the fetus develops, calcification of the bone occurs as calcium salts are deposited and osteoblasts lay down bone to replace the cartilage.

There are variations in the rate of development between bones and parts of bones, for example:

- in the femur the distal epiphysis appears around 36 fetal weeks
- in the tibia the proximal epiphysis appears around 40 fetal weeks
- the metatarsal bones appear at 8–16 fetal weeks
- the calcaneus appears at 24–26 fetal weeks
- the talus bone appears at 26–28 fetal weeks.

Knowledge of these factors is useful in the treatment of disorders such as developmental dysplasia of the hip or clubfoot, where early intervention before the bone is fully developed may influence the outcome.

Ossification or osteogenesis is the formation of bone by osteoblasts. This process involves the synthesis of an organic matrix and the addition of mineral salts such as hydroxyapatite. It occurs in two ways.

1 **Intramembranous**: the formation of bone within connective tissue membranes.
2 **Endochondral**: the formation of bone from cartilage.

Intramembranous ossification

Osteoblasts formed from osteoprogenitor stem cells colonise connective tissue membranes. They secrete intercellular substances and form a bony matrix in centres of ossification. Trabeculae radiate out from each centre of ossification into a latticework of collagen fibres where inorganic salts are deposited. The original connective tissue becomes the periosteum and the ossified area becomes spongy (cancellous) bone with a covering of compact bone. Blood vessels and unspecialised cells become the bone marrow.

The majority of the bones of the skull and the clavicle develop in this way. In the newborn,

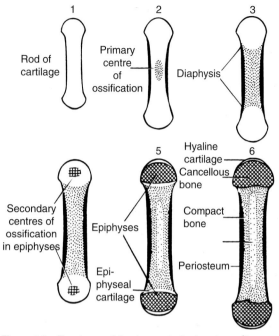

Figure 4.6   The stages of development of a long bone. (From Waugh & Grant 2001.)

membranous gaps (fontanelles) remain between the various bones of the skull. These close during the first year of life, allowing the bones to fuse together.

Endochondral ossification

Most of the bones of the body, including the base of the skull, are formed by endochondral ossification. Bone develops from a prototype of hyaline cartilage (Fig. 4.6). The cartilage is covered by a membrane called the perichondrium. This is invaded by numerous blood capillaries, stimulating osteoprogenitor cells to form osteoblasts. The layer of osteoblasts then forms osteocytes to make compact bone around the diaphysis. The surrounding membrane is then known as the periosteum.

During childhood the process continues mainly at the centres of ossification which allow the bone to grow. These centres of ossification are situated in the centre of bone (primary centre of ossification) and the extremities of long bones (secondary centre of ossification). At the primary centre of ossification the chondrocytes hypertrophy and the matrix becomes mineralised as the intercellular substance calcifies. The chondrocytes eventually die, leaving large lacunae for blood vessels to grow into. The spaces in the shaft of the long bone join together, forming the medullary cavity which fills with bone marrow.

In the long bone each extremity or epiphysis is separated from the shaft (diaphysis) by the epiphyseal line which is made of a layer of cartilage. Within the epiphysis, secondary centres of ossification lay down cancellous bone. Ossification continues until all the cartilage is replaced, where it covers the articular surfaces and in the epiphyseal plate. The articular cartilage and epiphyseal plate are directly formed from original embryonic tissue. Like the appearance of the various parts of bones, closure of epiphyses is variable and continues until adulthood. Once adulthood is reached this layer becomes calcified, the epiphysis and diaphysis fuse and there is no further bone growth.

Growth in the circumference of a bone occurs when osteoblasts lay down new bone under the periosteum, the tough fibrous covering of the bone.

BONE GROWTH

Bone grows by appositional growth or endochondral growth.

Appositional growth

This is the formation of new bone on the surface of existing bone. Most bones increase in diameter by this means. Appositional growth occurs along with growth in the length of a bone. Bone lining the marrow cavity is destroyed by osteoclasts, which originate from haematopoietic stem cells, enabling the cavity to increase in size. Simultaneously, osteoblasts from the periosteum produce new compact bone which covers the outer surface of the bone.

Endochondral growth

This is the growth of cartilage in the epiphyseal plate until its eventual ossification and fusion with the diaphysis between 12 and 25 years of age. This process of growth involves interstitial cartilage growth followed by calcification and replacement bone. Knowledge of this process has implications for treatment of the child and adolescent (Table 4.1).

REQUIREMENTS FOR BONE FORMATION AND GROWTH

Bone formation and resorption is a continuous process requiring an adequate intake of calcium

Table 4.1   Endochondral growth

Spine	Limbs
• Ossification in vertebrae is evident from the 8th embryonic week • Axial skeleton then changes with growth • The newborn infant has a large head and concave spine • At 3 months head control and a cervical lordosis develop • At 5 months sitting will produce a lumbar lordosis • At 1 year 50% total growth of the spine has occurred, height will be defined more by the lower limbs. Therefore spinal fusion is less stunting than premature closure of epiphyses of the lower limb	• Appear as buds about the 4th embryonic week • Joints are defined by the 6th embryonic week • Longitudinal growth is greatest around birth • As extremities grow longitudinally, they also change rotationally and angularly • Many rotational problems will be associated with pathological conditions, e.g. cerebral palsy • Some normal conditions, e.g. bow legs (genu varum), usually confined to the tibia and symmetrical, will correct by 18–24 months by walking

and vitamin D. The skeleton contains approximately 99% of the total body calcium which is equal to about 1 kg weight. The calcium within the cells is constantly changing with the calcium in the extracellular field; this is called dynamic equilibrium. This process, known as bone turnover, continues through life but is especially high during childhood. It is therefore important that the child is provided with an adequate diet to build good bone stock for later life. Calcium salts are present in greater quantities in adult bone than immature bone, which tends to be more elastic with a loose matrix. If trauma occurs in a child, it may result in a 'greenstick' or partial fracture, instead of a complete break that normally occurs in mature dense bones. In a freshly healed fracture, the bone matrix is less dense than normal, making the requirement for calcium higher than normal.

The formation of bone is affected by pituitary growth hormone, sex hormones (oestrogens and androgens) and thyroid hormone.

If resorption exceeds deposition, osteoporosis develops; in fact, many problems might develop if this fine balance is disrupted.

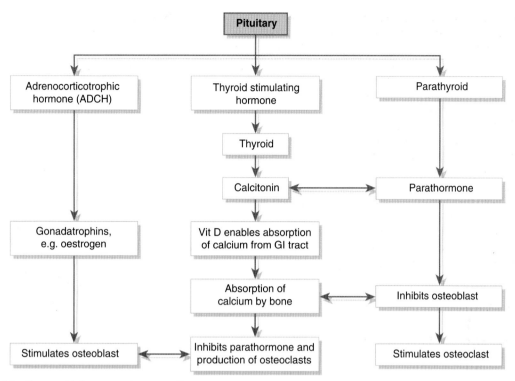

Figure 4.7 Hormonal influences on bone growth.

Repair and maintenance

Repair and maintenance of bone occurs as a result of several different stimuli.

- Remodelling during bone growth involves the replacement of old bone by new bone tissue.
- Additional bone is deposited in response to exercise and mechanical stress.
- The time taken for a fracture to repair will depend on the type of fracture. It will take longer in the elderly because of decreased blood supply and general inefficiency of the repair processes.

Remodelling

Remodelling takes place in bone growth, during an alteration in shape, in response to mechanical stress and in the repair process. Bone constantly remodels its matrix. The process allows worn or injured bone to be replaced and helps to regulate the storage of calcium for the rest of the body, as calcium is essential for the normal functioning of many of the body's tissues.

Normal bone replacement relies on sufficient dietary intake or production of:

- hormones
- calcium and phosphorus

- manganese and boron
- vitamin D which aids the absorption of calcium from the gastrointestinal tract into the blood, removes calcium from bone and reabsorbs calcium from the kidney tubules
- vitamin C which maintains the intercellular substance of bone and other connective tissue
- vitamin A which controls the activity, distribution and coordination of osteoblasts and osteoclasts.

Process of resorption

Osteoclasts are believed to be responsible for resorption. In the normal adult, homoeostasis is maintained between the removal and deposition of calcium and collagen. During this process it is thought that osteoclasts develop projections that secrete enzymes as well as lactic acid and citric acid. The acids cause bone to dissolve and the enzymes digest collagen and other organic substances.

Hormones

Human growth hormone, secreted by the anterior pituitary gland, is responsible for bone tissue growth (Fig. 4.7). Under- or oversecretion during childhood may result in dwarfism or gigantism, respectively. Growth hormone stimulates interstitial cartilage growth and appositional bone growth. The thyroid gland produces calcitonin, which is essential for normal growth. Calcitonin inhibits osteoclast activity and accelerates the absorption of calcium by bone.

Parathormone, produced in the parathyroid glands, increases osteoclast activity, releasing calcium and phosphate ions from the bones into the blood system.

Sex hormones stimulate bone growth. Oestrogen and testosterone increase the activity of osteoblasts and promote new bone formation. The burst of growth during puberty is due to a release of male and female sex hormones. These hormones stimulate ossification of the epiphyseal plate as skeletal growth is completed. Girls usually stop growing earlier than boys. The loss of bone density occurs as hormone levels decrease, especially in menopausal women, and may result in osteoporosis, thus increasing the risk of bone fracture.

Exercise

Bone is capable of altering its strength in response to a mechanical stress. Mechanical stress increases the deposition of mineral salts and the production of collagen fibres. An absence of this type of stress promotes the removal of mineral salts and collagen fibres.

Athletes whose bones are subjected to a high degree of stress have thicker bones than non-athletes. The effect of regular exercise is to stimulate bone growth and increase the production of calcitonin, thus inhibiting bone resorption.

FRACTURE REPAIR

Bones vary considerably in the length of time they require to heal. As a rule, in adults upper limb fractures take 6–8 weeks to heal and lower limb fractures require 8–12 weeks.

The following stages occur in the repair of a fracture (Fig. 4.8).

● **Stage 1**: inflammatory phase. As a result of a fracture, the bone ends and surrounding tissue bleed and a haematoma is formed. The bone ends are subsequently sealed by the fracture haematoma, where osteocyte and periosteal cell death occurs. This results in an inflammatory response with vasodilation and the gathering of polymorphonucleocytes and histiocytes.

● **Stage 2**: reparative phase. This stage is characterised by the formation of callus. External callus is produced by mesenchymal cells from the periosteum, forming a bridge between the bone ends. Direct endosteal proliferation also takes place on the exposed, broken surfaces of the diaphysis. The cells are gradually replaced by mineralised trabeculae of 'woven' bone. At this stage the callus is visible on X-ray.

● **Stage 3**: remodelling phase. Remodelling of the original structure takes place over a period of time. Any fragments of dead bone are resorbed by the osteoclasts and compact, lamellar bone replaces spongy bone around the fracture. On X-ray the surface of the bone will usually retain some evidence of the fracture site.

AXIAL AND APPENDICULAR SKELETON

The adult skeleton (Fig. 4.9) consists of 206 bones, which can be divided into two categories. The axial skeleton consists of 80 bones and the appendicular skeleton 126 bones.

The exact number of individual bones varies from person to person and may decrease with age owing to the fusion of some bones. The axial skeleton consists of the skull, hyoid bone, vertebral column, ribs and sternum. The appendicular skeleton consists of bones of the upper limbs and pectoral girdle, and the lower limbs and pelvic girdle. Movement takes place where two or more bones articulate with each other and is facilitated by a covering of smooth hyaline cartilage on each of the articulating surfaces.

CARTILAGE

Cartilage is made up of cartilage cells called chondrocytes. Cartilage consists of a dense network of collagenous fibres and elastic fibres within an extensive and fairly rigid matrix. The matrix, secreted by the chondrocytes, consists of protein fibres, a ground substance consisting of non-fibrous protein such as proteoglycans, and fluid. The proteoglycans are capable of trapping large quantities of water like a sponge, enabling the cartilage to spring back after it has been compressed, while the collagen fibres give cartilage its considerable strength.

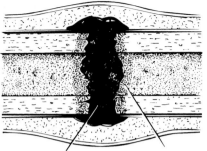

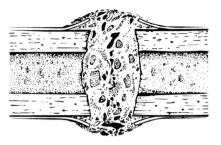

Figure 4.8 Stages in bone healing. (From Waugh & Grant 2001.)

Haematoma and bone fragments   Inflamed area

Phagocytosis of clot and debris. Growth of granulation tissue begins

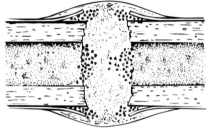

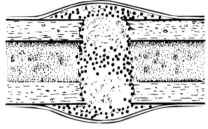

Osteoblasts begin to form new bone

Gradual spread of new bone to bridge gap

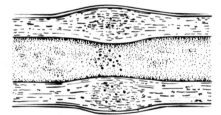

Bone healed. Osteoblasts reshape and canalise new bone

GROWTH OF CARTILAGE

Cartilage grows in two ways.

1 **Interstitial growth**: this is a rapid increase in size through the division of existing chondrocytes and the continual deposition of increasing amounts of intercellular matrix by the chondrocytes. This growth pattern occurs during childhood and young adolescence.

2 **Appositional growth**: this occurs as a result of activity within the inner chondrogenic layer of the perichondrium. Fibroblasts divide and differentiate into chondroblasts and chondrocytes. The matrix is deposited beneath the perichondrium on the surface of the cartilage. Appositional growth takes over from interstitial growth and continues throughout life.

TYPES OF CARTILAGE

There are three types of cartilage.

1 **Hyaline cartilage**: this is a resilient structure which covers the surface of bones where they articulate within a joint (Fig. 4.10). It is also found at the ends of the ribs, nasal septum, larynx, trachea, bronchi and bronchial tubes. It appears as a smooth bluish-white shiny substance; the cells are grouped together and the matrix is solid (Fig. 4.11). Hyaline cartilage does not have a direct blood supply but gains its nutrients from the vasculature of surrounding vessels. These nutrients are carried to the cartilage by the synovial fluid in the joint, which also removes the byproducts of metabolic activity within the cartilage. The continuous gliding motion of joints occurs due to the friction, lubrication and

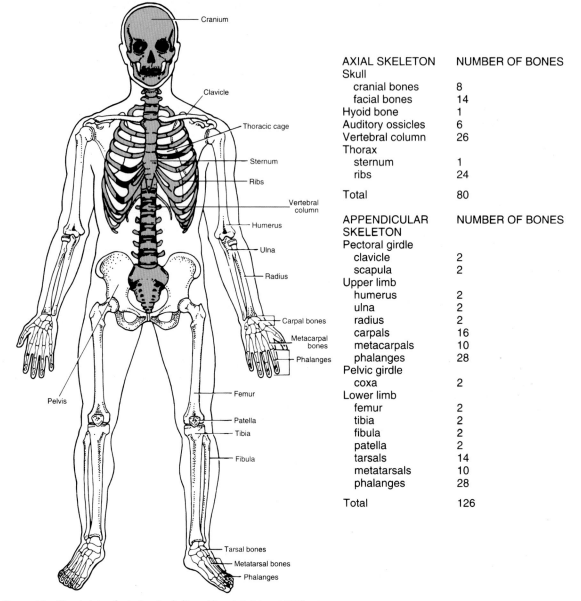

AXIAL SKELETON	NUMBER OF BONES
Skull	
cranial bones	8
facial bones	14
Hyoid bone	1
Auditory ossicles	6
Vertebral column	26
Thorax	
sternum	1
ribs	24
Total	80

APPENDICULAR SKELETON	NUMBER OF BONES
Pectoral girdle	
clavicle	2
scapula	2
Upper limb	
humerus	2
ulna	2
radius	2
carpals	16
metacarpals	10
phalanges	28
Pelvic girdle	
coxa	2
Lower limb	
femur	2
tibia	2
fibula	2
patella	2
tarsals	14
metatarsals	10
phalanges	28
Total	126

Figure 4.9 The skeleton (anterior view). (From Waugh & Grant 2001.)

wear characteristics of articular cartilage. It absorbs shock and spreads load to the subchondral bone and will last for 70–80 years under normal physiological load. The solid matrix consists of collagen fibres, which have great tensile stiffness and strength with little resistance to compression. Within this structure proteoglycan aggregates are trapped as a gel; hyaline cartilage in this way may contain 65–80% water. Compression or a pressure gradient causes water to be squeezed out or moved through the cartilage as the

joint moves, subsequently lubricating the joint and reducing friction. In osteoarthritis these properties are lost as the collagen fibrils break and fissures develop on the surface of the cartilage (Fig. 4.12).

2 **Fibrocartilage**: this is flexible and capable of withstanding considerable pressure and may therefore act as a 'shock absorber'. Thick dense collagen fibres are arranged in layers with a matrix similar to that of hyaline cartilage (Fig. 4.13). Fibrocartilage is found in the symphysis pubis, in the knee joint as

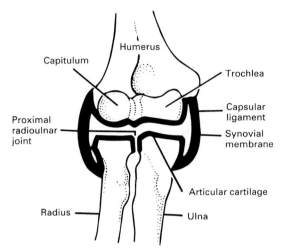

Figure 4.10   The elbow joint. (From Waugh & Grant 2001.)

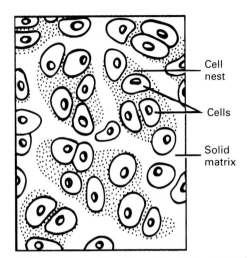

Figure 4.11   Hyaline cartilage. (From Waugh & Grant 2001.)

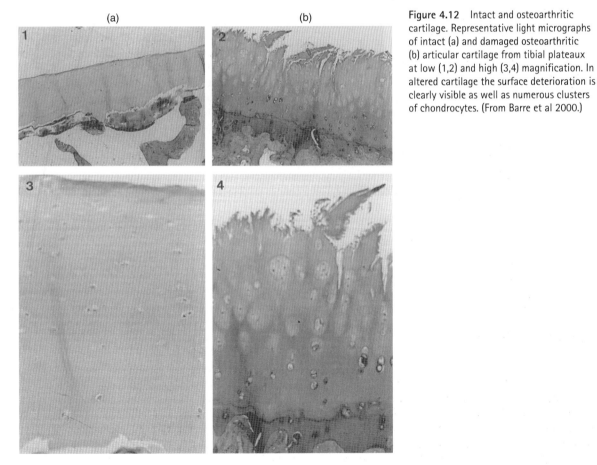

Figure 4.12   Intact and osteoarthritic cartilage. Representative light micrographs of intact (a) and damaged osteoarthritic (b) articular cartilage from tibial plateaux at low (1,2) and high (3,4) magnification. In altered cartilage the surface deterioration is clearly visible as well as numerous clusters of chondrocytes. (From Barre et al 2000.)

menisci and between the vertebrae as intervertebral discs (Fig. 4.14).

3 **Elastic cartilage**: this is found in the epiglottis, the larynx, the pinna of the ear and the eustachian tubes. The elastic fibres form a thread-like network which provides strength and flexibility while maintaining the shape of organs (Fig. 4.15). Otherwise, the structure is similar to that of hyaline cartilage.

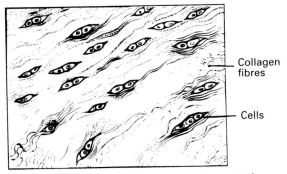

Figure 4.13   Fibrocartilage. (From Waugh & Grant 2001.)

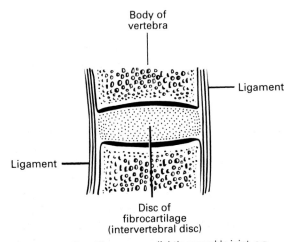

Figure 4.14   A cartilagenous or slightly moveable joint, e.g. between the vertebral bodies. (From Waugh & Grant 2001.)

SKELETAL MUSCLE TISSUE

Muscle tissue consists of highly specialised fibres for the active generation of force from contraction. This characteristic in muscles is responsible for movement, maintenance of posture and heat production.

Muscle tissue can be classified according to its structural and functional characteristics into three types:

1 skeletal or striated voluntary muscle
2 cardiac or striated involuntary muscle
3 smooth or non-striated involuntary muscle.

Only skeletal muscle tissue is described in detail in this chapter. This tissue provides force and power for the body to work and produces movement by acting in partnership with other muscles.

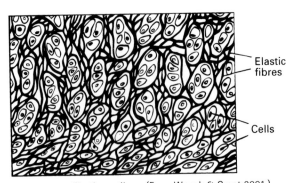

Figure 4.15   Elastic cartilage. (From Waugh & Grant 2001.)

CHARACTERISTICS

Muscle tissue has four principal characteristics.

1 **Contractility**: muscle contractions are responsible for the body's movements. Contractility is the ability of muscle tissue to actively generate force by shortening and thickening as a result of a stimulus.
2 **Excitability**: muscle is termed excitable when it responds to stimuli from nerves, hormones and injury. A stimulus is a change in the internal or external environment which is strong enough to initiate an impulse.
3 **Extensibility**: this is the ability of muscle to be stretched. Muscles work in opposing groups: while one is contracting and shortening, the other is relaxing and extending.
4 **Elasticity**: muscles are elastic and recoil to their original shape if they are stretched.

FUNCTIONS

Skeletal muscle comprises approximately 40% of body weight. In conjunction with the skeleton, muscle performs three functions.

1 **Motion (reflex and voluntary)**: movement relies on a partnership between the bones, joints and skeletal muscles attached to the bones.
2 **Maintenance of posture**: the contraction of skeletal muscles holds the body in stationary positions.
3 **Heat production**: skeletal muscle contractions produce most of the body's heat and therefore assist in the maintenance of normal body temperature.

EMBRYONIC DEVELOPMENT

All muscles are derived from the mesoderm. During the development of the mesoderm a portion becomes arranged in columns on either side of the developing nervous system. These columns segment into a series of blocks of cells known as somites. Except for the head and extremities, which develop from the general mesoderm, skeletal muscles develop from the mesoderm of somites.

The cells of a somite differentiate into three: myotome, dermatome and sclerotome. Skeletal muscle develops from a myotome of a somite.

SKELETAL MUSCLE STRUCTURE

Skeletal muscles are composed of muscle fibres and some connective tissue such as blood vessels and nerves. Muscle fibres develop from multinucleated cells called myoblasts. The myoblasts are converted into muscle fibres as contractile proteins accumulate within their cytoplasm. As the myoblasts form, nerves grow into the area and innervate the developing muscle fibres.

Muscle cells remain constant in number following birth. The enlargement of muscles is then dependent on an increase in the size of muscle fibres rather than their number. Skeletal muscle fibres have a striated appearance due to the arrangement of the myofilaments.

Surrounding each muscle fibre is an external lamina comprising reticular fibres which are indistinguishable from the muscle fibre's cell membrane, the sarcolemma. Outside the lamina is a delicate network of fibres called the endomysium. Each bundle of muscle fibres, called a fasciculus, is surrounded by a heavier layer, the perimysium.

A muscle consists of several fasciculi surrounded by a third layer, the epimysium, covering the entire surface of the muscle (Fig. 4.16). Individual muscles are separated by fascia, a layer of fibrous connective tissue, an important factor in the development of compartment syndrome.

Structure of muscle fibres

Each muscle fibre is composed of several layers (Fig. 4.17). Skeletal muscle fibres are composed of cylindrical structures called myofibrils. These are thread-like structures running from one end of the muscle to the other. Myofibrils consist of two kinds of smaller structures:

- actin or thin myofilaments, which contain two additional proteins (tropomysin and troponin) involved in the regulation of muscle contractions
- myosin or thick myofilaments composed of the protein myosin.

The actin and myosin myofilaments are arranged in compartments called sarcomeres. Certain areas within a sarcomere can be distinguished. A dense area called the anisotropic (dense band) or A band represents the length of the thick myofilaments. Each isotropic (light band) or I band is composed of thin myofilaments only.

PHYSIOLOGY OF SKELETAL MUSCLE

Skeletal muscle contracts in response to electrochemical stimuli. Through the central nervous system, nerve cells control and coordinate this muscle contraction.

The neuromuscular junction

The axons of motor neurons, motor nerve cells, enter skeletal muscle along the same pathway as arteries and veins. The axon may be as long as 3 feet or more. At the level of the perimysium the axon branches towards a muscle fibre, forming a neuromuscular junction or synapse (Fig. 4.18). Each axon innervates more than one muscle fibre. The area adjacent to the axon in the muscle cell membrane or sarcolemma is called the endplate or postsynaptic terminal. The neuromuscular junction refers to the space between the axon terminal of the motor neuron and the endplate.

The axon terminal is enlarged and forms the presynaptic terminal; the space between this and the muscle fibre is the synaptic cleft. The presynaptic terminal contains sacs, the synaptic vesicles, which store chemicals called neurotransmitters that stimulate or inhibit an action potential.

The neurotransmitter released in skeletal muscle is acetylcholine. Acetylcholine diffuses across the synaptic cleft, combining with the receptor sites of the sarcolemma of the muscle fibre. At this point the permeability of the sarcolemma to sodium (Na) and potassium (K) ions is increased. When two acetylcholine molecules bind to the receptor it opens channels. As a result there is an inward movement of sodium ions which depolarize the membrane to below threshold level, causing the muscle fibre to contract. This principle is used widely in the action of neuromuscular blocking agents, causing muscular relaxation for the duration of orthopaedic surgery.

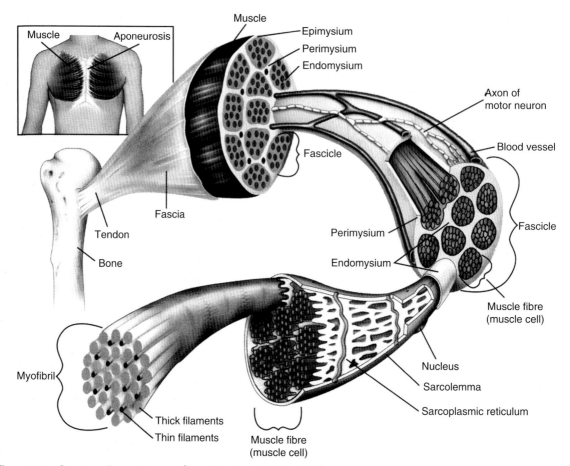

Figure 4.16   Structure of a muscle organ. (From Thibodeau & Patton 1999.)

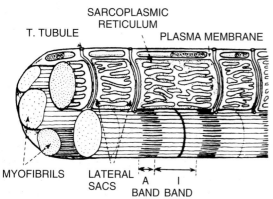

Figure 4.17   Three-dimensional drawing of skeletal muscle fibre. (From MacKenna & Callander 1990.)

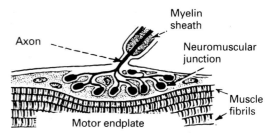

Figure 4.18   Neuromuscular junction. (From MacKenna & Callander 1990.)

the muscle fibre so that another impulse may be transmitted.

Acetylcholinesterase or cholinesterase inactivates acetylcholine by breaking it down into its components, acetate and chlorine. In this way it allows time for repolarisation of the membrane of

Energy source

Muscle contraction and relaxation require energy. Adenosine triphosphate (ATP) is the immediate source of energy for contraction. Within our bodies, 400 skeletal muscles use ATP to produce movement in a universe activated by force, gravity, friction and inertia.

Skeletal muscle fibres contain a high-energy molecule called phosphocreatine. Phosphocreatine and ATP constitute the phosphagen system which provides enough ATP for bursts of activity, of approximately 15 seconds. If activity is to be sustained for longer, the body's supply of phosphagen becomes depleted. Glucose then becomes the source of energy, derived from the breakdown of glycogen. Glycogen is stored in the muscles and the liver.

The breakdown of glycogen is known as glycolysis. This may occur with or without the continued presence of oxygen. Once the immediate oxygen stores have been used for aerobic respiration then anaerobic respiration occurs and lactic acid is produced. This glycogen–lactic acid system will provide sufficient ATP for 30–40 seconds of vigorous muscular activity. After this the muscles will need to rest or drastically reduce their activity in order to repay the oxygen debt they have built up.

In prolonged, less vigorous activity the metabolic process of cellular respiration must take place in the continuous presence of oxygen. This aerobic system combined with glycolysis will continue as long as nutrients and adequate oxygen are available.

Type of muscle contraction

Skeletal muscle contractions are either isometric or isotonic. Isometric contractions occur when the muscle length does not change but the amount of tension increases during the contraction, for example with the contraction of postural muscles. Isotonic contractions occur when the muscle length becomes shorter but the amount of tension produced by the muscle is constant during the contraction. Most muscle contractions tend to combine isometric and isotonic contractions.

SKELETAL MUSCLES AND BODY MOVEMENT

Body movement is produced by the coordinated action of the muscles, bones, nerves and joints. As a muscle contracts in response to a nerve impulse, a force is applied to a tendon which pulls on a bone. In body movement, bones act as levers and joints function as the fulcrum or pivot points. This process

allows a force to be transferred along a lever to some other point on that lever. Muscles provide the force to move the lever.

Levers

Levers may be categorised into three types (Fig. 4.19).

- **First-class levers**: the fulcrum is located between the force (effort) and the weight (resistance); for example, a seesaw or the head resting on the atlas where the atlantooccipital joint is the fulcrum, the skull is the weight and the muscles at the back of the neck the force.
- **Second-class levers**: the weight (resistance) is between the force (effort) and the fulcrum; an example is a wheelbarrow or standing on one's toes where the body is the weight, the ball of the foot is the fulcrum and the contracted calf muscle is the force.
- **Third-class levers**: the weight and the fulcrum are at opposite ends and the force is in between. This is the most common form of leverage in the body. An example is someone carrying a weight with the forearm flexed at the elbow, when the hand holds the weight, the elbow is the fulcrum and the biceps muscle acts as the force pulling on the forearm as the lever.

Origin and insertion of muscles

The origin of a muscle is normally the proximal attachment of the muscle and is attached to the more stationary of two bones (Fig. 4.20). The distal attachment, or insertion, is where the muscle inserts into the bone undergoing the greatest movement. Some muscles have multiple origins.

Group actions

Most skeletal muscles work in opposing groups, such as abductors and adductors, flexors and extensors. Muscles or groups of muscles working together to cause movement are known as synergists or agonists, while the opposing muscles or groups of muscles are called antagonists. A muscle is termed a 'prime mover' if it is predominant in causing a movement. Occasionally prime movers and antagonists act together as fixators or stabilisers to provide a fixed position from which other prime movers can function. For example, the shoulder blade is often fixed in position by its muscles to enable movement of the shoulder joint. The principal terms used in muscle action are defined in Table 4.2.

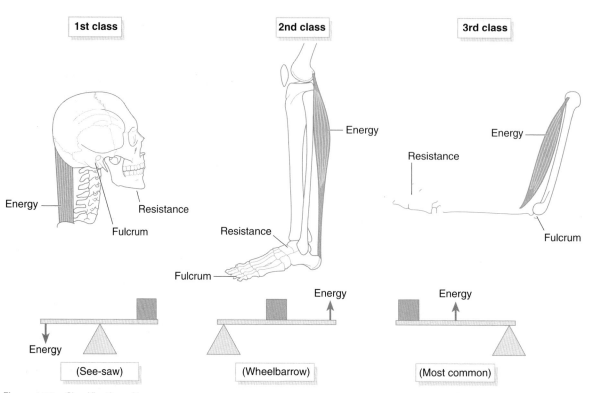

Figure 4.19   Classification of levers.

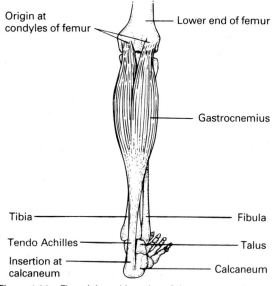

Figure 4.20   The origin and insertion of the gastrocnemius muscle.

JOINTS

Joints are found where two or more bones meet. A joint arises between adjacent bones or areas of ossification. Areas of ossification would include the

Table 4.2   Principal actions of muscles

Action	Movement
Abduction	Away from the midline
Adduction	Towards the midline
Depressor	Downward movement
Extension	Increases angle at a joint
Flexion	Decreases angle at a joint
Levator	Upward movement
Pronator	Turns palm (or sole) downwards
Rotator	Movement around the long axis
Supinator	Turns palm (or sole) upwards
Sphincter	Decreases the size of an opening
Tensor	Tightens the body part

sutures of the skull where, after ossification, no movement is possible.

CLASSIFICATION OF JOINTS

The classification of joints is based upon the presence or absence of a synovial cavity and the type of connective tissue that binds the bones together. There are three main classes:

● synovial

Table 4.3 Types of synovial joint

Type of joint	Examples	Movements possible
Ball and socket	Hip, shoulder	Flexion, extension, abduction, adduction rotation, circumduction
Condylar (uniaxial)	Knee, temporo-mandibular joint	Flexion, extension, rotation
Ellipsoid (biaxial)	Wrist, atlantooccipital joint	Flexion, extension, abduction, adduction
Hinge (uniaxial)	Elbow, ankle	Flexion, extension
Pivot (uniaxial)	Median atlantoaxial joint, odontoid process	Rotation
Plane	Sacroiliac, costovertebral, cubonavicular, sternoclavicular joints	Gliding

Table 4.4 Types of fibrous joints

Example of joint	Structures involved	Movement
Sutures of skull		
Coronal	Frontal and parietal bones	Fixed from age 2 years
Squamosal	Parietal and temporal bones	
Syndesmosis		
Tibiofibular	Tibia and fibula	Variable
Gomphoses		
Dentoalveolar	Teeth and alveolar process of maxilla and mandible	Minimal

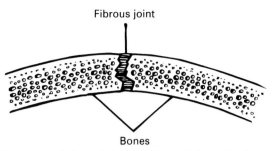

Fibrous joint

Bones

Figure 4.21 A fibrous joint. (From Waugh & Grant 2001.)

Table 4.5 Types of cartilaginous joints

Example of joint	Structures involved	Movement
Synchondroses		
Sternocostal	Ribs and sternum	Minimal
Epiphyseal	Diaphysis and epiphysis of a long bone	None
Symphyses		
Symphysis pubis	The two coxae	Variable
Intervertebral	Bodies of vertebrae	Variable

- fibrous
- cartilaginous.

Examples of synovial joints may be found in Table 4.3. There are three types of fibrous joints (Table 4.4); these have no joint cavity and are united by fibrous tissue and have little movement (Fig. 4.21). Cartilaginous joints also have no joint cavity as the articulating bones are united by hyaline cartilage or fibrocartilage; there are two types of cartilaginous joint (Table 4.5).

THE NERVOUS SYSTEM

The function of the nervous system is to coordinate and control all parts of the body. It works in close cooperation with the endocrine system to harmonise many complex body functions. Structurally it can be divided into:

- the central nervous system (CNS) comprising the brain and spinal cord
- the peripheral nervous system, comprising spinal and cranial nerves.

Functionally the nervous system can be divided into:

- the somatic or voluntary nervous system, which transmits impulses to and from non-visceral parts of the body; that is, the skeletal muscles, bones, joints, ligaments, skin, eyes and ears. Impulses carried in this way lead to activities which are conscious and willed
- The autonomic or involuntary nervous system, which transmits impulses concerned with activities of visceral organs, such as the muscles in organs, blood vessels and glands. These are not under conscious control.

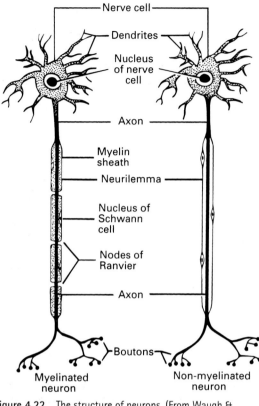

Figure 4.22 The structure of neurons. (From Waugh & Grant 2001.)

NEURONS

The functional unit of the nervous system is the neuron or nerve cell and its processes. It is composed of a nucleated cell body and cytoplasmic processes which include an axon and one or more dendrites (Fig. 4.22). The axon conducts nerve impulses from the cell body out towards the dendrites of other neurons or to muscles and glands. Large axons, and especially those of peripheral nerves, are covered by a white lipid protein sheath called myelin which assists the speedy passage of nerve impulses. Dendrites receive stimuli and carry impulses from the axons of other neurons towards the nerve cell body.

The junction between the axon of one neuron and the dendrite of another is called a synapse. Chemical neurotransmitters released at the synapse allow the transmission of the impulse from neuron to neuron (Fig. 4.23). Where a nerve fibre terminates in a muscle cell at the neuromuscular junction, the transmission process is similar to that at the synapse.

Neurons can be classified according to their function.

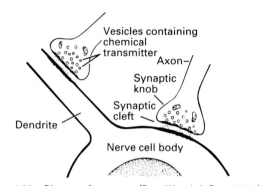

Figure 4.23 Diagram of a synapse. (From Waugh & Grant 2001.)

- In motor or efferent neurons, axons transmit impulses from the CNS to muscles or glands.
- In sensory or afferent neurons, axons transmit impulses from the periphery of the body to the brain or spinal cord.

NERVE IMPULSES

An impulse is the result of either a chemical, electrical or mechanical change to the neuron. This is called the stimulus. The stimulus alters the permeability of the cell membrane which allows the movement of sodium ions into the nerve cell and thus generates an electrical current. The speed of conduction of an impulse depends on the size of the nerve fibre and on whether it is covered by myelin. Myelinated fibres conduct impulses quicker than non-myelinated fibres.

CENTRAL NERVOUS SYSTEM

The central nervous system consists of the brain and spinal cord. The largest part of the brain is the cerebrum which is divided into two hemispheres. One hemisphere is dominant since it appears to take a 'lead' role, resulting in the limbs on one side of the body becoming dominant. Each hemisphere has a surface layer of grey matter with white matter below. This is in contrast to the spinal cord where the white matter encloses a core of grey matter.

The brain

The cerebral cortex contains:

- **primary sensory areas**: these are receptive areas for incoming impulses

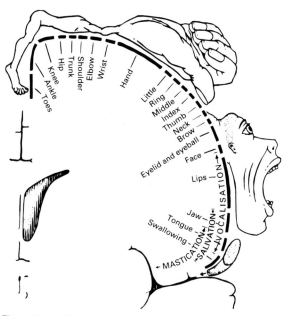

Figure 4.24 Motor area of the cerebrum. (From Waugh & Grant 2001.)

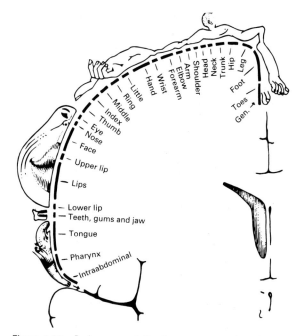

Figure 4.25 Body representation in sensory area of cerebrum. (From Waugh & Grant 2001.)

- **primary motor areas**: these send out impulses to stimulate action responses such as muscle contraction and glandular secretion
- **association areas**: which have a generalised function in the smooth working between sensory and motor centres.

The motor area initiates all voluntary movement of the body and is positioned in the frontal lobe, anterior to the cerebral fissure. In general, the motor area of one hemisphere controls the movement on the opposite side of the body. The body muscles are represented on the motor strip in the area of the longitudinal fissure (Fig. 4.24). The amount of brain surface related to a specific part of the body is proportional to the activity rather than the size of the part. Sensory impulses concerned with touch, pressure, pain, temperature and body position are transmitted to the parietal lobe which is posterior to the central fissure. Similar to the motor area, lower body sensations are received at the median portion of the sensory strip. Impulses from the head are received at the lowest part of the strip (Fig. 4.25).

Other key cerebral functions include the visual areas in the occipital lobe, auditory areas in the temporal lobe, memory, personality, emotional reaction, initiative and responsibility in the frontal lobe.

Basal ganglia are areas of grey matter embedded within the white matter of each cerebral hemisphere,

near the thalamus. Basal ganglia play a vital role in the control of voluntary motor activity. They have nerve connections with the motor cortical areas as well as the thalamus, which in turn has connections with the cerebellum. The ganglia give rise to extrapyramidal pathways to skeletal muscle. Basal ganglia appear to exert an inhibitory influence on muscle tone. Damage to them can cause motor disorders which lead to increased muscle activity.

Other parts of the brain include the midbrain, pons varolii, medulla oblongata and the cerebellum or hindbrain.

The brain requires a continuous flow of blood to provide the quantities of glucose and oxygen it needs to function. This need is the same whether the individual is mentally active or asleep. Brain cells are very sensitive to hypoxia, with irreversible brain damage occurring if the blood supply is interrupted for 2–6 minutes. The brain and spinal cord are surrounded by the meninges which protect and assist in the passage of nutrients to the brain cells.

The spinal cord

The spinal cord is a cylindrical structure composed of grey and white matter enclosed within the vertebral canal. It extends from the medulla oblongata at the base of the skull to the level of the first or second

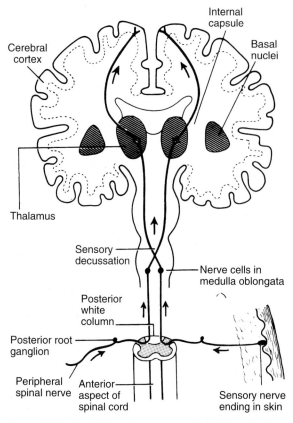

Figure 4.26   One of the sensory nerve pathways from the skin to the cerebrum. (From Waugh & Grant 2001.)

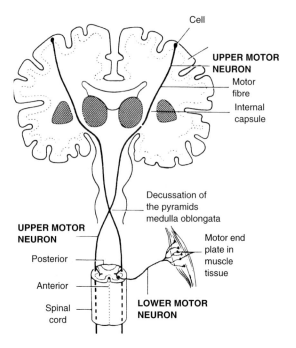

Figure 4.27   The motor nerve pathways. (From Waugh & Grant 2001.)

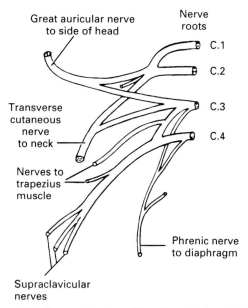

Figure 4.28   The cervical plexus. (From Waugh & Grant 2001.)

lumbar vertebra. A central canal extends the full length of the cord. It contains cerebrospinal fluid and is continuous with the ventricles of the brain. The functions of the spinal cord are:

- to carry impulses via sensory nerve fibres through ascending tracts to the brain (Fig. 4.26)
- to carry impulses from the brain via motor nerve fibres down the descending tracts to muscle or glands (Fig. 4.27)
- to act as a centre for reflex actions.

The cell bodies (grey matter) are found in the interior of the spinal cord in an H shape. The nerve fibres (white matter) are peripheral to the cell bodies. Afferent impulses are received by neurons in the posterior horn of the grey matter. Efferent impulses are discharged by neurons in the anterior horn of the grey matter. Neurons within the grey matter transmit impulses from one half of the cord to the other and to other levels of the CNS. Nerve impulses from the spinal cord leave via 31 pairs of posterior (sensory afferent fibres) and anterior roots (motor efferent fibres). At the intervertebral foramen the posterior and anterior roots meet to form a spinal nerve. The nerve fibres, on leaving the cord, form enlargements in the cervical and lumbar areas; these enlargements are called plexuses. The cervical plexus is associated with supplying the upper limb (Fig. 4.28). The lumbar plexus is associated with supplying the lower limb.

PERIPHERAL NERVOUS SYSTEM

The peripheral nervous system is composed of nerves and ganglia. There are two main groups of peripheral nerves – the cranial and spinal nerves.

Cranial nerves

There are 12 pairs of cranial nerves emerging from the inferior surface of the brain. Some of these nerves have mainly motor fibres, some have sensory fibres and some are mixed with both sensory and motor fibres. Cell bodies of the motor fibres form nuclei within the brainstem. Sensory fibres originate from groups of cells outside the CNS and are called ganglia. Exceptions are the olfactory fibres which originate from the nasal mucosa and the optic fibres which originate from the retina of the eyeball.

The origins and functions of cranial nerves are given in Table 4.6.

Spinal nerves

There are 31 pairs of nerves which arise from the spinal cord: eight cervical pairs, 12 thoracic pairs, five lumbar pairs, five sacral pairs and one coccygeal pair.

All spinal nerves are mixed nerves and have two origins: the anterior and posterior roots. After leaving the vertebral canal, each spinal nerve passes through the intervertebral foramen and divides into two branches called the anterior and posterior rami (Fig. 4.29). The posterior ramus then divides into smaller branches which supply the muscles and skin of the back portion of the head, neck and trunk. The anterior ramus divides into networks to supply all the structures of the extremities and the front portion of the trunk.

Four main plexuses are formed by the division of the anterior rami.

1 **Cervical plexus**: this supplies muscles of the neck and shoulder and the phrenic nerve supplies the diaphragm.
2 **Brachial plexus**: the median, radial and ulnar nerves supply the arms.
3 **Lumbar plexus**: the femoral, saphenous and obturator nerves supply the lower abdominal wall, external genitalia and part of the thigh and leg.
4 **Sacral plexus**: this supplies the buttocks, perineum and lower extremities. The largest and longest nerve in the body is the sciatic nerve arising from the sacral plexus.

THE AUTONOMIC NERVOUS SYSTEM

The autonomic nervous system carries efferent fibres and causes involuntary responses to control visceral function within the body. It exerts an influence on arterial blood pressure, sweating and body temperatures, gastric and intestinal mobility and secretion, plus urinary bladder emptying. It is controlled by groups of nerve cells in the brain stem, hypothalamus and spinal cord. It subdivides into the parasympathetic system and the sympathetic system.

Parasympathetic nervous system

The parasympathetic system has preganglionic and postganglionic fibres (Fig. 4.30). Postganglionic fibres are short and located within organs, for example the gastrointestinal tract. The effects of the parasympathetic system are associated with inactivity, restoring and conserving body energy and elimination of body waste.

Sympathetic nervous system

The sympathetic nervous system originates within the thoracic and lumbar regions of the spinal cord. Sympathetic nerves leave the spinal cord via the anterior roots and form the grey communicating rami of the thoracic and lumbar nerves. Immediately outside the spinal cord there are two interconnected chains of sympathetic ganglia (Fig. 4.31).

Stimulation of the sympathetic system results in stimulation of the medulla of the adrenal glands which increases the secretion of adrenaline (epinephrine) and noradrenaline (norepinephrine), thereby augmenting the body's defence response. The effects of the sympathetic system are generalised physiological responses to stress, strong emotion, severe pain, cold or any threat to the body. The purpose of such a response is mobilisation of body resources for defensive action.

The neurotransmitter that is released by the preganglionic fibres of both the sympathetic and parasympathetic systems is acetylcholine. At neuroeffector junctions the neurotransmitter differs in the two systems. In the parasympathetic system the postganglionic fibre releases acetylcholine and in the sympathetic system noradrenaline (norepinephrine) is released. The sympathetic and parasympathetic systems exert opposing influences upon their target organs.

Table 4.6 Origin and function of the cranial nerves (from Waugh & Grant 2001)

Name and number	Central connection	Peripheral connection	Function
I Olfactory (sensory)	Smell area in temporal lobe of cerebrum through olfactory bulb	Mucous membrane in roof of nose	Sense of smell
II Optic (sensory)	Sight area in occipital lobe of the: cerebrum cerebellum	Retina of the eyes	Sense of sight Balance
III Oculomotor (motor)	Nerve cells near floor of aqueduct of midbrain	Superior, inferior and medial rectus muscles of the eye Ciliary muscles of the eye Circular muscle fibres of the iris	Moving the eyeball Focusing Regulating the size of the pupil
IV Trochlear (motor)	Nerve cells near floor of aqueduct of midbrain	Superior oblique muscles of the eyes	Movement of the eyeball
V Trigeminal (mixed)	Motor fibres from the pons varolii Sensory fibres from the trigeminal ganglion	Muscles of mastication Sensory to gums, cheek, lower jaw, iris, cornea	Chewing Sensation from the face
VI Abducent (motor)	Floor of 4th ventricle	Lateral rectus muscle of the eye	Movement of the eye
VII Facial (mixed)	Pons varolii	Sensory fibres to the tongue Motor fibres to the muscles of the face	Sense of taste Movements of facial expression
VIII Vestibulocochlear (sensory) Vestibular Cochlear	Cerebellum Hearing area of cerebrum	Semicircular canals in the inner ear Organ of Corti in cochlea	Maintenance of balance Sense of hearing
IX Glossopharyngeal (mixed)	Medulla oblongata	Parotid glands Back of tongue and pharynx	Secretion of saliva Sense of taste and movement of pharynx
X Vagus (mixed)	Medulla oblongata	Pharynx, larynx, organs, glands, ducts, blood vessels in the thorax and abdomen	Movement and secretion
XI Accessory (motor)	Medulla oblongata	Sternocleidomastoid, trapezius, laryngeal and pharyngeal muscles	Movement of the head, shoulders, pharynx and larynx
XII Hypoglossal (motor)	Medulla oblongata	Tongue	Movement of tongue

REFLEXES

Reflexes are defence mechanisms with rapid auto-matic responses to painful and/or potentially harmful situations; for example, the blink reflex protects the eye from a foreign body. The reflex process functions via the reflex arc, an involuntary fixed motor response to a sensory stimulus (Fig. 4.32). The reflex arc consists of:

- a sensory or receptor neuron (afferent nerve) which is sensitive to specific stimuli and

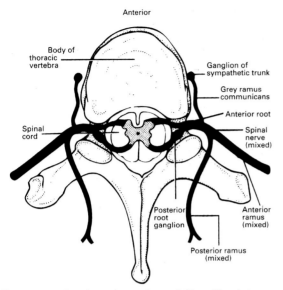

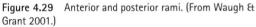

Figure 4.29   Anterior and posterior rami. (From Waugh & Grant 2001.)

integrates centres within the CNS at any level below the cerebral cortex

- a motor neuron (efferent nerve) within the muscular or glandular tissue.

The reflex process

A receptor is stimulated by a change in the environment, for example when stretching a tendon or there is a pressure or temperature change. This produces an impulse in the afferent nerve fibre. The impulse travels through the cell body of the sensory neuron and along its axon to the CNS. It may pass through a number of connecting neurons before it excites a motor efferent neuron whose axon transmits impulses out of the CNS to the efferent tissue or organ. Hence a muscle may then contract or a gland will produce a secretion.

The knee jerk is an example of a stretch reflex with two neurons involved. The cell of the lower motor neuron (a motor nerve cell with its cell body

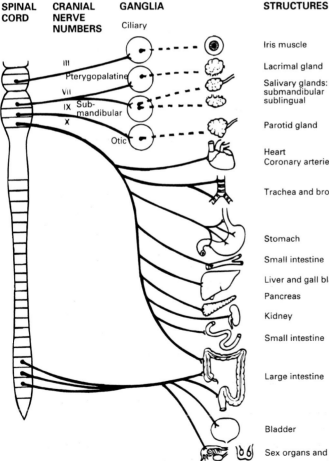

Figure 4.30   The parasympathetic outflow. (From Waugh & Grant 2001.)

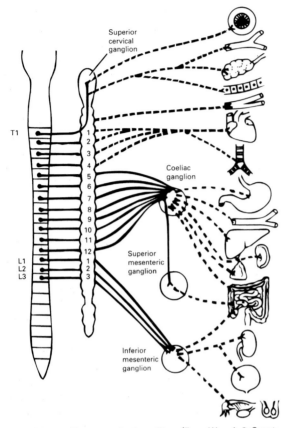

Figure 4.31   The sympathetic outflow. (From Waugh & Grant 2001.)

outside the central nervous system) is stimulated by the sensory neuron which responds to tapping of the stretched tendon below the knee. No connector neuron is involved. The lower motor nerve stimulates the muscle of the thigh, which contracts and therefore kicks the foot forward. The knee jerk is a test used in orthopaedics to assess the integrity of the reflex arc.

AGEING

Ageing is a normal and continual process occurring throughout life. Although it is generally accepted that there is some decline in the function of the organs and tissues of the body, ageing is not inevitably accompanied by disease or biological malfunction. Some of the decline is due to the progressive loss of body cells. This need not be significant in health terms since most body systems have considerable spare capacity. For example, we possess two kidneys when the body can adequately function with only one healthy kidney.

Demographic trends are resulting in an increasingly aged population and the present UK government is initiating standards for elderly care through the National Service Framework (DoH 2001). Within this, the sixth standard focuses on falls and the risk of osteoporotic fractures. Monitoring this group of the population will inevitably involve the orthopaedic nurse.

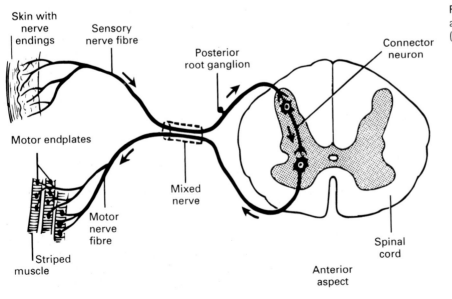

Figure 4.32   A single reflex arc involving one side only. (From Waugh & Grant 2001.)

In making a nursing assessment of an elderly person, it is essential that the orthopaedic nurse is meticulous in taking the patient's history and that an accurate physical examination is carried out. The nurse must be able to differentiate between the ageing process and pathological change.

AGEING THEORIES

Numerous theories have been put forward to explain ageing and the varied times of onset of the manifestations of ageing. Sociological, psychological and biological studies have been undertaken which provide different perspectives on the ageing process. Sociological studies on ageing cover changes in lifestyle, family roles and the individual's activities and interests. Psychological studies examine the individual's capacity to adapt to environmental demands. Biological studies cover time-related physical changes over which the individual has limited control.

Biological theories

From a biological perspective, the health of the individual depends on the efficient functioning of body cells and tissues in all body systems. In health, such functioning is ensured by a process called homoeostasis. However, with age, there is a decline in the adaptive ability of the body to cope with change. This means that the elderly person may maintain homoeostasis but with increasing difficulty as the years pass. Systems which normally function effectively may be less efficient under stressful conditions and the return to the normal state may be slower. Irreversible changes occur progressively and do not affect all body systems equally, nor are such changes chronologically related. External appearance can be misleading, masking major internal changes which may be the result of environment stressors or lifestyle.

Cellular change theory. Damage to the DNA, and faults which occur during cellular divisions, produce mutations. It has been postulated that ageing and death may be due to a build-up of such mutated cells so that the individual is no longer able to maintain life. Scientific evidence has established that chromosomal errors increase with age but no study has as yet identified them as being responsible for ageing. Some theorists have suggested that humans have a biological 'clock' programmed so the individual develops, ages and dies according to a personal timing device.

Immune theory. Theories associated with the immune system suggest that normal ageing is the result of a decrease in immunological efficiency, which then leads to general impairment of function throughout the body tissues. Various studies of the activities of different body cells have been undertaken and evidence suggests that major change occurs in T-cells and in the responsiveness of natural antibodies. There is a decline in both humoral and cell-mediated immunity with age and a loss of lymphoid tissue from bone marrow, the lymph nodes, the spleen and the thymus. Unfortunately, immune theories offer a perspective on ageing without fully explaining it.

Free radical theory. This theory, postulated by Harman in 1956, states that free radicals are central agents in producing changes at tissue, cellular and subcellular levels. Free radicals are produced normally during certain metabolic processes in the body. They are highly reactive and unstable due to the presence of unpaired electrons. With their production there is a large increase in free energy, leading to the damage of adjacent molecules. The accumulation of this damage leads to a decline in function seen in the ageing process. Organisms have developed enzymes for scavenging free radicals and destroying the potentially harmful products before further damage can occur. When molecules are attacked, fluorescent pigments are produced; hence the development of so-called 'age pigments'. The free radical theory suggests that ageing is potentially treatable, in that chemical antioxidants should be able to prevent oxidative damage. It is thought that the vitamins C and E are examples of chemical antioxidants capable of interrupting free radical reactions, although as yet there is no evidence to suggest these vitamins have any such benefit.

It is not yet possible to identify any one theory that can adequately explain ageing. What can be described are the signs of change observed in normal individuals as they age.

AGEING AND THE SKELETAL SYSTEM

The normal ageing process need not limit movement. Mobility is, to some extent, affected by personal lifestyle and the degree of activity that the individual has maintained throughout their life, although some limitation of mobility may occur as a result of fear, such as the fear of falling. Ageing does, however, lead to changes in balance, cartilage and bone tissue.

Changes in balance

The maintenance of balance relies on integrating responses from the visual system, vestibular system in the inner ear and the proprioceptors in muscles and joints. Older people require greater angular movement in joints for proprioception to be achieved.

Gait disorders are not usually a feature of ageing but are more likely to be an indicator of underlying pathology such as a stroke, peripheral neuropathy or vitamin B_{12} deficiency.

Cartilaginous changes

The normal elastic properties of cartilage may be lost because of an increase in water loss and the deposition of fibres. The increased fibre density in connective tissue and cartilage produces a 'mesh' for the deposition of calcium. This accounts for the increased calcification of cartilage with ageing.

Hyaline cartilage loses fluid and is converted to fibrocartilage. Articular cartilage changes with the elasticity being lost. Thinning occurs over weight-bearing areas, affecting the function; for example, changes in the menisci of the knee joint inhibit free movement. Many joints of the body become stiffened with age.

Loss of water from cartilage in the intervertebral discs leads to compaction of the vertebrae and shrinkage of the spinal column, seen as a loss in height. Height loss is also affected by joint changes and by the flattening of the arch of the foot.

Bone changes

Osteoporosis is an imbalance between bone reabsorption and formation and is a normal ageing process as androgens decrease. If severe, it may cause fractures, can lead to bowing of the long bones and to an increase in spinal curvature due to vertebral collapse.

AGEING AND MUSCLE

Most loss of lean body mass occurs in the muscle. Muscle cells display evidence of ageing with an increase in lipid content. Muscle fibres are reduced in number and size and such changes result in a degree of limitation in the range of movement produced by contraction. The size of individual muscles and the degree of loss of muscle strength vary among the muscle groups. The stiffening of joints and the cartilaginous changes mean that more muscular work

is required in many body functions, for example breathing. Periods of immobility, for example bed-rest, can lead to disuse atrophy and muscle wasting in the elderly.

AGEING AND THE NERVOUS SYSTEM

Brain weight and volume have been shown to decline with age, although this may not be significant. A reduction occurs in the cortical areas where the sulci broaden out and the gyri flatten. Cells are also lost from the cerebral cortex and the cerebellum, although this usually starts later in the cerebellum than in the cerebrum. Major cerebellar change affects the axons, with loss of myelin. Autonomic nervous system dysfunctions are also evident with age, for example postural hypotension, impaired thermoregulation and gastrointestinal function, urinary incontinence and impaired penile erection.

Cerebral blood flow decreases with age but oxygen extraction from the blood is increased as more oxygen is released from the haemoglobin. The vertebral arteries tend to become tortuous because of changes in the vertebral and intervertebral discs; they may become kinked with neck movement, leading to transient ischaemic attacks.

In the peripheral nerves, the number of large fibres reduces, especially in the dorsal roots of the lumbosacral region. As a result, the velocity of conduction of nerve impulses is reduced. Some reflexes, for example the Achilles tendon reflexes, are depressed and reaction time is longer. Part of this deterioration is due to nerve changes and part to a reduction of muscle power and stiffer joints.

REPAIR AND MAINTENANCE

Repair and maintenance of body tissues vary according to age and must be considered together with other aspects such as nutritional factors or the presence of infection. These are considered in other chapters and therefore are not covered in this brief section in spite of their importance in aiding recovery.

Bone

The adult skeleton is dynamic. The maintenance of this dynamic sequence relies on the coordinated action of osteoblasts and osteoclasts on the trabecular surfaces and in the Haversian systems previously described. Remodelling in each section of bone, first described by Frost in 1964 as a bone remodelling unit, takes between 3 and 4 months. Balance is dependent on optimum conditions in terms of such processes as hormonal control and kidney function. The repair of the damage incurred will increase demand for nutrients, especially calcium and vitamin D.

Cartilage

Articular cartilage is avascular, alymphatic and aneural, therefore maintenance of healthy cartilage is dependent on nourishment from synovial fluid. Disorders such as rheumatoid arthritis adversely affecting the joint synovium will inevitably lead to damage of the articular surface. The exact mechanism of this process is still being considered although recent research indicates that transport across the surface layer to the proteoglycines in the deeper layer can take place (Uesugi & Jasin 2000).

Ligaments

Ligaments are strong, inelastic structures which strengthen a joint. Normally there is a constant maintenance of tissues through homoeostasis in spite of high mechanical loads. When a ligament is damaged it is dependent on a complex system of molecular repair. This varies with different ligaments and the intraarticular environment is particularly harsh for healing. Therefore, normal tissue may be replaced by fibrous tissue with a subsequent loss in strength. A variety of techniques have been tried for repair and graft to ligaments but it is difficult to eliminate instability without excessive graft tension (Jaureguito & Paulos 1996). Repair and replacement of ligaments are therefore not as successful as other body tissues.

Muscle

Muscle tissue has a good blood supply and therefore heals well under normal conditions. Skeletal muscle is able to regenerate due to satellite cells, which act like reserve stem cells. If the basal lamina of the muscle remains intact, these stem cells fuse to form myogenic cells. These in turn fuse with existing fibres or each other to form tubes (Dop Bar et al 1997). Injuries occur at a variety of sites: the muscle belly, musculocutaneous junction, muscle insertions and the associated tendon. However, such injuries do require a balance of rest and stretching to allow for healing to take place and, as they are associated with activity, this may not always be to the individual's liking. Damage does act as a stimulus for muscle growth or repair and may also be affected by growth factors.

Nerves

Repair and regeneration of nervous tissue are largely dependent on the presence of a myelin sheath and the extent of damage. Maintenance of nerve function, like bone, relies heavily on calcium and the sudden depletion of calcium can result in tetany.

CONCLUSION

According to Powell (1986), nurses must develop an 'orthopaedic eye', an acute awareness of correct body posture and mechanics, so that they will notice anything that interferes with the patient's treatment. It is hoped that the orthopaedic nurse, using a basic understanding of the underlying anatomy and physiology of the locomotor system, will enhance the mobility of orthopaedic patients of all age groups.

GLOSSARY OF TERMS (BASED ON BRYAN 1996)

Skeletal terms

Anatomical position: the position assumed in all anatomical descriptions to ensure consistency and accuracy. The body is in an upright position with the head facing forward, the arms at the sides with the palms of the hands facing forward and the feet together

Anterior or ventral: the part being described is nearer the front of the body

Appendicular skeleton: the bones of the shoulder girdle, upper limbs, pelvic girdle and lower limbs

Axial skeleton: the bones of the skull, vertebral column, ribs and sternum

Coronal plane: a plane passing through the body from side to side at right angles to the sagittal plane

Distal: further from the axial skeleton

Inferior: indicates a structure further away from the head

Lateral: further from the midline

Medial: nearer the midline

Median plane: when the body in the anatomical position is divided longitudinally into right and left halves, it has been divided in the median plane

Posterior or dorsal: the part being described is nearer the back of the body

Proximal: nearer to the axial skeleton

Sagittal plane: when the body is divided horizontally into top and bottom, it has been divided in the saggital plane

Superior: this indicates a structure nearer the head

Transverse plane: any plane at right angles to the long axis of the body

Movement terms

Abduction: moving away from the midline of the body

Adduction: moving towards the midline of the body

Circumduction: a circular movement involving a combination of flexion, extension, abduction and adduction

Eversion: turning the sole of the foot away from the median plane

Extension: straightening

Flexion: bending, usually forward movement

Insertion: the end of a muscle that moves most, attaching to bone

Inversion: turning the sole of the foot towards the median plane

Origin: the end of a muscle that moves least in attachment to bone

Pronation: movement involving turning the palm of the hand posteriorly or rotating the sole of the foot outwards

Supination: opposite of pronation

Valgus and varus: these are not anatomical terms but orthopaedic terms indicating an abnormal deviation away from or towards the midline

Bony landmarks

Articulating surface: the part of the bone that enters into the formation of a joint

Articulation: a joint between two or more bones

Bony sinus: a hollow cavity within a bone

Border: a ridge of bone that separates two surfaces

Condyle: a smooth rounded projection of bone that forms part of a joint

Epicondyle: the bony prominence above the condyle

Facet: a small, generally rather flat articulating surface

Fissure or cleft: a narrow slit

Fossa (plural fossae): a hollow or depression, as is a notch

Foramen (plural foramina): a hole in a structure. Fenestra (meaning window) is also occasionally used

Lamina: a thin plate of bone

Meatus: a tube-shaped cavity within a bone

Septum: a partition separating two cavities

Spine, spinous process or crest: a sharp ridge of bone

Styloid process: a sharp downward projection of bone that gives attachment to muscles and ligaments

Sulcus: an elongated groove

Suture: an immovable joint, e.g. between the bones of the skull

Trochanter, tuberosity: roughened bony projections, for the attachment of muscles and ligaments

Trochlea: a pulley-shaped articular surface

Tubercle: a circumscribed bony projection

Further reading

Ebersole P, Hess P, Lugon AS 2003 Toward healthy ageing. Human needs and nursing response, 6th edn. Mosby, St Louis

Hinchliffe S, Montague S 1996 Physiology for nursing practice, 2nd edn. Baillière Tindall, London

Hubbard JL, Mechan DJ 1987 Physiology for health care students. Churchill Livingstone, Edinburgh

Redfern SJ 1999 Nursing older people, 3rd edn. Churchill Livingstone, Edinburgh

Sumbrook P, Schrieber L, Taylor T, Ellis A 2001 The musculoskeletal system. Churchill Livingstone, Edinburgh

Seeley RR, Stephens TD, Tate P 2003 Anatomy and physiology, 6th edn. McGraw-Hill, Boston

Smith EE, Nolen-Hoeksemas S, Fredrikson B 2002 Atkinson & Hilgard's Introduction to psychology, 14th edn. Harcourt, Brace & Jovanovich, New York

Tortora GJ, Grabowski SR 2003 Principles of anatomy and physiology, 10th edn. John Wiley, London

Walsh M 1997 Watson's clinical nursing and related sciences, 6th edn. Baillière Tindall, London

References

Barre PE, Redini F, Boumediene K et al 2000 Semiquantitative reverse transcription polymerase chain reaction analysis of syndecan − 1 and − 4 messages in cartilage and cultured chondrocytes from osteoarthritic joints. Osteoarthritis and Cartilage 8: 34–43

Bryan GJ 1996 Skeletal anatomy, 3rd edn. Churchill Livingstone, Edinburgh

Department of Health (DoH) 2001 National Service Framework for Older People. Department of Health, London

Dop Bar PR, Reijneveld JC, Wokke JHJ et al 1997 Muscle damage induced by exercise: nature, prevention and repair. In: Salmons S (ed) Muscle damage. Oxford University Press, Oxford

Frost HM 1964 Dynamics of bone remodeling. In: Bone biodynamics. Little, Brown, Boston

Gunn C 1996 Bones and joints, 3rd edn. Churchill Livingstone, Edinburgh

Harman D 1956 Ageing: a theory based on the free radical and radiation chemistry. Journal of Gerontology 11: 298–300

Jaureguito J, Paulos L 1996 Why grafts fail. Clinical Orthopaedics and Related Research 325: 25–41

MacKenna BR, Callander R 1990 Illustrated physiology, 5th edn. Churchill Livingstone, Edinburgh

Powell M 1986 Orthopaedic nursing and rehabilitation. Churchill Livingstone, Edinburgh

Thibodeau GA, Patton KT 1999 Anatomy and physiology, 4th edn. Mosby, London

Uesugi M, Jasin HE 2000 Macromolecular transport across the superficial layer of articular cartilage. Osteoarthritis and Cartilage 8: 13–16

Waugh A, Grant A 2001 Ross and Wilson's Anatomy and physiology in health and illness. Churchill Livingstone, Edinburgh

Chapter 5

Why move?

Peter S Davis

CHAPTER CONTENTS

INTRODUCTION

People accept and take mobility for granted, not realising the effect of temporary or permanent restrictions to mobility. The concept of mobility is central to orthopaedic nursing, to rehabilitation, adaptation to changed circumstances and the return to a normal lifestyle.

This chapter explores the concept of mobility by discussing it in relation to impaired physical mobility. In orthopaedic nursing, this process is aided by using mobility as a central theme in care and using mobility-based nursing diagnoses for identifying specific patient problems related to mobilising. The implications of mobility for good health, health promotion and ill health prevention are explored.

Within orthopaedic care, the terms mobility, reduced mobility and immobility are used quite specifically. Reduced mobility and immobility are perceived as being predominantly physical in origin but with physical, psychological and social effects. This is seen in a patient with rheumatoid arthritis who has altered physical function and physiology of their hands and wrists. Their impaired physical mobility, from the decreased range of movement, loss of muscle strength and pain, often results in their being unable to use their hands for long periods without having to stop due to pain (activity intolerance). These physical effects exacerbate the social effects, as the patient is less able or unable to take part in leisure activities. Psychological effects arise from issues such as the physical disfigurement, changed family and social roles and depression, which alter the patient's self-concept.

In other areas of healthcare, the terms reduced mobility and immobility are used differently. In mental health, for example, the causes of impaired physical mobility can include severe depression, anxiety or a catatonic state. Restricting the mobility of these patients may be social in origin because the results of the illness may produce antisocial behaviour, requiring the individual to be nursed in a secure environment. Orthopaedic wards often have patients with mobility problems that arise from mental health and orthopaedic causes. The experience of nursing these patients ensures that the nurse's skills and knowledge are tested to their limits. For example, patients with confusion and dementia often get up immediately after a hip arthroplasty without any of the encouragement necessary for the patient with no mental health problem. They may appear to suffer little pain; this is difficult to assess but leaving any patient in pain is unacceptable whatever the circumstances.

THE CONCEPT OF MOBILITY

The English language literature on mobility has only scant reference to mobility and mobilising, the bulk being devoted to the opposing terms, immobility and impaired physical mobility. Three elements are essential for mobility:

1 the ability to move
2 the motivation to move
3 an environment that is non-restrictive and provides freedom to move.

Impaired physical mobility may be considered a state in which the individual experiences a limitation in their independent physical movement (Kim et al 1991).

Nurses frequently misuse the term mobility; for example, when referring to 'mobility problems' they can mean impaired physical mobility or activity intolerance. Further confusion occurs when the term mobility is used in a very restricted sense to mean walking. The phrase 'mobilising well' occurs frequently in nursing and medical patient documentation when what is meant is that the patient is getting up and walking well. Accuracy in the use and interpretation of common terms is necessary (Box 5.1).

There are over 6.9 million disabled people of working age in the United Kingdom, one-fifth of the working age population. About 3.3 million disabled people are in employment, approximately 12% of the working population (RADAR 2003). About 10% of all disabled persons are aged under

Box 5.1	Common terms
Mobility:	This is when an object is 'free to move, able to move or flow easily'
Impairment:	A permanent or transitory psychological, physiological or anatomical loss or abnormality of structure or function (WHO 1980)
Disability:	Any restriction or prevention of the performance of an activity, resulting from an impairment, in the manner or within the range considered normal for a human being (WHO 1980)
Handicap:	A dynamic relationship between the individual and their environment. The degree to which a disability is handicapping depends on the situations experienced by the individual, the attitudes and the expectations of others and the intervention strategies and environmental modifications which are made
Rehabilitation:	The restoration of patients to their fullest physical, mental and social capability (Scottish Health Services Council 1972)

45 years, 30% are between 46 and 64 years and 60% are 65 years or older. More women are disabled than men but this effect is present only because of their greater life expectancy. The increase in the number of older people is leading to a greater need for orthopaedic nurses to develop skills and knowledge in the field of disability and rehabilitation.

NURSING DIAGNOSIS

Broadly speaking, physical disability and impaired physical mobility are the same in their effects. However, categories of physical disability have been derived from medical diagnoses and are perceived as disabling conditions, for example osteoarthritis, stroke, paraplegia and major congenital malformations. While a medical diagnosis is useful when caring for people with mobility problems, it is not always essential to nursing care.

Table 5.1 Directors of nursing care

Possible	Preferable
Medical assessment	Nursing assessment
Medical diagnosis	Nursing diagnosis
Planned therapy	Planned care
Implementation, e.g. surgery or prescribing medication	Implementation, e.g. pressure sore prevention, promoting compliance with drug therapy
Evaluation based on progression of disease	Evaluation based on progression of a person as a whole (holism)

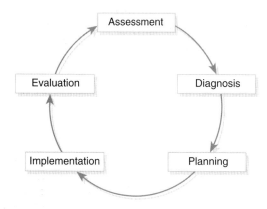

Figure 5.1 Elements of the nursing process.

Box 5.2   Comparison of nursing and medical diagnoses (NANDA 2003)

Medical diagnosis: Rheumatoid arthritis
Nursing diagnosis: Impaired physical mobility
Activity intolerance
Fatigue
Disturbed sleep pattern
Deficient of diversional activity
Ineffective health maintenance
Feeding self-care deficit
Bathing/hygiene self-care deficit
Dressing/grooming self-care deficit
Toileting self-care deficit
Impaired home maintenance

Box 5.3   Nine human response patterns

Exchanging: giving and receiving mutually
Communicating: sending messages
Relating: establishing bonds
Valuing: assigning relative worth
Choosing: selecting alternatives
Moving: changing position actively
Perceiving: receiving of information
Knowing: understanding the meaning of information
Feeling: being subjectively aware of information

The process of nursing should be directed by the elements of nursing (Table 5.1). A medical diagnosis indicates the disease an individual has and is used to plan their medical care. In comparison, a model of nursing, used to formulate a nursing diagnosis, provides a comprehensive picture of the patient's problems in order to plan nursing care. Using nursing diagnoses (Fig. 5.1) enables nursing practice to be problem finding and problem solving (Kirk 1986).

A helpful way of showing the differences between nursing diagnosis and medical diagnosis is to make a direct comparison between the two. Box 5.2 shows the nursing diagnoses, or patient problem categories, derived from the human response patterns to health and illness of 'moving' only. There are nine human response patterns (Box 5.3), of which moving is one. If, for example, an additional response pattern of 'feeling' is also considered, then further nursing diagnoses are identified in relation to mobility, for example pain, chronic pain and anxiety (NANDA 2003).

Woolley (1990) suggests that in order to provide an accurate nursing diagnosis, the nurse requires an understanding of three domains:

1 the central concepts of the nursing discipline, as reflected in a model of nursing
2 the processes of problem solving, illustrated by the nursing process
3 the foundation of theoretical knowledge on which to base practice.

The theoretical knowledge on which practice is founded will now be considered within a nursing diagnosis framework.

There can be little doubt that moving, mobility, mobilising, activity and other similar terms are important to orthopaedic nursing. The defining characteristics of impaired physical mobility are (McFarland & McFarlane 1993):

- inability to purposefully move within the physical environment, including bed mobility, transfer and ambulation
- decreased muscle strength, control or mass
- impaired coordination

> **Box 5.4   Aetiology or causes of impaired physical mobility (for a fuller description of these terms see Creason et al 1985)**
>
> - Intolerance to activity, decreased strength and endurance
> - Pain, discomfort
> - Perceptual/cognitive impairment
> - Musculoskeletal impairment
> - Neuromuscular impairment
> - Psychological impairment
> - Lack of knowledge

> **Box 5.5   Beliefs which lead to self-empowerment (adapted from Fenton & Hughes 1989)**
>
> - Each individual is unique, valuable and worthy of respect
> - Education, therapy and self-empowerment are value based
> - The more self-empowered a person becomes, the more they will be able to help others to be the same
> - Once individuals have learned to respect, love and value themselves, they will be able to respect, love and value others
> - It is helpful to differentiate the behaviours which encourage the developing parts of a person from those which serve to anchor them in states of depression, hostility, fear and/or insecurity
> - Taking risks and learning from mistakes is effective and valuable
> - Everyone has something to teach and something to learn

- imposed restrictions on movement, including mechanical or medical protocol restrictions
- range of motion limitations
- reluctance to attempt movement.

Consideration of the causes or aetiologies of a nursing diagnosis of impaired physical mobility demonstrates the importance of applying nursing diagnoses to orthopaedic nursing (Box 5.4). Using the same terminology as an agreed nursing language ensures that as a profession we communicate more accurately and clearly between ourselves and with our patients.

Mobility as a concept may be considered a blend of both activity and rest. Carrying out, or the potential to carry out, both of these elements of mobility is essential to a person's health. All nurses should understand the importance of exercise, rest, relaxation and sleep in appropriate quantities, as these are essential elements within health promotion. The maintenance or promotion of health is a vast topic that cannot be comprehensively covered in this text but must be considered as a fundamental component of the orthopaedic nurse's role.

SELF-EMPOWERMENT

Mobility and mobilising are essential to an individual's health irrespective of their age, gender and disabilities. Health, as with mobility, is often taken for granted and abused. An understanding of the essential concepts of health is essential for promoting mobility.

By promoting health and providing quality nursing care, the orthopaedic nurse is aiming to empower the patient but this may be difficult to achieve in environments as varied as the hospital and community or with individuals who are temporarily physically impaired or permanently physically disabled. To be able to empower others, the nurse must be capable of self-empowerment. Using self-empowerment will benefit the person with mobility problems, the nurse as a professional, the nursing profession and society in general, as many of the problems people encounter are due to actual or perceived powerlessness.

Self-empowerment is the process whereby the individual increasingly controls their life and becomes more independent (Fenton & Hughes 1989). They are able to choose to live within their inherent capacities and means, following their personal values and preferences. To facilitate self-empowerment, nurses need to develop appropriate beliefs and attitudes (Box 5.5). Table 5.2 lists characteristics of the more and less self-empowered individual, providing goals and directions for those seeking to promote self-empowerment.

NURSING MODELS AND MOBILITY

When identifying how three common models of nursing deal with mobility, it becomes evident that the physical and physiological elements of mobility predominate over the sociological and psychological elements.

- Orem's **self-care model** has a universal care requisite of the maintenance of a balance between activity and rest (Orem 2001).
- Roper's **activities of living model** includes the activity of mobilising (Roper et al 1996).

Table 5.2 Comparisons of more or less self-empowered individuals

More self-empowered	Less self-empowered
Proactive	Reactive
Open to change	Closed to change
Considers others in situations of change	Considers only self in situations of change
Assertive	Non-assertive or aggressive
Self-accountable	Blames others
Self-directed	Led by others
Uses feelings	Overwhelmed by or fails to recognise feelings
Learns from mistakes	Debilitated by mistakes
Confronts	Avoids
Realistic	Unrealistic
Seeks alternatives	Tunnel vision
Likes self	Dislikes self
Values others	Negates others
Considers others' needs	Selfish
Interested in the world	Self-centred
Enhances other people's lives	Restricts the lives of others
Can say no	Difficulty in saying no

- Roy's **adaptation model** involves the need for exercise and rest within the physiological mode (Reihl & Roy 1980).

Orem's model concentrates on the nurse–patient relationship, while Roy's concentrates on the individual and their response to their environment. These frameworks consider mobility in such a way that it is difficult to relate mobility meaningfully to other aspects of the model. Roper et al's activities of living model allows for the relationships between the other elements of the model and mobilising to be taken into account; for example, mobilising may be considered with respect to:

- factors influencing it such as physical, psychological, sociocultural, environmental and politico-economic aspects
- lifespan from conception to death
- a dependence to independence continuum
- other activities of living
- a systematic approach to individualising nursing.

Unfortunately, Roper's model tells us little about how the nurse should perceive the individual. However, by blending the activities of living model with an ethos of self-empowerment, it is possible to

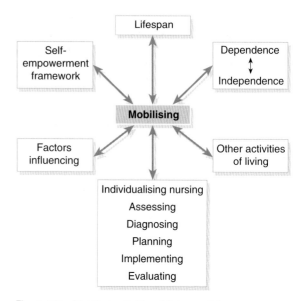

Figure 5.2 Modified activities of living model.

incorporate the essence of the goal of self-care from Orem's model and the essence of promoting the best possible adaptation choices by individuals in Roy's model. The addition of problem identification (nursing diagnosis) to Roper's systematic approach to individualising nursing, which has an inherent problem-solving approach, completes the new model (Fig. 5.2). The centralising of the activity of living of 'mobilising' makes the model specific to orthopaedic nursing. All other activities of living are to some extent dependent on mobilising within the field of orthopaedic healthcare and thus relate to it.

PATIENT PROBLEMS RELATED TO MOBILITY

The modified activities of living model of orthopaedic nursing is used here to provide an overview of the theoretical knowledge and practical skills that are fundamental to caring for patients with problems concerned with mobilising. All activities of living are affected by the impact that impaired physical mobility has on mobilising. In addition, the result of prescribed or unavoidable musculoskeletal inactivity increases the risk of disuse problems such as venous thromboembolism and pressure sores.

PRESSURE SORES

Impaired skin integrity is the potential or actual disruption or destruction of the skin layers, usually due to reduced or absent mobility, including the effects of extrinsic factors such as traction or a cast. The use of poor moving and handling techniques, long periods of sitting in a chair and inadequate pressure-relieving aids, such as mattresses and cushions, all exacerbate the problem. James (1995) identified these factors as particularly prevalent in the community. Kemp & Krouskop (1994) suggest that pain and depression produce activity intolerance and the patient is reluctant to change their position. The end result is a pressure sore (ulcer), which is a localised area of dead tissue resulting from the disruption and/or occlusion of the blood supply by pressure or other mechanical forces.

Size of the problem

Pressure sores are an ancient, extensive, significant and perennial problem. New pressure sores were found to occur in 4–10% of hospital patients in a UK general hospital study carried out by Clark & Watts (1994). The Touche Ross study (1993) found the cost of preventing pressure sores in a 600-bedded general hospital to be roughly between £600 000 and £3 million per year.

Versluysen (1986) found, in her one-hospital study, that 32% of patients in the three orthopaedic wards developed pressure sores, although this figure has been questioned. The size of the pressure sore problem has to be established before any action can be taken (Young 1997). To achieve this, two types of data collection are useful.

1 **Prevalence data**: provide the number of patients within the total patient population with pressure sores at any one time.
2 **Incidence data**: provide the number of patients developing pressure sores over a period of time, usually compared to the number of admissions in the same period.

Patient characteristics

Pressure sores are due to the interaction of many factors, divided into those characteristics specific to the individual patient and those derived from the patient's environment. Crow (1988) proposes that two of the most important patient characteristics are age and reduced physical activity.

Methods of calculating pressure sore risk are based on identifying the specific factors of the individual patient, which predispose him to pressure sore development (Table 5.3). Medical diagnoses do

Table 5.3 Factors predisposing to pressure sore development; ROM = range of movement

Related to	Problem/nursing diagnosis
Individual patient-specific factors	
Mobilising	Activity intolerance, pain, sensory alterations, decreased muscle strength, fatigue, lack of motivation, fear, limited ROM, imposed restriction of movement (e.g. splints, traction, prescribed bedrest, etc.), powerlessness, knowledge deficit
Eating and drinking	Feeding self-care deficit, altered nutrition (more or less than body requirements), fluid volume deficit
Eliminating	Altered patterns of urinary or faecal elimination; particularly incontinence
Sleeping	Fatigue and sleep pattern disturbance, e.g. leading to reduced movement caused by taking anxiolytics and narcotics
Cleansing and dressing	Bathing and hygiene self-care deficit
Breathing	Altered tissue perfusion (peripheral), e.g. due to smoking
Controlling body temperature	Hypothermia, hyperthermia
Environmental factors	
Compressive pressure	
Shearing pressure	

not specifically identify the nature of the patient problem but are useful as indicators of what the problems are likely to be. For example, the medical diagnosis of diabetes indicates that altered nutrition, peripheral tissue perfusion and sensibility, together with pain, are the likely potential or actual patient problems.

External loads

The most important external predisposing factor is the external load as this closes the microcirculation and lymphatic system. Cutting (1992) suggests that the body is capable of sustaining relatively high degrees of pressure, corroborating Crow's (1988) statement that patients can withstand pressures of 60 mmHg. Judd (1989) states that pressures greater than 32 mmHg on the skin for 1.5–2 hours can, in

Table 5.4   Incidence of pressure sores

Location	Incidence (%)
Sacrum	31
Buttocks	27
Heels	20
Trochanters	10
Lower limbs	5
Trunk	4
Upper limbs	3

immobile patients, lead to damage. However, capillary pressure varies with posture as well as with blood pressure fluctuations, so it is misleading to give a set figure for soft tissue ischaemic pressure; this probably accounts for the contradiction in the above figures.

There are three principal forms of mechanical force acting on body tissues.

1 **Compression**: the force exerted perpendicularly over a given area divided by that area. The greater the pressures on the skin, the more the tissues are distorted and the duration of the pressure is as important as its intensity. Short periods of very high pressure, for example sitting on a hard bedpan, can be as damaging as prolonged periods at lower pressures. The areas of the body where skeletal bony prominences are subjected to concentrated loading are the most likely sites of pressure sores. The incidence of pressure sores for each at-risk body location (Table 5.4) is based on the work of Locket (1983). It is interesting to note that 93% of pressure sores occur in the pelvic region or below and that Locket does not include the head. The omission of the head is an important error, as the occipital area in particular is prone to pressure sore development.

2 **Shear**: the force exerted parallel or at an angle to the skin surface, causing the skin layers and tissues to move laterally and producing severe distortion. This occurs where there is friction between the skin and, for example, the bed sheets. The frictional forces hold the upper layers of the skin stationary whilst the skeleton and the subcutis move. These forces stretch and squeeze the microvessels, leading to capillary and venule disruption as well as to tissue ischaemia. As the lymphatic system is also damaged, tissue necrosis is accelerated.

3 **Skin tension**: this has a similar effect to shear. It is seen when very tacky adhesive tape is used, causing blisters due to tension on the skin.

Box 5.6   Lowthian's (1987) classification of pressure sores

Grade 0 =	Potential sores	Inflammation with local heat, erythema, oedema and possible induration – more than 15 mm in diameter
Grade 1 =	Incipient sores	Blood under the skin or in a blister, or black (necrotic) discolouration under the skin – more than 5 mm diameter; or clear blister/bulla more than 15 mm diameter
Grade 2 =	Superficial sores (open)	A break in the skin (epidermis) which may include some damage to the dermis but without black discolouration (possibly a slough) – more than 5 mm diameter
Grade 3 =	Medium sores (open)	Destruction of the skin (epidermis and dermis) without an obvious cavity, but possibly with black discolouration (and possibly slough) – more than 5 mm diameter
Grade 4 =	Deep sores (open)	Penetration of the skin (epidermis and dermis) with a clearly visible cavity (with or without necrotic tissue) – more than 5 mm diameter at the surface
Grade 5 =	Sinus/bursal sores	Necrotic, possibly infected, possibly suppurating sore – more than 40 mm diameter overall but with either no skin opening or less than 15 mm diameter

Grading of pressure sores

A number of different grading systems are available for assessing pressure sores according to their location, size and severity, enabling accurate evaluation of pressure sores and documentation of the progressive deterioration or healing of the sore. The NHS

Centre for Reviews and Nuffield Institute (1995) conclude that 'the detection and grading of sores, particularly in their early stages, can be quite subjective and unreliable'. Lowthian (1987) probably provides the clearest, most usable classification for orthopaedic nurses (Box 5.6).

Pressure sore risk assessment

A variety of risk scales have been developed based on a range of clinical variables such as mobility, continence and activity. Most scales have been developed on relatively subjective opinions of the importance of the potential risk factors. Scales developed in one setting are not necessarily applicable to other settings and as yet there is no evidence to prove that risk scales provide better prediction than clinical judgement (NHS Centre for Reviews and Nuffield Institute 1995). Smith (2003) reviewed the evidence for identifying and establishing risk factors in the development of pressure ulcers and found variable evidence to support many of the currently accepted risk factors.

A review of the studies which used valid techniques to assess how well risk scales predict whether or not an individual will develop a pressure sore (predictive validity) has been produced (NHS Centre for Reviews and Nuffield Institute 1995). Many of the current popular scales are not included, as they have not had studies carried out on them. That is, there is no evidence to show that they work or make a difference. Of those that have been studied, Lowthian's (1989) Pressure Sore Prediction Score (PSPS) is rated very highly all round and specifically for its specificity and sensitivity. High specificity ensures that expensive resources are not wasted on patients who would not develop a sore. High sensitivity ensures that patients at risk of pressure sores, and in whom the risk of pressure sores will decrease if they receive effective preventive measures, are not missed. The PSPS has been developed for the orthopaedic setting, making it ideally suited to the demands of assessing risk in patients with impaired physical mobility (Fig. 5.3).

The potential of these risk scales is far reaching (NHS Centre for Reviews and Nuffield Institute 1995). They can be used to:

- aid the rational allocation of limited resources, such as special beds, to those who are likely to benefit most
- structure patient assessments and act as a reminder of the risk factors

- act as a case-mix adjuster to help make sensible comparisons of the incidence of pressure sores between units and/or over time.

The frequency with which pressure sore risk assessments are made depends on the patient's general condition and whether there are any sudden changes to them or their environment, such as having a general anaesthetic and surgery. These assessments can be made using risk calculators in any environment, including in hospital, community and long-stay units, and whenever possible patients should be taught to identify their own risks and take appropriate action.

Relieving pressure

Boore et al (1987) identify two mechanisms for relieving pressure:

1 those aiding natural behaviour
2 devices which redistribute pressure.

Devices that mechanically alter the patient's position should be added to Boore's categories.

Aiding natural behaviour. The nurse may aid natural behaviour by teaching and assisting the patient to move. It is essential the nurse assesses the patient's ability to move themselves and enables them to do this whenever possible, rather than automatically moving or transferring them and putting both the nurse and the patient at risk of injury.

Graham (1997), in his discussion of the role of patient education in preventing risks of pressure in the spinal cord-injured patient, emphasises its importance but questions its effect. Care must be taken not to overload and overwhelm the patient with the enormity of the problems. Equally, if too little information is given the patient will be ill informed and underestimate the importance of pressure sore risk. If the individual is to be motivated to be responsible for preventing their own pressure sores, they will require an internal locus of control; this should be encouraged and supported wherever possible. Maylor (2001) emphasises the importance of the nurse's locus of control, showing that the more the nurse believed they rather than the patient controlled pressure sore prevention, the higher the prevalence of sores.

The effect of movement is to relieve pressure from one area and to transfer it to another; this must be continued day and night. Lowthian (1979) developed a 24-hour turning clock for bedbound and chairfast patients. The previous position of the patient must be recorded to ensure that each area

	NO	NO but	YES but	YES
SITTING UP?	0	1	2	3
UNCONSCIOUS?	0	1	2	3
POOR GENERAL CONDITION?	0	1	2	3
INCONTINENT?				

	YES	YES & NO	NO
LIFTS UP?	0	1	2
GETS UP & WALKS?	0	1	2

A total of 6 or more = danger

DEVELOPED BY THE ROYAL NATIONAL ORTHOPAEDIC HOSPITAL TRUST

Explanatory notes for PSPS

Sitting up?
Yes: Propped up in bed most of the day; sits up both day and night
Yes but: For short periods only, although spends long periods in fixed chair; lies down for long periods
No but: Occasionally sits in a chair; sits in a self-propelled chair (long periods) but flat when in bed
No: Bedfast and nursed flat; only sits up when in a chair – short periods

Unconscious?
Yes: Deeply unconscious; does not respond to pain
Yes but: Rousable – responds to commands or pain
No but: Confused; withdrawn; excessive sleeping; semiconscious at times
No: Fully conscious and orientated; fully conscious and slightly confused

Poor general condition?
Yes: Seriously or critically ill; terminal (acute) illness; recent paraplegic; recent hemiplegic; quadraplegic; emaciated and cachectic; severe general infection; severe multiple sclerosis; iliac thrombosis; severe uraemia; severe injuries including legs or pelvis; on narcotics; Hansen's disease; extensive loss of pain or sensibility; limited mobility plus great age
Yes but: General condition could be worse; fair condition but some injuries to lower half of body; severe injuries but free movement of lower half of body; young paraplegic; active hemiplegic; well-established disease or disability
No but: Elderly and thin or obese; restricted movement of lower extremities; recent operation under general anaesthetic; on steroids; on chemotherapy; pyrexial; anorexic; arthritic; diabetic; some neuropathy; some arterial disease
No: Fairly good general condition – awaiting minor operation; fairly fit – awaiting discharge; minor local or mental disease; disease confined to upper extremities

Incontinent?
Yes: Continual dribble or leak; frequent urine or faecal incontinence or both
Yes but: Small amounts at infrequent intervals; urine only and infrequent; faecal (infrequent) but leaks from catheter or urinal
No but: Sometimes wets bed or spills urinal; occasional 'accidents' with attached urinal; occasional leaks from indwelling catheter; occasional faecal accidents
No: No incontinence or 'accidents' recently; indwelling catheter or stoma, but no leaks or 'accidents'

Lifts up?
Yes: Lifts all of body clear of support; easily lifts pelvis clear
Yes and No: Can only lift pelvis with some efforts, and soon tires; seldom lifts self; can lift with help; lifts slightly – shuffles into new position
No: Unable to lift pelvis; can neither help with lift nor shuffle

Gets up and walks?
Yes: Fully ambulant; slight impediment; uses walking aids with no difficulty
Yes and No: Has difficulty walking with aid; walks with help and encouragement; soon tires; can only walk to toilet
No: Bedfast or chairfast; stands and shuffles – with help and encouragement

Figure 5.3   Elements of the PSPS.

of the body is subjected to the minimum period of pressure possible. The use of these schedules is strongly recommended for high-risk patients. Although these positions may be difficult to maintain, Barton & Barton (1981) have shown that once a pressure sore has developed, effective treatment requires a 50% increase in nursing time.

Nursing interventions to promote patient self-help may be as straightforward as providing an overhead trapeze device or encouraging wheelchair patients to adjust their position frequently by doing push-ups.

Devices to redistribute pressure or mechanically alter a position. These fall into three categories (Torrance 1981a, b):

1 surface area utilised to support the body is increased or the area being compressed is varied
2 aid is provided when the patient is turned
3 those designed to support specific areas.

Increasingly, researchers and authors are producing comparative lists of these devices to help the nurse and patient make an appropriate choice (Cowan 1997, NHS Centre for Reviews and Nuffield Institute 1995). While these are very useful resources, they are often incomplete and biased by personal preference or manufacturer's involvement (Table 5.5). Fletcher's (1997) proposed set of criteria to help make decisions about pressure-relieving equipment can be of additional value.

Devices that increase the surface area utilised to support the body may be in the form of foam mattresses, such as the combination foam mattress which has different densities of foam, or mattresses made from slashed foam or rigid egg-box type foam. Scales (1982) showed how these mattresses reduced the pressure around a load by 50%, compared to the standard NHS mattress.

Mattresses and cushions filled with other materials are also used, especially air, polystyrene beads, fibres, gels and water. For example, low air-loss beds support the patient on sacks of a flexible vapour-permeable material with air pumped into the sacks. Fluidised airbeds also require pumped air to function. Santy et al (1994) carried out a useful comparison of various types of mattresses for preventing pressure sores in elderly hip fracture patients. Tarpey et al (2000) demonstrated that the condition and type of trolley in accident and emergency departments is also crucial as pressure sores often develop at this time but do not become apparent until a few days later.

Devices that vary the area being compressed include alternating-pressure beds such as the ripple

Table 5.5 Examples of devices to redistribute pressure

Mode of action	Equipment
Beds, mattresses and cushions	
Can equalise pressure over most of the support surface	Water flotation bed, low air-loss bed, fluidised air bed (Clinitron), individually shaped foam or matrix support
Can spread the load over a large area	Low-pressure airbed, net suspension bed, water mattress, bed and cushion, slit foam mattress, Roho mattress and cushion, polystyrene beads, silicone gel cushion
Alter the area subject to pressure	Alternating pressure beds: ripple, pulsair, airwave
Other	
Prevent contamination with urine	Special incontinence sheets
Absorb moisture	Bead pads, sheepskin, absorbs water vapour only

mattress and airwave systems. Large air-cell, double-layer mattresses have been shown to be more effective than small-cell ones (NHS Centre for Reviews and Nuffield Institute 1995).

Various pads and devices have been developed from materials such as sheepskin and foam to protect specific areas of the body like the heels and elbows. Sheepskin will only reduce shear and tension forces and does little to reduce direct pressure.

Beds to aid turning can be motorised or manual and can turn the patient through the vertical or horizontal axis. Examples are the circo-electric bed, the wedge turning frame and turning and tilting beds.

Unfortunately, knowing about methods and devices to systematically prevent pressure sore development does not guarantee their use, although the ritualised practices of massaging with soap, which damages the skin (Torrance 1981a, b), and ill-informed use of harmful devices such as ring cushions to sit on (Crewe 1987) have ceased.

Treating and dressing pressure sores

The cost of treating pressure sores in the UK is estimated as ranging from £60 million to £420 million per year (McSweeney 1994). Under appropriate

Table 5.6 Aims of wound care and dressing options

Aim	Dressing option
For debridement	Hydrogel Hydrocolloid Semipermeable
To deslough	Hydrogel Hydrocolloid Xerogel
To control low–medium exudate	Foam Hydrocolloid Alginate New semipermeable
To control medium–high exudate	Extra-absorbent foam Extra-absorbent alginate Hydrocellular foam
To control odour	Alginate and carbon dressing Foam and carbon dressing
Cavity dressing	Pouring foam Alginate ribbon Foam fillers
To promote healing	Lyofoam Hydrocolloid Hydrogel New semipermeable
For overgranulation	Lyofoam

conditions pressure sores will heal, but all the preventive measures described in the previous section must be considered and implemented as necessary throughout the healing process to preclude a recurrence or the development of further sores.

For the successful treatment of a pressure sore, an understanding of wound healing is necessary. Before wound healing can occur, any necrotic tissue should be removed to produce a healthy granulation bed. This wound debridement can be achieved surgically, enzymatically or chemically (Table 5.6). Other therapeutic measures include ultrasound, infrared, ultraviolet and laser treatment.

For a successful outcome, the prevention and treatment of pressure sores must be carried out within an holistic framework. The skin and underlying tissues are unlikely to remain healthy or to heal readily if the patient's nutritional status is poor or if they are suffering from sleep disturbance, as sleep is important in the restorative and repair processes of the body (Oswald & Adam 1983).

Organising and monitoring care

The process of risk management involves the identification of risks and/or potential hazards, plus the implementation of strategies to eliminate and prevent them. Kiernan (1997) suggests the need for the process to be proactive as this would minimise any potential financial loss. Financial loss is usually through litigation due to complaints about the standard of care. Fear of litigation should not dictate any initiatives to prevent pressure sores, which should be motivated by the desire to provide the best quality of care through acceptable patient outcomes. On analysing pressure sore cases and complaints, Tingle (1997) found that most could easily be avoided with little or no expense.

Accurately and comprehensively estimating the cost of preventing pressure sores, as opposed to their treatment and litigation costs once they occur, continues to be a problem. Costs and benefits involved, at all levels, need to be assessed (Brooks & Semlyen 1997). Costs should include those to the health service, patients and families plus the external costs to the rest of society including, for example, the implementation of moving and handling regulations.

If pressure sores are to be prevented and treated effectively, a systematic approach must be adopted. In practice, this is reflected in the development and implementation of decision-making flow charts, algorithms and protocols. There are numerous examples of these in the literature but they require full and appropriate implementation to be effective.

The success, or otherwise, of the management of the prevention and treatment of pressure sores can only be determined through evaluation, for example through:

- prospective research in which new elements are introduced to determine if they make a difference
- retrospective audit in which established elements are investigated once they have occurred.

Setting standards and auditing their implementation is another simple means of changing practice (Lizi 2000).

Orthopaedic nurses are at the forefront of pressure sore management due to the nature of the specialty. Currently there is little 'good' evidence to support a coherent, consistent and comprehensive approach to the problem. However, the majority of nursing care relevant to pressure sore management relates to simple, timely, cost-effective and knowledgeable interventions provided consistently by experts 24 hours a day.

DEEP VEIN THROMBOSIS (VENOUS THROMBOEMBOLISM)

Nurses are essential in preventing identifying and managing the care related to a deep vein thrombosis (DVT) and subsequent pulmonary emboli (PE). This requires knowledge of the pathophysiology, incidence, risk factors, methods of risk assessment, diagnostic presentation, treatment and, of course, prevention strategies.

Impaired physical mobility may give rise to circulatory stasis. If injury or trauma to the circulatory system and an alteration in blood chemistry have also occurred, the patient is at risk of developing a deep vein thrombosis. If the thrombus or part of it becomes dislodged and begins to float in the venous system, a potentially fatal pulmonary embolism may occur with the clot blocking one of the pulmonary vessels.

Obtaining accurate data on the incidence of DVT is difficult due to the inability to make a diagnosis by clinical signs alone and it is often asymptomatic (Griffin 1996). In the general population, a DVT of the lower limbs presents with clinical signs in approximately 1 per 1000 annually (Nicolaides et al 1997). Incidence rates in the hospital population are much higher than this, due to a combination of acute injury, surgery and immobilisation. For example, the incidence of a clinical DVT in orthopaedic surgery is thought to be in the region of 4% (THRiFT II 1998), although DVT rates as high as 60% have been reported in patients undergoing knee replacement surgery (Warwick & Whitehouse 1997). Prevalence rates of DVT of 58% have been documented in cases of major trauma (Geerts et al 1994). Further, an overview of the results of major studies (Bergqvist 1990) suggests that the risks of DVT are greatest with orthopaedic surgery involving the leg and lowest with minor and endoscopic surgery.

The three factors responsible for the development of DVT – venous stasis, vein injury and blood chemistry changes – were first described by Rudolph Virchow, a German pathologist, in 1856 and are commonly referred to as Virchow's triad (Fig. 5.4). It is now generally accepted that a combination of these factors usually causes a thrombosis, rather than one factor in isolation.

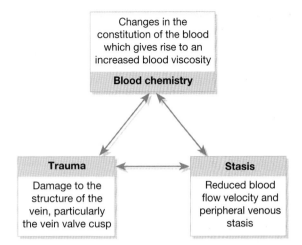

Figure 5.4 Virchow's triad.

A combination of these factors occurs in some patients in virtually all hospital specialties, including all types of surgery, trauma, obstetrics, oncology, medical and paediatrics (Donnelly 1999, THRiFT II 1998). For example, as a result of surgery the blood chemistry changes occur as a protective mechanism to prevent wounds bleeding excessively, venous stasis occurs due to the anaesthesia and inactivity in the postoperative period and vein injury may occur as a direct result of the surgical procedure.

Risk factors

Calculation of a patient's risk of developing a DVT is based on assessing the patient's individual characteristics. Age and reduced physical activity are important factors that increase the risk (Table 5.7) while environmental factors include:

- compressive pressure, particularly in specific regions of the body, for example long socks with garter supports
- surgery of more than 1 hour's length and in certain regions of the body
- the surgical technique used.

Stamakis et al (1977) showed that during total hip replacement surgery the femoral vein becomes distorted, leading to 51% of the 160 patients studied developing a DVT in the femoral vein.

Risk assessment

The recognition of predisposing factors is important in identifying at-risk patients. Autar (1996, 2003)

Table 5.7 Factors predisposing to deep vein thrombosis (DVT)

Related to	Problem/nursing diagnosis
Individual patient-specific factors	
Mobilising	Activity intolerance, pain, decreased muscle strength, fatigue, lack of motivation, fear, limited ROM, imposed restriction of movement (e.g. splints, traction, prescribed bedrest, etc.), powerlessness, knowledge deficit
Eating and drinking	Altered nutrition (more than body requirements, causing obesity), fluid volume deficit
Breathing	Ineffective breathing pattern
Controlling body temperature	Hypothermia
Expressing sexuality	Altered hormonal status, e.g. due to contraceptive pill, pregnancy
Other	Presence of malignancy, previous history of DVT
Environmental factors	
Compressive pressure	
Surgery: length and nature	

suggests that a nursing diagnosis of a 'potential problem of DVT' is insufficient; the risk needs to be objectively assessed for each patient. His scale consists of seven distinct categories identified following a literature review of the pathogenesis of DVT (Fig. 5.5).

1 **Age**: probably the most important general factor (Bergqvist 1990) as the risk of a DVT increases exponentially with advancing age (Rosendaal 1997). Any patient over the age of 40 years should be considered to be at significant additional risk of surgical thromboembolism.
2 **Mobility**: is related to aspects of impaired physical mobility and leads to a significant increase in the risk of DVT (Autar 1996). This is due to the diminished pumping action of the leg muscles through not walking and of the foot pump through not weight bearing.
3 **Build and body mass index**: this is not identified by many researchers as a risk factor.

The evidence for these is far from conclusive although obesity causes venous dilation, resulting in venous stasis (Herzog 1992) and some impairment in fibrolytic action (Poller 1993).

4 **Special risk**: this applies to women on contraceptive therapy or in the puerperium.
5 **Trauma**: specifically referring to those patients with an injury to the lower limbs or spine.
6 **Surgical intervention**: as discussed earlier.
7 **High-risk diseases**: including inflammatory bowel disease, blood dyscrasias, cardiovascular diseases and a previous DVT.

Autar (2003) developed a simple scoring system, based on these categories, to produce a patient risk category grouping that enables nurses to make decisions about respective actions.

Detection

As an undetected DVT may lead to pulmonary embolism, early recognition of its occurrence is essential. Love (1990a, b) identifies four methods for the detection of DVT that are substantially a part of nursing care (Table 5.8).

The clinical diagnosis of DVT is unreliable. As many as 50% of patients have no symptoms or signs in their legs and only 50% of patients with leg symptoms are found to have DVT on further investigation (Bergqvist 1990). Iodine labelling and scanning, phlebography and Doppler ultrasound investigations help to confirm and gauge the extent of the thrombosis. Unfortunately, in up to 80% of affected patients, the pulmonary embolism is not detected.

Methods of prevention

The debate regarding thromboembolic prophylaxis in orthopaedic patients continues. The basic question of whether any prophylaxis should be given is still unanswered (CEPOD 1999), leading to controversy over the different methods and duration of prophylaxis. Consensus statements have given unequivocal recommendations that thromboembolic prophylaxis must be used for hip fracture patients. These are at odds with the more recent analyses which, whilst confirming that thromboembolic prophylaxis will reduce the risk of thrombotic events, fail to establish whether this benefit is offset by other adverse events affecting overall mortality (CEPOD 1999). For the foreseeable future thromboembolic prophylaxis will remain a controversial topic.

Name: Unit No: Ward:		Age: Type of admission: Diagnosis:		

AGE SPECIFIC GROUP (years)   **Score**

10–30	0
31–40	1
41–50	2
51–60	3
61–70	4
71+	5

BUILD/BODY MASS INDEX (BMI)

Wt (kg)/ht (m^2)

Build	BMI	Score
Underweight	16–18	0
Average/desirable	19–25	1
Overweight	26–30	2
Obese	31–40	3
Very obese (morbid)	41+	4

MOBILITY   **Score**

Ambulant	0
Limited (uses aids, self)	1
Very limited (needs helps)	2
Chairbound	3
Complete bedrest	4

SPECIAL RISK CATEGORY   **Score**

Oral contraceptives:	
20–35 years	1
35+ years	2
Hormone replacement therapy	2
Pregnancy/puerperium	3
Thrombophilia	4

TRAUMA RISK CATEGORY
Score item(s) only preoperatively   **Score**

Head injury	1
Chest injury	1
Spinal injury	2
Pelvic injury	3
Lower limb injury	4

SURGICAL INTERVENTION
Score only one appropriate surgical intervention   **Score**

Minor surgery <30 min	1
Planned major surgery	2
Emergency major surgery	3
Thoracic	3
Gynaecological	3
Abdominal	3
Urological	3
Neurosurgical	3
Orthopaedic (below waist)	4

CURRENT HIGH-RISK DISEASES
Score the appropriate item(s)   **Score**

Ulcerative colitis	1
Polycythaemia	2
Varicose veins	3
Chronic heart disease	3
Acute myocardial infarction	4
Malignancy (active cancer)	5
Cerebrovascular accident	6
Previous DVT	7

ASSESSMENT INSTRUCTION
Complete within 24 hours of admission

Scoring: Ring out the appropriate item(s) from each box, add score and record total below.

Total score:

Assessor:

Date:

ASSESSMENT PROTOCOL

Score range	Risk categories
≤10	Low risk
11–14	Moderate risk
15≥	High risk

Please record any other clinical observations that may supplement this DVT risk assessment.

VENOUS THROMBOPROPHYLAXIS

Low risk:	Ambulation + graduated compression stockings
Moderate risk:	Graduated compression stockings + heparin + intermittent pneumatic compression stockings
High risk:	Graduated compression stockings + heparin + intermittent pneumatic compression

International Consensus Group recommendation 2001
© R Autar 2003

Figure 5.5   New Autar (2003) DVT risk assessment scale. (Reproduced with permission from Elsevier Ltd.)

Table 5.8 Methods for the detection of deep vein thrombosis (DVT) (adapted with permission from Love 1990a, b)

Test	Purpose and method	Advantages	Disadvantages
Visual examination of the limb	Perform a daily visual assessment for discoloration of the skin and signs of redness in the distribution of the tibial, popliteal and femoral veins. A mirror can be used if visual access is made difficult by restricted positioning	Non-invasive procedure which can be carried out by nurses	Cannot be done if the lower limb is bandaged or encased in a cast
Assessment of pain and/or discomfort	Regularly assess the patient's level of comfort. Ask the patient to specify the exact location of pain or discomfort. Identify sources of discomfort or pain in the distribution of the tibial, popliteal, femoral and iliac veins. Locate pain source to calf muscle, behind the knee, at the back of the leg or in the groin region	Non-invasive procedure which can be carried out by nurses	The patient's complaint may not be fully appreciated. Delay in identifying the cause may occur if the first recourse is to administer analgesic agents. The patient may have other sources of pain which are confusing the situation
Four-hourly temperature	Be suspicious of all unexplained low-grade pyrexia	Non-invasive procedure which can be carried out by nurses	There are many causes of low-grade pyrexia other than DVT
Homan's sign	Examine for sharp pain or discomfort in the calf when the patient's foot is dorsiflexed. Eliminate the possibility of pain or discomfort arising from other sources such as a Baker's cyst	Non-invasive procedure which can be carried out by nurses	DVT needs to be in an advanced stage before the test is positive. Can only be used to detect calf vein thrombosis. Does not detect potentially fatal femoral and iliac vein thromboses. Cannot be done if the lower limb is bandaged or encased in a cast. There are other causes of calf pain, such as a Baker's cyst
Calf measurement	Take and record measurements of the calf in cm. A baseline measurement needs to be established preoperatively. The same position needs to be used on each occasion. Take measurements daily throughout the risk period. Eliminate the possibility of swelling arising from other sources	Non-invasive procedure which can be carried out by nurses	Cannot be done if lower limb is bandaged or encased in a cast or there are other causes of calf swelling. Distortions occur unless the same position on the calf is used each time. A baseline measurement needs to be known

Nurses are essential in dealing with the problem of DVT and subsequent PE. For this they require knowledge of pathophysiology, incidence, risk factors and risk assessment, diagnostic presentation, treatment and prevention (Davis 1998). Love (1999) has produced an in-depth review of preventive measures for DVT.

Interventions in common use generally fall into several broad categories:

- pharmacological agents: aspirin, heparin, warfarin
- antiembolism stockings (graduated compression antiembolic stockings)

- intermittent compression devices: calf garments and foot garments
- early mobilisation
- lower limb elevation
- hydration.

Pharmacology. Low-dose, 150 mg enteric-coated aspirin, started before surgery and continued for 35 days, is recommended for orthopaedic patients undergoing total hip and knee replacement surgery and surgery for a hip fracture (SIGN 2002a, b, guidelines 62 and 56). This is based on studies such as the PEP Trial (2000) in which 13 356 patients undergoing surgery for hip fracture were treated with 160 mg enteric-coated aspirin daily for 5 weeks, producing a 43% reduction in pulmonary embolisms. Low-dose aspirin has a low risk of increased bleeding.

Generally unfractionated heparin or low molecular weight heparin should only be used in those patients at high risk. Salvati et al (2000) have emphasised that the mortality risk from bleeding due to heparin may exceed that due to pulmonary embolism, that low molecular weight heparin needs monitoring and bleeding complications exceed those of warfarin.

In summary, prophylactic pharmacological agents are best assessed by their overall death rate, accounting for both risks and benefits. The proponents advocating that prophylaxis should not be used routinely are not necessarily negligent.

Aspirin has accumulated an excellent safety track record and its use may be indicated in conjunction with epidural or spinal anaesthesia in patients with no additional risk factors (Salvati et al 2000).

Antiembolism stockings. Many clinical trials support the use of graded compression stockings in general surgery. However, Best et al (2000) found that 98% of stockings failed to produce the 'ideal' pressure gradient of 18, 14 and 8 mmHg from the ankle to the knee, while 54% produced a 'reversed gradient' on at least one occasion.

Intermittent pneumatic compression (IPC). This is achieved through calf or foot pumps (Davis & O'Neill 2002). These offer advantages over pharmacological methods because patients have a high tolerance of these devices. There is no associated risk of bleeding, no laboratory monitoring and there is stimulation of endogenous fibrinolytic activity.

Decreased blood flow or even stasis due to lack of the pump action of large muscle groups is a

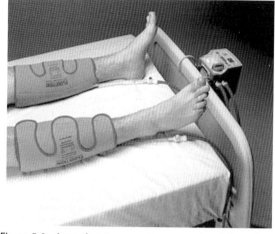

Figure 5.6 Intermittent pneumatic compression of the calf. (Reproduced with permission from Huntleigh Healthcare.)

major factor in the development of DVT. It seems logical to compensate for this by simulating this pumping action mechanically. IPC is applied by wrapping an inflatable garment around the leg or foot and a section of the garment is inflated with air via a pump. The garment is deflated after a few seconds. This sequence of inflation and deflation of the garment continues for the duration of therapy, providing cyclic mechanical compression to the venous system of the leg or foot.

Calf garments (Fig. 5.6) operate at low pressures, for example 40 mmHg, with a short inflation period, 12 seconds, and a long deflation period, 48 seconds, to allow venous refilling to occur (Huntleigh Healthcare 1998). The inflation forces blood in the superficial veins into the deep veins of the leg, increasing venous blood velocity and preventing venous stasis.

Foot garments (Fig. 5.7) utilise the venous foot pump in the sole of the foot, which consists of the venae comites of the lateral plantar artery (Binns & Pho 1988). Applying IPC to the foot causes a flattening of the plantar arch similar to that caused by weight bearing (Gardner & Fox 1983). This causes emptying of the lateral plantar veins into the deep veins of the leg. Gardner et al (1990) have subsequently shown that machines used to produce impulse pumping have such a marked effect on the microcirculation that they produce other benefits such as a reduction in swelling, prevention of compartment syndrome and relief of pain as well as prevention of deep venous thrombosis. Foot pump

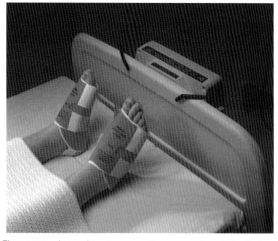

Figure 5.7 Intermittent pneumatic compression of the foot. (Reproduced with permission from Huntleigh Healthcare.)

systems operate at higher pressures than calf and thigh systems with shorter inflation and deflation periods. The garments should be applied and worn continuously during the pre-, intra- and postoperative phases of surgery for a minimum of 72 hours postoperatively or until the patient is fully mobile (Huntleigh Healthcare 1998).

Early mobilisation. More attention is being paid to physiological exercises performed in bed as unassisted active movement of the ankle increases femoral venous flow by more than 75% (Salvati et al 2000). There is, however, little evidence to demonstrate the benefits of early mobilisation. Early mobilisation and elevation of the foot of the bed have obvious benefits but need more evidence to support them as interventions.

Hydration. Adequate hydration is essential but again has little good evidence to support its benefit, as is the case with deep breathing exercises.

Treating deep vein thrombosis

Once detected, the patient with a DVT or pulmonary embolus will require anticoagulation therapy and possibly surgical or other interventions to disperse or remove the thrombus. Anticoagulation is a prophylactic measure to ensure that no further episodes of DVT occur but it creates potential problems for the patient, so they must be well informed about the possible side effects, recommendations and contraindications while on long-term therapy (Box 5.7). Similar information must be incorporated

---

Box 5.7 Information for patients on anticoagulant therapy

Because the medication you are taking reduces your blood's ability to clot, you must take special precautions.

- Wear a Medic Alert bracelet or carry a card with information that you are taking anticoagulants
- Take your medication at the same time each day, as prescribed
- Keep all appointments for blood tests
- Increase or decrease your medication only as directed by your doctor
- If you do cut yourself, immediately apply pressure to the wound with a clean dressing or cloth for 5–10 minutes. If possible, elevate the part cut. If the bleeding does not stop, go to your nearest hospital accident and emergency department immediately
- Tell your dentist you are on anticoagulants on each visit
- Always check with your doctor before taking any new medications
- Never take aspirin or other medication that contains aspirin. Read all labels carefully
- Avoid alcoholic beverages – they may alter your blood clotting time. Ask your doctor for specific advice
- Immediately report any of the following to your doctor:
  Nosebleeds
  Coughing up red to black mucus
  Bruises that persist longer than usual or that increase in size
  Bleeding gums
  Blood in your urine or stools (which might be bright red or tarry)
  Weariness
  Dizziness, faintness
  Anxiety, apprehension
  Irritability
  Confusion

---

into care plans to ensure nurses are able to detect complications at an early stage, promote desirable patient behaviours and ensure compliance by empowering the patient.

The International Consensus Statement (1997) reports that patients who have developed a DVT may

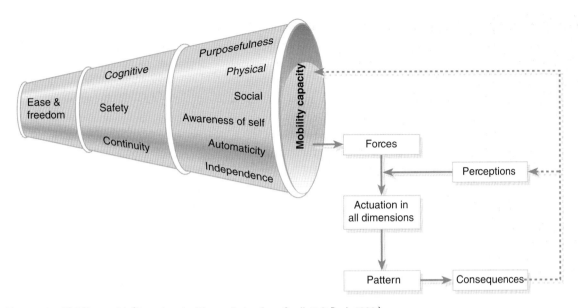

Figure 5.8 Mobility model. (Reproduced with permission from Ouellett & Rush 1998.)

also suffer a long-term complication known as postthrombotic syndrome, affecting the blood supply of the lower limb and leading to possible leg ulcers. They report the incidence of postthrombotic syndrome as being 35–69% at 3 years after DVT and 49–100% at 5–10 years. In addition, venous ulcers develop in at least 300 per 100 000 of the population and the proportion due to DVT is approximately 25%.

PROBLEMS RELATED TO THE LOCOMOTOR SYSTEM

Creason et al (1985), in their research on the nursing diagnosis of impaired physical mobility, identified what may be termed its causes or effects. Ouellett & Rush (1998) suggest that mobility is predominantly viewed from a physical perspective and has been addressed only when deficits arise. Their model (Fig. 5.8) depicts mobility as having multiple components. The element 'mobility capacity' refers to the possibility for movement and all the components are interrelated in a dynamic manner. Other elements such as 'forces' are then affected by or affect the mobility capacity of the client.

Reluctance to move

There are many reasons why a patient feels reluctant to move. If the patient is experiencing pain, it must be managed effectively and reduced to a level

acceptable to the patient. Frequently the patient is afraid that moving will cause further pain, damage or harm. A knowledgeable, confident and reassuring nursing approach is required to encourage and support the patient at these times. Persuasion and support rather than coercion are needed. If the patient feels in control of the situation because they understand the reason for movement and its therapeutic effect, then progress is often accelerated and complications reduced. The patient must have the desire to move; the motivation for this has to come from them, but may be promoted or extinguished by the nurse.

Maslow's (1954) theory of man's drive to meet physical, social and psychological needs based on the individual's motivation to achieve their potential can be related to Ouellett & Rush's (1998) 'qualities' of mobility. It is relatively straightforward for a nurse and patient to identify and satisfy basic physiological needs, such as eating and drinking or breathing, but it is more difficult to satisfy psychological needs such as a high self-esteem. Nurses can help the patient satisfy both basic and more complex psychological needs by empowering them with the drive and desire to meet these needs and then allowing them to achieve their potential. For example, an arthritic patient may allow the nurse to do everything for them as this is easier and quicker for both the patient and nurse; however, the patient will tend to become demotivated and dependent.

Limited range of movement

Joints that are not put through a range of movement at regular intervals will become stiff and eventually a joint contracture will occur due to the ligaments and tendons not being stretched and instead becoming denser, contracted and less elastic. For example, wearing shoes with high heels for a period of time reduces the range of dorsiflexion of the ankle; the Achilles tendon shortens and contracts, causing ankle stiffness. When flat shoes are worn again, stretching of the Achilles tendon can often be felt. If the contraction is significant or the individual elderly, the tendon may become painful, damaged or even torn when full dorsiflexion is imposed by wearing flat shoes.

Generally, the patient's joints should be rested in a neutral, functional position as far as possible, to prevent damage from prolonged hyperextension or flexion. The wrist, for example, has a neutral position of 30° of extension, so splints used for immobilising the wrist in neutral should produce this degree of extension with slight ulnar deviation and allowing the metacarpophalangeal joints to rest in a position of 90° of flexion, as though the patient was gripping a tumbler. These neutral positions are therefore not only optimum for the prevention of joint contractures but are also functional as patients will still be able to feed themselves and take a drink.

Decreased muscle strength, control and mass

Many of the patient problems so far discussed require a close working relationship between the nurse, physiotherapist, occupational therapist and patient, but as Ouellett & Rush (1998) identify, there is a tension between these professionals and the role of the nurse. The skill of the healthcare professional is in getting the balance between activity and rest right, at any point in time, so that the patient can achieve an optimum rate of recovery and degree of comfort, with minimal complications.

Powell (1986) proposes that active exercises have four main purposes.

1 To retain movement to prevent stiffness in joints and maintain normal tone in the muscles controlling them.
2 To restore movements which have been lost owing to disuse, injury or disease.
3 To redevelop muscles and to restore muscle balance that has been lost through disuse, injury or disease.

4 To retain the memory of movement patterns and to regain functional control in general.

These exercises all require patient cooperation and participation. They may be classified according to the degree of participation and the degree (or lack) of movement required.

- **Free active exercises**: carried out by the patient on their own, the aim being to gain or retain joint movement and strengthen muscles. They also stimulate and assist the circulatory system to prevent circulatory stasis.
- **Isometric exercises (static contractions)**: these are performed by the patient and involve muscular contractions without movement of the joint(s). The patient performs them, for example, when their leg is immobilised in a plaster cast, to maintain the tone and strength of the quadriceps muscles. Thus recovery is speeded up and circulatory stasis reduced.
- **Assisted active exercises**: active movements performed by the patient but with the assistance of a healthcare professional such as the physiotherapist or nurse, or a mechanical device or the patient's sound limb.
- **Resisted active exercises**: carried out by the patient against a resistance such as a footboard or weight attached to a limb or against the physiotherapist or nurse.

Individuals should be provided with written instructions on their exercise programme, to prevent joint and muscle deterioration due to disuse and to enable them to continue progressive rehabilitation once discharged from hospital. Many day centres now provide exercise classes for the elderly to enable them to maintain muscle strength and their range of joint movement and so help them avoid the potential problems of reduced physical mobility and improve their quality of life. For instance, to strengthen a patient's shoulder, they are given a programme of exercises they are expected to perform twice daily (Box 5.8).

Passive movements. The patient does not perform these; instead, the physiotherapist, nurse or a mechanical device such as a continuous passive mobiliser puts the patient's joint(s) through a range of movement and stretches their muscles. These movements are necessary for patients with impaired physical mobility due, for example, to polyneuritis, multiple sclerosis or motor neuron disease. They aim to prevent tightness and contractures of joints and muscles. The nurse is usually instructed and

1 Standing upright, with your arms straight by your sides, raise your right arm forward and upward above your head, as far as possible. Return to resting position and repeat with your left arm
2 Standing upright, with your arms straight by your sides, raise your right arm sideways and upwards above your head, as far as possible. Return to resting position and repeat with your left arm
3 Standing upright, with your arms straight by your sides, raise your right arm sideways to shoulder level. Then bring your arm across your body, bending your elbow at the same time, to touch your left shoulder if possible. Return to resting position and repeat with your left arm

assisted by the physiotherapist to ensure continuity and consistency and that appropriate movements are used. Downie & Kennedy (1980) emphasise that care must be taken when carrying out passive movements because the joints and tissues are easily damaged by excessive vigour or overextension of the range of movement of relatively unprotected joints and muscles because all the soft tissues are weakened by disuse.

PROBLEMS WITH ELIMINATION

Impaired physical mobility may cause a toileting self-care deficit, such as inability to maintain or achieve continence, leading to constipation, renal calculi or a urinary tract infection. These problems are further exacerbated by therapies or nursing interventions such as the drugs given for pain management, premedications or restricted fluid intake before and after surgery. The lack of privacy and the discomfort of using bedpans, commodes and urinals while confined to bed only add to the patient's difficulties.

Whether the patient is at home or in hospital, the inability to eliminate without assistance leads to an inevitable loss of privacy and dignity and causes discomfort. Anderson (1978) paints a vivid picture of these problems. 'There you sit, enveloped in the array of white screening that surrounds your bed, but offers no privacy whatsoever. Perched in an uncomfortable and impossible position, the great trial of concentration and effort begins.'

Western culture and basic human anatomy and physiology ensure that patients are unprepared for eliminating while in bed, in the presence of others and into strange receptacles. Postures such as lying and restriction of movement and position due to casts or traction add to the problem. This makes it difficult for the individual to relax sufficiently to urinate. As defaecation occurs best in a squatting position, this function is also inhibited by environmental and positioning restrictions which therefore may lead to constipation.

Psychological stimuli such as running water may help a patient to urinate but other interventions should also be carried out to help alleviate inhibiting factors:

- ensuring maximum privacy for the patient when they are using a bedpan
- allowing the patient to communicate that they have finished or need assistance, for example by giving them a call bell rather than keep checking on them
- ensuring the patient is comfortable and feels safe
- providing toilet paper and leaving it within reach
- whenever possible, allowing the patient to use the toilet or commode rather than bedpan or urinal
- providing hand-washing facilities.

Constipation

This is the reduction in the frequency of defaecation from what is normal for the individual, with an associated difficulty in passing faeces (Boore et al 1987). It is said to occur when an individual displays two or more of the following symptoms (Thompson 1992):

- straining for at least a quarter of the time
- lumpy or hard stool for at least a quarter of the time
- a sensation of incomplete evacuation for at least a quarter of the time
- two or fewer bowel movements per week.

There can be little doubt that constipation is a significant problem both for the patient with reduced mobility and for the orthopaedic nurse. For the former it is uncomfortable and distressing; for the latter it consumes both time and resources.

In patients with orthopaedic conditions, reduced mobility and therapeutic interventions often lead to reduced food or fluid intake; for instance, if a patient has difficulty in eating and drinking owing to pain on movement or a limited range of movement. Medication such as antibiotics may also lead to anorexia, nausea and even vomiting. The insufficient food intake will not stimulate peristalsis and dehydration produces small, hard, dry stools that irritate the colon, causing spasm and a failure to stimulate normal colonic motility.

A nursing assessment based on bowel motions and habits will establish any deviation from the individual's norm. A nursing diagnosis identifies the probable cause of the problem and a care plan in the form of dietary modifications, such as increasing fibre or daily fluid intake to approximately 2 litres for adults, may be all that is necessary. Alleviation of the problem may be achieved directly by assisting the patient with eating and drinking or through the provision of aids or patient education. In some cases it may be necessary to alleviate constipation with laxatives or enemas such as bulking agents, stimulants, softeners and those that have an osmotic effect by drawing fluid into the bowel (Hicks 2001). However, their regular use is not recommended.

Diarrhoea

As this is often due to a change in diet or to antibiotic therapy, simply altering the diet or reducing the patient's anxiety by informing them that antibiotics are causing the problem may be all that is required. However, if diarrhoea is profuse and lasts for more than a day or two, urgent action must be taken as the resultant dehydration may be life-threatening.

Diarrhoea as a result of conditions such as pseudomembranous colitis induced by antibiotic therapy must be suspected if the onset is sudden and severe. Seal & Borriello (1983) explain that *Clostridium difficile*, the infective organism in pseudomembranous colitis, occurs from disruption to the gastrointestinal flora resulting from antibiotic therapy. As the majority of orthopaedic patients undergoing surgery have prophylactic antibiotic cover, this infection can spread quickly through a ward of susceptible patients.

Retention and difficulties in micturition

Difficulties in defaecating generally develop over days and do not require urgent nursing interventions. On the other hand, micturition problems and urinary retention often develop over minutes or hours and require more immediate attention.

Urinary tract infection due to urinary stasis and urinary retention as a result of surgery or a general anaesthetic are common in patients with orthopaedic conditions and are the commonest problem following orthopaedic surgery, with 11% of patients suffering from them (Slappendel & Weber 1999). The effects of urinary stasis can be minimised by ensuring an adult patient drinks at least 2 litres of fluid per day, providing that no other medical or nursing diagnosis contraindicates this. If, however, the patient is unable to urinate, then urethral catheterisation may be necessary. The use of diagnostic bladder ultrasound can dramatically reduce the number of catheterisations by ensuring only those with sufficiently full bladders are catheterised (Frederickson et al 2000). There is a high risk of infection from both the catheterisation procedure and from leaving an indwelling catheter in situ. As 19% of catheterised patients develop urinary tract infections (Moore & Edwards 1997), all other reasonable nursing interventions must be attempted before this is carried out.

Urinary incontinence as a consequence of impaired physical mobility due to an orthopaedic condition, together with the potential for ill health in elderly patients, is not an uncommon combination. It is essential orthopaedic nurses develop the skills necessary in caring for the elderly with continence problems and they should form close links with nurses directly involved in the healthcare of the elderly.

PROBLEMS OF EATING AND DRINKING

Good nutrition is fundamental to physical well-being and is important for many activities of living, including elimination. However, poor nutrition must not be confused with self-care deficits in feeding which are more specific in nature and related to problems of mobility. The importance of a balanced diet, the nutrients needed for growth, healing and good health are discussed in Chapter 8. Self-care deficits in feeding relate mainly to physical disability, motivational factors, the patient's position and the availability of assistance.

Physical disability

To overcome the individual's self-care deficit, the orthopaedic nurse must have empathy, patience, resilience and common sense. Arthritic patients, for example, suffer from joint deformity and pain. If these are severe and involve the joints of the hand, the grip strength is reduced and holding cutlery is difficult. Arthritic patients tend to use both hands to support cups while drinking and built-up handles on cutlery can help a weak grip. Mandelstam (1990) offers valuable information on assessing the disabled individual, for decisions on and obtaining appropriate aids to help them eat and drink in hospital and the community, along with details on the rights of disabled individuals. The provision of sandwiches and other finger foods for some meals offers a simple, effective solution (Wainwright 1978) but can lead to a restricted diet.

Motivational factors

Henley (1987) warns that we should not underestimate the psychological importance of giving the patient familiar food or food they consider healthy. Compliance with cultural and religious customs, such as eating and fasting at set times, and the presentation and prohibition of certain types of food and drink need consideration; for example, a devout Muslim would not feel able to eat a salad from which a slice of ham had merely been removed. It is essential the nurse obtains as much information as possible from the patient and is prepared to be flexible and innovative in providing nutritional support. An individual's appetite may have been good or bad throughout their life and may remain unchanged with age but their illness may cause anorexia or nausea. They will have their own food and drink likes and dislikes which must be taken into account.

Positioning for eating and drinking

As eating and drinking are social events, efforts must be made to enable the patients to eat together or with their family if at home. However, coercion must not be used on those individuals who do not wish to eat with others as this can be stressful and embarrassing for them. The patient's position will impose further restrictions. Poor positioning, for example balancing a plate on the lap, not sitting upright in bed or when forced to lie flat to eat or drink, can create ingestion and swallowing problems (Roper et al 1996). Special chairs and beds are available to ease these problems but common sense and a few carefully positioned pillows suffice in many instances.

Assistance

Some patients require assistance varying from arranging and cutting up food to inserting food into the patient's mouth. Whenever possible, the patient's ability to feed themselves must be maintained, which requires the orthopaedic nurse to use all their knowledge and skills. A patient who has

undergone spinal surgery and is confined to a supine or prone position is still able to use their arms. With mirrors, careful selection and preparation of food and drink and the use of suitable utensils and aids, these patients are able to feed themselves. This gives them more control over their situation and is psychologically beneficial.

PROBLEMS OF PERSONAL CLEANSING AND DRESSING

Bathing, grooming and dressing are all personal and private aspects of everyday life. One of the stabilising and often pleasurable aspects of daily living is removed if the individual is unable to carry out these activities. Dressing, in particular, is one way for people to demonstrate individuality and show they have control of their lives and possess decision-making capabilities. All these activities reflect, to some extent, people's social and economic position and niche in life.

The inability to perform personal cleansing and dressing activities is predominantly due to impaired physical mobility as a result of:

- pain on movement
- prescribed restrictions, such as plaster of Paris casts or bedrest
- limited range of movement
- reduced muscle strength
- the lack of a desire to move.

Personal cleansing

Whenever possible, the individual must be enabled to perform personal cleansing activities independently. The use of equipment and aids often makes this possible (Mandelstam 1990); for example, using a wide-handled toothbrush or glove flannel to give a patient with arthritic hands greater independence.

The patient may not be able to take a bath independently; Roper (1988) describes a variety of aids and equipment available to assist such patients and nurses to perform this activity, including bath seats, handrails, hoists, special baths and shower units. However, some orthopaedic patients are unable to move or be moved from their beds. In hospital and the community this problem demands imagination, tact and time. Each patient will have individual needs, idiosyncrasies and levels of dependence. It may be that a towel bath, as described by Wright (1990), is more appropriate and comforting to the patient than the usual bed bath. Special basins are available for washing patients' hair while they are in bed.

Sexuality is often expressed through the way people groom, dress and maintain their hygiene. The male patient who wishes to but cannot shave daily must be given assistance or be shaved by the nurse. Mirrors should be available to enable women and men to groom, apply make-up or shave themselves if possible or to see the results of the nurse's attention.

Menstruation may create problems for women, for example when on traction or in a hip spica cast. Sensitive assistance with the positioning of sanitary pads is required.

Dressing

The majority of able-bodied people dress daily without giving a thought to the strength, suppleness, stamina and agility required. For orthopaedic patients, clothing and footwear may need to be adapted or specially manufactured. The individual's need can be temporary, for example following foot surgery, or permanent, for example when an artificial limb is fitted or the individual has rheumatoid arthritis. Often simple advice is needed; for example, a person with a frozen shoulder should be encouraged to put garments over the unaffected arm first (Roper et al 1996).

The Disabled Living Foundation, Royal Association for Disability and Rehabilitation (RADAR) and other similar bodies provide a wealth of information on availability, designs and costs of clothing and footwear. In addition, there are aids to assist dressing such as shoehorns and stocking aids.

Patients in hospital or at home should, when possible and appropriate, wear their own clothing and maintain their own routines of dressing and undressing.

General principles to consider when assisting the patient to decide on appropriate clothing and footwear are:

- ease of putting on and removing
- cost
- aesthetic quality and style
- comfort
- ease of washing and cleaning
- safety
- non-restrictiveness, for general mobility and therapeutic exercises
- warmth, but not excessive
- versatility, adaptability and reparability.

Developments such as Velcro fastening, elastic laces and the style of many of today's clothes and shoes help to ensure, with careful selection and adaptation, that dressing and undressing are potentially easier, less painful and less frustrating for those with impaired physical mobility. The mass production of sports and leisure wear has meant that stylish, comfortable, washable and relatively cheap clothing and footwear are now available for all ages. The latest developments in materials, particularly for shoes, enable orthotists to produce items that are comfortable and acceptable to wear.

PROBLEMS OF BREATHING

The absence of breathing is obviously serious, as in respiratory arrest or apnoea. Other problems may occur with breathing and the gaseous exchange in the lungs owing to:

- the quality of breathing
- the quality of the breathed air
- the condition of the individual's lungs and cardiopulmonary system.

The activity of breathing

Ideally the lungs should be able to expand easily on inspiration and the lung bases should be aerated regularly by taking deep breaths. There are several reasons why this may not occur in orthopaedic patients.

- Impaired physical mobility: this can be local, such as when wearing a tight plaster jacket, or general, for example owing to conditions such as rheumatoid arthritis or from a prescribed therapy such as bedrest.
- Posture: lung expansion is easiest in the upright position.
- Pain and its management.
- Physical deformity.
- Surgery.

Pain prevents deep breathing and coughing. Also some analgesics, such as morphine, depress the respiratory centre and reduce the depth and rate of breathing. Physical deformities such as scoliosis and the effects of ankylosing spondylitis reduce lung expansion. General anaesthetic agents reduce respiratory function by depressing breathing and paralysing the cilia of the respiratory tract that keep the lungs clear of mucus and debris.

By encouraging regular deep breathing, more oxygen enters the bloodstream to respond to increased metabolic demands, especially following injury or surgery. Additionally, the lung bases are aerated by dilation of the bronchioles and alveoli, preventing the mucus secretions stagnating in them. If secretions do collect, they can solidify and act as a mucus plug in the bronchioles. This plug is difficult to expectorate; the air distal to the plug is absorbed but fluid still exudes from the walls of the alveoli, providing an ideal medium for bacterial growth. The resultant chest infection further reduces gaseous exchange. Deep breathing also reduces the negative pressure in the thorax, thus drawing venous blood back to the heart more effectively and reducing the risk of DVT.

The orthopaedic nurse needs to work closely with, and often under the guidance of, the physiotherapist in teaching patients deep breathing exercises and helping them to maintain these. Powell (1986) advises that the nurse should place their hands on either side of the patient's thorax and instruct the patient to breathe in so as to push the hands away, and then breathe out and relax. After each deep breath, taken slowly, there should be complete relaxation and the procedure should be repeated 5–6 times. The patient can place their own hand below the sternum and if the exercises are performed correctly, they should feel a significant movement of the hand as compared to shallow breathing. Once taught, these exercises can be performed hourly by the patient at home or in hospital, with monitoring by the nurse.

More specialised breathing exercises may need to be taught by the physiotherapist or the patient may need to be assisted by equipment such as patient-activated positive pressure ventilation or spirometers that gauge lung ventilation improvements and allow the patient to see their progress, adding a competitive and fun component to the exercises.

The upright position allows greater diaphragmatic freedom and thus encourages increased ventilation of the lungs with less effort from the patient, as the abdominal contents drop with the assistance of gravity on inspiration. As Boylan & Brown (1985) describe clearly, inspiration is an active process whereas expiration is passive. Therefore, inspiration requires greater energy and motivation from the patient and is more tiring. Often the orthopaedic nurse needs to be innovative and flexible, as the patient's condition or therapy may prevent or make difficult the achievement of this posture. The patient must be encouraged to be up and walking as soon as possible. Sitting upright, well supported, in a chair is also beneficial.

However, if the patient is confined to bed, then the upright sitting position, well supported by pillows, may be the only possible solution. The patient must be upright, as the slumped position is even more detrimental to diaphragmatic freedom than lying flat. To help minimise the risk of the patient sliding down the bed, the foot of the bed should be elevated by 5–10°. This not only maintains the patient in a more upright position but reduces the risk of sacral pressure sore development, as shear forces are markedly reduced. Heavy bedclothes tucked in tightly around the chest also impede good lung ventilation. Therefore, bedclothes should be loose and light and should allow freedom of movement.

An environment that is airy, well ventilated and with a constant warm temperature is pleasant and psychologically beneficial to the individual. The opposite can be harmful to physical, social and psychological health. For example, a hot, stuffy, smoky atmosphere for even a short time can cause coughing, a sore throat, headache, tiredness and lethargy. Impaired physical mobility may reduce the patient's ability to control their environment and thus makes them dependent on the nurse. However, whenever possible, they should be encouraged to be outside in the fresh air as this will have psychological benefits as well.

Good ventilation keeps unpleasant odours to a minimum and reduces the prevalence of airborne bacteria and viruses. Pleasant-smelling aromas from oils will encourage deep breathing and have therapeutic benefits. The use of aromatherapy essential oils, such as lavender which helps relaxation and promotes sleep, dates back to the ancient Egyptians who used oils for religious and medical reasons.

The patient may have a breathing problem that is exacerbated by their orthopaedic condition or its therapy. Many are elderly with a risk of:

- respiratory conditions, such as chronic bronchitis
- poor lung ventilation from the normal ageing process. In the elderly there is a reduction of vital capacity by 25%, a reduction of maximum breathing capacity by 50% (between 20 and 80 years of age), increased rigidity of the chest wall and reduction of the thoracic volume due to a tendency to stoop, kyphosis and/or scoliosis.

A patient who smokes should be given information, encouragement and support to stop or reduce their smoking, although the decision to do so has to be the patient's. The patient's health would benefit generally and ensure a quicker, more efficient therapy and better quality of life if recovery or cure were not possible.

Adult respiratory distress syndrome (ARDS) results from interference with the gaseous exchange in the lungs, leading to interstitial fibrosis and hyaline membrane formation. This can be associated with severe soft tissue injury and fat emboli caused by fractures. Treatments such as massive blood transfusions, excessive fluid administration and prolonged artificial ventilation may also cause ARDS.

PROBLEMS OF SLEEP AND REST

Undoubtedly, sleep pattern disturbance causes discomfort and interferes with the desired lifestyle; it may also lead to ill health or be the result of ill health. Recovery from orthopaedic conditions and their treatment is hindered or prevented by a lack of adequate sleep and rest.

Since nurses tend to spend more time in close contact with orthopaedic patients than do other healthcare professionals, the responsibility for dealing with sleep pattern disturbance rests largely with them. A limited understanding of the nature of sleep and rest, reinforced by general attitudes which belittle their importance can lead to nursing and medical staff providing inappropriate or inadequate care for patients with a sleep pattern disturbance.

Many arthritic patients are woken several times a night by their joint pain and find changing their position, relaxation and rest are impossible to achieve. The anxieties of having arthritis and not knowing what the future holds further affect sleep and rest. Closs et al (1997) showed that sleep was shorter and more fragmented for orthopaedic patients in hospital than at home, with pain being the main cause of night-time waking.

Functions of sleep

Sleep and rest are essential to functioning and preparation for periods of mobility. Although there is still much debate about the exact nature and function of sleep, there are areas of general agreement. Sleep is considered restorative, is important in tissue renewal and in the growth of body cells in children (Closs 1988a, b, Webster & Thompson 1986). Horne (1983) suggests that sleep is necessary only for brain cell restitution and that physical rest will suffice to allow the restoration of other body cells. In either case, sleep and rest are fundamental activities of living.

Individuals vary in the length and quality of the sleep and rest that they require. However, sleep

---

Box 5.9   Effects of sleep pattern disturbance
• Difficulty falling asleep
• Awakening earlier or later than desired
• Interrupted sleep
• Not feeling well rested
• Malaise
• Tiredness
• Lethargy
• Restlessness
• Irritability
• Sensitivity to pain and discomfort
• Listlessness
• Apathy
• Slow reaction

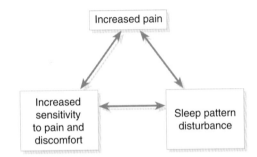

Figure 5.9   Pain and sleep pattern disturbance.

pattern disturbance in all individuals leads to specific adverse effects (Box 5.9) and although these may vary in importance for each patient, the healthcare team must identify how each aspect affects the patient and try to overcome it. Sleep pattern disturbance often forms part of an interrelated complex cycle of cause and effect; for example, many patients state that they would be able to cope with the pain and discomfort of their condition, such as rheumatoid or osteoarthritis, if only they could get a good night's sleep. Somehow this cycle of pain, lack of sleep and rest must be overcome (Fig. 5.9).

Promoting sleep and rest

Pain is probably the most significant cause of sleep pattern disturbance (Closs et al 1997). Medications, such as hypnotics, are not a suitable solution to the long-term chronic pain and sleep disturbance for many orthopaedic patients, owing to the effects of increased tolerance, dependence and side effects. However, immediately prior to surgery or for a few days post trauma, they can help promote sleep and rest. Interventions such as relaxation techniques, aromatherapy, massage and instructions on self-relaxation are preferable and can be used with pain-reducing medication.

Increased relaxation will often reduce the necessity for analgesia. If further sleep-promoting interventions are encouraged (Box 5.10), the quality of sleep may improve dramatically, obviating the need for medication.

Closs (1988a, b), in her review of the research on sleep disturbances in hospital, showed that 78% of patients were woken at least once during the night. The commonest cause of significant sleep disturbance was noise, along with routines such as drug rounds and the lights going out late.

If sleep is accepted as important to the patient's health, recovery and well-being, then orthopaedic nurses must be more knowledgeable and systematic in their nursing care. Patients vary significantly in their sleep needs and the factors that promote or hinder them. Indeed, the same person's sleep pattern will change throughout their life and from day to day depending on their situation and life events.

Short-term sleep disturbances lasting a few days, such as those due to the discomfort caused by orthopaedic surgery, are not a significant problem, especially if the patient is reassured that their diminished sleep will have no long-term effects. More important are chronic sleep problems and the cause should be identified and interventions planned and implemented to reduce or eradicate the problem. The orthopaedic nurse will find it difficult to gauge the extent of the problem or whether interventions were successful unless information is obtained from and about the individual.

Assessing sleep pattern disturbance and evaluating nursing interventions may be achieved relatively easily. Subjective methods used are similar to those for pain management:

- visual analogue scales
- questionnaires
- interviews
- daily sleep charting.

Self-assessment of sleep using a daily sleep chart can produce useful information about changes and gives the individual more control over their care (Church & Davis 1998). Recording this information requires little time and effort and is easy to carry out (Fig. 5.10). It is also important to accept that patients are satisfied or dissatisfied with their sleep when they say they are, no matter what others may think or feel.

In many cases the nurse and patient must make the best sleep and rest environment despite adverse situations. Positioning patients wearing casts and splints or in traction can be restricted; however, imaginative use of pillows and supports together with pain and anxiety-reducing interventions and a quiet, warm, well-ventilated environment will all help to promote and ensure better quality sleep.

Box 5.10   Sleep-promoting interventions

- Reduce or eliminate pain
- Reduce or eliminate anxiety and depression
- Assist patient to achieve comfortable position
- Ensure warmth and dark
- Minimise noise
- Ensure satisfaction of basic needs such as hunger or desire to eliminate
- Encourage regular circadian clock, i.e. awaken at same time each day

---

Figure 5.10   Examples of sleep assessments.

What time did you go to bed?   Before 21.59
22.00–22.59
23.00–23.59
24.00–24.59
01.00–+

What time did you get up?   Before 04.59
05.00–05.59
06.00–06.59
07.00–07.59
08.00–+

How well did you sleep?

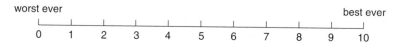

worst ever   best ever

0   1   2   3   4   5   6   7   8   9   10

Table 5.9 Examples of aetiology of body changes in orthopaedic patients

Aetiology	Example of body change
Congenital	Muscular dystrophy, spina bifida
Hereditary	Osteogenesis imperfecta
Medical/disease	Arthritis
Trauma	Spinal injury
Surgery	Amputation

PROBLEMS OF SELF-IMAGE

The musculoskeletal system is an important and very visible component of the human body so many patients with orthopaedic problems have noticeable body changes due to a variety of causes and origins (Table 5.9). Physical changes to the body may not impair a patient's mobility significantly but their perception of how their body appears may give rise to significant problems. A patient may not be pleased with their self-perception and may not accept their altered body image, whether real or apparent. Disturbances to this self-image make it very difficult for the patient to feel good about themselves and reduce the extent to which self-empowerment, and hence their ability to overcome or accept their altered body image, can be achieved. These difficulties are compounded in our present society because, as Salter (1997) suggests, the mass media appear continually to confront society with the suggestion that it is essential to have a healthy, pleasant appearance. An inability to achieve this leads to dissatisfaction, a poor self-image and low self-esteem.

Body image loss can be due to a combination of a change in appearance and impaired physical ability. How a person responds to their altered body image is also affected by society's response to and acceptance of them. The stigma sometimes attached to disabled people can affect their social identity and social encounters. For sufferers of chronic orthopaedic conditions, the disabilities experienced often accelerate their adaptation to ageing and diminishing function (Maycock 1988). 'Feeling older than one's years' is a phrase often used and applies to perceived physical, social and psychological age but bears little relationship to chronological age.

Many see the process of adjusting to altered body image as a grieving process. The fact that a patient advances through certain stages when experiencing a change such as an alteration in body image is a useful framework on which patients and nurses can build (Davis 1997). It enables the patient to realise they are not the only one who feels and reacts in these ways and provides an end goal of acceptance or adjustment to the loss. Weeks (1999) provides a graphic case study of a patient with an old congenital dislocation of the hip undergoing surgery which gives an illustration of the above and many other elements of altered body image. Crowther's article (1982) on new perspectives in nursing lower limb amputees reveals some interesting insights on limb loss and altered body image from the amputee's view.

CONCLUSION

An examination of the concepts of mobility and mobilising provides an indication of why being able to move is fundamental to people's health. It is important for nurses to understand the effects of impaired physical mobility so they can make a nursing diagnosis and then plan care. From this a high standard of care is provided, which can be demonstrated through evaluation and audit.

Nurses are becoming increasingly more assertive and empowered. This serves to improve their professional status and clarify their roles and responsibilities within a multidisciplinary team without alienating their healthcare colleagues. With this increased sense of professional worth and self-esteem, the orthopaedic nurse is in a better position to empower patients to make their own decisions and act appropriately in relation to their health and illness.

References

Anderson E 1978 The bedpan and the commode. Nursing Times 74(16): 684

Autar R 1996 Nursing assessment of clients at risk of deep vein thrombosis: the Autar scale. Journal of Advanced Nursing 23: 763–770

Autar R 2003 The management of deep vein thrombosis: the Autar DVT risk assessment scale re-visited. Journal of Orthopaedic Nursing 7(3): 114–124

Barton A, Barton M 1981 The management and prevention of pressure sores. Faber and Faber, London

Bergqvist D 1990 Thrombosis clinical practice and perspectives: fatal pulmonary embolism. Oxford Clinical Communications, Oxford

Best AJ, Williams S, Crozier A et al 2000 Graded compression stockings in elective orthopaedic surgery. Journal of Bone and Joint Surgery 82B(1): 116–118

Binns M, Pho WH 1988 Anatomy of the venous foot pump. Injury 19: 443–445

Boore JRP, Champion R, Ferguson MC 1987 Nursing the physically ill adult. Churchill Livingstone, Edinburgh

Boylan A, Brown P 1985 Respiration. Nursing Times 81(11): 35–38

Brooks R, Semlyen A 1997 Economic appraisal in pressure sore management. Journal of Wound Care 6(10): 491–494

CEPOD 1999 National Confidential Enquiry into Perioperative Deaths: extremes of age. CEPOD, London

Church L, Davis P 1998 Sleep: the gentle healer. Journal of Orthopaedic Nursing 2(4): 226–231

Clark M, Watts S 1994 The incidence of pressure sores within a National Health Service trust hospital during 1991. Journal of Advanced Nursing 20: 33–36

Closs J 1988a Patient's sleep–wake rhythms in hospital, Part 1. Nursing Times 84(1): 48–50

Closs J 1988b Patient's sleep–wake rhythms in hospital, Part 2. Nursing Times 84(2): 54–55

Closs J, Briggs M, Everitt V 1997 Night-time pain, sleep and anxiety in postoperative orthopaedic patients. Journal of Orthopaedic Nursing 1(2): 59–66

Cowan T 1997 Pressure-relief seating. Professional Nurse 12(11): 809–818

Creason NS, Pogue NJ, Nelson AA et al 1985 Validating the nursing diagnosis of impaired physical mobility. Nursing Clinics of North America 20(4): 669–683

Crewe R 1987 Problems of rubber ring nursing cushions and a clinical survey of alternative cushions for ill patients. Care: Science & Practice 5: 9–11

Crow R 1988 The challenge of pressure sores. Nursing Times 84(38): 68, 71, 73

Crowther H 1982 New perspectives on nursing lower limb amputees. Journal of Advanced Nursing 7: 453–460

Cutting KF 1992 Pressure sores: a case to answer. Nursing Standard 7(4): 9–14

Davis P 1997 Spinal cord injury and changes to body image. In: Salter M (ed) Altered body image: the nurse's role, 2nd edn. Baillière Tindall, London

Davis P 1998 The hidden threat: deep vein thrombosis. Journal of Orthopaedic Nursing 2(1): 45–52

Davis P, O'Neill C 2002 The potential benefits of intermittent pneumatic compression in the prevention of deep venous thrombosis. Journal of Orthopaedic Nursing 6(2): 95–100

Donnelly KM 1999 Venous thromboembolic disease in the paediatric intensive care unit. Current Opinion in Pediatrics 11(3): 213–217

Downie A, Kennedy P 1980 Lifting, handling and helping patients. Faber and Faber, London

Fenton M, Hughes P 1989 Passivity to empowerment. Royal Association for Disability and Rehabilitation, London

Fletcher J 1997 Pressure-relieving equipment: criteria and selection. British Journal of Nursing 6(6): 323–328

Frederickson M, Neitzel JJ, Miller EH et al 2000 The implementation of bedside bladder ultrasound technology: effects on patient and cost postoperative outcomes in tertiary care. Orthopaedic Nursing 19(3): 79–87

Gardner AMN, Fox RH 1983 The venous pump of the foot – preliminary report. Bristol Medico-Chirurgical Journal July: 109–112

Gardner A, Fox R, Lawrence C et al 1990 Reduction of post-traumatic swelling and compartment pressure by impulse compression of the foot. Journal of Bone and Joint Surgery 72-B(5): 810–815

Geerts WH, Code KI, Jay RM et al 1994 A prospective study of venous thromboembolism after major trauma. New England Journal of Medicine 331: 1601–1606

Graham A 1997 The development of pressure sores in patients with spinal cord injury. Journal of Wound Care 6(8): 393–395

Griffin J 1996 Deep vein thrombosis and pulmonary embolism. Office of Health Economics, London

Henley A 1987 Caring in a multiracial society. Bloomsbury Health Authority, London

Herzog J 1992 Deep vein thrombosis in the rehabilitation client. Rehabilitation Nursing 17(4): 196–198

Hicks A 2001 The prevention and management of constipation. Journal of Orthopaedic Nursing 5(4): 208–211

Horne JA 1983 Human sleep and tissue restitution. Clinical Science 65(6): 569–578

Huntleigh Healthcare 1998 Flowtron excel protocol for use of external intermittent pneumatic compression for deep vein thrombosis prophylaxis. Huntleigh Healthcare, Luton

International Consensus Statement 1997 Prevention of venous thromboembolism. Med-Orion Publishing, London

James H 1995 Preventing pressure sores in patients' homes. Professional Nurse 10(10): 649–650, 652

Judd M 1989 Mobility. Heinemann Nursing, London

Kemp MG, Krouskop TA 1994 Pressure ulcers: reducing incidence and severity by managing pressure. Journal of Gerontology Nursing 20(9): 27–34

Kiernan M 1997 Pressure sores: adopting the principles of risk management. British Journal of Nursing 6(6): 329–332

Kim MJ, McFarland GK, McLane AM 1991 Pocket guide to nursing diagnosis, 4th edn. Mosby, St Louis

Kirk LW 1986 Framework. In: Hurley ME (ed) Classification of nursing diagnosis. Mosby, St Louis

Lizi D 2000 Setting the standard for pressure sore prevention on a trauma orthopaedic ward. Journal of Orthopaedic Nursing 4(1): 22–25

Locket B 1983 Prevalence and incidence in pressure sore disease. Symposium at the Royal Hospital and Home for Incurables, London

Love C 1990a Deep vein thrombosis. Nursing Times 86(5): 40–43

Love C 1990b Deep vein thrombosis. Nursing Times 86(6): 52–55

Love C 1999 A focused review of nursing and the effectiveness of preventative measures for deep vein thrombosis. Journal of Orthopaedic Nursing 3(2): 73–80

Lowthian P 1979 Turning clocks system to prevent pressure sores. Nursing Mirror 148(21): 30–31

Lowthian P 1987 The classification and grading of pressure sores. Care: Science & Practice 5(1): 5–9

Lowthian P 1989 Letter. Care: Science & Practice 7(27)

Mandelstam M 1990 How to get equipment for disability. Jessica Kingsley Publishers & Kogan Page, London

Maslow AH 1954 Motivation and personality. Harper, New York

Maycock J 1988 The image of rheumatic disease. In: Salter M (ed) Altered body image: the nurse's role. John Wiley, Chichester

Maylor M 2001 Control beliefs of orthopaedic nurses in relation to knowledge and prevalence of pressure ulcers. Journal of Orthopaedic Nursing 5(4): 180–185

McFarland GK, McFarlane EA 1993 Nursing diagnosis and intervention. Mosby, St Louis

McSweeney P 1994 Assessing the cost of pressure sores. Nursing Standard 8(52): 25–26

Moore D, Edwards K 1997 Using a portable bladder scan to reduce the incidence of nosocomial urinary tract infections. Medsurg Nursing 6: 39–43

NHS Centre for Reviews and Nuffield Institute 1995 The prevention and treatment of pressure sores. Effective Health Care 2(1)

Nicolaides AN, Bergqvist D, Hull R 1997 Consensus statement on prophylaxis of venous thromboembolism. International Angiology 16: 3–38

North American Nursing Diagnosis Association (NANDA) 2003 Available online at: www.nanda.org/

Orem DE 2001 Nursing: concepts and practice, 6th edn. Mosby, St Louis

Oswald I, Adam K 1983 Get a better night's sleep. Martin Dunitz, London

Ouellett LL, Rush KL 1998 Conceptual model of client mobility. Journal of Orthopaedic Nursing 2(3): 132–135

Poller L 1993 Recent advances in blood coagulation. Churchill Livingstone, Edinburgh

Powell M 1986 Orthopaedic nursing and rehabilitation, 9th edn. Churchill Livingstone, Edinburgh

Pulmonary Embolism Prevention (PEP) Trial 2000 Prevention of pulmonary embolism and deep vein thrombosis with low dose aspirin. Lancet 355: 1295–1302

Reihl J, Roy C 1980 Conceptual models for nursing practice. Appleton-Century-Crofts, Norwalk, Connecticut

Roper N 1988 Principles of nursing in process context, 4th edn. Churchill Livingstone, Edinburgh

Roper N, Logan WW, Tierney AJ 1996 The elements of nursing. Churchill Livingstone, Edinburgh

Rosendaal FR 1997 Thrombosis in the young: epidemiology and risk factors: a focus on venous thrombosis. Thrombosis and Haemostasis 78(1): 1–6

Royal Association of Disability and Rehabilitation (RADAR) 2003 Available online at: www.radar.org.uk

Salter M 1997 Altered body image: the nurse's role, 2nd edn. Baillière Tindall, London

Salvati EA, Pellegrini VD, Sharrock NE et al 2000 Symposium: recent advances in venous thromboembolic prophylaxis during and after THR. Journal of Bone and Joint Surgery UK 82A(2): 252–270

Santy JE, Butler MK, Whyman JD 1994 A comparison study of 6 types of hospital mattress to determine which most effectively reduces the incidence of pressure sores in elderly patients with hip fractures. Northern & Yorkshire Regional Health Authority, Leeds

Scales J 1982 Pressure sore prevention. Care: Science & Practice 1(2): 9–17

Scottish Health Services Council 1972 Medical rehabilitation. HMSO, Edinburgh

Scottish Intercollegiate Guideline Network (SIGN) 2002a Prevention and management of hip fracture in older people. Available online at: www.sign.ac.uk

Scottish Intercollegiate Guideline Network 2002b Prophylaxis of venous thromboembolism. Available online at: www.sign.ac.uk

Seal DV, Borriello SP 1983 Management and treatment in control of hospital-acquired infections. Update Publications, London

Slappendel R, Weber EW 1999 Non-invasive measurement of bladder volume as an indication for bladder catheterization after orthopaedic surgery and its effect on urinary tract infections. European Journal of Anaesthesiology 16(8): 503–506

Smith M 2003 A comprehensive review of risk factors related to the development of pressure ulcers. Journal of Orthopaedic Nursing 7(2): 94–102

Stamakis JD, Sagar S, Nairn D 1977 Femoral vein thrombosis and total hip replacement. British Medical Journal 2(6081): 223–225

Tarpey A, Gould D, Fox C et al 2000 Evaluating support surfaces for patients in transit through the accident and emergency department. Journal of Clinical Nursing 9: 189–198

Thompson WG 1992 Functional bowel disease and functional abdominal pain. Gastroenterology International 5: 75–91

THRiFT II 1998 Risk of and prophylaxis for venous thromboembolism in hospital patients. Phlebology 13: 87–97

Tingle JH 1997 Pressure sores: counting the legal cost of nursing neglect. British Journal of Nursing 6(13): 757–759

Torrance C 1981a The perennial pressure sore, part 3. Nursing Times 77(12): 9–12

Torrance C 1981b The perennial pressure sore, part 4. Nursing Times 77(16): 13–16

Touche Ross & Co 1993 The costs of pressure sores. Report to the Department of Health, London

Versluysen M 1986 Pressure sores in patients admitted for hip operations. Geriatric Nursing 6(2): 20–22

Wainwright H 1978 Feeding problems in elderly disabled patients. Nursing Times 74(13): 542–543

Warwick DJ, Whitehouse S 1997 Symptomatic thromboembolism after total knee replacement. Journal of Bone and Joint Surgery 78B: 780–786

Webster RA, Thompson DR 1986 Sleep in hospital. Journal of Advanced Nursing 11: 447–457

Weeks M 1999 Altered body image in a patient with an old congenital dislocated hip requiring total hip replacement surgery: a case study approach. Journal of Orthopaedic Nursing 3(3): 133–137

Woolley N 1990 Nursing diagnosis: exploring the factors which may influence the reasoning process. Journal of Advanced Nursing 15: 110–117

World Health Organisation (WHO) 1980 International classification of impairments, disabilities and handicaps. WHO, Geneva

Wright L 1990 Bathing by towel. Nursing Times 86(4): 36–39

Young T 1997 Pressure sores: incidence, risk assessment and prevention. British Journal of Nursing 6(6): 319–322

Chapter 6

Why restricting movement is important

Brian Lucas, Peter S Davis

INTRODUCTION

Orthopaedic nursing is concerned with enabling patients to maximise their mobility but there are occasions when mobility needs to be restricted for reasons of health, therapy or safety. Such restrictions may be freely chosen, such as an individual with back pain choosing to lie flat, or they are recommendations or prescription from others, usually healthcare professionals. This chapter addresses the important aspects related to restricted movement that orthopaedic nurses need to understand, namely:

- when and why restriction of movement is in the patient's best interest
- the methods by which restriction can be achieved and the nursing role in this
- the effects on the individual of restriction on movement
- why restricting movement has consequences for patients beyond the merely physical
- the legal and ethical implications of restricting movement that must be considered
- the principles of restricting movement in order to provide high-quality, safe and evidence-based care
- how nurses can, through education and support, help patients to minimise the effects of restricted movement.

IMMOBILITY

Immobility can be described as the inability to move about freely. This restriction of movement can be for physical, emotional, intellectual or social reasons; for example, psychological immobility may develop when an individual is unable to mobilise self-defence mechanisms in a stressful event.

Within orthopaedic nursing immobility is usually considered from a physical perspective, although the important psychosocial effects should not be forgotten. In nursing diagnosis terms it is described as 'impaired physical mobility' (NANDA 2001, p117) and defined as a 'limitation in independent, purposeful physical movement of the body or of one or more extremities'. The related factors include: reluctance to initiate movement, decreased muscle strength, control and/or mass and factors relating to prescribed restrictions of movement, including those due to mechanical and medical protocols.

Physical immobility can develop suddenly, as in patients who sustain a fracture in a road traffic accident, or it can develop slowly, as in a patient with rheumatoid arthritis who gradually finds it more difficult to use their hands to carry out self-care activities. In scope it can vary from immobility in unconscious patients to immobility of part of the body due to illness or a fracture.

Orthopaedic nursing is often concerned with helping to enforce the prescription of restricted movement; for example, the application of traction following a fracture or bedrest following fractured pubic rami.

RESTRICTING MOVEMENT

An individual's freedom of movement is usually restricted for either protective or therapeutic reasons; the whole or part of an individual may be affected.

PROTECTIVE AND THERAPEUTIC RESTRICTIONS

Protective restrictions prevent injury or damage from occurring and are related to aspects of safety. Generally, individuals accept imposed or recommended limitations to their movement. On a global scale this includes the use of passports to control entry and exit from countries. Nationally, countries have speed restrictions on roads in an attempt to reduce the number of accidents, together with legislation regarding such matters as the use of seatbelts. Some individuals use their own protective restrictions; for example, sports participants often use strapping, supportive braces and similar appliances to limit the movement of joints.

Therapeutic restrictions promote healing and prevent further damage or injury from occurring. The most common ones in orthopaedic care are covered in this chapter: traction, casts, bandages, splints, orthoses, internal fixation and external fixation. These restrictions are initiated by intrinsic patient choice or external prescription by healthcare professionals. This raises the issue of control and has a number of legal and ethical implications.

Intrinsic choice

Some therapeutic restrictions are chosen and controlled by the patient: an intrinsic choice. For example, a patient with rheumatoid arthritis who has developed tenosynovitis in the wrist may believe that wearing a splint provided by the nurse will help reduce the pain. However, such a restriction of movement does not exist in isolation and the patient must also consider what effects this may have on their lifestyle. Will it mean that certain activities are harder, if not impossible, to carry out? The patient makes a choice, which may not be the one the nurse believes is in the patient's best interests. Dines (1994), when talking about health education, argues that patients can be helped to make health decisions but that other factors such as environment and gender mean that choice may in fact be limited. In the case of the patient with rheumatoid arthritis, for example, if the person is a carer who needs to use their hands in household chores such as washing up and cleaning, they may feel the splint is not appropriate to wear in these situations and therefore not wear it.

Extrinsic prescription

Restrictions of movement directed and controlled by the healthcare professional are considered extrinsic. The control is outside the patient, although some control can remain with the patient if care is planned and carried out sensitively. Control can be defined as 'the individual's perception that he or she can execute (or has the potential to execute) some actions that change an aversive stimulus' (Miller et al 1989, quoted by Smith & Draper 1994, p884).

Each patient will react differently to the same control situations because of the way they interpret the situation. The literature on this subject is summarised by Smith & Draper (1994). They cite Folkman (1984) who proposes that this interpretation of the situation has two stages. The first stage is primary appraisal, when the person judges whether the event is a threat to their well-being, based on their beliefs about the controllability of the situation and their ability to influence outcomes (locus of control). A person with an internal locus of control believes that their own behaviour or attributes dictate what happens to them. Those with an external locus of control believe that luck, fate or the actions of powerful others (such as healthcare professionals) dictate what happens. In secondary appraisal the person assesses available options and coping responses, influenced by individual coping strategies and the extent to which the person believes they can behave in a way that will produce desirable results (self-efficacy).

Thus a person with an internal locus of control may not acknowledge the worth of non-weight bearing after lower limb surgery and decide that it would not be beneficial for them, whilst someone with an external locus of control may accept the medical advice and the need for it. As Williams (1997) points out, we must be aware that patients will have differing needs with regard to control; some will automatically accept external control and be happy with it whilst others will want more control themselves.

Control when movement is restricted has many facets. There is the physical restriction itself; for example, a patient on bedrest to reduce swelling in the leg following injury, who desires control, may feel that it is embarrassing to use a bedpan and would like to go out to the toilet. Those for whom the physical restriction cannot be removed (such as a cast) should be given the appropriate information so they can care for it properly and maximise their potential for independence. This links to the control of information, an example being that when practitioners communicate with each other in technical language, they exclude the patient from the discussion and from being involved in the decision-making process. Information then becomes the exclusive property of healthcare professionals and the patient loses any control they may have been able to have.

Nurses should also be aware that patients with restricted movement might express mobility behaviours in alternative ways (Ouellet & Rush 1992). In other words, those with restricted movement may use devices such as controlling behaviour and increased use of speech as substitutes for not being able to mobilise, as ways of retaining some control over their lives.

ETHICAL IMPLICATIONS OF RESTRICTING MOVEMENT

Ethics and healthcare is a complex subject and one that cannot be covered in depth here. However, orthopaedic nurses need to consider the ethical implications of restricting a person's movement through external means such as a cast, traction, surgery, external fixation or internal fixation.

One common approach to healthcare ethics (Beauchamp & Childress 1989, Gillon 1994) is using the four principles of:

- respect for autonomy
- non-maleficence (not doing harm)
- beneficence (where possible being of benefit)
- justice (considering the interests of all those affected).

Autonomy involves respect for persons and the idea that each of us has an intrinsic value and is more than an object. Taken to its logical extreme, true patient autonomy would mean that a patient could refuse treatment for a fractured limb and the health professionals would have to respect this. However, for a person to be autonomous they have to be aware of the options and be able to understand the consequences of their actions. Nurses may feel that patients will harm themselves by not agreeing to restriction of movement such as traction and that it would be to their benefit to accept this extrinsic prescription. This would link with the NMC *Code of Professional Conduct* (NMC 2002, p3) which states that a registered nurse should 'protect and support the health of individual patients and clients'. A nurse could therefore argue that persuading a patient to accept restricting treatment was in the patient's best interest and in the interests of those caring for them both in hospital and during or after treatment (the principle of justice).

Ethical decision making is not easy and orthopaedic nurses need to consider whether patients are given enough information and guidance to make a decision about accepting restrictions on their movement for therapeutic reasons. This will include knowledge about the possible harm that could arise from not having movement restricted, for example the non-union of a fracture, and from restriction, for example a plaster cast sore or nerve stretching from traction. This knowledge is vital to consent, an important component of the legal implications to restricting movement.

LEGAL IMPLICATIONS OF RESTRICTING MOVEMENT

Any mentally competent adult has, in the UK, the legal right to consent to any touching of their person; if they are touched without consent or other lawful justification, they can sue for trespass in the civil courts. Trespass can be classed as battery, where the person is actually touched, or assault where the person feels that they will be touched (Dimond 1995). This has obvious implications for patients who are subject to therapeutic restrictions of whatever type.

Consent can be expressed, in the form of writing or word of mouth, or it can be implied. For internal and external fixation, written consent is usually obtained but what if the nurse feels that the patient has not been given sufficient information about the procedure, that the consent is not 'informed consent'? Acting in the patient's best interests, the nurse should arrange for the doctor or other person who will be carrying out the procedure to give the patient more information; the person who will be carrying out the procedure should be the one obtaining consent. However, a doctor need only act in accordance with practice accepted as proper by a responsible body of medical opinion, the 'Bolam' test. In the United Kingdom this does not usually mean that full disclosure has to be given but rather that the patient is told as much as would have been accepted as proper by a body of skilled and experienced doctors (Tingle & Cribb 1995).

It is good nursing practice to seek verbal consent for procedures to be carried out on patients, which includes application of traction or casts. It could be argued that a patient implies consent by remaining a patient on the ward for treatment but it may not mean they are consenting to specific modes of treatment.

Another basic legal principle in the United Kingdom is that a mentally competent adult has the right to refuse treatment for whatever reason or for no reason at all (Cox 2001). This can lead to conflict between the professional duty of care and patient autonomy. For example, a patient may be adamant that they cannot wear a plaster cast for 6 weeks and therefore refuse one. The medical and nursing staff have no right to insist. All that can be done is to present all the available information and allow the patient to choose. This could obviously be a difficult situation and is another reason why patients need to be kept informed about the importance of their therapeutic restrictions. When we consider the patient's needs when restricting movement, education to overcome knowledge deficits is an important component of care.

METHODS OF RESTRICTING MOVEMENT

There are many ways of restricting movement for therapeutic reasons. These are usually prescribed by the doctor but are often applied, maintained, altered and removed by nurses. The orthopaedic nurse must have an in-depth understanding of the methods of restricting movement and be able to relate this to relevant nursing care. The remainder of this chapter will describe the general principles of these methods, focusing on those areas related to nursing care. Methods of restricting movement are considered with reference to:

- drawing (i.e. traction)
- casting
- bandaging and strapping
- internal fixation, the restriction of movement following bone damage
- external fixation of fractures with pins or wires placed in the bone and attached to an external bar or ring
- applying an external device – an orthosis.

As many of these methods are used following trauma to bones and joints, a brief description of the principles of trauma management in restricting the movement of damaged limbs is necessary.

PRINCIPLES OF RESTRICTING MOVEMENT AFTER TRAUMA

The principles of fracture management are:

- reduction of the fracture, to align the bone ends and allow healing to take place
- immobilisation of the fracture fragments long enough to allow union. As a rough guide this takes 6–8 weeks for a lower limb, less for an upper limb and for fractures in children
- rehabilitation of the soft tissues and joints.

Reduction and immobilisation of fractures can take place by any or a combination of methods. The choice of restriction for particular fractures depends on many factors; these are discussed in more detail in the chapters dealing with specific injuries.

Trauma does not result only in fractures; damage can also occur to other structures, such as ligaments and muscles. As with fractures, the mainstay of treatment for these injuries has often been therapeutic restriction through methods such as a cast following torn ligaments of the knee. However, it has been questioned whether restricting movement is necessarily the most appropriate way of treating trauma in all cases. Woo & Hildebrand (1997) suggest that ligament injuries in stable joints benefit from early mobilisation but in unstable joints early motion appears detrimental to healing. Kalimo et al (1997) reviewed the literature on muscle injuries in sports and concluded that active mobilisation should begin as soon as the risk of re-rupture is over (3–5 days for partial ruptures) because it induces good orientation of the regenerating muscle fibres, recapillarisation, scar resorption and restoration of strength. Therapeutic restriction of movement may not always be in the patient's best interests; each case should be judged on its own merits based on the available evidence.

NURSING DIAGNOSES AND CARE: PATIENTS WITH RESTRICTED MOVEMENT

Although there are varying methods of restricting movement, common patient care needs can be identified (the nursing diagnoses) and plans of care should be devised with the patient to ensure their needs can be met. This section will outline the most common nursing diagnoses related to restricting movement; specific application will then be made to particular methods of restriction. The nursing diagnoses are adapted from the North American Nursing Diagnosis Association (NANDA 2001) definitions and classification.

Knowledge deficit

Patients may not be familiar with many aspects of care related to restricting movement. Care can be divided into three aspects or stages.

1 What happens when the restriction is applied, for example before a cast is applied, before a patient goes to theatre for internal fixation or prior to application of external fixation.
2 The care required for restriction methods in place for a specified period of time.
3 Rehabilitation and adaptation to a potentially changed level of mobility.

The goal of care in all these instances is for the patient to indicate that they have sufficient knowledge to cope with the situation, to be able to repeat facts or reproduce behavioural actions related to the information provided. For example, a patient with external fixation for malunion of a fracture needs to be able to explain why pin-site care is important and to demonstrate the practical skills of care prior to discharge.

Nursing interventions. The nursing actions to achieve this goal can be varied; there is a great deal of research on information giving and the effect it has on patient behaviours. Some factors to consider are as follows.

● **Patient information**: information for patients is important for a variety of reasons as outlined by Gammon & Mulholland (1996). There is an increasing emphasis on self-care, patients wish to take more control over their healthcare and treatment, the average stay in hospital is shorter and government policies such as The NHS plan (DoH 2000) mean that patients have an expectation that they will be informed about their care. Research has also demonstrated many psychological and physical benefits (Gammon & Mulholland 1996).
● **The timing of information giving**: research has not yet established the most appropriate time to begin patient education. Levesque et al (1984) suggested that timing of preoperative education did not have an effect on anxiety, ventilatory function, well-being, pain or length of hospitalisation. Mavrais et al (1990) also found there was little difference between patients prepared the day before surgery as opposed to 2 weeks before, in terms of variables such as anxiety and length of stay.

Some studies have looked at when patients themselves prefer to receive information. Schoessler (1989) found that patients preferred to receive education in the short time between admission and surgery, although it is acknowledged that this may be because patients were unaware of the complexity of preoperative education and therefore the time required. In this study the patients were asked to fill in the questionnaire the morning after surgery when they may not have been in a position to adequately assess their preference for the timing of information giving. Wallace (1985) found that over two-thirds of her sample of 131 gynaecology patients preferred to receive preparation 6–8 weeks prior to hospital admission. None of this research is specifically orthopaedic related although this is no reason to suppose that patients undergoing orthopaedic surgery will have strikingly different needs or views.

Gammon & Mulholland's study (1996) involved patients undergoing total hip replacement (THR). They found that those given patient teaching and preparatory information the day before surgery, plus teaching before discharge, were significantly less anxious and depressed than those who received advice and support that would 'normally' be given to THR patients by ward staff, which is said to be often minimal and sometimes non-existent. The normal level of teaching is not made more explicit, making comparisons between the groups difficult. The study does not examine if preparation before the evening of surgery would have resulted in an even more significant reduction in patient anxiety and depression. Shuldham (1999) concludes from a review of the literature that the appropriate timing of education remains unclear.

- **The content of information given**: McDonnell (1999) concluded from a systematic review of the effectiveness of preparatory information that there is insufficient research to assess the impact on post-procedural outcomes. However, her review only included studies that used preparatory information alone and not those where personal teaching and/or psychosocial elements were also used. Devine (1992) undertook a metaanalysis of psychoeducational care (defined as relevant healthcare information, the teaching of exercises and psychosocial support) and found beneficial effects on recovery, pain experienced, psychological distress and length of hospital stay.

- **The format of information**: Mitchell (2000) outlines a variety of formats for giving information including written, video and oral. Mitchell argues that each patient should be assessed to determine the most appropriate method(s) to be used. Arthur (1995) reviewed the literature on written patient information and found that few studies have evaluated its effectiveness.

- **Patient reactions**: nurses know intuitively that patients are individuals and some will desire to know everything about their forthcoming experience whilst others will be happy for the doctors to do what they think best. This is of course linked with locus of control; those with an external locus of control may not feel that knowing about a procedure to restrict movement will necessarily help them to cope with it. The nurse may not have the option to choose when a patient receives information; for example, a trauma patient going to theatre for internal fixation

will have only a limited amount of time for receiving information preoperatively. For others, more time is available and it is important for informed consent that the patient receives the information they need. This includes information for patients when they are discharged from regular care, for example a patient leaving the ward or clinic with a plaster cast in situ.

Self–care deficit

Restricting movement may impose self-care deficits for the patient with regard to toileting, bathing, dressing, preparing and eating food. The goal of care is to help patients to make up this deficit, by educating them how to do it themselves, providing help, for example by teaching a family member to help the patient, or arranging for help to be provided, for example meals on wheels on discharge. Depending on the type of restriction imposed on the patient, the degree of self-care deficit will vary; for example, a patient on traction will not be able to prepare their food or wash without assistance, while a patient in a below-knee cast may have fewer self-care deficits.

Nursing interventions.   Nursing actions will include:

- a thorough assessment of the patient to determine what self-care activities they want and need to carry out
- education on practical matters such as choosing appropriate clothing
- advice on help available.

Risk of disuse syndrome

A patient is at risk of deterioration of body systems as the result of therapeutic restrictions. This deterioration might be systemic, with restrictions such as traction leading to the risk of pressure ulcers, constipation and urinary tract infection, or more localised, with restrictions imposed by a cast or orthosis causing muscle atrophy and joint stiffness.

The goals of care are to reduce the risk of these arising, with continued monitoring and observation of the patient enabling the early detection of any problems. The nursing interventions will depend on the potential or actual problems that arise.

Risk of peripheral neurovascular dysfunction

Restricting movement, whether through internal fixation, a cast, external fixation or bandaging, may, through increased pressure, cause temporary or permanent damage to nerves and blood vessels.

Table 6.1 Assessment of sensation and motor function

Nerve	Assessment of sensation	Assessment of motor function
Peroneal	Touch the web space between the great and second toe	Ask the patient to dorsiflex their ankle and extend the toes at the metatarsal and phalangeal joints
Tibial	Touch the medial and lateral surfaces of the sole of the foot	Ask the patient to plantar flex their ankle and toes
Radial	Touch the web space between the thumb and index finger	Ask the patient to hyperextend their thumb, the wrist, and the four fingers at the metacarpophalangeal joints
Ulnar	Touch the distal fat pad of the small finger	Ask the patient to abduct all their fingers
Median	Touch the distal surface of the index finger	Ask the patient to oppose the thumb and small fingers and note whether they can flex the wrist at the joint

A particular risk is compartment syndrome, increased pressure within a limited anatomic space, which leads to compromised circulation and function of tissues within that space. Compartments within the body are areas where muscle, nerve and blood vessels are confined within inelastic boundaries composed of skin, fascia and/or bone. It is the compartments within the extremities that are particularly prone to compartment syndrome. Fractures are the most common risk factor for compartment syndrome but therapeutic restrictions to treat these fractures such as casts, splints and traction may also increase compartmental pressure. The pressure is relieved by a fasciotomy which involves an incision through the overlying skin and subcutaneous tissues into the fascia, allowing the swollen muscle to bulge out. Without this, ischaemia and necrosis of muscles, nerves and other tissues can result. In cases where compartment syndrome is not treated, the result can be a severely contracted and functionally useless distal extremity.

Nursing interventions. The goal of care is to reduce the risk of neurovascular dysfunction occurring and to detect early signs of development.

Neurovascular observations Not all blood vessels or nerves supplying a particular hand or foot may be affected by constriction; therefore each digit must be checked separately for any neurovascular deficit. This should be carried out and recorded, at least 2–4 hourly post-trauma or after restriction has been applied. It is important that the limb being observed is compared with the opposite limb, to ensure that what is the norm for the particular patient is known. The following observations should be carried out.

● **Colour and warmth**: is the extremity pale and cold below the fracture or restriction, indicating arterial insufficiency? Warmth with a bluish tinge could indicate venous stasis. Capillary refill can be checked by pressing the nailbed; return to its original colour should occur within 3–5 seconds.

● **Sensation**: the patient should be asked to report any changes in sensation such as reduced sensation, hypersensation, tingling, numbness or loss of sensation. Assessment should ensure that all areas of the extremity are checked so the functions of each nerve serving the limb are recorded (Table 6.1).

● **Movement**: knowledge of the nerves supplying the extremity being observed is necessary so the nurse can accurately assess and test appropriate movements (Table 6.1).

Compartment syndrome For suspected compartment syndrome pain is the most common and important presenting symptom; it is caused by muscle ischaemia and necrosis. The patient describes pain out of proportion to the magnitude of the injury or restriction, which is poorly localised, not relieved by analgesia and can be elicited on passive movements such as extending the fingers or toes. These signs do not usually occur until neurovascular damage is well advanced and they can be difficult to elicit in unconscious or uncooperative patients. Compartment monitoring is a much more effective method of early detection.

Compartment monitoring Normal compartment pressure ranges from 0 to 20 mmHg (Good 1992). Pressure within a compartment can be measured using a transcutaneous Doppler or ultrasound or percutaneously using a wick or slit catheter. These devices provide an instantaneous report on the local compartmental pressure (Love 1998).

Recommended thresholds for decompression by fasciotomy vary from 30 to 45 mmHg. McQueen & Court-Brown (1996) suggest, however, that using absolute measures may lead to an unnecessary fasciotomy in patients with tibial diaphyseal fractures and that using differential pressure monitoring reduces the number of unnecessary fasciotomies and does not lead to any missed cases of acute compartment syndrome. Differential pressure is diastolic blood pressure minus compartment pressure; McQueen & Court-Brown conclude that only patients with a differential pressure of 30 mmHg or less require a fasciotomy.

Reducing the risks In addition to monitoring, nurses can reduce the risk of neurovascular deficit occurring. In many instances this can be achieved by careful application of the therapeutic restriction, for example by following the principles of cast application to reduce the risk of increased pressure on the limb.

The use of the four RICE measures (rest, ice, compression and elevation) to reduce swelling in an injured limb is beneficial particularly where there is intramuscular haemorrhage. However, if compartment syndrome is suspected, ice, compression and elevation above heart level must be stopped immediately as there is research evidence to suggest that they can exacerbate the condition by further impairing oxygenation of muscle tissue through reducing local arterial blood flow (Love 1998).

Deep vein thrombosis Peripheral neurovascular dysfunction can also lead to the formation of a thrombus in the deep veins of a patient whose ability to walk has been restricted.

Altered body image (body image disturbance)

Body image can be defined as the way people see themselves and how they think others see them (Salter 1997). Price (1995) has developed a model of body image, which suggests that normal body image is maintained by the person's coping strategies and social support network. A person who adapts well to change and who has a good social support network will maintain their body image when changes occur due to trauma or ageing. Their body ideal, for example norms of appearance, is influenced by society and cultural norms, while body presentation is influenced by the way the body is presented to the outside world such as how a person dresses or their limitations of movement or dexterity.

Price (1995) therefore characterises altered body image as a state of personal distress, indicating that the body no longer supports self-esteem and that coping strategies are overwhelmed by injury, disease, disability or social stigma. This personal distress leads to limited social engagement with others. Price suggests that using this definition enables

nurses to assess patients more effectively because it removes the assumption that a particular body change will necessarily cause altered body image; the threats, responses and coping mechanisms the individual demonstrates are the key factors in altered body image.

For patients undergoing therapeutic restriction of all or part of their body, altered body image may or may not be an issue; they should be assessed as individuals. The environment has additional factors that affect the patient. Limb (M Limb, unpublished work, 1998) found that patients with external fixators were less concerned about appearance whilst an inpatient in an environment where other patients were having the same or similar treatment than when they were discharged with the external fixator and were exposed to the gaze and curiosity of other people.

Price (1995) suggests some assessment steps for identifying altered body image.

- A preliminary assessment when potential body image threats are known, such as deformity and rheumatoid arthritis or the application of external fixators or casts.
- Assessment of normal body image, the usual coping style and social support.
- Assessment of body image constructs now and in the future.
- Assessment and care are inseparable; questioning patients may have a therapeutic or non-therapeutic impact.

The goal of care for altered body image will usually be formulated in terms of what the patient expresses about their feelings, mood or confidence (Price 1990). It is helpful if the diagnosis specifies which of the five body image components (body reality, body ideal, body presentation, coping strategies and social support network) are affected. For example, a patient may have a change in body reality following a fractured tibia which requires external fixation, the external fixator may then affect the body ideal and the patient may feel that they have lost control over part of their body, the affected lower limb (requiring new coping strategies). In this instance the goal of care may be that in 7 days the patient will state that he is able to care for the external fixator and demonstrate this care, thus indicating that he has accepted the altered body image. Davis (1997) discusses this in relation to spinal cord injuries but the issue is relevant to other injuries and therapeutic restrictions. The psychosocial aspects of the injury or restriction may not be of paramount importance to the patient in the immediate postinjury period but take on increasing priority during rehabilitation.

Nursing interventions.   These will depend on the assessment and nursing diagnosis. They may include some or all of the following.

- **Communication**: the nurse should endeavour to be open and honest with the patient, making it easier for the patient to talk about any body image changes they are uncomfortable with.
- **Independence**: maintaining and developing the patient's independence ensures the patient's coping strategies are strengthened. This could include educating the patient in the physical care of, for example, an external fixator or in how to maintain self-care whilst in a cast.
- **Support**: involving the patient in a social support network, with their consent, during rehabilitation can be beneficial, especially when body image changes may be long-lasting, for example, when an external fixator will be in place for 18 months to 2 years or there are prominent surgical scars following internal fixation. This can involve a formal support group or the opportunity for the patient to meet someone who has had a similar experience. For example, a patient about to have an external fixator for non-union of a fracture may find it beneficial to talk with someone who has already had, or is in the middle of, this treatment.
- **Counselling**: provide access to more formal counselling if necessary.

TYPES OF THERAPEUTIC RESTRICTION

TRACTION

Orthopaedic traction occurs when a pulling force is applied to a part or parts of the body. Countertraction, that is, traction in the opposite direction, is also necessary. Hippocrates, in 350 BC, when describing the use of traction in the reduction of a fractured leg, gave the example of two strong men pulling in opposite directions: the pull in one direction was traction and that in the opposite direction, countertraction. Countertraction is usually provided by the patient's body weight within orthopaedic practice.

Traction can be used to:

- reduce and maintain fractures
- control movement of an injured part of the body, thus facilitating bone healing
- lessen the muscle spasm that occurs following fractures and dislocations

- prevent or correct deformity, for example a flexion deformity that may occur following inflammation of the hip joint due to infection
- prevent or correct soft tissue contracture that would reduce the range of movement in the joint
- prevent contraction of healing soft tissues following joint surgery
- rest diseased or injured joints, such as in tuberculosis, thus minimising pain and facilitating initial healing.

Traction is used less often within orthopaedic nursing than in the past, particularly following trauma, and as a result many skills in applying it have been lost. Alternative methods, particularly internal fixation, have become more widespread as a result of technical developments and their perceived benefits, particularly in reducing the amount of time patients have to remain in bed post injury. The use of traction for pain relief has been challenged and found not to be as effective as previously imagined, for example for patients with a fractured neck of femur (Draper & Scott 1998). Parker & Handoll's (2001) systematic review of preoperative traction for fractures of the proximal femur found no research evidence that conclusively demonstrates the benefit of traction for the outcome measures of pain relief or ease of fracture reduction at the time of surgery. Kahle et al (1990) suggest that prior to treatment of developmental dysplasia of the hip (DDH) by open or closed reduction, the routine use of skin traction, which aims to stretch the contracted soft tissues around the hip and decrease the pressure on the reduced femoral head, does not reduce the incidence of osteonecrosis of the femoral head.

There are occasions when traction is required and for these, orthopaedic nurses need to have a basic understanding of the principles of traction and the ability to apply the most common types, particularly straight leg traction, Hamilton-Russell traction and a Thomas splint.

METHODS OF APPLYING TRACTION

To apply traction a satisfactory grip must be obtained on a part of the patient's body through the skin or bone, for short or long periods of time.

Manual traction

This is applied by the hands, for example when a doctor reduces a fracture or holds an alignment

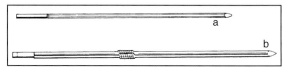

Figure 6.1   Pins for skeletal traction. (a) Steinmann pin; (b) Denham pin. (From Dandy & Edwards 1998.)

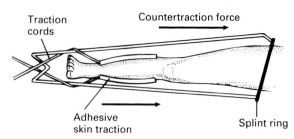

Figure 6.2   Fixed traction using a Thomas splint.

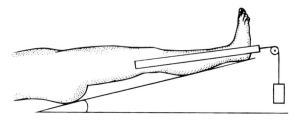

Figure 6.3   Sliding traction using skin traction and weights.

whilst a cast or more permanent form of traction is being applied.

Skin traction

The application of a traction force over a large area of skin, which is transmitted via the soft tissues to the bone. The maximum pull should not exceed that recommended by the manufacturers of the traction appliance, usually 10–15 lb (4.5–6.7 kg). Skin traction can be adhesive or non-adhesive. The adhesive type is not recommended for patients with friable or damaged skin, as removal of the adhesive strips may cause further damage. Non-adhesive types are preferred if the traction has to be on for only a short period of time.

Skeletal traction

Here the traction force is applied directly to a bone, commonly through metal pins or wires. Two types of pin are used.

1   The Steinmann pin, which has a trocar point and smooth sides (Fig. 6.1a).
2   Threaded pins, such as the Denham pin, which have threads standing proud of the pin shaft (Fig. 6.1b).

Threaded pins are particularly useful for soft cancellous bone such as the calcaneum. Sites for insertion of skeletal pins include the proximal end of the tibia, the calcaneum, the distal femur, the skull or the olecranon. Skeletal traction is preferred if the traction is to be maintained for a long time or when more pull is required, as a greater weight can be applied.

Countertraction

With any traction, the whole body is pulled in the direction of the traction force if countertraction is not present. Countertraction is achieved in two ways.

1   Fixed traction is the application of countertraction acting through an appliance, which obtains purchase on a part of the body. To apply a force against a fixed point on the body, an appliance such as a Thomas splint is used. The ring of the splint snugly encircles the root of the limb, i.e. the groin and hip. Traction cords are tied to the distal end of the splints and the countertraction force passes along the sidebars of the splint to the ring, as indicated on Figure 6.2 by the arrows. The grip on the leg is achieved by adhesive skin traction.

2   Sliding or balanced traction relies on the patient's own body weight to produce the necessary countertraction (Nichol 1995). For instance, the bed is tilted so that the patient tends to 'slide' or move in the opposite direction to that of the traction force (Fig. 6.3). The pull of gravity should equal that of the traction so the two are 'balanced' and the patient remains stationary. The traction force is produced by weights and may be applied through a cord passing over a pulley.

Suspension is not traction, as no countertraction is necessary. It occurs when part or all of the body is suspended to increase the mobility of the patient. It may be used on its own or as part of a traction and suspension system. It is sometimes confused with traction as the same types of equipment are used and both may be carried out at the same time as part of the patient's treatment.

COMMON TYPES OF TRACTION

Straight–leg traction

Also known as Pugh's traction, this method allows the traction cord to be fixed by tying it to, for example, the end of the Thomas splint or used as sliding

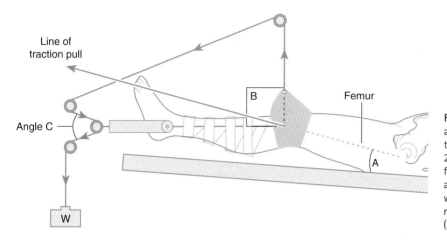

Figure 6.4 Recommended angles and forces for Hamilton–Russell traction. When the bed is elevated 25 cm, angle A is 20° of hip flexion from the horizontal, angle B is 90°, angle C is 40°, combined with a weight (W) of 2.3 kg (5 lb), the resultant force on the leg is 4.8 kg. (From Draper & Scott 1996.)

traction using a pulley and weights (Fig. 6.3). It is used as a temporary measure for fractured neck of femur injuries, to rest the hip or relieve pain or muscle spasm (Heywood Jones 1990); however, its efficacy has been questioned.

Hamilton–Russell traction

This has traditionally been used for fractures of the neck and the shaft of femur. The arrangement of the foot pulleys multiplies the traction force by 100%; for example, 5 kg of weights applied would lead to 10 kg of traction force along the line of the femur. This is generally believed to be useful both in maintaining the position of femoral fractures and in relieving the pain of muscle spasm in the quadriceps, although the latter is now disputed. Draper & Scott (1996) suggest that more attention needs to be paid to the direction and size of the theoretical force if Hamilton-Russell traction is to be effective in maintaining the pulling force along the line of the femur (Fig. 6.4). They admit, however, that for short-term traction this may not be so crucial but if alignment of the bony fragments to promote healing is the aim, then incorrect alignment can lead to angulation at the fracture site along with deformity.

Draper & Scott (1998) found there was no increased incidence of pressure ulcers for patients with Hamilton-Russell traction; in fact, there was less susceptibility to pressure ulcers on the heel of the uninjured leg, possibly because, when patients attempt to sit up the traction supports the injured leg, making it easier for patients to move in bed without causing friction from the heel slipping against the sheets.

Thomas splint for fixed traction

This is less commonly used now in the care of adult patients, except for restricting the movement of a femoral shaft when transferring a patient, between hospitals for example (Fig. 6.2). In paediatric orthopaedics the Thomas splint is still used in the treatment of fractures of the shaft of femur; its use in this context is discussed further in Chapter 13.

SETTING UP AND MANAGEMENT OF THE TRACTION SYSTEM

Whilst the exact nature of the traction may differ, the principles of maintaining the traction system are similar. For more detailed information on the safe and effective use of traction and patient care, readers are referred to *A traction manual* (RCN/SOTN 2002).

- The weights used must be known and recorded in the nursing documentation.
- The traction system should be thoroughly checked at least once every shift (6–8 hours) and always after interventions such as moving a patient, physiotherapy and radiographic examination, as the system may be inadvertently altered.
- The cords must be attached securely by standard knots that will not move or come undone, for example a clove hitch or two half-hitches (Figs 6.5–6.8).
- The ends of the cords should be short (5 cm) and bound back onto themselves with adhesive tape to prevent fraying of the cord end and possible slipping and accidental disruption of traction. The knot itself should not be covered.

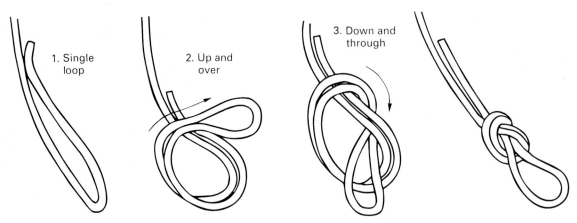

Figure 6.5 Overhand loop knot for attaching weights.

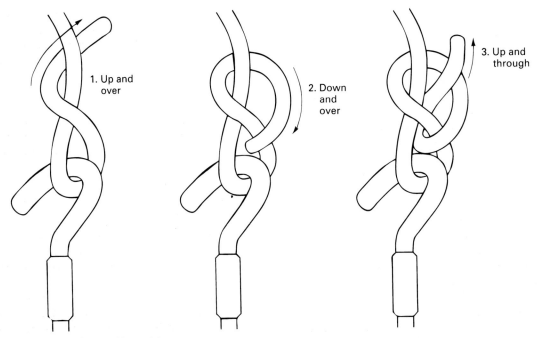

Figure 6.6 Slip knot for attaching weights.

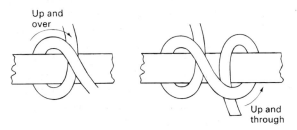

Figure 6.7 Clove hitch for attaching to an appliance such as a Thomas splint.

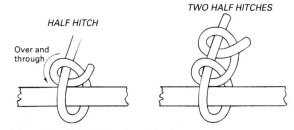

Figure 6.8 Half hitches for reinforcing.

- Short cords should not be joined by knots; these would stop the cord running freely through pulleys and if incorrectly tied, would slip and come undone.
- Cords should be checked daily for fraying, particularly where they pass over pulleys, or for rubbing against each other. If these occur the system's efficiency is reduced or the cord may break.
- The line of pull of the cords should be correct and regularly checked. This ensures the appropriate pulling force is applied for optimal therapeutic effect at all times.
- Pulleys must be free-running and oiled as necessary to prevent squeaking. Friction is then minimised, efficiency maintained and the patient is not disturbed by the noise. The majority of pulleys now have plastic components requiring minimal maintenance.
- The cords must rest comfortably in the pulley, one cord to each pulley wheel. This reduces friction and fraying of the cord.
- The weights must hang free and not rest on the floor; otherwise the efficiency of the system is not maintained.
- To minimise discomfort for the patient, the weights should not catch or jam, particularly on the bed ends when the patient moves.
- Weights should not be hung over the patient. If this is necessary, an extra safety cord must be used.
- Weights should be securely attached by a fishhook (S-hook) where available. This aids safe but easy removal of the weights if necessary, for example during physiotherapy.
- Pointed ends of pins or wires, used in skeletal traction, should be covered to prevent injury to the patient and staff.
- The patient should be on a firm-based bed to give full support and comfort and which will allow efficient action of the traction system.
- Bed aids, such as cradles, should be used to keep bedclothes away from the patient, for comfort and to ensure free running of the traction cords.
- Countertraction, if required, should be applied at all times.

NURSING DIAGNOSES AND CARE: TRACTION

Risk of impaired skin integrity

As well as the general risk of pressure ulcers developing due to reduced mobility, patients on traction are at risk from the traction system itself, for example the area in contact with the ring of the Thomas splint and the skin underneath skin traction.

Nursing interventions.   The goal of care is for the skin to remain intact.

- With a Thomas splint, a separate cord can be tied to the distal end of the splint and a weight attached to this cord, to relieve the pressure on the ischial tuberosity of the pelvis (Nichol 1995).
- If using adhesive skin traction, consider the use of skin protection such as a semipermeable film dressing to which the adhesive can stick, rather than to the skin.
- Ensure bony prominences are protected, such as the head of fibula and malleoli, with the use of a semipermeable film dressing or protective wool. If used, ensure these do not slip and cause additional pressure.
- Skin covered by the traction system should be assessed daily for signs of dryness or allergic reaction. This ensures the early detection of, for instance, patients who have an allergy to the adhesives in adhesive skin traction.

Risk of infection

A patient with skeletal traction is at risk of infection because the skeletal pins have broken the skin's integrity.

Nursing interventions.   The goals of care are to reduce the risk of infection and the early detection of a developing infection.

- Inspection for looseness of the pins or wires and signs of infection at the sites of insertion of skeletal traction should be performed at least daily. Infection at the site of insertion may be indicated by a purulent discharge, redness or inflammation. An infection can easily spread to the bone itself, leading to osteomyelitis (Ward 1998). Infections can be graded using a classification system; this also aids audit of the effectiveness of pin-site care protocols (Sims et al 2000).
- Reducing the risk of infection at pin-sites is a controversial topic and there is no overwhelming evidence on which to base practice. Until large-scale, multicentre randomised controlled trials are undertaken, only a range of treatment options and their rationale can be offered. However, a consensus conference has produced best practice guidelines based on the available literature and expert opinion (Lee-Smith et al 2001).
- Identification of risk factors will include poor nutritional status, smoking, poor patient

understanding of pin-site care regimes, pins being sited too close to joints and loosening or motion between the pin and the surrounding tissues.

● Cleaning of pin-site entry sites: a number of solutions have been suggested for cleaning the pin-site wound, including alcohol, hydrogen peroxide and povidone-iodine (Rowe 1997). However, the potentially damaging effects of these on healthy skin should be considered. Normal saline is not harmful and may therefore be used safely. Pin-sites should be cleaned once daily but only if there is exudate present (Lee-Smith et al 2001).

● Removal of pin-site crust should be encouraged as it allows visualisation of the wound and free drainage of the exudate (Lee-Smith et al 2001).

● Covering pin-sites: gauze is a common dressing used to cover pin-sites (Mandzuk 1991), although it has been suggested that woven gauze is preferable to non-woven gauze because the fibres are less likely to lodge in the pin-tract. If there is no exudate the pin-sites may be left exposed.

BANDAGING AND STRAPPING

The term 'bandaging' will be used to refer to the application of extensible bandages for the purpose of compression or support of an injury, to prevent oedema or to keep dressings in place. The term 'strapping' will be used to refer to the application of non-extensible strapping for the purpose of support and protection of an injury, to retain dressings in place and to hold lacerated skin edges together.

Bandaging is now used less within orthopaedic nursing but orthopaedic nurses need to understand the principles of bandaging and how to choose the correct bandage.

Strapping is used widely in the prevention and treatment of sports injuries.

USES OF BANDAGING

Compression to either control or prevent oedema is a common reason for bandaging in orthopaedic care. For example, a stump bandage applied after amputation will control oedema, while a Robert Jones bandage applied immediately after surgery or injury to the knee will prevent oedema (Brodell et al 1986). Whatever the reason for bandaging, it must be remembered that, if applied incorrectly or inappropriately, bandages can easily and quickly cause further injury to the patient. By understanding

and putting into practice the basic principles of application and care, the nurse is able to minimise risks to the patient and promote rapid healing and recovery.

TENSION AND PRESSURE

Love (2000) points out that correct bandaging involves the application of three concepts, namely magnitude of pressure, distribution and duration of pressure and the application of Laplace's Law.

The magnitude of pressure refers to the subbandage pressure measured at the skin–bandage interface in mmHg. The desired subbandage pressure is usually achieved by stretching the bandage one-third of its resting length and by using a 50% overlap at each turn (Love 2000). The resulting subbandage pressure will depend on the extensibility of the bandage, ranging from 5–8 mmHg for a dressing retention bandage to 25–35 mmHg for a high compression bandage. Distribution of pressure is safely achieved through the application of Laplace's Law (Love 2000). This states that:

$$P = (N \times T) \div (W \times C)$$

where
P = subbandage pressure
N = number of layers. A complete overlap doubles the subbandage pressure. Expected subbandage pressures are calculated according to a 50% overlap
T = tension. Correct tension is achieved in an extensible bandage by stretching it one-third of the resting length
W = bandage width. Narrow bandages produce a higher subbandage pressure than wide bandages
C = limb circumference. Wider limbs produce a lower subbandage pressure.

Duration of pressure refers to the length of time the appropriate subbandage pressure is achieved. All bandages tend to lose their tension over a period of time from application. This 'relaxation' can be as much as 50% in less than 20 minutes from application but again there is marked variation in the rate of relaxation of different bandage types (Thomas et al 1980).

The nurse should always read the manufacturer's instructions when gauging tension to find out how much the bandage should be stretched in application. Stretching a bandage can be practised by unrolling about 2 m of new bandage and marking it with a pen across its width at 15 cm intervals.

Low pressure	Moderate pressure	High compression
5–20 mmHg	20–35 mmHg	35–50 mmHg
Dressing fingers	Shoulder spica	Joint injuries involving damage to either muscles or ligaments
Limb dressing retention	Minor sprains and strains	
Securing backslabs in acute injuries	Control of oedema	Major sprains or soft tissue injuries
	Specialty dressing, e.g. splinting	Minor fractures
	Robert Jones bandaging	Amputation stumps
		Tenosynovitis
		Corrective bandaging, e.g. club foot

Figure 6.9 Bandage types and possible uses.

The bandage is then applied and the distance measured between the marks. If, for example, the distance between the marks is now 20 cm the bandage has been stretched by a third, the desired amount. Uniformity of the increased intervals will indicate that the tension has been applied evenly.

TYPES OF BANDAGE

The choice of bandage type will depend on how and for what it is being used. The required amount of pressure or compression is a key factor in its selection (Fig. 6.9). Moderate pressure will improve or increase circulation, thus aiding healing. High compression is most frequently used to prevent oedema and increase venous return but may also be useful in protecting injured areas and preventing injury by limiting joint movements.

Common types of bandage are listed below in order of their potential to apply increasing pressure.

Conforming bandages

These are used primarily for dressing retention (Orford 1989). They tend to be light, absorbent and have a two-way stretch. Common types are cotton BPC and equivalents made from viscose or rayon.

Tubular bandages

Tubular bandages have a wide variety of uses and are popular because of their ease of application (Love 1989). The simple sizing charts enable the user to select the size of dressing most appropriate to the patient's needs with a choice of high, medium or low pressure on application. Thomas et al (1980)

recommend Tubigrip-type bandages in situations where low to moderate pressures are desirable.

Lightweight stretch bandages

These are probably the most widely used type of bandage (Love 1989). They may be employed to achieve a moderate pressure. There are two main types: those with twisted cotton, wool or rayon threads, for example crepe bandages, and those containing elastomer, such as Lycra or rubber.

Heavy compression bandages

These bandages contain varying amounts of elastomeric thread. They are used to apply moderate to high compression over long periods for support and the prevention of oedema. They are usually removed at night.

BANDAGING TECHNIQUES

There are many ways to bandage and the choice of technique will depend on the purpose, the area of the body to be bandaged and personal preference. Some techniques may be quite complex. As yet, little research has been carried out on the effectiveness of bandaging in specific situations, which makes it difficult for the nurse to decide whether or not to bandage and which techniques or type of bandage to use.

There are three basic turns that can be used when bandaging (Fig. 6.10).

1 A circular turn to anchor a bandage.
2 A spiral turn used to bandage a long straight part of the body or a part of the body of increasing circumference.

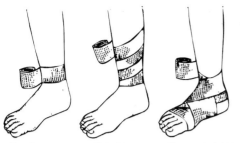

| Circular turn | Spiral turn | Figure of eight turn |

Figure 6.10   Basic bandaging turns.

3   A figure-of-eight turn to bandage a part of the body of increasing or decreasing circumference.

Dale et al (1983) found the figure-of-eight technique appeared to give a better graduated pressure than a simple spiral when applied above the ankle for moderate-pressure bandaging.

General principles of bandaging

The following principles should be remembered when bandaging.

- A bandage of appropriate type, width and length should be chosen. Where possible, new bandages should be used as elastic bandages in particular lose their elasticity after use or washing.
- Seek assistance if the part of the body affected needs to be supported during the bandaging process.
- Bandage the part of the body in the position you want it maintained.
- Secure the ends of the bandage, ensuring that the patient cannot injure themselves. If the bandage is likely to slip, secure it with extra strapping across all the turns.
- Record the details of the bandaging in the patient's documentation.

USE OF STRAPPING

Strapping is used to (Austin et al 1994):

- support an injured structure
- limit harmful movements
- allow pain-free functional movement
- allow early resumption of activities.

For examples of common strapping techniques, see Austin et al (1994).

TYPES OF STRAPPING

There are two common types of strapping.

Elastic cohesive strapping

These possess a limited amount of elasticity and stick only to themselves and not to skin or hair (Jamieson 1989). They are an alternative to adhesive strapping as they do not cause allergic reactions or skin trauma on removal. They should be used for contractile tissue injuries of muscles and tendons because they give strength, support and a graduated resistance, yet limit the full stretch of the muscle or tendon (Austin et al 1994).

Adhesive strapping

These are coated on one side with an adhesive (Jamieson 1989) but possess little elasticity. Skin preparation is usually necessary prior to application or the bandage may be applied over stockinette, a semipermeable membrane dressing such as Opsite or a conforming bandage. They should be used to support injuries of non-contractile structures such as ligaments.

General principles of strapping

The nurse should follow these guidelines when carrying out strapping.

- Select strapping of appropriate type and width. The more irregular the surface and the more acute the angles, the narrower the strapping should be. For example, for hands use 1.25–2.5 cm strapping and for ankles use 3.72–5 cm strapping.
- Ensure that the patient's skin is clean and dry.
- If adhesive strapping is applied directly to the skin, remove hair from the affected part to prevent discomfort on removal of the strapping.
- Strap the affected part of the body in the position required for support.
- Avoid encircling turns if possible, as further swelling may occur.
- Check that overlap strapping has not separated during activity and damaged the skin trapped between the edges.
- Inspect the skin carefully each time the strapping is removed.
- Record the details of the strapping in the patient's documentation.

NURSING DIAGNOSES AND CARE: BANDAGES AND STRAPPING

Knowledge deficit

The aim of care is for the patient to articulate their understanding of why bandaging or strapping is necessary and the implications for their life.

Nursing interventions. Patients and carers may need education in the reapplying of bandages or strapping if they become loose and in the importance of neurovascular observations, including the actions to take if the limb becomes swollen.

Risk of peripheral neurovascular dysfunction

The goal of care is to prevent neurovascular damage occurring and the early detection of any changes.

Nursing interventions. In addition to general principles of care for potential neurovascular deficit, the following should be considered.

- If possible, apply the bandage or strapping in the direction of venous blood return to prevent blood pooling.
- Keep an even tension on the bandage or strap. Ensuring the unrolled part of the bandage is kept close to the body surface helps this. If strapping is used, consider using strips rather than encircling a limb to reduce the risk of neurovascular impairment.
- Ensure that overlaps of the bandage are even with no creases or wrinkles that may become a focus for increased pressure.
- Be sure to bandage or strap the body part above and below the affected area but leave the fingers or toes exposed for neurovascular observations to be performed.
- Only use the length of bandage or strapping needed. Cut if necessary rather than applying extra turns as a double layer may increase pressure.
- Bandage from smaller to larger circumferences for closer shaping of the bandage to the affected body part.

Risk of impaired skin integrity

The patient may be at risk of skin damage from the bandage or strapping due to increased pressure.

Nursing interventions

- Ensure that the patient's skin is clean and dry before applying the bandage or strapping, as moisture predisposes the skin to breakdown.

- Cover any wounds before bandaging or strapping the injured area.
- If appropriate, add padding to areas at risk of pressure.
- The skin beneath the bandage or strapping should be inspected carefully each time it is removed for signs of damage due to pressure. Ulcers can occur very rapidly if the bandage or strapping is too tight.
- Ensure that the skin is washed each time the bandage or strapping is removed.

CASTING AND PLASTER CASTS

Casting in many different materials has been used to immobilise fractured limbs due to injury for centuries. Hippocrates in about 350 BC used cloth stiffened by waxes and resins to immobilise fractures. In the 16th century, Cheselden, an English surgeon, used bandages soaked in egg white and flour to form a cast. Matthysen, a Dutch military surgeon, was the first to record the use of plaster of Paris bandages in 1852. The bandages were made by rubbing dry plaster of Paris into coarsely woven cotton bandages; these were then soaked in water before application. It is only in the recent past that a range of materials with different properties to suit specific purposes has been developed and produced commercially.

The decision to apply a cast is a medical one but nurses are involved in their application. Fitting a cast is a highly skilled task and should not be undertaken lightly as a poor cast rapidly causes temporary or permanent injury to the patient. The orthopaedic nurse should understand the principles of casting and be able to:

- recognise good and bad casts
- identify and prevent potential problems
- act swiftly and appropriately if problems do occur, including safely removing a cast
- educate the patient in living with a cast, including what problems to look for and what actions to take if they should occur.

The orthopaedic nurse who is not regularly applying casts will not have the skills to do so independently and must consider the implications if they do so without guidance or supervision. As the NMC (2002, p8) states, 'You must acknowledge the limits of your professional competence and only undertake practice and accept responsibilities for those activities in which you are competent'. Equally, all nurses who are regularly applying casts must maintain and improve their skills as part of their professional development. Guidelines have been produced setting out the desired educational and training standards for casting and the role of nurses with management responsibilities for plaster technicians (RCN 1999).

USE OF CASTS

To make a cast, the casting material is applied to the patient's limb or trunk and held in position until it hardens sufficiently. Materials are chosen which can be moulded to fit closely to the bone contours. The functions of casts in therapeutic restriction following traumatic injury and orthopaedic surgery are (Prior & Miles 1999):

- the treatment of fractures, through the support of fractured bones
- after surgery, for example after nerve or tendon repair until healing has occurred
- to correct deformities, by wedging the cast or by application of serial casts
- for support
- to provide pain relief, through resting of an infected or injured joint
- to aid in the healing of pressure ulcers, especially foot ulcers in diabetic patients.

MATERIALS USED FOR CASTS

Casts are made from plaster of Paris or a range of synthetic materials that are resin based (RCN/ SOTN 2000). There have been more recent developments in adjustable focused rigidity casts, which can be reapplied and adjusted during the treatment process (Large 2001, Petty & Wardman 1998).

Plaster of Paris

Plaster of Paris bandages are manufactured by heating gypsum powder and suspending it in a solvent. The slurry is used to coat gauze cloth and the solvent is then removed by drying the cloth in an oven. The bandages are cut, rolled and wrapped in moisture-resistant packets. They will last for about 2–3 years if stored appropriately. Plaster of Paris consists of the compound calcium sulphate.

When the bandage is immersed in water and then removed, heat is given off and quickly growing solid crystals of mouldable gypsum are produced:

$$2(CaSO_4\tfrac{1}{2}H_2O) + 3H_2O \Leftrightarrow 2(CaSO_42H_2O) + Heat$$
$$\text{Plaster of Paris} + \text{Water} \Leftrightarrow \text{Gypsum} + \text{Heat}$$

This reversible reaction explains the properties of plaster of Paris. The patient must be warned that the plaster will feel warm when first applied. Additional heat, usually from the patient's body and surrounding air, drives off water from the gypsum, producing plaster of Paris. The patient must therefore be advised that the plaster will feel cold during the drying process and that they must not cover the cast, to allow for evaporation of the water.

Resin–based casts

These are lighter but non-absorbent. The small molecules of resin undergo polymerisation (linking to form long-chain polymers), a process usually activated by submerging the bandages in water.

Adjustable focused rigidity primary casts

The cast is adjustable to accommodate swelling or atrophy, reducing the risk of neurovascular impairment or ensuring sufficient support for a limb. A trial comparing adjustable focused rigidity casts (the experimental group) with traditionally applied synthetic or plaster of Paris casts (the control groups) found there was no difference in fracture healing between the two groups; however, the ability to carry out activities of living was greater in those patients with the focused rigidity casts (Petty & Wardman 1998).

Selection of appropriate casting material

Ideal attributes of casting materials are listed in Box 6.1. The specific attributes of plaster of Paris and synthetic casts are as follows.

- Plaster of Paris has better moulding properties than synthetic casts and is cheaper. It interferes with the visualisation of bony detail on X-ray more than synthetic casts but it can be split or windowed if tension increases due to swelling or for dressings. It can be bivalved to make splints.
- Synthetic casts have a greater resistance to wear than plaster of Paris. When immersed in water, they recover 90% of their strength within 24 hours whereas plaster of Paris casts deform permanently when immersed (Wytch et al 1991). Synthetic casts are lighter and may therefore help patients in maintaining their independence with

---

Box 6.1   Ideal attributes of casting materials

- Suitable to apply directly to the patient
- Easy to mould to the body contours
- Non-toxic to the patient and user during application, while worn and when removed
- Unaffected by fluids such as water
- Transparent to X-rays
- Easy to alter and modify, quick setting
- Easy and safe to remove
- Permeable to air, odour, water and pus
- Light but strong
- Non-inflammable
- Clean to use and remove
- Cheap and easily available in a variety of sizes

Box 6.2   Contents of a basic casting trolley (Prior & Miles 1999)

- Stockinette, if required
- Synthetic padding and/or felt
- Plaster of Paris bandages and slabs, if necessary, or synthetic cast bandages
- Plaster strips or waterproof tape to finish
- Marking pencil
- Knife
- Scissors
- Elbow or knee rest
- Protective plastic sheeting
- Plastic aprons
- Plastic-covered pillows
- Bucket or bowl of water
- Bowl of water for washing the patient's skin
- Towel
- Rubbish bag
- Patient information leaflet

---

activities of living, especially if they are elderly. However, they cannot be used with patients who have a history of allergic reactions: gloves must be worn by the person applying the cast and by the assistant when using synthetic materials. Protection is needed as they have sharp edges that may damage skin.

Herzig et al (1999) found that synthetic casting materials had a lower replacement need and a lower application time than plaster of Paris casts in a survey of 2698 casts applied at 32 hospitals in five countries.

APPLYING A CAST

Many different techniques are used in applying a cast but the basic principles remain the same whether the cast is made from plaster of Paris or synthetics (Miles & Barr 1991).

The nurse should check the patient's documentation for relevant information, treatment details and casting instructions before application.

Preparation of equipment and the patient

All equipment and materials should be prepared and assembled before application commences; this ensures that the patient has the cast applied as quickly and smoothly as possible. The contents of a basic casting trolley are listed in Box 6.2.

Cast application

Stockinette should be fitted only if there is no likelihood of any swelling, as it is difficult to cut through and may crease, causing further localised pressure.

The following guidelines on fitting a plaster of Paris cast apply to any type of casting material.

- Apply wool padding, usually as a single layer but with extra layers around bony prominences. This allows for swelling, reduces friction of the cast against the skin and acts as a protective barrier when shears and saws are used to remove the cast.
- Soak the bandage in lukewarm water, 25–30°C. Cold water slows and hot water quickens the setting process.
- Remove the bandage when the bubbles stop, squeezing very gently; only soak one bandage at a time.
- Roll the bandages on, maintaining contact between the roll of the bandage and the body part.
- Start from one end of the affected part, covering approximately one-third of the previous turn; tension on the bandage is not required.
- Allow the bandage to form tucks to fit the contours of the body; never twist the bandage as this creates ridges.
- Apply all the bandages successively, continuously smoothing and rubbing to enable the cast to bond and laminate.
- Trim the edges when the cast is complete and has set, to allow all joints not encased to move freely; this should be carried out on a pillow with a waterproof cover to prevent any indenting.

- Handle the cast at all times during setting and drying with the palms of the hands and not fingers; otherwise, indentations will be formed with the risk of pressure ulcer development.
- Turn back the stockinette, if used, over the edges of the cast and hold it in place with strips of plaster of Paris bandage. For synthetic casts use waterproof tape.
- Clean the patient's skin and supply any necessary supports or give the patient any aids such as arm slings, collar and cuff or crutches.

Knowledge deficit

The patient should fully understand the procedure about to take place so the principles of informed consent can be met. Ideally the patient should be given time to assimilate the information and ask any questions.

Pain

The patient may have pain if the cast is being applied to support fractured bones or support damaged joints or soft tissues. The goal of care would be for the patient to articulate that they were pain free before the casting begins. This can be achieved by the administration of appropriate analgesia, allowing sufficient time for it to take effect, and correct positioning of the patient and affected part of the body.

Potential for skin impairment and peripheral neurovascular damage

The skin should be checked for ulcers, abrasions and bruising; these should be cleaned, washed or dressed according to local guidelines. The patient should be protected with plastic sheeting. Any rings or jewellery, if not removed previously, should be removed and stored safely so that swelling after the cast is applied will not lead to neurovascular impairment.

NURSING DIAGNOSES AND CARE: AFTER CAST APPLICATION

Patients in a cast will have many of the core problems identified at the beginning of the chapter. Specific care issues and nursing diagnoses are addressed below.

Knowledge deficit

Few, if any, patients are receiving regular attention or visits from healthcare professionals whilst wearing a cast. It is vital they are fully educated to safely take control of their care, including detecting when problems are developing. The patient should be able to articulate the principles of care and what measures to take if complications develop.

Nursing interventions. Any information given should be reinforced and supported by written guidance, which should contain information similar to that in Box 6.3. Whenever necessary, this guidance should be given to any other relevant carer, such as parents and relatives, so they can reinforce and be aware of the principles of care.

Some patients may experience a claustrophobic reaction to the presence of the cast, not relieved by education; relaxation exercises or the prescription of a mild tranquilliser may be necessary.

Box 6.3   Information for patients with a cast

Report back to the hospital if at any time you experience any of these:

- Toes or fingers become blue, swollen or difficult and painful to move
- The limb becomes painful
- You feel 'pins and needles' or numbness
- You have 'blister-like' or 'burning' pain
- You see any discharge or wetness or detect an unpleasant smell from the cast
- If you drop anything under the cast
- If you are worried at all about yourself or your cast

THE TELEPHONE NUMBER TO RING IS ....

- Keep the cast dry and allow it to dry naturally, leave it uncovered
- Do not apply external heat such as a hairdryer or by sitting in front of a fire
- If an irritation occurs under the cast, never poke anything down the cast
- Wash the skin around the cast daily, checking for redness or sores
- Never try to pad the edges of the cast if it is rubbing, but seek advice
- Do not let the limb hang down, especially in the first few days
- Carry out the exercises you have been shown for your fingers or toes and other joints of your body for 5 minutes every hour during the day
- Do not misuse your cast, for instance by weight bearing before you have been instructed to do so

Self-care deficit

Patients with a cast may find that everyday activities suddenly become difficult, if not impossible. It is important that nursing staff undertake a comprehensive assessment to ensure that a person will be able to cope with the cast. The goal of care is for the patient to maintain everyday activities to a level acceptable to them. The patient may need help to achieve this level.

Nursing interventions

- Assessment of the patient's capabilities. This will depend on a number of factors, including the site of the cast, the previous level of independence and the support available from family or friends. Referral to a social worker may be required.
- Provision of practical advice such as how to bath with a leg cast (see Smith & Nephew 1991 for such advice). Pearson (1987) found that patients wearing below-knee casts had difficulty in carrying out activities of living not anticipated by nurses. Most patients experienced some difficulty with activities related to hygiene. Over 90% of those not given specific information about how to take a bath were unable to do so. However, of those given information on how to prevent the cast getting wet, 90% were able to take a bath.

Peripheral neurovascular impairment

The goal of care is to reduce the risk of neurovascular impairment and identify any early complications.

Nursing interventions.   Neurovascular observations must be carried out. If neurovascular impairment, including compartment syndrome, is suspected some or all of the following interventions should be carried out.

- Inform the medical staff immediately.
- Cease elevation of the limb, as elevation may increase the compartment pressure.
- The cast should be split down to the skin; a few threads of padding left uncut could impair circulation.
- If there is local pressure on a nerve, a window needs to be cut or the cast bivalved.
- Compartment syndrome requires immediate surgery to relieve the pressure built up in the muscle compartment before irreversible damage occurs to the ischaemic muscle.

Traditionally, backslabs have been used after a fracture when swelling is anticipated, as the bandaging will expand to accommodate any oedema and reduce the risk of neurovascular impairment. Similarly, full casts are often split down to the skin and a bandage applied to the exterior of the cast to accommodate swelling. However, after an experiment carried out on forearm casts with different modifications (split down to soft dressing, split through cast and soft dressing, a split and spread cast, and a backslab), Younger et al (1990) suggest that only the split and spread cast will accommodate a wrist circumference increase of 5 mm (which they postulated would be the increase after fracture reduction) at an acceptable internal pressure of less than 40 mmHg. They found that a backslab would not expand by 5 mm until there is an internal pressure of 135 mmHg and that applying a crepe bandage to a split cast reduces its ability to expand. They conclude that the best method of accommodating swelling is to split a cast fully down to the skin and spread it widely (1 cm). This may, however, reduce the ability of the cast to maintain the position of a fracture.

Impaired skin integrity

Localised pressure within the cast may cause pressure or cast sores, which can be identified by the following signs (Powell 1986):

- itching beneath the plaster
- a characteristic burning pain; this should not be ignored as the tissues quickly become ischaemic, leading to numbness and disappearance of the pain
- disturbed sleep, restlessness and fretfulness in children
- local areas of heat on the plaster
- swelling of the fingers or toes after the immediate swelling has subsided
- a characteristic offensive smell due to tissue necrosis
- the appearance of discharge.

The aim of care is to prevent damage to the skin integrity.

Nursing interventions

- The edges of a cast can be eased or trimmed but should not have extra padding inserted, as this will increase the pressure or the padding could fall further down into the cast.
- Cotton wool should not be used for padding as it tends to be compressed into hard small pellets that cause further problems when the pellets fall into the cast and become lodged.

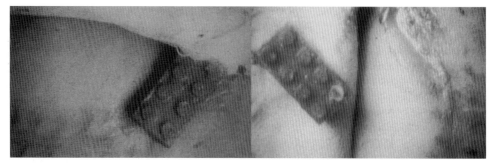

Figure 6.11 Plaster sores.

- A window should be carefully cut and removed as a whole piece for inspection of a potential sore site. To prevent local oedema the window must be replaced.
- Foreign objects inside the cast (Fig. 6.11) can be detected by radiography and the cast may have to be removed.
- No objects, such as knitting needles, must be pushed down the cast to scratch itching areas as skin damage can easily occur.
- When observing casts that are stained by oozing of blood or pus, the nurse may find it useful to mark the edges of the stain with a pen and put the date and time next to it. When subsequent observations are made, a comparison with any further oozing can be made.

Drying the plaster

The goal of care is for the cast to dry, ensuring the required position is maintained. A plaster of Paris cast takes minutes to set firmly enough to maintain the affected part of the body in the required position. However, it will take from 24 hours for a small arm cast to 96 hours for a total body cast to dry and reach its full strength. As the cast dries it will change from a matt grey colour, with a musty smell, to a shiny white colour with no odour. Synthetic casts dry much more quickly, within 20–30 minutes.

Nursing interventions. In order to ensure that the cast dries thoroughly without damage to it or to the limb, the following principles should be borne in mind.

- The cast should be well supported, to prevent sagging; a fracture board can be used for large casts such as hip spicas.
- To prevent pressure on bony prominences, the affected part should be rested on pillows with waterproof coverings.

- To aid drying:
  —the pillows should be covered by towelling or similar absorbent material, which should be changed every few hours
  —the cast must be exposed to the air in a warm dry atmosphere and not covered by clothing or bedclothes
  —the use of artificial heat, such as from lamps or hairdryers, is not recommended as the cast may crack if it dries too rapidly; there is also a danger of burning the patient as the cast stores heat and transmits it only slowly through to the body surface, which means that the wet skin surface may be at a high temperature even after the heat source is removed.
- Patients in large casts should change position by turning every few hours so the complete cast is dried. This may require the assistance of a nurse(s).
- Limbs in casts should be elevated using pillows, footrests or slings to aid venous return and, if trauma has occurred, to prevent or reduce oedema.
- The cast should be observed regularly for cracking, softening and breakdown at the edges and acute angles. Observations should be continued by the nurse and later the patient once the cast is dry.

Risk of disuse syndrome (stiffness of the joint)

Stiffness will occur in joints held in a cast and in adjacent joints if the patient is unwilling to move them. The aim of care is to ensure that the adjacent joints retain their normal range of movement.

Nursing interventions. Patient education is vital in relation to the importance of using adjacent joints; this should be included in the written patient information (Box 6.3).

Potential allergic reaction

Plaster of Paris or other synthetic casting material rarely produces an allergic reaction for patients but the padding may. The possibility of an allergic reaction may be anticipated from the patient's past history and the patient should be instructed in what to observe for. The aim of care is to prevent reactions in patients known to have had a reaction in the past and for early detection of any reaction occurring in other patients.

Nursing interventions. The nurse needs to check before applying a cast that the patient has no known allergies. The nurse and patient need to observe for signs of reaction: itching, a non-localised burning pain, rashes and blistering of the skin. If these occur, the medical staff should be informed and the cast will need to be removed. The skin is cleaned, treated and a new cast applied using other materials.

PRINCIPLES OF REMOVING A CAST

The removal of a cast is a skilled task and is usually achieved by bivalving it: deliberately cutting it in half. Staff undertaking this procedure should ensure they have the requisite skills and knowledge (Miles 1997). The following principles should be applied.

- Clear instructions should be obtained from the medical staff, unless an agreed protocol is in place allowing nurses to make decisions regarding cast removal.
- The patient should be positioned appropriately, for example lying supine with a knee rest for the removal of a lower leg cast.
- A clear explanation should be given to the patient with, if necessary, a demonstration of the procedure and how the equipment is used.
- Equipment and techniques used should not damage the patient's skin.
- The patient should be comfortable and not subjected to any pain.
- The bivalved cast should be kept on to support the limb until it is decided that it can be discarded.

Casts may be cut with shears or oscillating electric saws. Synthetic casts require special shears and saws with tungsten-hardened blades. Generally, shears are used for casts on children, small casts and upper limb casts. Oscillating saws must not be used on unpadded casts, as the skin beneath will be cut.

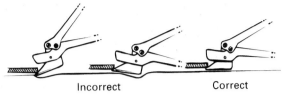

Incorrect   Correct

Figure 6.12   Bivalving with plaster shears.

Bivalving casts

The technique and equipment used to remove casts should at all times be safe for the patient and operator. The lines along which the cast is to be cut should be marked with a pen or pencil. The lines should avoid bony prominences to reduce the risk of skin damage; for example, a lower leg cast should be marked down either side with lines passing in front of the lateral malleolus and behind the medial malleolus.

Using shears. The blade of the shears passes between the cast and the padding and should be kept parallel to the limb. This prevents the point of the heel of the shears digging into the patient's skin and pinching it (Fig. 6.12). After both sides have been cut, the plaster is eased open with spreaders and the padding cut with bandage scissors.

Using an oscillating saw. The saw has an oscillating circular blade; the blade does not rotate but vibrates back and forth at high speed, rubbing its way through the cast. It should be used only on dry padded casts. The blade is held at right angles to the cast and applied with light pressure to make a cut. It is then removed and reapplied slightly higher or lower down the cast along the line to be cut (Fig. 6.13). The blade must not be dragged along the cast as the skin may be cut. As with all electrical appliances, the saw should not be handled by someone with wet hands. The blade may become very hot and burn the skin if it is used continuously for a long period of time, particularly on synthetic materials. To reduce the risk of inhalation of fine dust particles and to comply with safety regulations, a vacuum removal system should be used with the saw.

Skin care

When a cast is worn for any length of time the upper layers of skin cannot be shed as normal, so collect as flaky yellow scales. In addition, the muscles lose tone and bulk because of disuse. Before the nurse finally removes any part of the cast she must warn the patient of this scaly, withered appearance.

The skin can be washed gently and patted dry. The skin flakes should not be picked off, as this may

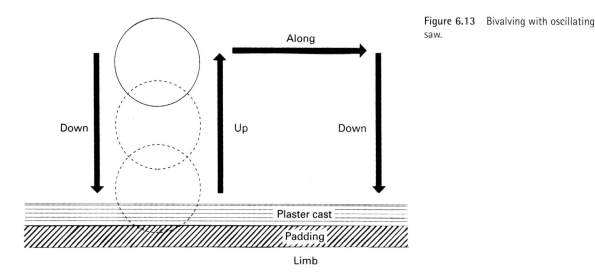

Figure 6.13 Bivalving with oscillating saw.

damage the skin underneath. Oil or cream should be applied if the skin is dry. Some support such as bandages or shaped support stockings may be necessary to control swelling, particularly for lower limbs. The patient then begins a progressive, gentle exercise programme.

INTERNAL FIXATION

Internal fixation is a method of reducing and maintaining the position of fractures to aid bone healing. Bone fragments can be held in position with screws, plates, wires and nails. Dandy & Edwards (1998) suggest that the main indications for internal fixation are:

- fractures that cannot be managed in any other way
- patients with fractures of more than one bone
- to protect vessels in fractures where the blood supply is threatened
- and for intraarticular, displaced fractures.

They suggest that the disadvantages of internal fixation are: the increased risk of infection at the time of operation and the additional trauma of an operation when wide exposure devitalises some of the bone and soft tissue.

TYPES OF INTERNAL FIXATION

Screws

Screws can be used to compress plates against bone or bone against bone (Fig. 6.14). Although there are specific screws for different situations, there are two main types:

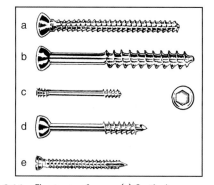

Figure 6.14 Five types of screw. (a) Cortical screw. (b) Cancellous screw. (c) Herbert scaphoid screw – note the different pitch of the threads at each end. (d) Malleolar screw with pointed tip. (e) Self-tapping screw – note the flutes at the tip. (From Dandy & Edwards 1998.)

- cortical screws which are tapped into the bone after a hole has been drilled
- cancellous screws which have a wide thread to grip soft cancellous bone.

Plates

These are used to hold bones in the correct position and to compress the bone ends together.

Intramedullary nails

These are placed in the medullary canal of the long bone (Fig. 6.15). The medullary cavity varies in width; it is narrowest at the centre of the bone, which means that the cavity must be reamed carefully otherwise the nail can break the bone when inserted. The nails hold length and alignment but

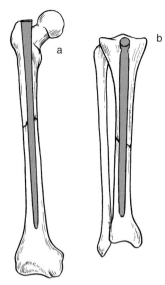

Figure 6.15   Intramedullary nails. (From Dandy & Edwards 1998.)

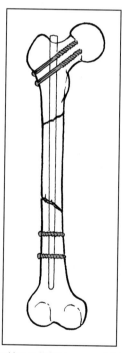

Figure 6.16   Locking nail for a segmental fracture. Screws are passed through the bone and nail above and below the fracture to hold the bone length. (From Dandy & Edwards 1998.)

they are less effective in controlling rotation unless cross screws are used.

Locking intramedullary nails have screws that fix the bone fragments to the nail itself (Fig. 6.16). Intramedullary nails can be inserted by a closed

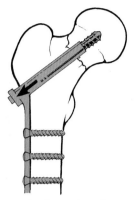

Figure 6.17   Compression from a dynamic screw and plate for fixation of femoral neck fractures. (From Dandy & Edwards 1998.)

technique using an image intensifier; this avoids exposing the bone and devitalising it (Wicker 1992).

Nail plates or screws and plates

These are used particularly for trochanteric fractures of the femur. The nail or screw grips the proximal fragment and the plate is screwed to the femoral shaft (Fig. 6.17).

Wires

Wires can be used to fix fractures in two ways.

- Tension band wiring where the wire is applied as a loop to the outer side of a fracture so that it comes under tension when the joint is flexed. This is used for fractures of the patella and olecranon in particular.
- Circlage wiring is used for spiral fractures with minimal displacement (Fig. 6.18).

NURSING DIAGNOSES AND CARE: INTERNAL FIXATION

The majority of internal fixation is applied following trauma; the principles of nursing care are the same for patients pre- and postoperatively. Particular attention should be paid to the following issues.

Knowledge deficit

The majority of patients will have internal fixation of fractures as an emergency, with little or no time to educate them preoperatively, even if they are receptive to information at that time. Postoperatively, however, it should be the goal of care to ensure the patient can explain why internal fixation was necessary and what can be done to ensure it is successful.

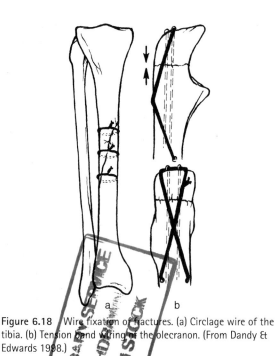

Figure 6.18 Wire fixation of fractures. (a) Circlage wire of the tibia. (b) Tension band wiring of the olecranon. (From Dandy & Edwards 1998.)

Self-care deficit

Patients who have internal fixation to either their upper or lower limb may have problems with maintaining self-care. The goal of care is for the patient to be able to carry out the activities of living important to them, either independently or with the support and help of others. The nursing interventions are similar to those for patients with other forms of therapeutic restriction, such as casts, and involves ensuring patients are taught how to perform tasks whilst their mobility is reduced.

Neurovascular impairment

The surgery necessary for inserting the internal fixation may lead to neurovascular impairment, through bleeding at the operation site or the position of the patient on the operating table can stretch nerves and blood vessels. Postoperative bandaging or casts following internal fixation may also increase the pressure within a limb. Neurovascular observations are therefore vital following internal fixation.

Impaired skin integrity

If a patient has a closed internal fixation the resulting surgical incision will be small, while open internal fixation requires a larger incision. Appropriate wound care is needed for all surgical and trauma wounds.

Altered body image

A scar from the surgery involved in internal fixation may affect the body image of the patient, especially if it is visible in everyday life.

Impaired physical mobility

Internal fixation for fractures of the lower limb usually results in a secure fixation on which the patient can fully bear weight. However, a patient might not be allowed to fully bear weight in the first 4–6 weeks if the fracture is particularly severe or the fixation technically difficult. The goal of care should be determined with the physiotherapist and medical staff. It should be described in terms of the distance to be mobilised, what aids might be used and the support required from others.

Nursing interventions. These are to ensure the patient is using any aids correctly. Patients must be encouraged to wear the correct size of footwear, with non-slip soles that provide support for the foot. The nurse should walk with the patient until they are, and feel, safe and have regained their confidence.

EXTERNAL FIXATORS

Bone fragments can be held in place with external fixators. These are threaded pins set in the bone fragments with a scaffold or gantry attached (Fig. 6.19). The main indications for their use are for:

- stabilising open fractures with extensive soft tissue loss
- non-union of fractures, for example non-union of tibial fractures treated with an Ilizarov frame (Ebraheim et al 1995)
- reconstructive surgery for congenital and posttraumatic deformities of long bones and joints, for example leg lengthening using an Ilizarov frame
- the treatment of some closed fractures, such as the pelvis (Olerud 1990) and wrist (Pennig & Gausepohl 1996).

Depending on their function, external fixators may remain in place for as little as 6 weeks, for example for the treatment of a wrist fracture, or for up to 2 years for the treatment of non-union of a fracture.

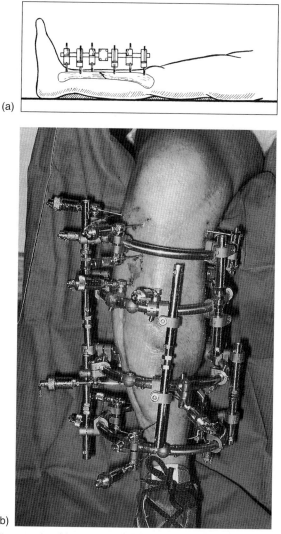

(a)

(b)

Figure 6.19 (a) External fixation of the tibia. (b) An external ring fixator in position. (From Dandy & Edwards 1998.)

NURSING DIAGNOSES AND CARE: PATIENT WITH AN EXTERNAL FIXATOR

The nursing diagnoses and associated nursing care for a patient with an external fixator are closely interlinked. For example, a knowledge deficit will include knowledge about pin-site care, which is linked with impaired skin integrity, while the ability or willingness to carry out this pin-site care is linked to altered body image.

Knowledge deficit

Few patients will have experienced having an external fixator; many will not even have seen one on another person. Patients need knowledge not only of what the treatment entails but what part they play in the care of the pin-sites on discharge from the acute care setting. The goals of care will be for the patient to demonstrate knowledge of the treatment goals and associated care of the fixator.

Nursing interventions. For patients having planned application of external fixators, education will commence prior to hospital admission and can include meeting patients who have, or have had, treatment involving external fixators. Assessment of whether the patient will cope with the fixator is advisable because the treatment can be a complex, lengthy and demanding experience (Sims et al 1999).

If a patient will need to be involved in cleaning and dressing the pin-sites, they are assessed preoperatively to ensure they are willing and able to carry this out. The patient initially observes the pin-site care, then practises it under supervision and finally carries it out independently before discharge from hospital.

Self-care deficit

Patients who have external fixation to either their upper or lower limb can have problems in maintaining their self-care activities. The goal of care is for the patient to be able to carry out the activities of living important to them, either independently or with the support and help of others.

The nursing interventions are similar to those for patients with other forms of therapeutic restriction, such as casts, and involve ensuring patients are taught how to perform tasks whilst their mobility is reduced or providing them with help until it is restored. Advice should be given about clothing to wear around the external fixator and about any adaptations necessary in the home, such as a raised toilet seat (Sims et al 2000).

Peripheral neurovascular impairment

The application of an external fixator may lead to damage to nerves or blood vessels at the time of surgery. If the fixator is being used in the distraction (lengthening) of shortened limbs, care is needed as too fast a distraction can lead to local ischaemia that in turn will slow osteogenesis. Neurovascular observations to identify this early are essential.

Impaired skin integrity

The patient with an external fixator has impaired skin integrity where the skeletal pins are applied.

Many patients are capable of carrying out pin-site care and doing so may lead to reduced infection rates (Haines 2000). This may not be feasible for some patients, requiring primary care nurses to be involved when the patient is discharged. It is important that primary care staff are aware of the correct techniques of pin-site care to ensure continuity of nursing care and to reduce the risk of infection.

Altered body image

External fixators are very visible forms of therapeutic restriction; they are not commonplace so other people feel inquisitive about them. Patients may feel very vulnerable in terms of their body image whilst the fixator is in place.

Impaired physical mobility

The external fixator can reduce a person's ability to mobilise. Fortunately weight bearing is often allowed as it is considered to aid the healing process. The goals of care should be determined with the physiotherapist and medical staff. These should be clearly recorded and articulated in terms of the distance to be mobilised, the mobility aids and the support required from others.

Nursing interventions. These ensure the patient is using any aids correctly. Patients must be encouraged to wear the correct footwear and be accompanied by a nurse until they are, and feel, safe and have regained their confidence in walking.

ORTHOSES

An orthosis is a device added externally to the patient, in contrast to a prosthesis which replaces a missing part of the body. Orthoses can be used for the following purposes.

- To immobilise a limb, thus reducing pain and promoting rest; for example, a hand splint to promote rest in a person with an acute episode of rheumatoid arthritis involving the hand.
- To provide fixed or balanced traction, for example a Thomas splint.
- To prevent or correct a mild deformity or maintain correction of a deformity when this has been achieved; for example, a splint to prevent foot drop or a brace post surgery for scoliosis.
- To relieve weight; for example, a hip brace to relieve weight on a healing femoral neck fracture.

- To stabilise joints and protect weak muscles; for example, a knee brace following a knee arthroplasty.
- To maintain correct posture when the individual is weight bearing by maintaining extension of the spine, hip or knees; for example, a lumbar corset or brace.

NURSING DIAGNOSES AND CARE: PATIENT WITH AN ORTHOSIS

Many of the principles of nursing care for a patient with an orthosis are similar to those for a patient in a cast. However, there are some particular points to be borne in mind.

Knowledge deficit

It is important that a patient understands how to wear the orthosis correctly and safely. Although they are usually made and fitted by an orthotist or occupational therapist, it is a nursing role to ensure the patient can demonstrate this understanding. Written information should be given to reinforce verbal advice (Box 6.4).

Impaired skin integrity

An orthosis can cause skin breakdown in the form of a pressure ulcer. The care outlined for patients in casts should be considered for a patient in an orthosis, the goal of care remaining the same, namely that the skin remains intact. In addition, the following should be considered.

Box 6.4   Instructions for patients with orthoses

Report back to the hospital if at any time you experience any difficulties.
The telephone number to call is ....

- Always handle your orthosis with care, avoid dropping it or leaving it where it may get damaged
- Examine your skin at least twice a day for signs of pressure or damage due to your orthosis. Contact the hospital or your GP if this occurs
- Keep up the simple maintenance schedule given to you, e.g. clean locks and oil joints weekly
- Inspect all moving parts regularly for wear and tear
- Clean your orthosis and skin as directed
- Keep the heels and soles of footwear in good condition to prevent falls

Nursing interventions

- The skin should be kept clean and dry, as dampness, usually due to sweating, is a contributory cause of pressure ulcers.
- Talcum powder should be used only in moderation as it may clump and become a source of pressure and irritation.
- When the splint is applied initially, the areas of skin beneath it subjected to pressure should be observed every 2 hours. Once the skin has hardened and got used to pressure, the number of observations may be reduced.

Orthotic designs are continually changing as new materials and techniques are developed and expertise increases. Nurses need to be aware of developments so that they can continue to educate patients.

Altered body image

Aesthetically acceptable orthoses can now be made but wearing an orthosis can affect an individual's body image and self-esteem.

WALKING AIDS

Aids to walking are required at all stages of life, from the use of push-walkers for children to the use of sticks in the elderly with decreased muscle strength and balance. Those who have sustained injury to their lower limbs may also require a walking aid (Figs 6.20, 6.21).

Crutches and walking sticks are commonly used when walking restrictions are prescribed, for example when a lower limb cast is applied and the patient has to be non-weight bearing or when the stresses through a joint need to be reduced due to diseases such as osteoarthritis.

Stewart & Hallett (1983) identify four criteria to be considered when a walking aid is selected.

1 The stability of the patient.
2 The strength of the patient's upper and lower limbs.
3 The degree of coordination of movement of the upper and lower limbs.
4 The degree of relief of weight bearing required.

CRUTCH WALKING

Crutches are generally used when the patient is not allowed to put any weight through one or both legs or when only minimal weight bearing is allowed.

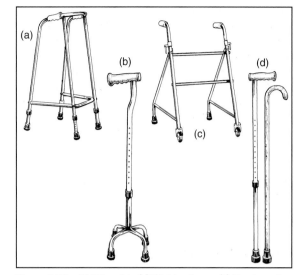

Figure 6.20   Walking aids. (a) Walking frame. (b) Quadrupod walking stick. (c) Wheeled walking frame or Rollator. (d) Metal and wooden walking sticks. (From Dandy & Edwards 1998.)

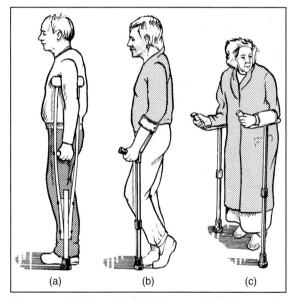

Figure 6.21   Walking aids. (a) Axillary crutch. (b) Elbow crutch. (c) Gutter crutch. (From Dandy & Edwards 1998.)

Elbow crutches are preferred as axillary crutches have a potential risk of arterial and nerve injury, such as axillary nerve palsy (Love 2001).

Measurement for elbow crutches

When elbow crutches are adjusted correctly, the tips of the crutches are on the ground 15 cm in front of and lateral to the tips of the toes when the patient is standing up straight, their shoulders depressed and elbows in 30° of flexion. The armband is correctly positioned when the gap between the top of the armband and the flexor crease of the elbow is 5 cm.

NURSING DIAGNOSES AND CARE: FOR CRUTCHES

Knowledge deficit

It is important that patients have a full understanding of how to use crutches correctly and safely. Whilst the physiotherapist normally demonstrates this, it is the orthopaedic nurse who supervises patients using their crutches until they feel confident; in some areas the nurse also measures the patient for and demonstrates the use of the crutches. For these reasons it is important that the orthopaedic nurse is familiar with the techniques of walking, sitting and standing, plus going up and down stairs so they can educate the patient.

Nursing interventions. The goal of care is for the patient to demonstrate the safe use of crutches by teaching the following.

• **Standing position**: when first using the crutches, the patient should be allowed the time to feel stable in the upright position. With the crutches, a balanced or tripod position is achieved with the foot of the crutch about 10 cm in front and 15 cm to the side of the outside edge of each foot. All walking starts from this position. The weight must rest on the hands.

• **Walking**: there are several types of gait that may be used for crutch walking.
  —Swinging crutch gait; fast, needs good balance.
  —Four-point crutch gait; slow, for poor balance.
  —Three-point crutch gait; fairly fast, needs reasonable balance.
  —Two-point crutch gait; fairly fast, needs good balance.
Which gait to use will depend on the amount of weight the person can put through each or both feet. This may range from non-weight bearing through partial weight bearing to full weight bearing.

• **Three-point crutch gait**: the commonest gait used by a patient needing to be partial or non-weight bearing on one leg, as the weight will be supported by the stronger leg and the two crutches; for example, after unilateral surgery or injury to the lower limb.

Starting from the balanced or tripod position, the crutches are simultaneously moved forward a short

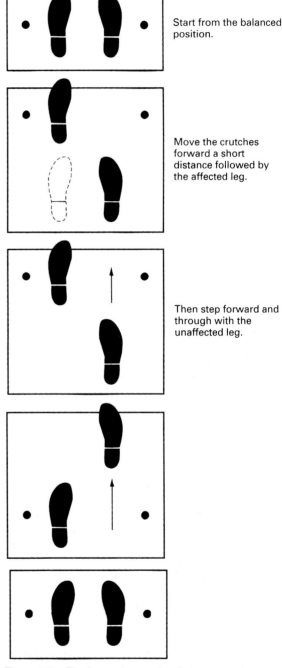

Start from the balanced position.

Move the crutches forward a short distance followed by the affected leg.

Then step forward and through with the unaffected leg.

Figure 6.22 The three-point crutch gait.

distance, about 30 cm. The patient must be advised not to attempt large distances at each movement. The affected leg is swung forward to be level with the crutches, then the patient steps forward with the unaffected leg; this is then repeated (Fig. 6.22). This

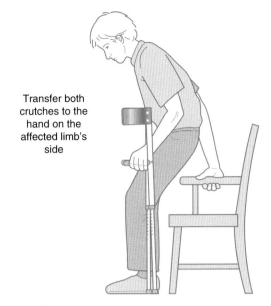 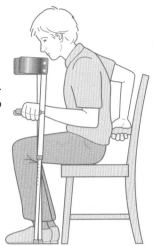

Transfer both crutches to the hand on the affected limb's side

Use the other hand to grasp the arm rest and sit down

Figure 6.23 Sitting in a chair.

type of crutch walking requires a great deal of effort on the part of the patient, with the heart and respiration rate rising as much as 48% above the normal (Love 2001). Patients must therefore be assessed as to the correct use of the crutches and to ensure they have sufficient physical capability and cardiovascular strength to use them safely (Love 2001).

• **Sitting and standing**: there are several ways for a patient to sit on and rise from a chair safely. The simplest way to sit down is for the patient to stand with their back to the chair, the unaffected leg just touching the seat of the chair. Both crutches are then transferred to the hand on the affected limb's side while the other hand is used to grasp the armrest and sit down (Fig. 6.23). The crutches are then placed within reach in a safe position. The reverse procedure is carried out when standing.

• **Going up and down stairs**: in going up and down stairs the crutches are always moved with the affected leg. To go upstairs the patient stands in front of the first step, both crutches are transferred to the hand opposite the wall or handrail. Pushing down on the crutches and supported by the wall or handrail, the patient lifts the unaffected leg onto the first step (Fig. 6.24). Remember the slogan 'up with the good' leg first. The affected leg and crutches are then lifted onto the first step and the process repeated.

To go downstairs the same procedure is followed except the affected leg and crutches are the first to be moved onto the first step down, followed by the

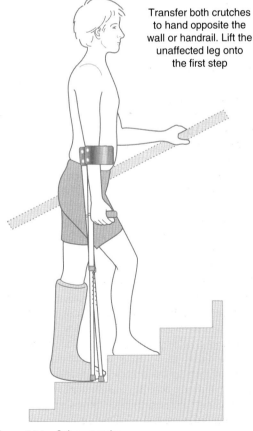

Transfer both crutches to hand opposite the wall or handrail. Lift the unaffected leg onto the first step

Figure 6.24 Going up stairs.

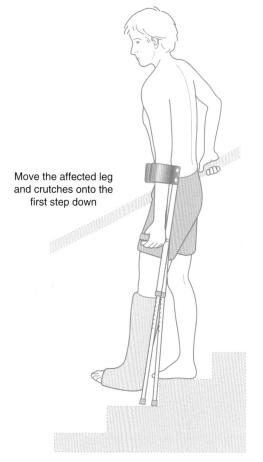

Move the affected leg and crutches onto the first step down

Figure 6.25   Going down stairs.

unaffected leg (Fig. 6.25). Remember, 'down with the bad' leg first.

● **Care of the crutches: instructions to patients**: written instructions to patients should contain information similar to that in Box 6.5. To promote safety, crutches must be checked regularly to ensure the wood or metal is not cracked, to tighten all adjusting nuts and ensure any spring-loaded double-ball catches are working properly, to ensure the rubber tips (the ferrules) are in good condition and change them if badly worn and to ensure handgrips and axillary pads are in good condition.

Self-care deficit

Using crutches means a patient will find it difficult to carry out many activities important for self-care, such as carrying food to the table and shopping. Kay (1990) describes some of the problems encountered from personal experience such as being

---

Box 6.5   Information for patients using crutches

Report back to the hospital if at any time you experience any difficulties.
The telephone number to ring ....

Generally
● Stand with the crutches about 4 inches (10 cm) to the side of your feet and 6 inches (15 cm) in front, making a triangle
● Always take small steps, be careful on slippery or wet floors
● Wear tie shoes with low heels
● Check the rubber tips for wear twice a week
● Your hands should take the weight on the handgrips
● Your elbows should be slightly bent

Walking
● Move both crutches in front of you
● Move the affected leg forward
● Move the unaffected leg through

Sitting in a chair
● Stand with your back to the chair
● Put both crutches into the hand on the side of the affected leg
● Use the other hand to grasp the armrest and sit down
● Place the crutches safely and within reach
● Reverse the procedure to stand up

Going upstairs
● Move to the bottom of the stairs
● Put both crutches into the hand opposite the wall or handrail
● Lift the unaffected leg onto the first step
● Move the crutches and your affected leg onto the same step and repeat

Going downstairs
● Move to the top of the stairs
● Put both crutches into the hand opposite the wall or handrail
● Move the affected leg and crutches onto the first step
● Move the unaffected leg down onto the same step and repeat

---

dependent on others and needing someone to carry her handbag. The goal of care is for the patient to be able to carry out activities important for self-care or to receive appropriate help to do so.

STICK AND FRAME WALKING

Sticks and walking frames are for use by patients who are permitted to weight bear, such as those who have had stable internal fixation of a fracture. A walking frame can provide maximum stability but has to be lifted forwards in order for the patient to take a step (Fig. 6.20a) which requires some effort and coordination. A frame with wheels at the front can overcome this (Fig. 6.20c) but is difficult to manoeuvre on carpets.

Walking sticks are usually made of wood with a C-curved handle and a rubber tip on the lower end. Adjustable sticks made from aluminium alloy tubing are also available (Fig. 6.20d), as are multilegged sticks (Fig. 6.20b) which provide a higher level of stability. Walking sticks are lighter and more easily stored than crutches but are only able to assist balance slightly and to provide moderate support for the lower limb. They cannot be used unless the person can partially or fully bear weight on the affected limb. They can be used to decrease the amount of body weight taken through the lower limb by up to 25%, compensating for weakness and providing pain relief.

Measurement for sticks and walking frames

The length of the walking stick is measured by placing the handle of the stick on the floor. With the patient standing upright and wearing walking shoes, the lower end of the stick must be adjusted to be level with the wrist. To check, reverse the walking stick and ensure the patient's elbow is flexed to 30° when standing in the stable position. This degree of elbow flexion is also required for the correct use of a walking frame.

NURSING DIAGNOSES AND CARE: USE OF STICKS AND WALKING FRAMES

The patient with a stick or frame has a potential knowledge deficit similar to patients with crutches. Walking with two sticks using a three-point gait requires the same technique as used with crutches.

A patient using one stick needs to be educated to hold the stick correctly. The stick needs to be carried in the hand opposite to the affected lower limb, although some patients may find holding the stick on the same side gives more relief in knee or ankle injuries. The technique is similar to the three-point gait used with crutches (Fig. 6.26). For frame walking the patient should be taught to lift the frame forward

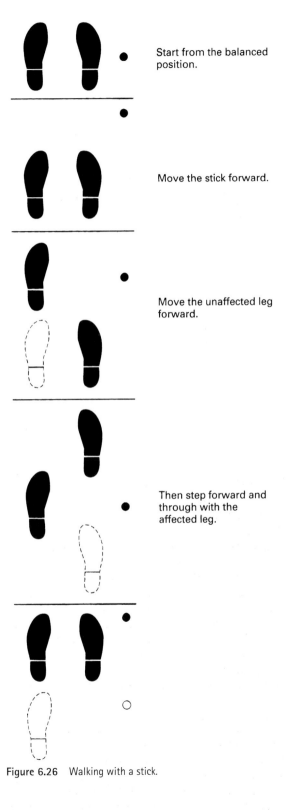

Start from the balanced position.

Move the stick forward.

Move the unaffected leg forward.

Then step forward and through with the affected leg.

Figure 6.26   Walking with a stick.

and then step into it, unless it has wheels in which case it can be moved without lifting.

CONCLUSION

With the continuing emphasis on patients' rights and their participation in care, it is important that nurses are aware how potentially damaging therapeutic restrictions can be. This is not just in a physical sense but also in the way in which it may remove patients' independence and lead them to become passive recipients of care. Orthopaedic nurses need to have an understanding of the legal and ethical implications of restricting movement in order to strive to ensure the patient is involved as much as possible in their care. They also have a responsibility to ensure they have adequate knowledge so that they can apply restrictions safely.

Further reading

Austin K, Gwynn-Brett K, Marshall S 1994 Illustrated guide to taping techniques. Mosby-Wolfe, London

Bourret EM, Bernich LG, Cott CA, Kontos PC 2002 The meaning of mobility for residents and staff in long-term care facilities. Journal of Advanced Nursing 37(4): 338–345

Royal College of Nursing (RCN) Society of Orthopaedic and Trauma Nursing (SOTN) 2002 A traction manual. RCN, London

Salter M 1997 Altered body image: the nurse's role, 2nd edn. Baillière Tindall, London

References

Arthur VAM 1995 Written patient information: a review of the literature. Journal of Advanced Nursing 21(6): 1081–1086

Austin K, Gwynn-Brett K, Marshall S 1994 Illustrated guide to taping techniques. Mosby-Wolfe, London

Beauchamp TL, Childress JF 1989 Principles of biomechanical ethics. Oxford University Press, New York

Brodell JD, Axon D, McCollister Evarts C 1986 The Robert Jones bandage. Journal of Bone and Joint Surgery 68B(5): 776–779

Cox C 2001 The legal challenges facing nursing. Journal of Orthopaedic Nursing 5(2): 65–72

Dale JJ, Callam MJ, Ruckley CV 1983 How efficient is a compression bandage? Nursing Times 79(46): 49–51

Dandy DJ, Edwards DJ 1998 Essential orthopaedics and trauma, 3rd edn. Churchill Livingstone, Edinburgh

Davis P 1997 Spinal cord injury and changes to body image. In: Salter M (ed) Altered body image: the nurse's role. Baillière Tindall, London

Department of Health (DoH) 2000 The NHS plan. Stationery Office, London

Devine EC 1992 Effects of psychoeducational care for adult surgical patients: a meta-analysis of 191 studies. Patient Education and Counselling 19: 127–142

Dimond B 1995 Legal aspects of nursing, 2nd edn. Prentice Hall, London

Dines A 1994 What changes in health behaviour might nurses logically expect from their health education work? Journal of Advanced Nursing 20(2): 219–226

Draper J, Scott F 1996 An investigation into the application and maintenance of Hamilton Russell traction on three orthopaedic wards. Journal of Advanced Nursing 23(3): 536–541

Draper P, Scott F 1998 Using traction. Nursing Times 94(12): 31–32

Ebraheim NA, Skie MC, Jackson WT 1995 The treatment of tibial nonunion with angular deformity using an Ilizarov device. Journal of Trauma: Injury, Infection and Critical Care 38(1): 111–117

Gammon J, Mulholland CW 1996 Effect of preparatory information prior to elective total hip replacement on psychological coping outcomes. Journal of Advanced Nursing 24(2): 303–308

Gillon R 1994 Principles of health care ethics. John Wiley, Chichester

Good LP 1992 Compartment syndrome, a closer look at etiology, treatment. Association of Operating Room Nurses Journal 56(5): 904–911

Haines D 2000 My Ilizarov experience. Journal of Orthopaedic Nursing 4(4): 191–193

Herzig, Muller J, Schuren J 1999 A comparative study of the number of replacements required and application times for synthetic casts, Combicasts and plaster of Paris casts. Journal of Orthopaedic Nursing 3(4): 193–196

Heywood Jones I 1990 Making sense of traction. Nursing Times 86(23): 39–41

Jamieson E 1989 Strength and stability. Nursing Times 85(27) (suppl): 13–15

Kahle K, Anderson MB, Alpert J et al 1990 The value of preliminary traction in the treatment of congenital dislocation of the hip. Journal of Bone and Joint Surgery 72A(7): 1043–1047

Kalimo H, Rantanen J, Jarvinen M 1997 Muscle injuries in sports. Clinical Orthopaedics 2(1): 1–24

Kay J 1990 Trying to keep a balance. Nursing Times 86(19): 37

Large P 2001 A 'new focus' in casting – an introduction to the concepts of focus rigidity casting. Journal of Orthopaedic Nursing 5(4): 176–179

Lee-Smith J, Santy J, Davis P et al 2001 Pin-site management. Towards a consensus: part 1. Journal of Orthopaedic Nursing 5(1): 37–42

Levesque L, Grenier R, Kerouac S, Reidy M 1984 Evaluation of a presurgical group program given at two different times. Research in Nursing and Health 7: 227–236

Love C 1989 The light touch. Nursing Times 85(27) (suppl): 9–12

Love C 1998 A discussion and analysis of nurse-led pain assessment for the early detection of compartment syndrome. Journal of Orthopaedic Nursing 2(3): 160–167

Love C 2000 Bandaging skills for orthopaedic nurses. Journal of Orthopaedic Nursing 4(2): 84–91

Love C 2001 Using assisted walking devices. Journal of Orthopaedic Nursing 5(1): 45–53

Mandzuk L 1991 External pin-site care: a review of the literature and nursing practice. Canadian Orthopaedic Nursing Association Journal 13(1): 10–15

Mavrais R, Peck C, Coleman G 1990 The timing of pre-operative preparatory information. Psychology in Health 5: 39–45

McDonnell A 1999 A systematic review to determine the effectiveness of preparatory information in improving the outcomes of adult patients undergoing invasive procedures. Clinical Effectiveness in Nursing 3(1): 4–13

McQueen MM, Court-Brown CM 1996 Compartment monitoring in tibial fractures. The pressure threshold for decompression. Journal of Bone and Joint Surgery 78B(1): 99–104

Miles S 1997 The removal business: safely removing a cast. Journal of Orthopaedic Nursing 1(4): 195–197

Miles S, Barr L 1991 Principles of casting. In: A practical guide to casting. Smith and Nephew Medical, Hull

Mitchell M 2000 Nursing interventions for pre-operative anxiety. Nursing Standard 14(37): 40–43

Nichol D 1995 Understanding the principles of traction. Nursing Standard 9(46): 25–28

North American Nursing Diagnosis Association (NANDA) 2001 Nursing diagnoses: definitions and classification 2001–2002. North American Nursing Diagnosis Association, Philadelphia

Nursing and Midwifery Council (NMC) 2002 Code of professional conduct. Nursing and Midwifery Council, London

Olerud S 1990 External fixation of pelvic fractures. Current Orthopaedics 4: 33–39

Orford J 1989 Keeping things in place. Nursing Times 85(27) (suppl): 4–8

Ouellet LL, Rush KL 1992 A synthesis of selected literature on mobility: a basis for studying impaired mobility. Nursing Diagnosis 3(2): 72–80

Parker MJ, Handoll HHG 2001 Pre-operative traction for fractures of the proximal femur. Cochrane Library, Issue 2. Update Software, Oxford

Pearson A 1987 Living in a cast. Royal College of Nursing, London

Pennig D, Gausepohl T 1996 External fixation of the wrist. Injury 27(1): 1–15

Petty AC, Wardman C 1998 A randomized, controlled comparison of adjustable focused rigidity primary casting technique with standard plaster of Paris/synthetic casting technique in the management of fractures and other injuries. Journal of Orthopaedic Nursing 2(2): 95–102

Powell M 1986 Orthopaedic nursing and rehabilitation, 9th edn. Churchill Livingstone, Edinburgh

Price B 1990 A model for body-image care. Journal of Advanced Nursing 15: 585–593

Price B 1995 Assessing altered body image. Journal of Psychiatric and Mental Health Nursing 2: 169–175

Prior M, Miles S 1999 Principles of casting. Journal of Orthopaedic Nursing 3(3): 162–170

Rowe S 1997 A review of the literature on the nursing care of skeletal pins in the paediatric and adolescent setting. Journal of Orthopaedic Nursing 1(1): 26–29

Royal College of Nursing (RCN) 1999 Issues in nursing and health no. 50. Education and training in casting. Royal College of Nursing, London

Royal College of Nursing (RCN), Society of Orthopaedic and Trauma Nursing (SOTN) 2000 A framework for casting standard. Royal College of Nursing, London

Royal College of Nursing (RCN), Society of Orthopaedic and Trauma Nursing (SOTN) 2002 A traction manual. Royal College of Nursing, London

Salter M 1997 Altered body image: the nurse's role, 2nd edn. Baillière Tindall, London

Schoessler M 1989 Perceptions of pre-operative education in patients admitted the morning of surgery. Patient Education and Counselling 14: 127–136

Shuldham C 1999 A review of the impact of pre-operative education on recovery from surgery. International Journal of Nursing Studies 36: 171–177

Sims M, Bennett N, Broadley L et al 1999 External fixation: part 1. Journal of Orthopaedic Nursing 3(4): 203–209

Sims M, Bennett N, Broadley L et al 2000 External fixation: part 2. Journal of Orthopaedic Nursing 4(1): 26–32

Smith R, Draper P 1994 Who is in control? An investigation of nurse and patient beliefs relating to control of their health care. Journal of Advanced Nursing 19(5): 884–892

Smith Nephew 1991 A practical guide to casting. Smith and Nephew Medical Limited, Hull

Stewart JDM, Hallett JP 1983 Traction and orthopaedic appliances, 2nd edn. Churchill Livingstone, London

Thomas S, Dawes C, Hay P 1980 A critical evaluation of some extensible bandages in current use. Nursing Times 76(26): 1123–1126

Tingle J, Cribb A (eds) 1995 Nursing law and ethics. Blackwell, Oxford

Wallace LM 1985 Surgical patients' preferences for pre-operative information. Patient Education and Counselling 7: 377–387

Ward P 1998 Care of skeletal pins: a literature review. Nursing Standard 12(39): 34–38

Wicker P 1992 Orthopaedic trauma: perioperative care. Nursing Standard 6(20): 24–27

Williams S 1997 Quantitative study into the relationship between a patient's locus of control and their subsequent clinical outcome following joint replacement surgery. Journal of Orthopaedic Nursing 1(3): 137–143

Woo SL-Y, Hildebrand KA 1997 Healing of ligament injuries: from basic science to clinical practice. Baillière's Clinical Orthopaedics 2(1): 63–79

Wytch R, Ashcroft GP, Ledingham WM, Wardlaw D, Ritchie IK 1991 Modern splinting bandages. Journal of Bone and Joint Surgery 73B(1): 88–91

Younger ASE, Curran P, McQueen MM 1990 Backslabs and plaster casts: which will best accommodate increasing intracompartmental pressures? Injury 21: 179–181

Chapter 7

Pain management and orthopaedic care

Julie Gregory

INTRODUCTION

Orthopaedic patients commonly experience pain, particularly when moving (Davis 1997). The pain is a consequence of surgery and trauma and may lead to serious complications.

As pain is an individual subjective experience, it is difficult to define and describe. Many factors influence the acute pain experience, including the site and nature of the injury or surgery, personality, age, gender, social and cultural factors (Allcock 1996). Nurses provide the essential link in the provision of adequate pain relief, the principles of which include reducing anxiety, regular assessment of pain, appropriate administration of analgesics to achieve optimum pain relief (Buck & Paice 1994) and evaluation of its effectiveness.

The multidisciplinary approach to pain management involves the whole care team, including the pharmacist, physiotherapist, occupational therapist, orthopaedic medical and nursing staff, and the acute and chronic pain teams. They need to communicate effectively to manage the patient's pain in a coordinated and effective way. Lack of education and knowledge among health professionals about pain management is often cited as one of the reasons for inadequate pain relief (Thomas 1997), along with the inappropriate or underprescribing of analgesia and nurses' reluctance to challenge such prescriptions.

The aim of this chapter is to increase orthopaedic nurses' knowledge and understanding in order to empower them to provide a holistic approach to pain management.

CONSEQUENCES OF UNRELIEVED PAIN

Fear of pain and pain itself lead to immobility in orthopaedic patients, the implications of which include deep vein thrombosis, pressure ulcers and chest infections.

Pain can slow the return of normal gut activity and cause nausea, leading to a reduced fluid intake and dehydration. If fluids and diet are restricted for medical reasons or the patient is vomiting, then intravenous fluids are required, occasionally for longer than normal until the patient's pain and nausea symptoms subside.

Tachycardia and hypertension caused by pain can increase the risk of myocardial ischaemia or an infarction, especially if the patient has an existing heart disease. Poor pain relief impairs respiratory function, potentially leading to chest infections, hypoxia, respiratory failure and a longer hospital stay.

Metabolic and endocrine changes occur in response to the stress of major surgery or trauma. The response depends on the amount of damage to the tissues, although other factors such as pain, anxiety, nutritional state and cardiovascular changes are important. Reducing these factors can decrease the extent of the stress response which, if excessive, could lead to an infection or deep vein thrombosis, among other effects.

Psychologically, reactions to unrelieved pain include increased anxiety, fear, sleeplessness and fatigue (MacIntyre & Ready 2001). In turn these can lead to distrust and anger in patients and their relatives.

Effective pain relief is a basic human right and an essential element of good-quality care. It is no longer acceptable to see pain as a natural consequence of injury or trauma that will gradually reduce over time, as unrelieved pain can lead to the above complications, increased hospital stay and distress. Good pain relief will reduce the potential harmful effects and improve patients' outcomes (MacIntyre & Ready 2001). Patients who are pain free and comfortable will take a more active role in their nursing, physiotherapy and rehabilitation care.

WHAT IS PAIN?

The International Association for the Study of Pain (1986) views pain as an unpleasant sensory and emotional experience that is associated with actual or potential tissue damage or described in terms of such damage. This definition takes the interaction of the mind and body into account when trying to describe pain.

The other well-known nursing definition takes into account the subjective individual experience of pain by stating that 'Pain is what the experiencing person says it is and exists whenever he says it does' (McCaffery 1968, cited in McCaffery & Beebe 1989, p7).

ACUTE PAIN

This is characterised by a well-defined onset, accompanied by a stress response, resulting in sweating, vasoconstriction, raised heart rate and blood pressure. Acute pain from fractures, dislocations, traumatic injuries or postoperative joint replacement surgery normally responds well to analgesia and treatment of the underlying cause (Hawthorn & Redmond 1998). Acute pain has a protective warning function to avoid further damage and is one of the reasons people seek help.

CHRONIC OR LONG-TERM PAIN

In contrast, chronic pain is defined as having lasted for 3 months or more. Constant long-term pain changes the central nervous system, resulting in the individual no longer displaying the signs that accompany pain such as sweating and a raised pulse. This can lead to health professionals doubting the individual's pain (Hawthorn & Redmond 1998). At this point, the pain has stopped serving a useful purpose (Thomas 1997). Low back pain, osteoarthritis and rheumatoid disease are common examples of long-term chronic pain.

The individual with chronic pain is affected physically and psychologically. The pain results in inactivity, leading to decreased suppleness in the joints, progressive muscle weakness and fatigue. This can lead to loss of income, social withdrawal, demoralisation and preoccupation with the pain. Personal relationships become impaired, affecting families; this in turn leads to tension, arguments and feelings of hopelessness (Hawthorn & Redmond 1998).

The treatment of chronic pain involves the multidisciplinary team in helping the individual to resume activity. Conventional analgesia is reviewed and may be adjusted. Complementary therapies are often tried by patients, including acupuncture, transcutaneous electrical nerve stimulator (TENS), reflexology and aromatherapy.

Physiotherapy is used to reeducate the muscles and joints and to gradually increase the level of activity. Occupational therapy helps with pacing activities, to set realistic goals, plus advice on relaxation and coping strategies.

Psychology helps the individual to accept their pain by addressing negative beliefs and illness behaviour; these aspects are explored on an individual basis. Counselling can help some individuals.

Pain management programmes are becoming more available with suitable individuals attending for intensive help over a 2-week period or regular attendance at the clinic with the frequency of contact being reduced as the patient becomes more able to manage their pain.

THE MULTIDIMENSIONAL NATURE OF PAIN

Pain is a complex phenomenon involving the mind and body. Everyone has experienced pain at some time, each experience being individual and unique. Consequently, the reaction to pain differs between patients even when the injury is the same. The cause does not predict the amount of pain each person experiences, nor how they will tolerate or cope with the painful experience. It should also be remembered that individuals react differently to the treatment of pain.

There are a range of factors influencing perceptions and reactions to pain.

- The age of the individual. Younger people tend to exhibit pain behaviour, grimacing, rolling around and crying, whereas older people are less likely to move around when in pain and generally tend to be more stoical.
- A previous pain experience influences the individual's sense of control. A positive experience results in confidence, while a negative experience can result in apprehension and distrust.
- The fear and anticipation of pain lead to anxiety, with patients who have increased emotional distress reporting more pain. Consequently, allowing a sense of control helps a patient to cope with a stressful situation (Hawthorn & Redmond 1998).
- A lack of knowledge influences a person's belief about whether they have control over the situation. This is demonstrated by the provision of information prior to surgery which is known to have a positive effect on pain, with less analgesia being required (Heywood 1975).

- Pain is influenced by cultural values. Generally Western cultures value the scientific approach to pain and the importance of finding a medical diagnosis and cure. This can lead to unrealistic expectations of cure and relief from pain, especially for chronic pain sufferers. Other cultures are more accepting and find a meaning in their pain. In some cultures it is acceptable to openly demonstrate pain while in others the patient tends to withdraw and become silent. Practitioners need to be aware of their own and their patients' cultural values, in order to avoid finding different behaviours unacceptable or demanding (Hawthorn & Redmond 1998).
- Do women perceive and express pain more than men? Generally women are more aware of health problems and are more willing to accept help, whereas men may be less willing to report pain, especially to mainly female nurses. A macho or stoic attitude to pain tends to be valued amongst men (Hawthorn & Redmond 1998) but it does not mean that they experience less pain than women.

PHYSIOLOGY OF PAIN

The perception of pain is a function of the sensory nervous system. The nervous system is a communication system involving a two-way process, transmitting messages between the brain and the body with the interpretation of the pain sensation occurring in the higher brain centres.

The two types of nerve fibres, motor and sensory, are involved in the normal transmission and reaction to pain.

NOCICEPTIVE PAIN

Nociceptors are free nerve endings that are specialised pain receptors. They are located extensively in the dermal layer of the skin, periosteum of the bone, the articular surface of joints, walls of arteries and the dura mater. Deeper tissues have fewer nociceptors; hence, deeper tissue and organ trauma is less painful compared to dermal trauma. Fortunately, cutaneous pain receptors have a high threshold, otherwise all cutaneous sensations could be perceived as pain; instead a strong stimulus is required to generate the electrical signal initiating the pain pathway.

Somatic pain is defined as that arising from injury or surgery to bone, joints, muscles, skin or connective tissue. This pain is localised and decreases over time (Hall 2000).

Visceral pain arises from visceral organs such as the heart and bowels (Buck & Paice 1994). It tends to be poorly localised, can be referred to other parts of the body and is associated with nausea and vomiting (Hall 2000).

NEUROPATHIC PAIN

Neuropathic pain is associated with an injury or disease of the peripheral or central nervous system (MacIntyre & Ready 2001). Following an injury, changes occur peripherally or in the spinal cord, such as hyperexcitability of the peripheral nerves.

The symptoms for neuropathic pain include a delay in the onset of pain after injury and pain in the area of sensory loss. Patients experience and describe different sensations, for example shooting, burning, stabbing or an electric shock. This type of pain responds poorly to opioids.

The amputation of a limb leads to altered sensations commonly referred to as phantom limb pain, with the sensations being in the missing limb. Treatment for this requires a combination of pharmacological, physical and behavioural therapy (MacIntyre & Ready 2001).

PAIN FIBRES

There are two main pain nerve fibres: A delta and C fibres.

A delta fibres

These are small myelinated fast fibres conducting pain at 2.5–20 metres a second. They carry sharp prickling pain, which is precisely located (Park et al 2000). A delta pain is not affected by opiates (Carr & Mann 2000), meaning that the tenderness and pain carried by these fibres will not be masked following opiate analgesia, as traditionally thought. As a result, trauma patients continue to experience pain on movement after the administration of opiate analgesia.

C fibres

C fibres are unmyelinated slow fibres conducting pain at less than 2.5 metres a second, causing pain described by patients as dull, burning, aching, throbbing, persistent and poorly localised. This pain responds well to opiates.

The two types of nerve fibres work together, giving different sensations; for example, the immediate pain of surgery is due to A delta fibres but it becomes more widespread from the effect of C fibre transmission.

PAIN-PRODUCING SUBSTANCES

Tissues damaged by injury release histamine, prostaglandin and bradykinin. These combine with the nociceptor receptor sites to initiate neural transmission. The brain interprets the intensity of pain according to the number of pain impulses received within a period of time. The more impulses there are, the greater the intensity of pain experienced.

Prostaglandin is produced following the breakdown of phospholipids that make up the cell wall. They are amongst the most important mediators of pain and are synthesised from arachidonic acid by the enzyme cyclooxygenase. The prostaglandins sensitise nociceptors and enhance the effects of other pain-producing substances, including keeping the level of bradykinin high.

As part of the inflammatory response to trauma, bradykinin is produced from the kininogens in the small blood vessels and the nearby tissues. This stimulates the nociceptor receptor binding sites, initiating the chain of events in the perception of pain.

Histamine is also released in the immune response to damaged tissues. Histamine is a potent inflammatory agent that causes swelling by producing oedema and trapping waste products locally. At low levels, histamine activates an itching sensation but at high concentration, it evokes painful sensations.

The presence of substance P, a pain neurotransmitter, precipitates the release of bradykinin, serotonin and histamine. Other substances stimulate the pain pathway when they are released from damaged tissues, for example potassium.

Each individual produces different amounts of pain-producing substances and inhibitory neurotransmitters.

THE PAIN PATHWAY

There are four stages involved in pain physiology: transduction, transmission, perception and modulation.

Stage one: transduction

The nerve endings, or nociceptors, detect the stimulus from one or more processes.

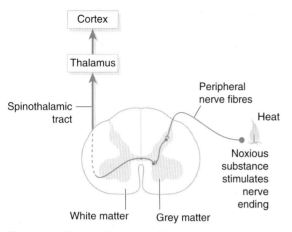

Figure 7.1   Cross-section of dorsal horn.

1 Mechanoreceptors are stimulated by a mechanical stimulus such as compression or stretching.
2 Temperature variations from heat and cold stimulate thermoreceptors.
3 Chemical stimulation of nociceptors by bradykinin, lactic acid, potassium or prostaglandin released from tissues damaged by injury, inflammation or surgery.

Once the stimulation of the nociceptors attached to the distal end of the primary afferent pain fibres reaches a certain level, it is converted into an electrical impulse.

Stage two: transmission

The electrical impulse is transported along the fibres to the central nervous system, entering the spinal cord in the grey matter at the dorsal horn (Fig. 7.1). Here the pain fibres synapse and the pain impulse passes from the dorsal horn to the opposite side of the spinal cord before ascending the spinothalamic tract to the thalamus in the brain (Buck & Paice 1994).

Stage three: perception

The higher pain centres in the brain interpret the electrochemical impulses. From the thalamus, the pain fibres synapse with more neurons, which transmit to the basal areas of the brain and the somatosensory cortex. Pain is felt in the midbrain but appreciation of its unpleasant qualities depends on the cerebral cortex (Buck & Paice 1994).

Stage four: modulation

Descending nerve tracts are mainly inhibitory, responsible for modulating pain perception (Park et al 2000). Descending control from the higher centres in the brain, involving the brainstem, reticular formation, hypothalamus and cerebral cortex, can modify the pain (see Fig. 7.2).

Endogenous opiates, the body's natural analgesics, are released in the dorsal horn of the spinal cord by the descending neurons. These endogenous opiates or neuron modulators bind to opiate receptor sites on the presynaptic membranes of pain fibres and inhibit the production of substance P.

The psychophysiological aspects of pain management, such as distraction, counselling and placebo effects, are explained by modulation.

The pathway cannot explain different pain experiences because each individual has a unique range of anatomical, physiological, social and psychological identities. Individualised pain relief, based on knowledge of the patient's background, progress of illness, pain behaviours and personal interpretation of the situation, is relevant to successful pain management (Buck & Paice 1994).

THE GATE CONTROL THEORY

Melzack & Wall (1965) proposed that the substantia gelatinosa in the grey matter of the spinal cord is the principal site of pain control. This site of control, referred to as a 'gate', is influenced by internal and external factors. The gate is symbolic of synapses between the afferent neurons and the various ascending and descending tracts. It explains some of the multidimensional aspects of pain and the wide variation of reactions to a painful experience.

Information about pain can only pass through when the gate is opened by the release at the synapse of a pain impulse, an excitatory neurotransmitter (Fig. 7.2). It is closed by the release of inhibitory neurotransmitters and neuromodulaters (Clancy & McVicar 1998).

More simply, imagine a garden gate. People entering through the gate represent pain impulses and when the gate is open they pass through easily. If the gate is partially open fewer people can enter; likewise less pain is transmitted. If a larger or faster impulse travelling along a thicker myelinated A beta fibre passes through the gate, it is harder for the pain impulse to pass through. These fibres are stimulated by rubbing or changes in temperature on the skin,

Pain perception involves the cascade of various chemicals irritating the nerve endings, resulting in the messages being relayed along the nerve to the central nervous system (CNS), initially to the spinal cord then to the brain. Once this impulse is interpreted, the response can be physical or emotional, the stimulation and perception depending on numerous factors as described. This helps to explain the wide range of reactions by individuals who have similar injuries.

PAIN ASSESSMENT

Good assessment is the cornerstone of effective symptom control.

ATTITUDES TO PAIN ASSESSMENT

For orthopaedic patients, pain is often very different when they move compared to sitting or lying still. Hence, during a medicine round, a pain assessment that only asks 'Do you have any pain, Mr Jones?' is often answered negatively as the patient is sitting still. Equally, there is no time to assess their pain in depth if the answer is yes; neither is an evaluation of the effectiveness of their analgesia appropriate at this time. Assessment of pain should be frequent, regular and part of routine practice so that the treatment of pain is approached in a logical, methodical and professional manner (Lovett 1994).

Both the absence of, and an inaccurate assessment of, a patient's pain are major obstacles to achieving effective pain management (Briggs 1995). Despite many research studies highlighting the lack of pain assessment (RCS/RCA 1990), there is evidence that use of pain tools and regular documentation of pain rarely occur in everyday practice (Hollingsworth 1994), with the patient's pain often being recorded inaccurately, incompletely and inconsistently.

Nurses have a professional responsibility to ensure the correct assessment of pain and to make appropriate decisions for interventions based on that assessment (Davis 1997). The use of analgesia cannot be planned without accurate knowledge of the nature and severity of the pain experienced. As a result, each nurse must take responsibility for systematically assessing pain and pain relief and recording this assessment. By doing so they expand the nurse's role in a truly nursing, rather than technical area (Seers 1987).

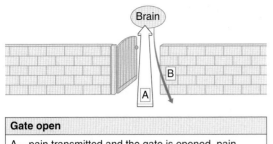

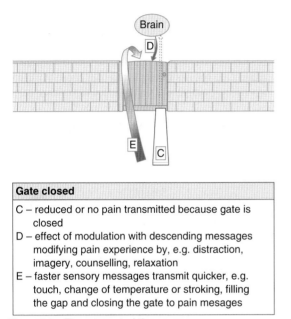

Gate open

A – pain transmitted and the gate is opened, pain messages pass freely
B – pain behaviours seen as a result, e.g. guarding, crying, anxiety

Gate closed

C – reduced or no pain transmitted because gate is closed
D – effect of modulation with descending messages modifying pain experience by, e.g. distraction, imagery, counselling, relaxation
E – faster sensory messages transmit quicker, e.g. touch, change of temperature or stroking, filling the gap and closing the gate to pain mesages

Figure 7.2   The gate control theory.

hence pinching an area prior to an injection helps to activate the A beta fibres, reducing or inhibiting the pain signals from the needle. Equally, heat or ice applied to the skin will send a temperature change message through the gate rather than the pain message. When people enter the gate from the other side, fewer people or no one can get through. Descending impulses from the brain, brainstem, cerebral cortex and thalamus also have an effect on the gate. An inhibitory signal from the cortex due to feeling confidant and in control helps to decrease pain perception. Likewise, modulation by distraction with guided imagery prevents or reduces the amount of pain felt.

One issue affecting pain assessment is the attitude of the nurse towards the person in pain. It is important to acknowledge the pain experience and spend time with the patient and never use the type of surgery or the number of days since the operation to indicate the type of analgesia required.

NURSES' PERCEPTIONS OF PAIN

Nurses' perception of pain is often very different from that of patients. Nurses usually underestimate patients' pain and overestimate the effectiveness of interventions. One simple question will not provide an accurate assessment of the patient's pain (Carr & Mann 2000, Hawthorn & Redmond 1998); neither will the physical signs and behaviours, which are relied upon by some nurses.

Seers' (1987) study showed that nurses infer less pain than the person experiencing it does, with 54% of nurses scoring pain lower than the patient, compared to 13% overestimating it. Three-quarters of the nurses said the analgesia was effective, yet a third of the patients had not been able to have analgesia when they wanted some. These results arose from patients waiting for nurses to ask them if they had pain or to provide analgesia, while at the same time nurses were waiting for the patient to 'complain of pain'. This indicates the need for nurses to be proactive and assess pain regularly.

According to Hollingsworth (1994), British nurses find it particularly difficult to cope with expressive patients. This does not mean that nurses in other countries find this aspect of practice easier or that they cope with it any better. It does show the importance of nurses realising their own values and attitudes when assessing pain (Sofaer 1992), as non-judgemental nurses carry out more accurate pain assessments (Thomas 1997). In the United States pain scores are recognised as the fifth vital sign and recorded along with temperature, pulse, respiration and blood pressure (Joint Commission for the Accreditation of Healthcare Organisations 2000). This approach ensures pain is taken more seriously and should be considered when developing pain management practices.

Readers should consider their own reactions. For instance, do colleagues admire people who persevere despite pain or who refuse analgesia, saying they can manage without? As some patients may feel they are treated more favourably if they do not complain of pain, nurses need to be aware of how their personal values and perceptions affect their judgement of patients.

An initial accurate pain assessment establishes a baseline identifying the location, nature and severity of the pain, helps in the selection of appropriate interventions and provides a measure of a patient's response to treatment (Thomas 1997). In doing so it gives the patient's description of the pain, quantifies it, helps nurses to understand the nature of the individual's experience and makes the healthcare professional responsible and accountable for pain management (Thomas 1997).

PAIN ASSESSMENT TOOLS

A simple assessment tool can eliminate some of the problems associated with assessing a very subjective phenomenon. Only patients can measure their pain accurately, so nurses need to provide them with the means to help them assess and communicate their pain (Baillie 1993). The assessment tool then conveys to the patient that the nurse has a genuine concern and interest in their pain and provides the basis for communication between the patient and the healthcare team, helping to build the therapeutic relationship.

It could be argued that this oversimplifies the pain by reducing it to a single number or word. To some extent, it does; there is no single ideal measure of pain. The intensity of the pain experience cannot be directly measured, neither can the profound emotional aspects that alter the patient's perception of their own pain. The patient's expression of pain is the most reliable index; after all, they are the experts.

The use of a tool reduces the chance of bias and error. Thomas (1997) suggests that a subjective assessment reflecting the multidimensional aspect of pain is appropriate, with the assessment being carried out with the patient, not on the patient (Seers 1987), thereby actively involving the patient in their pain management (Hawthorn & Redmond 1998).

Visual analogue scale (VAS)

This scale consists of a straight line, usually 10 cm long (Fig. 7.3). One end is marked 'no pain', the opposite end marked 'worst possible pain'. It is used vertically or horizontally, with the patient being asked to put a mark on the line at the point that represents their level of pain at that moment.

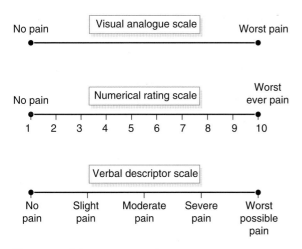

Figure 7.3 Pain assessment scales.

This method is used widely, especially in research. The advantages of a VAS are that:

- patients can mark exactly their level of pain
- it results in a sensitive measure that reflects changes over time and with different interventions. For example, an initial mark at the 7.25 cm point, as measured from the no pain end of the scale, will change to a lower point with an effective intervention
- it is quick and easy to use, easily reproduced and universally used to measure pain and the effectiveness of pain relief.

The limitations of a VAS are that it:

- is a one-dimensional measure of pain
- reflects the pain experienced only at that moment
- is difficult for confused, elderly patients, children and those with impaired cognitive function as it requires a degree of abstract thinking to use a VAS
- requires adequate vision
- it is felt to be irrelevant by patients in severe or chronic pain.

Numerical rating scale (NRS)

With a NRS, patients are asked to rate their pain with a number, generally on a 0–10 scale where 0 is no pain and 10 is unbearable or the worst pain experienced (Fig. 7.3). Some units use a 0–3 or 0–5 scale on the same basis. Careful instructions are required, particularly if the pain is severe.

The advantages are that it allows greater sensitivity and avoids misunderstandings that occur when words are used. The limitations relate to people who have difficulty in imagining their pain as a number.

Verbal descriptor scale (VDS)

Here words are used to describe the level of pain, for example no pain, mild, moderate or severe pain (Fig. 7.3). The advantages of a VDS are that they are quick and easy to use, can be easily adapted and often combined with a numerical score. Baillie's (1993) review of pain assessment tools, comparing VAS, NRS and VDS tools, showed that patients preferred VDS. Patients with limited intelligence, impaired motor skills or severe pain tend to find VDS more suitable.

The main limitations of a VDS relate to the words used and assumptions that there are similar intervals between the words. However, patients will describe their pain in different ways at different times and different patients will describe the same experience in different ways. As a result, VDS tools lack sensitivity as the terms can be misinterpreted and patients can find it hard to express small changes in their pain.

Verbal descriptor numerical scores

Here a number is added to the description used to express the pain; for example, 0 = no pain, 1 = mild pain, 2 = moderate pain and 3 = severe pain. These have some of the advantages and limitations of a VDS and NRS as described above.

Postoperative pain is best assessed by a simple scale such as a VAS, VDS or verbal descriptor numerical score as they are quick and easy to use in an acute surgical setting (RCS/RCA 1990).

Questionnaires

A McGill questionnaire contains 78 adjectives reflecting the dimensions of:

- sensory aspects: flicking, stabbing, burning and stabbing
- affective terms: tension, fear and punishment
- autonomic aspects: exhausting, frightening, punishing and sickening
- evaluative descriptions: miserable, annoying and unbearable.

A shortened form of the questionnaire is used clinically and in research to obtain information in a shorter time than a standard McGill questionnaire (Fig. 7.4).

PLEASE SELECT FROM THE LIST BELOW WORDS THAT YOU WOULD USE TO DESCRIBE YOUR PAIN
(Tick the appropriate column for each word):

	NONE	MILD	MODERATE	SEVERE
Throbbing				
Shooting				
Stabbing				
Sharp				
Cramping				
Gnawing				
Hot-burning				
Aching				
Heavy				
Tender				
Splitting				
Tiring-exhausting				
Sickening				
Fearful				
Punishing-cruel				

CIRCLE A NUMBER BELOW TO INDICATE THE INTENSITY OF YOUR PAIN: between 0 = NO PAIN and 10 = WORST PAIN

a) **RIGHT NOW:**

NO PAIN   0 1 2 3 4 5 6 7 8 9 10   WORST POSSIBLE PAIN

b) **AT ITS WORST IN THE LAST MONTH**

NO PAIN   0 1 2 3 4 5 6 7 8 9 10   WORST POSSIBLE PAIN

c) **AT ITS BEST IN THE LAST MONTH**

NO PAIN   0 1 2 3 4 5 6 7 8 9 10   WORST POSSIBLE PAIN

PRESENT PAIN INDEX:

Which of the following words explains your present pain (tick one only):

0	NO PAIN	
1	MILD	
2	DISCOMFORTING	
3	DISTRESSING	
4	HORRIBLE	
5	EXCRUCIATING	

Figure 7.4 Short-form McGill questionnaire. (Reproduced with permission from the Bolton Hospitals NHS Trust.)

PAEDIATRIC PAIN ASSESSMENT

In paediatric care, a child's inability to speak or express their pain leads to reliance on behaviour and physiological changes. Infants' facial expressions provide obvious evidence of pain, along with crying which clearly conveys distress, the cry is generally at a higher pitch if they are in pain compared to crying due to hunger.

Behavioural changes, including movements, depend on the age of the child. Toddlers from the age of 18 months to 3 years can express pain as a hurt (Thomas 1997). Parents are reliable sources of information in identifying behavioural changes that enable assessment of their child's pain.

Paediatric pain assessment scales

There are a wide range of assessment tools available (Figs 7.5, 7.6), the most commonly used being the 'Oucher' scale or the smiley faces developed for children aged 3–12 years (Thomas 1997).

Pain drawings (Fig. 7.7) involve the child colouring in a body outline using different colours for varying intensity of pain. The child chooses the colours that reflect different levels of their pain; red and black are commonly associated with severe pain.

Numerical and descriptor scales are useful for older children.

ASSESSING PAIN

The assessment needs to be carried out as early as possible. It is a two-way process involving listening to the patient and providing information about the importance and benefits of effective pain relief. Patients may worry that reporting pain will increase their length of time in hospital or they may be afraid of what the pain may signify.

Assessment strategies

Effective communication is vital in all aspects of assessment. This involves carefully listening to the patient, asking clear questions and believing what is said. Difficulties that arise include patients' reluctance to discuss their pain, a lack of vocabulary, inability to speak the same language and a cognitive impairment. Some patients do not use the word 'pain'; they may describe a heaviness, discomfort or unpleasant feeling.

As part of the assessment, the patient should be asked what they think is causing their pain, as they may associate it with factors other than those obvious to the healthcare professionals. Additional factors that need to be established are listed in Box 7.1.

Often asking is not enough so observing patients' behaviour provides clues that are essential to identify if the patient is unable to express their pain.

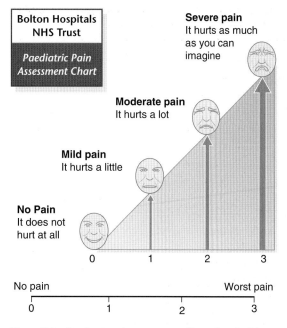

Figure 7.5 Paediatric pain assessment. (Reproduced with permission from the Bolton Hospitals NHS Trust.)

According to Carr & Mann (2000), observations indicating pain include:

- **body language**: keeping still, guarding, rocking, restlessness and changes in walking gait
- **facial expression**: tears, grimacing, muscle tension, look of alarm, squinting or clenching teeth
- **vocalising**: sighing, crying, moaning, change in pitch, impaired speech, calling out
- **distance**: quiet, withdrawn or uncommunicative
- **emotional**: worried, angry, sad or a change in mood.

ACTION OF ANALGESICS

The transduction, transmission, perception and modulation of pain signals lead to its interpretation by the brain. Analgesia aims to block these signals at some point along the pathway. It may stop the formation of prostaglandins, block the transmission along the nerves or alter the perception of pain in the cerebral cortex.

OPIOIDS

The effects of opioids occur mainly within the CNS; these are grouped as depressant and stimulant effects (Table 7.1). The fear of addiction, dependence, tolerance and respiratory depression can stop patients asking for analgesia. Underprescribing by medical staff and underadministration by nurses compound this (see Table 7.2 for opioid drugs and their equivalent doses). Patients also have fears about opiates, particularly morphine, leading to their reluctance to take adequate analgesia and failing to report pain (Day 1997).

Eyes
Tightly shut, despite the baby being wide awake. Often the effort involved will make the eyelids flutter

Brow
Tight lines across the brow or around the eyes indicate discomfort

Mouth
Tight lines around the mouth, also shape of the mouth and position of the tongue can show problems

Thumbs
Clenched tightly inside the fist, showing stress

Toes
Big toe is held apart from others. Also other toes can be held rigidly apart

Bolton Hospitals NHS Trust
Pain Assessment Tool

This tool is based on a modified version of the Neonatal Infant Pain Scale (NIPS) devised by the Children's Hospital of Eastern Ontario (1989)

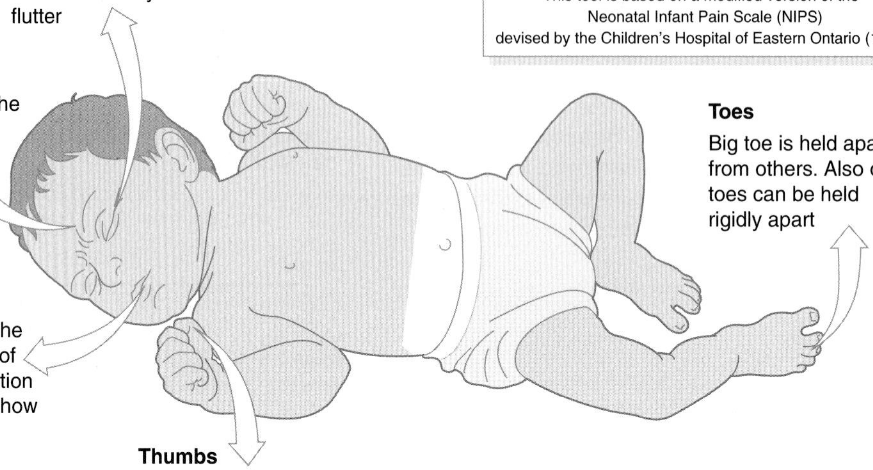

A **Cry**

    0 Quiet
    1 Whimper
    2 Vigorous

B **State of arousal**

    0 Calm   Quiet, peaceful. Sleeping or awake but settled
    1 Fussy   Restless, fretful

C **Facial expression**

    0 Restful   Relaxed facial muscles, neutral expression
    1 Grimace   Tight facial muscles, furrowed brow, chin and jaw

D **Breathing pattern**

    0 Relaxed   The usual pattern for this baby
    1 Changes in breathing Inspirations irregular, faster than usual, breath holding

E **Arms**

    0 Relaxed   No muscular rigidity. Occasional random movements
    1 Tense   Rigid and/or rapid flexion/extension

F **Legs**

    0 Relaxed   No muscular rigidity. Occasional random movements
    1 Tensed   Rigid and/or rapid flexion/extension

G **Fingers/hands**

    0 Normal   Normal grasp for this baby
    1 Tensed   Thumb folded into palm, difficult to uncurl fingers

Figure 7.6   Neonatal pain assessment. (Reproduced with permission from the Bolton Hospitals NHS Trust.)

Morphine is the cornerstone of analgesia for severe pain (Buck & Paice 1994). It is naturally derived from opium poppies and has been used for over 2000 years. Morphine acts on special opiate receptors in the nervous system, mainly in the midbrain and the posterior horn of the spinal cord. It binds with these receptors and activates them, mimicking the action of the endogenous opiate enkephalin. Once morphine binds with the receptors, transmission of the pain impulse is suppressed, thus relieving pain.

When given by injection, the analgesic effect occurs quickly. After absorption morphine is metabolised in the liver into morphine-6-glucuronide, which is the active analgesic constituent of morphine; this is later excreted by the kidneys. Repeated administrations are effective as the kidneys slowly excrete the morphine-6-glucuronide. The amount of morphine required to achieve pain relief varies widely between patients, depending on the severity of their pain, the sensitivity of the patient to the drug and the dose.

Diamorphine is rapidly diffused into the brain and converted to morphine: 5 mg diamorphine is equivalent to 10 mg morphine.

Fentanyl has a short duration of action and little cardiovascular depression. It is used mainly intra-operatively and for critically ill patients in the ICU and is administered into the epidural space to provide an epidural analgesia.

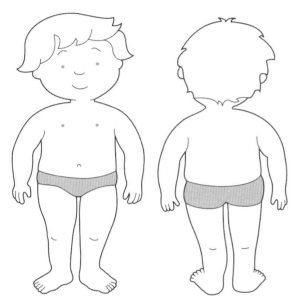

Figure 7.7   Pain drawings. (Reproduced with permission from the Bolton Hospitals NHS Trust.)

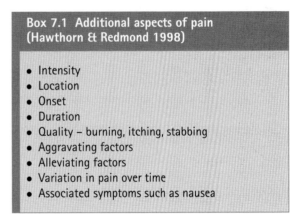

Box 7.1   Additional aspects of pain (Hawthorn & Redmond 1998)

- Intensity
- Location
- Onset
- Duration
- Quality – burning, itching, stabbing
- Aggravating factors
- Alleviating factors
- Variation in pain over time
- Associated symptoms such as nausea

Table 7.1   Effect of opioids

Depressant effects	• Depress the appreciation of pain by the brain. If pain is felt it seems to have lost its unpleasant nature • Reduce anxiety and is euphoric • Depress respiration by acting on the respiratory centre in the medulla oblongata, to reduce its responsiveness to carbon dioxide. Result is a slow respiratory rate with a large tidal volume • Depress the cough centre and thus damp down the cough reflex. This is related to codeine and diamorphine, rather than morphine • Are mild hypnotics and may produce drowsiness and sleep; this may also be from pain relief (Park et al 2000)
Stimulating effects	• Stimulate the chemoreceptor trigger zone in the brainstem, causing nausea and vomiting in about 30% of patients. This effect is enhanced on movement • Constriction of pupils as a result of stimulating the ocular motor nerve • Increase the tone of smooth muscle throughout the gastrointestinal tract. Gastric emptying and transit time are delayed, leading to constipation • Contraction of smooth muscle in the bladder and urinary sphincter which may lead to retention of urine • Stimulate the vagus nerve, may slow the pulse and lower the blood pressure • Morphine releases histamine, producing allergic reactions. This can lead to vasodilation, flushing, itching and can cause bronchoconstriction (Park et al 2000)

Table 7.2 Doses of commonly used drugs equivalent to morphine 10 mg and the delivery mode (adapted from Park et al 2000)

Drug name	Adult dose	Paediatric dose	Onset of action	Duration
Morphine	2–5 mg IV 5–15 mg IM 30–40 mg orally	0.02 mg/kg IV 0.2 mg/kg IM	5–10 min IV 15–20 min IM	3 h
Diamorphine	2–5 mg IV/IM	0.1 mg/kg IM	2–5 min IV 5–10 min IM	3 h
Pethidine	10–20 mg IV 50–150 mg IM 50–300 mg orally	Not recommended	10–15 min IM 15–30 min orally	2 h
Fentanyl	50–200 μg IV	1–3 μg/kg IV	1–2 min IV	30–60 min
Methadone	5–10 mg IM 10–15 mg orally	Not recommended	10–15 min IM 30–60 min orally	6–8 h
Codeine	30–60 mg IM 30–60 mg orally	3 mg/kg IM daily in divided doses	10–15 min IM 30–60 min orally	4–6 h
Tramadol	50–100 mg IV/IM/orally	Not recommended		

Pethidine is a poor analgesic, especially for orthopaedic pain. It has a short duration of action with its metabolite, norpethidine, becoming toxic with larger doses and repeated administration. It is used when a patient is allergic to morphine.

Methadone is a synthetic opioid with a prolonged duration of action and slow elimination. The duration of the analgesic effect is 6–8 hours. Like pethidine, methadone is not licensed for paediatric pain. It is not commonly used for its analgesic properties but can be used to prevent withdrawal symptoms for drug-using patients.

Codeine is obtained from opium. It can be given orally or by intramuscular injection but is not given intravenously as it causes a profound histamine release. About 10–14% of a dose of codeine is converted to morphine but approximately 10% of the population lack the enzyme required for this conversion. Dihydrocodeine is similar to codeine, given in smaller doses (Park et al 2000).

Tramadol is a synthetic opioid effective for moderate to severe pain. It is effective for some orthopaedic pain, especially if codeine is ineffective. It is not licensed for paediatric care. Tramadol is given orally or as an injection and can be used as a patient-controlled analgesic if the patient has a high risk of respiratory depression. In comparison to morphine, respiratory depression is not a problem. It is less constipating and it is not subject to controlled drug regulations. The main side effect is nausea and vomiting, although this appears to be less troublesome with the longer-acting slow-relief tablets. Some patients, particularly the elderly, experience confusion while taking tramadol.

The nursing actions related to the care of the patient on opioids are listed in Table 7.3.

Intramuscular opioids

Traditionally opioids were administered intramuscularly (IM) 4–6 hourly as required but this provides poor-quality analgesia as it fails to take into account wide variations in requirements and the time taken from experiencing pain to pain relief (Fig. 7.8). Subcutaneous and IM routes are the least reliable methods of administration as the rate of absorption is variable with the peak effect taking up to 1 hour to occur. They also inflict pain from the injection and may deter patients from requesting further analgesia (Buck & Paice 1994).

Complications of IM injection include bruising, especially in anticoagulated patients, and damage to the sciatic nerve if injected into the buttock. It is less effective and potentially dangerous if the patient is hypovolaemic because their low circulatory volume prevents its absorption, giving a low analgesic effect

Table 7.3   Monitoring of patients on opioid therapy

Nursing diagnosis	Nursing action
Altered sedation level	Monitor sedation levels for all patients receiving opioid drugs
Altered respiratory rate and potential changed oxygen levels	Opioids reduce the respiratory rate; this must be monitored with the sedation level. A respiratory rate of less than 8 per minute in an unresponsive patient requires immediate intervention. Pulse oximetry allows oxygen saturation of haemoglobin monitoring. Normal saturation is 95–100%. This is useful in detecting hypoxia; however, if a patient is on oxygen therapy a low saturation may not be detected and if the patient is anaemic low oxygen levels may not be detected
Changes to pain score	Regular assessment and evaluation of the analgesia is required
Changed observations from pain	Pulse and blood pressure monitoring for hypotensive effects of the opioids
Nausea from pain	Monitor any nausea and prevent vomiting by administering appropriate antiemetic
Potential side effects from opioid analgesia	Measure urinary output to detect early signs of retention. Observe for itchiness or a rash indicating a histamine reaction and treat with antihistamine as prescribed. Monitor for constipation, a common problem that can be anticipated with the use of appropriate laxatives and a high fluid and fibre intake

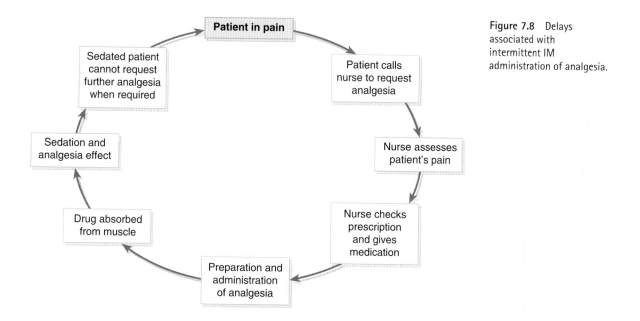

Figure 7.8   Delays associated with intermittent IM administration of analgesia.

and resulting in repeated doses being given. As the patient's circulation to the muscles improves, the sudden absorption of the opioid causes unexpected, delayed or adverse effects (Park et al 2000).

Once the patient is tolerating oral fluids, severe pain is best treated with an oral opioid as there is little difference between the speed of onset of pain relief with oral and IM administration, with the dose being titrated against the patient's pain relief (Day 1997).

Respiratory depression is reversed by the use of naloxone, which binds to the opioid receptors. Unfortunately, it also reverses the analgesic effect, causing ventricular arrhythmias, pulmonary oedema and sudden death, so warrants extreme caution (Buck & Paice 1994). Naloxone is given diluted to 0.4 mg in 10 ml of normal saline, with 1 ml being slowly administered every 2 minutes.

Intravenous opioids

The intravenous (IV) route is the most rapid and predictable route for opiates, with the slow

---

Box 7.2   Advantages and disadvantages of patient–controlled analgesia (Park et al 2000)

Advantages	Disadvantages
• Patient feels in control of their pain • Flexible pain relief • Overcomes the wide variation of opioid requirement for individuals • Lowers the requirement for morphine • Bypasses delays in administration by traditional intermittent IM analgesia • Linked to earlier mobilisation • Safe method of IV administration • Can be used with children from 4 years upwards	• Patient suitability needs careful selection • Education and explanation required • Some individuals do not want control, preferring nurses to administer analgesia • Electronic devices are initially expensive and require maintenance

---

administration of morphine, titrated against the individual's pain, providing relief within minutes. It is unusual to use a continuous infusion of morphine on busy trauma wards, as constant monitoring is required.

Patient–controlled analgesia (PCA)

PCA provides the means of infusing analgesia on demand using morphine or other drugs in a disposable or electronic device. It provides analgesia tailored to the individual patient's analgesic requirements, avoiding dependence and delays from waiting for oral or intramuscular analgesia to be given.

It is ideal for patients in severe pain or when oral fluids are restricted. Although normally used for postoperative pain management, it can be used for trauma patients prior to any surgical intervention. Disposable PCA devices introduced for trauma patients in A & E have ensured continued pain management when admitted to the trauma wards (J Gregory 2002, presentation at RCN Society of Orthopaedic Nursing Conference). The main advantage is that the patient is in control of their pain and analgesia (Box 7.2).

An initial loading dose is given to provide initial pain control. This is a variable amount depending on the severity of the pain and the individual's requirement. Once this has taken effect the patient is given the button to use as they need. The PCA allows the patient to administer a small preset dose by activating the button attached to the syringe pump or disposable device. The initial demand is usually high, followed by stable maintenance doses with the demand naturally declining as the patient recovers from their injury or surgery.

The patient must be alert enough to press the demand button. If the patient becomes sedated, demand reduces but they may still experience severe pain on waking. The device has a lock-out period of usually 5 minutes, during which no drug is delivered despite any demands made by the patient. Only the patient must press the button; relatives and staff must be informed not to use the device.

Patient education and teaching is vital to ensure the PCA is effective (Park et al 2000). Practitioners must understand the rationales, processes and philosophy behind the use of a PCA system. To ensure good practice, standards in prescribing and clearly written protocols or guidelines are required (MacIntyre & Ready 2001).

NON-STEROIDAL ANTIINFLAMMATORY DRUGS (NSAIDs)

Non-steroidal antiinflammatory drugs act peripherally at the site of injury (Park et al 2000), by interrupting the inflammatory response. By lowering the body temperature, they act as antipyretic analgesics.

NSAIDs are used for headache, migraine, dysmenorrhoea, injuries, for the pain and inflammation of arthritis, musculoskeletal disorders and postoperative pain (White 2001). They are much less likely to cause sedation, respiratory depression or mood change than opioids. Given orally, they are very effective for moderate to severe postoperative pain. Indeed, as McQuay & Moore (1998) point out, it can be difficult to distinguish between the analgesic effects of intramuscular morphine and oral NSAIDs.

Physiological effect of NSAIDs

This group of drugs inhibits the enzyme cyclooxygenase, of which there are different types (Park et al 2000).

• COX 1 is involved in producing prostaglandins with a regulating function; for example, they

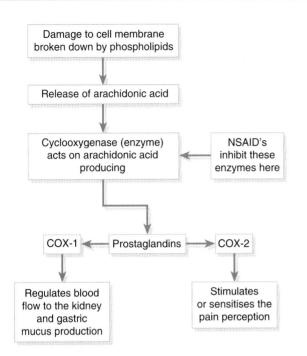

Figure 7.9 Mechanism of prostaglandin inhibition.

regulate the blood flow to the kidneys and the production of gastric mucosa.

- COX 2 is produced as a response to cellular damage and is responsible for prostaglandins causing nociceptor sensitisation.

As NSAIDs block the formation of both COX 1 and COX 2 (Fig. 7.9), they result in unwanted side effects. Cyclooxygenase is necessary for the production of prostaglandins, which protect the gastrointestinal mucosa. With the absence of prostaglandins, some patients will experience dyspepsia, peptic ulceration and gastric bleeds, with 10–30% of people who take long-term NSAIDs having gastrointestinal damage (White 2001). The effects on the stomach are more marked in the elderly due to thinning of the gastric mucosa with age.

Inhibition of prostaglandins also leads to bleeding abnormalities, which affect the platelets' ability to aggregate and increase the bleeding times (Buck & Paice 1994).

In addition, NSAIDs cause acute renal nephritis from decreased renal blood flow and glomerular function. They cause sodium retention, due to the inhibition of renal prostaglandins, which enhances the reabsorption of sodium. Those particularly at risk are elderly patients, dehydrated patients and those on diuretics.

One in 10 asthmatics may have acute bronchospasm as an allergic reaction to NSAIDs. Additionally, at high doses, NSAIDs produce tinnitus and impaired hearing.

The risks of the side effects have to be balanced with the potential benefits. The use of NSAIDs has been shown to reduce the amount of opiates required postoperatively by improving the quality of pain relief; patients can move more freely, are less sedated and have fewer nausea, vomiting and respiratory problems. For nursing implications see Box 7.3.

Bone metabolism has a complex regulatory system that involves prostaglandins. Animal studies suggest that the presence of prostaglandins improves bone healing. However, a randomised controlled trial study by Rueben (2001) on patients with Colles' fractures taking NSAIDs found they had no effect on bone healing. A study of 32 patients (Giannoudis et al 2000) suggested that NSAIDs inhibited fracture healing but this was a retrospective study of unhealed fractures. No other studies of unhealed fractures have identified NSAIDs as a cause (Bandolier 2002) and according to Bandolier, there is currently no strong evidence that NSAIDs have a detrimental effect in bone healing.

Types of NSAID drugs

There are a large number of NSAIDs available, diclofenac (Voltarol) and ibuprofen being the most commonly used. Diclofenac is administered orally, rectally or intramuscularly, although as there is a risk of abscesses with IM administration, this method is avoided. Ibuprofen is widely available without prescription, in syrup, tablet and meltlet form. There is no significant difference between ibuprofen and diclofenac; both drugs work well for postoperative pain (McQuay & Moore 1998).

Feldene (piroxicam) is a beneficial drug to use as a meltlet immediately after surgery when patients are not eating or drinking.

Injectable versions include mobiflex and ketorolac. There is no evidence that injection or the rectal route is any quicker or more effective than orally administered NSAIDs (McQuay & Moore 1998). The oral route is the simplest and preferred by patients.

The topical drugs, for example ibuprofen, ketoprofen and piroxicam, are valuable for both acute and chronic pain as this method has a low incidence of adverse effects (McQuay & Moore 1998).

Newer antiinflammatory agents act more specifically on the COX 2 pathway. Celecoxib is used for chronic or long-term pain and has a lower incidence of gastric ulcers in comparison to ibuprofen and diclofenac. Rofecoxib also has significantly fewer gastrointestinal problems in comparison to naproxen but in trials the rofecoxib group was found to have an unexpected excess of cardiovascular events (Medical Control Agency 2002). The National Institute for Clinical Excellence has emphasised the use of these newer, though expensive, drugs for patients with a high risk of gastrointestinal bleeds (Jones 2002).

PARACETAMOL

Paracetamol is an effective analgesic for mild pain, being weaker than non-steroidal analgesia with less inhibition of cyclooxygenase. Its specific method of action is not clear but it is known to act centrally to lower the body temperature. It is a widely used but often undervalued analgesic for mild pain that can be given orally, rectally or by injection.

Schug et al (1998) suggest that paracetamol should be used in combination with an opioid wherever possible. Dolbos & Boccard (1995), who demonstrated a significant reduction in pain scores and morphine demand from a PCA after knee ligament surgery, support this.

Codeine is frequently combined with paracetamol to increase the analgesic effect (McQuay & Moore 1998).

Paracetamol also enhances the analgesic efficiency of NSAIDs (Hyllested et al 2002). Hyllested et al's review found the combination of paracetamol and ketorolac reduced patients' pain scores at rest and on

movement following surgery, with a notable 33–46% reduction in the use of opioids when both drugs were used compared with paracetamol alone.

LOCAL ANAESTHETICS (LA)

Local anaesthetics act by directly inhibiting nerve conduction, giving a very effective method of controlling pain. Bupivacaine is commonly used, as its effects are generally longer acting (12–24 hours) than those of lidocaine (lignocaine) (1–2 hours).

The potential side effects of LA are associated with high blood concentrations. This can occur after accidental injection of local anaesthetic into a blood vessel or absorption of large amounts. Numbness of the tongue and mouth are early indicators, along with ringing in the ears and a light-headed sensation. If blood levels continue to rise, generalised convulsions occur followed by respiratory depression and cardiac arrest. The effect on heart rhythms is seen when a bradycardia occurs from a LA given at a very high rate through an epidural.

EPIDURAL ANALGESIA

The epidural route has been widely accepted as the most effective way of providing acute pain relief. It is especially good for managing pain associated with activity such as on movement and coughing (MacIntyre & Ready 2001).

The anaesthetist initiates the choice of an epidural for pain management. Epidural analgesia is used for labour and caesarean sections, postoperative pain relief following major abdominal and joint replacement surgery, chest injuries, trauma, chronic and cancer pain.

The advantages of epidural analgesia are noticeable when practitioners assess and document the patients' pain scores and pain relief and evaluate the effectiveness of the intervention. The patient is less sedated and has better pain control than if they are having intramuscular opioids; they can participate in their nursing and rehabilitation care, allowing more comfortable chest physiotherapy and earlier mobilisation.

The disadvantages relate to the potential complications of any epidural: nerve damage, a dural tap, headache, backache, urinary retention, respiratory depression, nausea and vomiting. The potential risks must be weighed against the advantages for individual patients (MacIntyre & Ready 2001).

The aspects to be considered in the safe use of epidural analgesia are:

- appropriate patient selection
- having appropriate standing orders, nursing procedures or protocols
- education of nursing and other healthcare staff in the care and management of the patient
- regular review of patients by the nursing and pain management team as appropriate
- availability of anaesthetists to manage any complications.

The two main agents used in the epidural space for analgesia are local anaesthetics and opioids (Cox 2001).

Drugs given via an epidural

Local anaesthetics (LA) act by stopping the action potential along the nerve fibres transmitting pain. A LA can be used alone when opioids are contraindicated, for example using 0.125–0.25% of bupivacaine. As a LA causes vasodilation, it often results in a low blood pressure, which is compounded if the patient is hypovolaemic. In such cases the hypotension usually responds to intravenous fluids.

The LA can affect the motor nerves, especially if administered in high concentrations. This means patients are unable to move their lower limbs and may experience urinary retention. It is unlikely to cause sedation, nausea and vomiting or pruritus. In very high doses or accidental intravenous administration, bradycardia and hypotension may occur; in the extreme this can result in cardiac arrest.

When used in an epidural, opiates act by attaching themselves to the opiate receptors found in the spinal cord. The drug is then absorbed into the blood vessels, resulting in the normal side effects of opiates, although these are less severe than when opiates are given intramuscularly or intravenously.

Epidural analgesia is usually prescribed as a combination of low concentration local anaesthetic and opiate agents to achieve a minimum motor block and good analgesic effect. Less is required of both agents and therefore an effective level of analgesia is maintained while reducing the potential side effects of respiratory or motor depression. Examples of commonly used mixtures are:

- 0.1% bupivacaine and 2 mg fentanyl or 20 mg morphine

- 0.125% bupivacaine and 5 mg fentanyl or 40 mg morphine.

The infusion rate will vary according to the concentrations, site of insertion, injury and type of surgery (MacIntyre & Ready 2001).

Preprinted prescription forms are generally used with standard mixtures of local anaesthetic and opiates. Prefilled bags are available commercially to reduce the risk of calculation errors and potential contamination risks. Specific forms (Fig. 7.10) are used to document observations and ensure regular monitoring of pain and sedation scores.

Patient-controlled epidural analgesia (PCEA)

This is a rarely used application of epidural analgesia, combining effective epidural analgesia with a patient control system. A loading dose is required and a background or continuous infusion is used. An example of a PCEA would involve bupivacaine 0.1% with fentanyl 5 µg, started with a bolus dose and continued with a background infusion and further small pre-set doses via the patient-controlled system.

Nursing management of an epidural infusion

It is important to advise the patient of the implications relating to the insertion of the epidural, analgesia effect and nursing care implications (Box 7.4). Information should be verbal and in writing; for elective patients this should be in the preadmission clinic to give the patient time to consider the implications and make an informed choice.

Having an epidural should not restrict movement, as patients with an epidural analgesia in progress can sit out of bed and mobilise. This should be done slowly as the patient may have postural hypotension and potentially weak legs (MacIntyre & Ready 2001).

Compartment syndrome can be masked by epidural analgesia. However, the pain from compartment syndrome is generally very severe; if patients complain of unexpectedly restricted movement or severe pain, this must be investigated and appropriate action taken.

Infection control is vital to prevent infection in the epidural space which could lead to meningitis or an epidural abscess. Prevention must include regular recording of temperature, ensuring asepsis when changing infusion bags and when changing dressings, observation of the insertion site, and observation of any motor or sensory changes, complaints of backache or tenderness.

Sedation scores	**Leg movement**	**Pain score**

1 = awake
2 = drowsy, easy to rouse: eyes open to
    speech or light shake
3 = sedated, difficult to arouse: eyes open
    only to vigorous shaking
4 = unconscious, unrousable
S = normal sleep
	0 = no movement
	1 = moves ankles only
	2 = bends knees
	3 = able to straight leg raise
	4 = unable to move legs due to surgery
		0 = no pain
		1 = mild/slight pain
		2 = moderate pain
		3 = severe/unbearable pain

Comments

N = nausea	U = urinary retention	R = respiratory depression
V = vomiting	C = catheterised	N = Naloxone given
I = itching	B = bolus dose given	

Date/time	R	BP	P	Sedation score	Pain score	Leg movement		Dermatome level		Infusion rate	Comments	Initials
						R	L	R	L			

Figure 7.10 Epidural observation charts.

ENTONOX

Entonox is a mixture of 50% nitrous oxide and 50% oxygen, inhaled by the patient for a rapid analgesia especially for emergency or procedural pain relief. It is commonly used in maternity and accident and emergency units and by paramedics in pre-hospital care. The benefit of Entonox has led to its increased use in orthopaedics for the application of casts, traction, change of dressings and removal of drains.

The analgesic effect of the gas is felt within one minute and is quickly eliminated. Patients feel light-headed and relaxed but as they are awake throughout the procedure they can cooperate with nursing actions. The patient remains in control of the amount of gas inhaled and the effects felt. The main side effect for some patients is nausea due to the nitrous oxide.

Entonox must never be used by patients with a pneumothorax or haemothorax or with those who cannot cooperate or understand the use of the gas and instructions. It must not be used instead of stronger analgesia or to avoid a general anaesthetic if this is required (Sealey 2002).

NEFOPAM

Nefopam (Accupan) is an effective analgesic for moderate to severe pain. It is occasionally used when NSAIDs are contraindicated (Day 1997) and has the advantage of being less constipating than codeine but can cause confusion.

ANTICONVULSANTS

Oral anticonvulsant drugs are given for peripheral nerve syndromes; hence, they are often used in chronic pain. Carbamazepine reduces the excitability of the nerve and sodium valproate raises the stimulation threshold so that a greater stimulus is required for the nerve to fire (Day 1997). They can cause sedation and dizziness.

ANTIDEPRESSANTS

Antidepressants are useful as an adjunct in neuropathic pain; they improve mood and sleep. Amitriptyline is commonly used in low doses, initially 10–25 mg at night. Patients need to be warned that it can take 7–10 days or longer to take effect. The main side effects include a dry mouth and hypotension.

CORTICOSTEROIDS

Some patients with bone pain or following a nerve injury find corticosteroids effective. Dexamethasone is given intravenously or intramuscularly to reduce inflammation following a nerve or spinal cord compression. If used in the short term, the side effects of fluid retention, hypertension and hyperglycaemia are generally avoided (Buck & Paice 1994).

NON-PHARMACOLOGICAL PAIN THERAPIES

Many patients find that more than one method of pain control is needed to manage their pain. This does not always mean changing their drugs but rather adding adjuvant therapies. Patients with chronic pain particularly find these additions valuable.

TEMPERATURE-BASED THERAPIES

Heat and warmth provide comfort, help muscles to relax and suppress the sensation of pain. Raising the temperature of an area increases the blood flow, reducing oedema, and accelerates repair by improving the oxygen supply to the area (Thomas 1997) and speeding up the elimination of pain-producing substances (Hawthorn & Redmond 1998). Heat appears therefore to close the gate by stimulating the large A beta fibres (Carr & Mann 2000).

Heat is useful in arthritic pain, back pain and abdominal pain but is not advisable immediately after injury as it can increase swelling. It can be applied using hot water bottles, gel packs and electric heat pads. Care is required to avoid skin burns by wrapping the packs in a towel (Hawthorn & Redmond 1998).

Cold therapy reduces the inflammatory response in some acute conditions. Vasoconstriction occurs from the reduced temperature, decreasing the inflammatory response and limiting further damage. The A beta fibres are again stimulated to induce pain modulation.

The use of cold water following some burn injuries can reduce the degree of damage as well as relieve pain. Crushed ice, gel-filled packs or, if at home, a bag of frozen peas can be applied to cool an area. They must be wrapped in a towel or cotton to prevent skin damage (Carr & Mann 2000). Cold should not be used for conditions where vasoconstriction increases the symptoms, for example Raynaud's syndrome or peripheral vascular disease (Hawthorn & Redmond 1998).

The use of heat and cold can be interchanged; patients will decide which they feel is most beneficial (Hawthorn & Redmond 1998).

TRANSCUTANEOUS ELECTRICAL NERVE STIMULATION

Transcutaneous electrical nerve stimulation (TENS) acts by stimulating A beta nerve fibres around the painful area, producing modulation. A small battery-operated device generates small electrical impulses via fine wires attached to electrodes placed on the skin. Initially healthcare professionals arrange the placements of electrodes and machine settings; thereafter the patient is encouraged to adjust the electrodes and settings to obtain maximum benefits (Thomas 1997).

TENS is effective for chronic pain (McQuay & Moore 1998), particularly musculoskeletal pain, amputation stump pain and neuralgia (Carr & Mann 2000). Although patients are very rarely admitted with acute back pain, TENS has been beneficial for patients in hospital but is more commonly used as an outpatient treatment through spinal assessment and physiotherapy clinics. The main advantage is that TENS has few side effects but it is not suitable for patients with cardiac pacemakers, if the skin is broken or there is a loss of sensation.

ACUPUNCTURE

Acupuncture involves the insertion of fine needles to specific points of the body following energy meridians. These points have been mapped and used systematically in traditional Chinese medicine. A stimulus is applied to the specific points either mechanically, by, for instance, rotating the needles, or electrically (Thomas 1997). Acupuncture itself can be painful as it stimulates endorphin release, enhancing the analgesic effect (Hawthorn & Redmond 1998).

Only qualified practitioners must use acupuncture. Its value is increasingly being recognised and it is gaining credibility in Western medicine as a valid treatment for different types of pain (Carr & Mann 2000).

INFORMATION

The provision of information is an important aspect of pain management. Anxiety is a recognised component of acute and chronic pain. Preparation for a painful procedure must involve giving information. This has a positive effect by reducing the anticipation of the pain, as knowing what a sensation will be like helps the individual to cope (Thomas 1997). In chronic pain management, provision of information helps to overcome some misconceptions patients have about their pain problem; for example, a degenerative back may be pictured as 'crumbling', especially when moving. Information also improves adherence to a treatment plan (Carr & Mann 2000).

DISTRACTION

This essentially takes the patient's mind off their pain. The focus of attention is redirected to the stimulus, banishing pain to the periphery of awareness. In children, play is used effectively to distract them away from a painful event.

There are four types of distraction.

1 **Imaginary inattention**: where the patient imagines doing something very pleasant, for example walking in a forest or floating on water.
2 **Guided imagery**: with the help of another person, the patient creates a mental picture either by distraction away from the pain, by focusing on somewhere pleasant and relaxing, or by focusing attention on the pain, by directly imagining they can fight or control the pain in some way (Hawthorn & Redmond 1998).
3 **Mental distraction**: the individual focuses on an activity such as counting or reciting poems.
4 **Task distraction**: frequently used by watching TV, listening to audio tapes, reading and talking with friends.

For effective distraction, the practitioner and patient need to explore which approach is most effective. After using distraction a patient may experience an increased awareness of pain, irritability and fatigue (Hawthorn & Redmond 1998); this is commonly seen on hospital wards once visitors leave.

COGNITIVE THERAPIES

Focusing cognitive coping technique differs from distraction, by imagining pain as an entity that is controllable. An example would be imagining the pain as heat radiating from an oven, then imagining that turning the oven off reduces or controls the pain (Hawthorn & Redmond 1998).

RELAXATION

Relaxation breaks the relationship between the pain, muscle tension, autonomic hyperarousal and anxiety. Simple relaxation techniques can be brief and simple to use, such as deep breathing. Progressive muscle relaxation is more complex as it involves systematically focusing on a group of muscles in the body and getting the patient to tense and then relax each muscle group in turn. This should be avoided in postoperative settings or with patients prone to cramp or muscle spasm. It may not be useful in frail or confused patients (Hawthorn & Redmond 1998).

PAIN MANAGEMENT FOR OLDER PEOPLE

According to Thomas (1997), pain has been seen as an inevitable part of growing old. Arthritis, osteoporosis, injuries from falls, cancer, cardiovascular and respiratory disease are health problems seen as causes of pain in older people. Pain and disability associated with osteoarthritis, for example, has far-reaching consequences for the individual, their family and society as a whole, yet it is not considered a national health priority.

There is no evidence that pain sensitivity changes with age but older people seem to cope better with chronic pain (Thomas 1997). There are a number of myths associated with pain in older people (Box 7.5), which result in poor pain management and less postoperative analgesia being given to the elderly compared to younger adults.

To improve pain management in older people, there needs to be an increase in health professionals' knowledge of analgesia, increased use of appropriate pain assessment, more communication about pain between patients and healthcare staff and the development of individual pain management plans. There is also a real need to educate the patients about the benefits of analgesia to improve concordance with treatment.

PAIN ASSESSMENT AND THE ELDERLY

There is underreporting of pain in the older population as they do not volunteer reports of pain (MacIntyre & Ready 2001), leading to the degree of pain being underestimated (Carr & Mann 2000). This is particularly evident in cognitively impaired patients where dementia, confusion and memory loss can result in impaired thinking and poor

> **Box 7.5   Myths about older people and pain**
>
> - Old age and pain go together
> - Pain is a consequence of old age and must be tolerated
> - Old people have a higher pain threshold
> - Older people need less analgesia
> - Older people cannot tolerate opiates
> - The effects of analgesia are enhanced in old age
> - The failure to express pain equals an absence of pain

conception of the painful experience (Carr & Mann 2000, MacIntyre & Ready 2001). In some circumstances, for instance with confused elderly patients, the assessment of pain is more reliant on interpretation of non-verbal behaviours, such as facial grimaces and body language (Carr & Mann 2000). There is currently little research into pain assessment in cognitively impaired patients.

When communication is impaired it is important to be creative in assessing and managing the older person's pain (Carr & Mann 2000). If in doubt, it should be assumed to exist when the situation is potentially painful (MacIntyre & Ready 2001) as older people are more susceptible to the harmful effects of undertreated pain, particularly chest infections, pressure ulcers and cardiac problems.

ANALGESIA IN OLDER PEOPLE

Older people respond more quickly to drugs generally. However, age, along with other diseases such as atherosclerosis and heart failure, can lead to a lowered ability to process drugs and a poor ability to correct the adverse effects caused by the drugs (Farhaquar 2002, presentation at RCN Pain Forum Conference).

There is no increased risk with age in relation to taking paracetamol but the side effects of NSAIDs are increased in older people. An increased sensitivity to the side effects of opioids can occur, including low blood pressure, confusion and drowsiness which result in falls, while nausea and constipation can lead to weight loss (Hawthorn & Redmond 1998). Confusion can occur for many reasons, including fluid and electrolyte imbalance, hypoxaemia, severe pain, alcohol withdrawal and multiple medical problems. When confusion occurs opioids tend to be withdrawn but these other factors need to be considered and if present, reducing the dose of opioids, rather than withdrawal, is a more appropriate option (MacIntyre & Ready 2001).

OPIATE-DEPENDENT PATIENTS

Effective pain relief in opiate-dependent patients is very difficult and challenging. There is a wide variation in the amount of opioids individuals require and when a patient has developed a dependency on drugs (Box 7.6), an effective dose is difficult to titrate. Such patients will be tolerant of the drug concerned, so require larger doses to obtain effective pain relief (MacIntyre & Ready 2001).

MacIntyre & Ready (2001) describe three groups of opioid-dependent patients:

- those with cancer pain, admitted for example with a metastatic fracture
- those with chronic non-malignant pain, such as osteoarthritis, who are admitted for joint replacement surgery
- those with a past or current addiction to opioids who are admitted with trauma or infections as a result of their lifestyle.

The principles of treating acute pain in all three groups are to provide effective analgesia and to prevent or manage any withdrawal symptoms.

Patients with a prior addiction will report higher pain scores so pain assessment scores may not be useful for these patients. To help avoid making value judgements, an objective assessment of their ability to breath deeply, cough and mobilise and information about the site of pain and their description of the pain need to be obtained (McCreadie & Davidson 2002).

A balanced approach to pain management is necessary, including the use of paracetamol and NSAIDs where there are no contraindications. An epidural infusion with local anaesthetic alone is very effective. When this is ineffective, short-acting opioids used frequently can be beneficial. If a patient is nil by mouth, a PCA is useful and avoids staff–patient conflicts about analgesia (McCreadie & Davidson 2002). In general, intramuscular and intravenous routes should be avoided in illicit drug users to avoid needle rush (McCreadie & Davidson 2002).

It is important to maintain the opioid user with their regular doses of opioids or a maintenance dose of methadone. In registered addicts, it is advisable to confirm the dose of methadone with their normal prescriber to avoid conflicts of information.

Additional analgesia is required for acute pain (MacIntyre & Ready 2001). Drug addicts have an extended duration of pain and a greater need for analgesia after surgery than non-addicts (McCreadie & Davidson 2002).

If an illicit drug user is not on a methadone regime, an open non-judgemental approach is required. The drug team can advise on the dose of methadone required to prevent withdrawal with additional help, support and advice being available from the acute pain team, pharmacists and local drug and alcohol teams (Carr & Mann 2000).

CONCLUSION

In understanding the physiology of pain and the mechanism of delivering analgesia, the nurse is able to appreciate how and why relevant drugs are used. Along with appreciation of the importance of pain assessment options and the need to evaluate the effectiveness of analgesic interventions, this enables the quality of patient care to be improved.

By understanding the physiology of pain and where the different drugs act, it becomes more apparent why combining different analgesics is more effective than using one. Non-steroidal antiinflammatory drugs block the prostaglandins that sustain the release of chemicals initiating the pain signal. Local anaesthetics stop the transmission of pain to the spinal cord, while opiates act within the spinal cord and the brain to alter the perception of pain. The use of distraction, providing information and allowing the patient choice and a degree of control all help to modulate pain signals.

These important aspects of effective pain management should not be underestimated.

References

Allcock N 1996 The use of different research methodologies to evaluate the effectiveness of programmes to improve the care of patients in post-operative pain. Journal of Advanced Nursing 23: 32–38

Baillie L 1993 A review of pain assessment tools. Nursing Standard 7(23): 25–29

Bandolier 2002 Do NSAIDs inhibit bone healing? Available online at: www.jr.ox.ac.uk/bandolier/booth/painpag

Briggs M 1995 Principles of acute pain assessment. Nursing Standard 9(19): 23–26

Buck M, Paice JA 1994 Pharmacologic management of acute pain in the orthopaedic patient. Orthopaedic Nursing 13(6): 14–22

Carr CJ, Mann EM 2000 Pain: creative approaches to effective management. Macmillan, Eastbourne

Clancy J, McVicar A 1998 Neurophysiology of pain. British Journal of Theatre Nursing 7(10): 19–27

Cox F 2001 Clinical care of patients with epidural infusions. Professional Nurse 16(10): 1429–1432

Davis P 1997 Pain when we move. Journal of Orthopaedic Nursing 1(3): 147–153

Day R 1997 A pharmacological approach to acute pain. Professional Nurse 13(1) (suppl): S9–S12

Dolbos A, Boccard E 1995 The morphine sparing effect of propacetamol in orthopaedic postoperative pain. Journal of Pain and Symptom Management 10(4): 279–286

Giannoudis PV, MacDonald DA, Mathews SJ et al 2000 Non union of the femoral diaphysis. The influence of reaming and non-steroidal anti-inflammatory drugs. Journal of Bone and Joint Surgery 82B: 655–658

Hall A 2000 The nature of pain. Nursing Times 96(24): 37–40

Hawthorn J, Redmond K 1998 Pain causes and management. Blackwell, Oxford

Heywood J 1975 Information: prescription against pain. The study of nursing care. Project report series 2 number 5. Royal College of Nursing, London

Hollingsworth H 1994 No gain? Nursing Times 90(1): 24–27

Hyllested M, Jones S, Pederson JL et al 2002 Comparative effects of paracetamol and NSAIDs or their combination in postoperative pain management: a qualitative review. British Journal of Anaesthesia 88(2): 199–214

International Association for the Study of Pain (IASP) 1986 Classification of chronic pain. Description of chronic pain syndromes and definitions of pain terms. Pain 3 (suppl): S1–S226

Joint Commission for the Accreditation of Healthcare Organisations (JCAHO) 2000 Accreditation manual. JCAHO, Washington DC

Jones R 2002 Efficiency and safety of COX 2 inhibitors. British Medical Journal 325: 607–608

Lovett PE 1994 Prevention and control of pain in children. A manual for health care professionals. BMJ Books, London

MacIntyre PE, Ready LB 2001 Acute pain management: a practical guide. WB Saunders, London

McCaffery M, Beebe A 1989 Pain: clinical manual for nursing practice. Mosby, St Louis

McCreadie M, Davidson S 2002 Pain management in drug users. Nursing Standard 16(19): 45–51

McQuay H, Moore A 1998 An evidence based resource for pain relief. Oxford University Press, Oxford

Medical Control Agency 2002 Non-steroidal anti-inflammatory drugs and gastrointestinal safety. Committee on Safety of Medicines Newsletter 28: 5

Melzack R, Wall PD 1965 Pain mechanisms: a new theory. Science 150: 971

Park G, Fulton B, Senthuran S 2000 The management of acute pain, 2nd edn. Oxford University Press, Oxford

Royal College of Surgeons and Royal College of Anaesthetists (RCS/RCA) 1990 Commission on the Provision of Surgical Services: report of the working party on pain after surgery. RCS and RCA, London

Rueben SS 2001 Consideration in the use of COX 2 inhibitors in spinal fusion surgery. Anaesthesia and Analgesia 93: 798–804

Schug S, Sidebotham DA, McGuinnety M et al 1998 Acetaminophen as an adjunct to morphine by patient controlled analgesia in the management of acute postoperative pain. Anaesthesia and Analgesia 87: 368–372

Sealey L 2002 Nurse administration of Entonox to manage pain in ward settings. Nursing Times 98(48): 28–29

Seers K 1987 Perception of pain. Nursing Times 83(48): 37–39

Sofaer B 1992 Pain: a handbook for nurses. Harper and Row, London

Thomas VJ 1997 Pain, its nature and management. Baillière Tindall, London

White JS 2001 Non-steroidal anti-inflammatory drugs: clinical issues. Nursing Standard 15(23): 45–52

Chapter 8

The importance of nutrition

Julia D Kneale

CHAPTER CONTENTS

INTRODUCTION

Nutrition plays a vital role in enabling the body to grow, fight infection and heal. This aspect of care must not be ignored. Good nutrition and good health are inextricably linked; we cannot have good health without taking the appropriate nutrition to support it. Despite a good nutritional intake we can still be ill but diet will affect the time taken to heal and return to an optimum health status.

The level of nutritional intake for a patient is variable depending on the reason for their admission, the health of the patient, how their nutritional status is assessed and the provision of food within the clinical setting. Unfortunately nutritional deprivation in hospital is not a new phenomenon but remains an issue inadequately addressed in many areas. Nutritional deprivation does not just imply a lack of food but the provision of a diet that does not meet a patient's physiological needs. These needs will vary throughout their period of admission, rehabilitation and long-term care.

In the case of orthopaedic patients, inappropriate nutritional support can lead to reduced callus formation and increased healing times for both bone and soft tissues and affects the level of activity during rehabilitation. The patient can potentially be affected by loss of weight, muscular weakness, increased susceptibility to infection, lowered morale and accentuation of underlying disease processes. The delayed recovery time leads to an increased length of time during which they are dependent on others in hospital and at home, a prolonged time away from work and increased costs to the health service, the individual and others.

Table 8.1   Benchmarks for food and nutrition (from DoH 2001)

Benchmark: patients are enabled to consume food (orally) which meets their individual need.

Factor	Benchmark for best practice
1 Screening or assessment to identify patients' nutritional needs	Nutritional screening progresses to further assessment for all patients identified as 'at risk'
2 Planning, implementation and evaluation of care for those patients who require a nutritional assessment	Plans of care based on ongoing nutritional assessment are devised, implemented and evaluated
3 A conducive environment (acceptable sights, smells and sounds)	The environment is conducive to enabling the individual patients to eat
4 Assistance to eat and drink	Patients receive the care and assistance they require with eating and drinking
5 Obtaining food	Patients and carers, whatever their communication needs, have sufficient information to enable them to obtain their food
6 Food provided	Food that is provided by the service meets the needs of the individual patients
7 Food availability	Patients have set meal times, are offered a replacement meal if a meal is missed and can access snacks at any time
8 Food presentation	Food is presented to patients in a way that takes into account what appeals to them as individuals
9 Monitoring	The amount of food patients actually eat is monitored, recorded and leads to action when cause for concern is identified
10 Eating to promote health	All opportunities are used to encourage the patient to eat to promote their own health

The King's Fund Report in 1992 showed that a high percentage of elderly patients with femoral neck fractures were malnourished or undernourished on admission. This is further affected by the limited use of nutritional assessment tools in orthopaedic areas, resulting in the low nutritional levels not being recognised and acted upon (Grimley Evans 1989). The *Orthopaedic clinical outcomes* document (RCN 1997) emphasises the need for quality care provision for orthopaedic and trauma patients, which has to include and be supported by good nutritional care. The orthopaedic nurse has to be aware of the effects that illness, age, disability, social implications and economic factors can have on the individual in hospital and their being able to purchase, prepare and eat food at home.

Eating matters (Bond 1997), the aptly named resource for developing an integrated approach to the provision of good nutrition in hospital, explains the importance of nutritional elements, the need for health professionals to be educated about nutritional needs, the value of patient assessment and the role of evaluative audits. Within this resource, McLaren's (1997) case study of a patient with a fractured neck of femur illustrates the positive benefits of a coordinated multidisciplinary approach to

nutrition in hospital. This is now supported by the *Essence of care* document (DoH 2001), which specifies food and nutrition as one of the eight vital aspects for benchmarking care provision (Table 8.1).

Collectively the literature demonstrates and supports the need for orthopaedic nurses to be aware of the nutritional status of patients and how to develop high-quality nutritional care. Yet it also demonstrates repeatedly that this is not being consistently achieved.

This chapter reviews the links between nutrition and musculoskeletal health, the assessment options for identifying patients at risk of nutritional deprivation and the provision of a balanced nutritional diet through the activities of the multidisciplinary team. It is then up to the individual practitioner to review their own practice and support the development of appropriate nutritional care for their clients.

NUTRITION AND HEALTH

To understand how nutrition affects musculoskeletal health, knowledge of the metabolic processes and the relevance of macro- and micronutrients is needed.

CHANGING METABOLISM

The effects of trauma and surgery change patients' metabolism and nutritional needs. The basal metabolic rate refers to the activity that maintains life, especially respiration, cardiac function and body temperature. In women, the lower percentage of lean body mass and higher percentage of the less metabolically active fat means that their basal metabolic rate is lower compared to that of men.

The metabolic rate is affected by three processes: metabolism, catabolism and anabolism.

Metabolism

The reactions that affect the processing of nutrients within the body. Changes that affect the metabolism and nutritional status include stress, age, infection, injury, catabolic and anabolic states. A simple fracture will raise the energy requirements by 15–25% above normal (D'Eramo et al 1994), while multiple fractures, burns or sepsis will rapidly raise this demand further. The patient's nutritional demands need to be met to ensure they have the nutrients for tissue healing and the muscle activity to enable their mobility and rehabilitation. This needs to be balanced by nutritional content and volume, otherwise the body will be compromised by trying to deal with an inappropriate nutrition state.

Catabolism

The reactions that release energy. A hypercatabolic state occurs after trauma or surgery as a stress response to maintaining homoeostasis; here the breakdown of protein exceeds the rate of intake and synthesis of protein. It generally peaks around 3–5 days post trauma or surgery, making the first week after the event particularly important for nutritional support.

Initially the body reacts to the incident by using stored glucose and fatty acids to cover the increased energy requirements. The amount of energy required depends on the severity of the injury; hence following complex major trauma the patient's energy stores can be quickly depleted. This leads to the breakdown of muscle tissue to release the glucose for energy use, the process known as glycogenesis. The combination of a raised metabolic rate, catabolism and not eating can lead to rapid muscle and weight loss within days of injury.

This is a high risk for all trauma patients, especially the elderly. The fast-track system for patients with a hip fracture, which aims to reduce the time taken from the patient's arrival in the A & E department until their admission to a ward, should enable this to be addressed by ensuring the patient is given intravenous fluids or commenced on oral fluids and diet if they are not having their surgery within the next 4 hours.

Anabolism

This is the building of new tissue by the combining of complex substances, making it a vital factor in tissue growth and repair. This relies on adequate calories, proteins, vitamins, minerals and trace elements being present for the formation of new cells and for storing energy for later use. A fine balance between catabolism and anabolism is vital for normal health. If anabolism exceeds catabolism there is weight gain with tissue growth exceeding tissue breakdown. If catabolism exceeds anabolism there is weight loss with tissue breakdown, further compromising the health of the patient (D'Eramo et al 1994).

REQUIRED NUTRIENTS

A balance of adequate and appropriate macro- (proteins and fats) and micronutrients (vitamins and minerals) is vital for maintaining health. The nutrients required for musculoskeletal health are described here along with the recommended daily intake (RDI) where appropriate. These are based on the average healthy adult so the amounts then need to be adapted to take into account the individual patient's needs, bearing in mind their age, health status and physiological changes. Table 8.2 provides a summary of the importance of each nutrient to musculoskeletal health and some of their dietary sources.

Protein need

The RDI of 18 g of protein per main meal or 50 g per day is too low for most orthopaedic patients. The exudate from wounds, including pressure ulcers, is protein rich. The loss of protein and amino acids from major trauma injuries and surgery reduces fibroblast activity and collagen synthesis, the result being the diminished tensile strength of the wound and delayed healing. Trauma patients are often protein depleted prior to admission and this is exacerbated for all patients by any periods of fasting, particularly before and after surgery.

Table 8.2   Role and sources of nutrients for musculoskeletal health

Nutrient	Role	Examples of dietary sources
Protein	Required for normal tissue growth and repair, support for the immune system and wound healing	Meat, poultry, fish, eggs, dairy products, beans
Fats	Needed for cell development, responsible for normal tissue function, transporting nutrients into cells and acting as an energy bank	Butter, margarine, oils
Carbohydrates	Required for cell metabolism, essential for involuntary and voluntary activities including growth and repair of tissues	Bread, cake, cereals, pasta, potatoes
Vitamin A (retinol)	Maintains healthy skin, epithelialisation and tissue repair. Needed for vision. Essential for the distribution and coordination of osteoblast and osteoclast activity for the formation and repair of bones and teeth	Fish, eggs, dairy products, green and yellow vegetables
Vitamin B_1 (thiamin)	Needed to release energy from food	Milk, dairy products, meat, vegetables
Vitamin B_2 (riboflavin)	Needed for cell respiration	Meat, milk, eggs, green vegetables
Vitamin B_3 (niacin)	Needed for skin, tongue and intestinal function	Dairy products, fish, fortified cereals, yeast extract
Vitamin B_6 (pyridoxine)	Needed for haemoglobin formation. Involved in protein metabolism and sensory nerve function	Bananas, fish, meat, nuts, pulses, potatoes
Vitamin B_{12} (cobalamin)	Needed with folic acid by rapidly dividing cells, e.g. bone marrow. Essential for synthesising fatty acids in nerve myelin, hence deficits present as neurological symptoms	Meat, fish, eggs, milk and dairy products
Vitamin C (ascorbic acid)	Required for wound healing, especially for collagen formation and maintenance of healthy connective tissues	Potatoes, green vegetables, citrus fruit, fruit juices
Vitamin D	Needed to maintain serum calcium and phosphorus levels	Margarine, butter, oily fish, eggs, fortified cereals
Vitamin E	Promotes wound healing and prevents scarring	Fresh nuts, seed oils and green leafy vegetables
Vitamin K	Required for coagulation	Dairy products, green vegetables and cereals
Calcium	Essential for teeth and bone structure and strength. Required for muscle contraction and nerve function, enzyme activity and normal blood clotting	Milk and dairy products, green leafy vegetables, fish with edible bones
Iron	Required for haemoglobin and red blood cell formation, optimises tissue perfusion, increases collagen synthesis	Red meat, cereals, egg yolk, green leafy vegetables
Magnesium	Required for skeletal development, nerve and muscle cell conduction	Dairy products, vegetables, meat, fish, hard water
Phosphorus	Combines with minerals to form phosphates which strengthen bones and teeth. Enables energy release from food	Cereal grains, eggs, fish, meat, vegetables
Potassium	Required for muscle and nerve function	Dairy products, meat, fruit, vegetables, grains
Sodium	Required for muscle and nerve activity	Table salt, bread, cereal products, cheese
Zinc	Required for wound healing, cell proliferation and protein synthesis	Red meat, fortified bread and cereals

The addition of a protein-rich diet would improve tissue healing and increase the patient's energy and motivation to participate in their care and rehabilitation. Porter & Johnson (1998) recommend protein supplements to minimise bone loss and reduce the rehabilitation time required. This can be achieved through consistent good advice on choice of meals once the patient is able to eat. By increasing the protein intake, the rates of secondary complications, length of inpatient stay and, potentially, mortality rates could be reduced.

Energy requirements

The energy provided by carbohydrate and fat intake is essential for maintaining life, voluntary and involuntary body function, growth, muscle and bone healing. It is often forgotten that the patient is expending energy while lying in bed and not doing any physical muscular activity.

For postoperative patients, an energy-rich diet is important for building up their reserves for tissue healing and rehabilitation activities. Such diets must be supported and encouraged in hospital.

If recommending a reduced fat intake as a long-term lifestyle health change, it is important that this is put into the context of the patient's normal diet and health to aid understanding. The patient must understand how their physical needs will change over time while the body repairs itself and that a lower fat intake for some patients will be more important once that healing is complete.

Vitamin replacement

A variety of vitamins are needed for tissue growth and repair. Vitamin deficiency in the elderly is very common so the addition of appropriate supplements will support and enable the healing process after trauma or surgery, as well as improving their general health. The principal vitamins are listed below in relation to the orthopaedic patient's needs.

- **Vitamin A** deficiency will increase the risk of a wound infection and slow the wound-healing process by reducing the rate of collagen synthesis and slowing the rate of tissue repair. The RDI of 600–700 µg therefore needs to be increased for patients with surgical and trauma wounds.
- **Vitamin B**, if absent from a patient's diet, will impair the normal function of most body systems. In particular, thiamin (B_1) deficiency has been specifically linked to postoperative confusion (Holmes 1996).

- **Vitamin C** is essential for wound healing; the RDI of 40–50 mg per day should be raised for most orthopaedic patients. The presence of extensive wounds, pressure ulcers or delayed healing are indicators for providing vitamin C supplements to prevent capillary fragility and wound breakdown.
- **Vitamin D** is needed for bone development and healing (RDI 10 µg). The elderly are more prone to vitamin D deficiency as they have a lower dietary intake. Solanki et al (1995) found that in the Asian elderly populations, the levels of vitamin D are lower than for a matched elderly white population, leading to their increased risk of osteomalacia. Solanki et al found no specific cause for this phenomenon but ruled out several misconceptions, namely that exposure to sunlight and dietary intake of vitamin D had no effect as they were similar between the two groups despite different cultural and religious influences. The effect of higher skin pigmentation diminishing vitamin D synthesis was not found when comparing young Asian and white adult groups. As the rate of photosynthesis is known to slow with age the study suggests that the higher pigmentation accelerates this decline. If confirmed, this puts the Asian population at continued risk of osteomalacia, necessitating appropriate health education and increased vitamin D intakes in the diet until an effective means of reducing the acceleration is found.

Mineral reserves

Calcium is an essential component in skeletal development and healing. The RDI of 1–105 g is mostly obtained through dairy-based products. Calcium is essential in achieving a high bone density in early adulthood which is generally at a peak around 30 years of age. The gradual loss of skeletal calcium is a normal ageing process, accelerated in women after the menopause.

The link between low childhood milk consumption and low bone density in adults (Murphy et al 1994) indicates the need to encourage an early calcium-rich diet in childhood or the use of calcium supplements to prevent or delay the onset of osteoporosis and osteoporotic fractures, especially for women. The importance of using alternative sources of calcium for children with milk intolerance and teenagers who have low milk consumption must be stressed for those families with a high risk of developing osteoporotic fractures.

Iron is one of the minerals most patients are aware of even if they do not know where a good dietary intake can be obtained from. The RDI is 8.7 mg for men and postmenopausal women and 14.8 mg for younger women. Vitamin C is needed for the body to absorb iron and the combination of iron and vitamin C is needed for collagen synthesis. An iron deficiency is indicated by anaemia, impaired cognitive function, impaired exercise tolerance, increased tissue ischaemia and wound breakdown caused by reduced collagen and wound tensile strength.

Sodium (RDI 1600 μg) is essential for cellular structure and function plus the maintenance of homoeostasis.

Potassium (RDI 3500 mg) is needed for muscle and nerve function, making it important in the rehabilitation of orthopaedic patients. The intracellular loss of potassium occurs as a direct result of cell lysis, fluid and electrolyte loss, a low potassium diet and the diuretic effect of alcohol. The effects of lower potassium include cardiac arrhythmias, mental apathy and muscular weakness, including slower gastrointestinal peristalsis.

Zinc. This is required for bone and wound healing, a deficiency leading to reduced wound strength and wound breakdown. The recommendation of 9.5 mg for men and 7.0 mg for women per day is attainable through a varied diet. Patients with a low appetite or on a restricted menu choice require supplements as a low appetite and loss of taste can be caused by a zinc deficiency. The use of zinc supplements benefits the patient after trauma and surgery by enabling wound healing and preventing tissue damage such as pressure ulcers.

Aluminium. The relationship between hip fractures and aluminium was explored in an epidemiological study based in Sydney, Australia (Cumming & Klineburg 1994). The links between patients with renal failure accumulating skeletal aluminium levels following exposure to aluminium sources and being unable to excrete it were used to initiate exploration of aluminium deposits in the hip and spine of non-renal failure patients who had hip fractures. The results are inconclusive but raise awareness of the potential increase in risk of hip fracture following increased indirect consumption and absorption of aluminium through the use of cooking utensils, antacids, deodorants, drinking water and foods that have high aluminium contents. The long-term effects of aluminium deposited in the bone and the possible increase in hip fracture risk require further research and the long-term follow-up of groups exposed to aluminium, such as those exposed to the aluminium

sulphate added to drinking water in Camelford, England (Eastwood et al 1990, Wood et al 1988).

Other necessary nutrients

Fibre. Many orthopaedic patients are at risk of bowel disorders, particularly constipation from analgesia, bedrest and reduced mobility, so a high-fibre diet needs to be considered. A balance is required though, as too much fibre can lead to incontinence.

Alcohol. This is high in calories but not in nutritional content, having no protein, vitamin or mineral value. The vitamin B complex is required to metabolise alcohol. Inappropriate consumption can lead to deficits in protein, folic acid, vitamin A and zinc. The diuretic effect increases the excretion of magnesium and potassium.

NURSING IMPLICATIONS

Malnutrition

Acute and chronic illness, trauma, stress and infection cause an increase in the metabolic rate. Quinn (1997) relates this effect to patients following major surgery, who experience a period of semistarvation during which the body requires an increased amount of protein and calories. If this is not met through diet, protein is acquired through glycogenesis and protein catabolism, causing increased muscle weakness and fatigue.

Preoperative fasting is often in excess of the recommended 2–3 hours for fluids and 6 hours for milk or food (Greenfield et al 1997, Jester & Williams 1998). This leads to the patient being undernourished preoperatively, an effect compounded by poor-quality postoperative nutrition.

If, as Holmes (1996) states, postoperative food consumption is providing only 50% of patients' requirements, the potential consequences of this will include poor wound healing and muscle atrophy with the loss of muscle function, which impairs cardiac, respiratory and skeletal muscle action. As a result, the patient can experience reduced mobility, cardiac failure, difficulty in coughing and expectoration and an increased risk of infections. Their recovery time will also be delayed by mental changes causing poor concentration, depression and apathy. Vomiting, diarrhoea and the increased toxicity of some drugs in malnutrition result in the reduced absorption of nutrients.

For trauma patients, the risk of protein and energy malnutrition is exacerbated if they are elderly, have cancer, a debilitating chronic condition, dysphasia, anorexia or a gastrointestinal tract compromise.

The presence of under- or malnutrition increases the risk of falls as coordination is impaired by reduced muscle and bone strength and reduced activity. If osteoporosis is present, the reduced mechanical strength of the bone increases the risk of fracture.

Reasons for malnutrition need to be explored as the presence of depression, social isolation or a disease process will affect the patient's dietary habits and intake. Psychological and social problems, for example posttraumatic stress syndrome, bereavement, depression, isolation, sensory changes and a prolonged or repeated hospital admission, frequently lead to a change of diet that is based on increased volume but of low nutritional value.

Overweight patients

Obesity is generally defined as when a person has a body mass index of 30 or more. It leads to health and nutritional problems, bringing risks of hypertension, shortness of breath and mechanical problems from the increased weight to be supported by the spine, hips, knees and feet with the possibility of exacerbating any joint conditions that are present.

What is less well recognised is that obesity can mask significant muscle tissue loss. Increased adipose tissue has a proportionally low vascular supply, increasing the risk of pressure ulcers and prolonging the skin and wound healing times. The overweight patient still requires an energy intake that matches their energy output but it needs to be from carbohydrates rather than fats.

Patient education

The orthopaedic nurse plays a vital role in patient education in relation to eating a healthy diet based on a balanced intake of nutrients and supporting supplements where relevant.

Supporting and empowering the patient and their family will increase the acceptance of a change in diet and sustain the changes in eating habits. The nurse can never be certain how long such changes will continue but for the patient, having an informed choice of how to break out of the cycle of having a poor diet, being overweight or malnourished can only be positive (Fig. 8.1). When a patient either chooses not to break these habits or finds it hard to do so, blame, being penalised or reprimanded are negative, unhelpful and damaging approaches to take. A supportive approach is needed at all times.

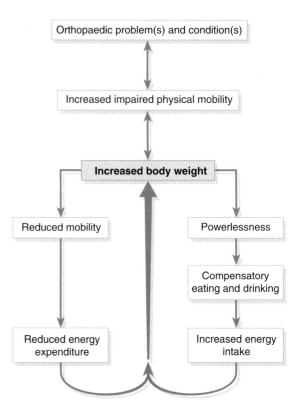

Figure 8.1 Cycle of increasing excess body weight.

Tissue healing

Wound breakdown and an increased risk of pressure ulcers occur from a lack of protein in the dermal layer. The risk of pressure ulcer development is increased by factors like immobility, inactivity, incontinence, reduced levels of consciousness and malnutrition, all of which are seen to some extent in orthopaedic patients. Reducing the risks of malnutrition can assist in the prevention of pressure ulcers and improve the healing process.

The presence of traumatic, surgical or chronic wounds increases the demand for energy and nutrient supply for tissue healing. This supply is taken from other body resources unless balanced by an increased and correctly supplemented nutritional intake.

Patients who are nil by mouth for periods of time, especially post trauma or during the pre-, intra- and postoperative phases, often have crystalloid fluid replacement that does not meet their energy requirements. There needs to be an early emphasis on nutritional support to promote bone and wound healing rates, tissue growth and repair and improve their rates of recovery and rehabilitation.

The evidence for slower healing rates, protracted hospital stays and increased complications following elective and trauma surgery on the undernourished patient is well recognised. Patient case studies by Handel (1997) illustrate the benefits of assessing nutritional needs preoperatively and show that when an assessment is not done or the findings are not acted upon, the implications include a longer admission time and prolonged healing periods. The ideal timing for these assessments is during the preoperative assessment for the elective surgery patient and on admission for the trauma patient. Health promotion, education and support can then be planned and implemented at appropriate points in their care.

NUTRITIONAL ASSSESSMENT

Ensuring adequate nutrition for all patients is essential. Where a patient's intake is poor a diet record covering assessment, summary of intake and supplementary support is vital to raise awareness of this aspect of care. Nursing models enable the assessment of a patient's needs and the planning, implementation and evaluation of care. These and most care pathways include an aspect of nutritional care but without the additional use of a nutritional assessment tool, this aspect can only be regarded as poor (Quinn 1997). Brown's (1997) audit of practice demonstrates that making the connection between the process of care and nutritional assessment is vital.

ASSESSMENT TOOLS

For most patients, a nutritional assessment is based on their weight, height, current health and normal eating habits, likes and dislikes. Less frequently carried out is a specific and continued nutritional assessment and evaluation of whether a patient's nutritional intake reflects their physiological needs. Yet a risk assessment tool allows the healthcare team to evaluate more accurately the patient's risk or current status of protein–energy match or mismatch, dehydration, potential risk factors, required dietary supplements or restrictions.

Choosing an assessment tool

The chosen assessment tool or risk score criteria must not be complex but needs to be research based, detailed enough to be valuable and reliable but convenient enough to use, easily interpreted and appropriate for the client group involved. McLaren et al's

(1997) summary of available assessment tools for their validity, reliability, sensitivity and practical use is a valuable resource for practitioners to begin evaluating such tools in relation to their clinical area.

The ideal assessment needs to include dietary and medical records, physical and anthropometric tests and laboratory assessments as relevant (Box 8.1).

Assessment scores and tools vary depending on what is regarded as important. Most include a height, weight or body mass index record plus questions about weight loss or gain, appetite, fluid and nutritional intake, ability to eat and potential risk factors. The variations can include the addition of scores for specific symptoms such as pain, skin condition, pressure ulcers, age and gender, physical stress and illness (Freebody 1998, Norton 1996). The addition of indicators of actions to be taken, including referral to specific members of the multidisciplinary team and an audit trail, is likely to improve the success of these tools in practice.

Using assessment tools

Nutritional assessments are not single, one-off events; it is the trend that repeated assessments identify which become important. Once an assessment has shown a patient is nutritionally compromised, the potential nursing diagnoses (Table 8.3) and plan of care need to be considered with appropriate actions being taken. Continued regular reassessment must follow for any patients identified as being at risk during an initial assessment. Continual assessment is a key to ensuring relevant nutritional support and should be evident in the patients' case notes. This will provide a continuous record reflecting changes in health status, risk factors and requirements from preadmission through to rehabilitation as appropriate.

Continual assessment can lead to a reevaluation of when surgery is appropriate. Delaying surgery can allow a metabolic imbalance to be corrected and enable the body to be in a better position to heal itself without a prolonged postoperative hospital admission (Handel 1997). This balance between the cost of a longer postoperative stay from delayed healing and higher risk of complications, versus improved preoperative care with the potential risks of delaying surgery has to be considered on an individual basis.

As with all tools, nutritional assessments are only accurate if they are used correctly and are understood by the practitioners involved. Forms such as daily

Box 8.1 Summary of components of nutritional assessments

Dietary and medical status
- Preadmission or preinjury intake habits and patterns, to determine the 'typical' daily regime, eating habits, appetite
- Previous medical history, current medications and history of allergies
- Record of cultural and religious implications, food and drink preferences
- Record of significant changes in eating, drinking or weight, especially recent unintentional rapid weight gain or loss
- Record of body weight on admission; repeated weekly
- Current medical and nursing diagnoses, especially relating to burns, trauma, infection, carcinoma, cerebral vascular disorders
- Record of changes in vomiting, pain, continence, tissue viability or mobility scores
- Assess and record effect of health status, medical or nursing care or treatment by nutritional problems such as positional restrictions, missed meals, time spent without food or fluid, e.g. prior to investigations
- Assessment of mental health including general mood, concentration, alertness, confusion, depression, motivation to eat and compliance with care
- Assess ability to shop, prepare and eat food with record of assistance required

Anthropometric tests
- Height (without shoes) and weight (in light clothing) using accurate calibrated scales, repeated weekly at the same time to show significant changes
- Body mass index indicating the proportion of lean body mass to body fat
- Triceps skinfold thickness with Harpenden skinfold callipers at the midpoint between the acromion and olecranon process
- Mid-arm circumference measured at the same point with a gently placed tape that does not squeeze the arm
- Observation of skin, oral and ocular mucous membranes, teeth, gums and eyes for visible changes such as:
  - dry hair indicating low protein, brittle and thick nails indicating low iron and protein
  - dry and red skin around the eyes indicating low riboflavin and niacin
  - dry, flaky skin on chest indicates low niacin
  - calf and shoulder pain indicating low magnesium, calcium or potassium
  - angular lip cracks from low riboflavin, B_6 and/or folate
  - reduced taste or 'it all tastes the same' comments, indicating low zinc
  - skin for wounds, abrasions and pressure ulcers
- Recording of temperature for signs of infection
- Observation of muscle wasting and loss of subcutaneous fat by, for example, reduced hand grip, poor cough reflex and changes in mobility

Laboratory assessments
- Estimates of haemoglobin and haematocrit to show signs of dehydration and lack of protein causing anaemia, though results could be due to blood loss
- Other serum indicators used are levels of vitamin B_{12}, folate, albumin, potassium, calcium, alkaline phosphatase levels, creatinine and electrolytes
- White blood cell and lymphocyte counts are lower in malnourishment but again this may reflect other underlying or associated problems
- Liver and renal function tests

diet charts tend to be completed only when the healthcare team, patient and their family are involved and actively support the assessment processes.

Practitioners using these assessments must understand the process, rigour and relevance of the assessment, be able to interpret the results correctly and initiate changes in patient care accordingly. This requires a practice framework which supports nutritional care at all levels, from the individual nurse assessing their patient's needs to the financial

Table 8.3 Nursing diagnoses and possible causes (adapted from D'Eramo et al 1994)

Nursing diagnosis	Possible cause
Nutrition inadequate to meet physiological needs	Ascertain the cause, especially if weight is less than 80% of normal. The cause can be related to anorexia, dry mucous membrane, mouth lesions, impaired swallowing, inability to ingest or digest food, nausea, vomiting or diarrhoea, increased metabolic rate with inadequate energy and protein-based intake
Nutritional intake more than body requires	This is evident when body weight is 20% over normal or falling into the overweight or obese percentiles on weight charts. This is usually related to changed or inappropriate dietary habits, including high fat and cholesterol intake with little or no exercise. The patient's knowledge on nutrition is either lacking or not actualised
Self-care deficit	Inability to shop, purchase, prepare or eat food. Difficulties in opening containers: requires assistance due to disability, position in bed, surgery or other dependency cause
Impaired tissue and skin integrity	Immobility, reduced mobility and incorrect patient handling can be contributory factors along with an altered nutritional intake and infection
Altered mucous membranes	Reduced or no oral intake, dehydration or side effect of medication
Fluid and electrolyte imbalance	Fluid loss through trauma, raised metabolic rate, altered nutritional intake before and after trauma or surgery, the presence of an infection or pyrexia

resources required for an integrated multidisciplinary approach to nutrition.

No single assessment is advocated in this chapter but the different assessments are described briefly to demonstrate the range available.

ANTHROPOMETRIC TESTS

These are physical body measurements that are simple, quick to use and an inexpensive means of providing regular serial patient assessments. Caution must be exercised as the tables used for comparison apply to average fit adults so the results for the elderly and for children must be considered within their age group. Many of these results can also be affected by a chronic illness and distorted by oedema, dehydration or obesity.

Body mass index

An accurate height to weight ratio can be compared to percentile charts for children or for adults. The body mass index (BMI) is determined by the equation:

BMI = weight in kg ÷ height in m^2

A BMI score of 19–25 is seen as desirable, a score of less than 19 indicates the patient is underweight, a score between 26–30 is classed as overweight and over 30 as obese.

Demiquet index

This is used as an alternative to BMI when measuring height is difficult or a BMI will be inaccurate. This involves the demispan measurement taken with the arm outstretched and in neutral rotation; it is from the sternal notch to the web between the middle and ring fingers. The equation is:

Demiquet = weight in kg ÷ demispan in cm^2

This gives a body mass related to skeletal size (Bond 1997).

Hand grip test

A simple hand grip test using, for example, the Harpenden hand grip dynamometer allows the practitioner to assess the skeletal muscle strength. The patient grips the dynamometer and squeezes it as hard as possible using the non-dominant hand; this is done on three occasions with the highest reading being recorded. This can indicate reduced muscle strength from malnutrition but the results can be distorted if the patient has a physical or neuromuscular hand disorder such as arthritis or carpal tunnel syndrome.

Skinfold tests

Skinfold tests or pinch tests are the measurement of the skinfold thickness in an area where adipose tissue is deposited, generally at the biceps, triceps, subscapular, suprailiac site, thigh and calf muscles. The measurement is taken in millimetres using callipers to establish the subcutaneous fat (energy) reserves.

Arm circumference

This is used in conjunction with a skinfold test. The combination of the triceps skinfold thickness (TSF) and mid-arm circumference (MAC) gives the mid-arm muscle circumference (MAMC):

$$MAMC = MAC - (0.314 \times TSF)$$

This gives an estimate of the skeletal body muscle (protein) reserves which are then compared to tables standardised for age and gender.

LABORATORY RESULTS

Biochemistry and haematology results may indicate the presence of malnutrition but any underlying disease process can also distort the results. A reduction in the level of serum albumin is recognised as an indicator of protein and energy malnutrition and a predictor of poor wound healing. However, the presence of infection and the body's reaction to trauma and the inflammatory response will alter the serum level without direct relationship to nutritional status. Hence laboratory results are unreliable as sole indicators of nutritional status but can be useful in conjunction with a full patient assessment.

FLUID IMBALANCE

For normal physiological function, homoeostasis, it is essential to maintain the body's fluid balance; any change will alter the patient's health and healing processes. Normally a person should drink 1.5–2 litres of fluid a day but in a ward environment, where the high temperature will increase insensible loss through perspiration, this should be increased. Additional fluid losses through vomiting, diarrhoea, serous fluid, haemorrhage, burn injuries and increased renal diuresis have to be countered by an appropriate compensatory intake. Dehydration occurs when there is a loss of extracellular water. The loss of fluids will also lead to an electrolyte imbalance.

Trauma patients have a high risk of fluid loss at the site of the accident, from the type of injury and being unable to access fluids possibly for several hours before admission. If these patients have a prolonged wait in the accident and emergency department before intravenous fluids are commenced, they will be further compromised before admission to a ward or transfer to the operating theatre. Urgent fluid replacement is vital as more patients will die from haemorrhage and loss of fluid volume than from fluid overload.

The provision of drinks has to be considered. Orthopaedic patients may not be able to lift a water jug, pour the water or lift the glass. The rheumatoid patient or a patient with upper limb incapacity may require half-filled glasses or mugs with wider handles in order to drink independently. This may necessitate returning more regularly to ensure the patient is able to drink, not neglecting them or seeing their additional needs as a burden.

PREOPERATIVE FLUID REPLACEMENT

When the patient has surgery they are exposed to pre- and postoperative dehydration. This risk is exacerbated if not identified or, if identified, is not acted upon. The risks of dehydration are exacerbated by the length of time the patient is nil by mouth preoperatively, the length of the surgical procedure and being unable to eat or drink properly for 12–24 hours or more after surgery due to sleep, nausea, pain and exhaustion.

Greenfield et al (1997) show that there is overwhelming evidence for patients to be allowed to drink clear fluids up to 2 hours prior to an anaesthetic or intravenous sedation. This practice is not consistently followed in many orthopaedic units. Jester & Williams (1998) examine an action research process they followed using audit and education to change practice successfully by reviewing practice and reducing nil by mouth times to an acceptable minimum. Similar practice changes could be implemented in other areas if the multidisciplinary team are willing to review and change practice appropriately. Benchmarking such practices is appropriate for reviewing this aspect of care and comparing outcomes between units or hospitals (DoH 2001).

NUTRITIONAL SUPPORT

All patients are entitled to good nutrition. If they are critically ill, their nutritional needs are low in priority in the initial resuscitation and treatment phases. In the subsequent days the multidisciplinary team must consider whether the patient's nutritional demands are being met and the options for addressing this through supported nutritional care. Ideally nutritional support is commenced within 24–48 hours of major trauma or surgery, especially if enteral or parenteral nutrition is required. Unfortunately, there is plenty of anecdotal evidence that this rarely happens.

Both enteral and parenteral nutrition should provide the patient with an appropriate balance of protein, energy normally in the form of carbohydrates, electrolytes, vitamins, minerals and other trace elements along with fluids.

ENTERAL FEEDS

By definition, enteral feeds pass through the gastrointestinal tract, whereas parenteral feeding bypasses it. Enteral feeding is preferable as it helps maintain normal gut function.

The use of small-bore nasogastric tubes is preferred as wider tubes cause more complications and are less well tolerated by patients. Placing the gastric feed tube in the jejunum or duodenum can increase the tolerance of enteral feeds.

Commercially prepared enteral feeds are usually used. If used with a continuous feeding pump, the rates of nausea and diarrhoea can be reduced. For gastric feeds there needs to be a 4–6 hour period of rest from the feed in each 24 hours. This allows the pH of the gastric contents to return from alkaline back to acid, killing any pathogens present, and it appears to reduce the rates of pneumonia (Zainal 1995). This rest period is not required with jejunostomy or duodenum tube feeds.

Sullivan et al (1998) found that giving enteral feeds overnight to patients following hip fracture resulted in a reduction in patient mortality rates at 6 months following injury. This has not been introduced as common practice but is worth considering for patients identified as being at high risk.

In the critically traumatised patient, if slower gastric motility or a paralytic ileus is present there is reduced absorption, with the gastrointestinal contents remaining stationary; this indicates that an enteral feed is inappropriate.

PARENTERAL FEEDS

Ideally the patient will be able to take oral nutrition but if the gastrointestinal function is poor or eating is not possible parenteral feeding is required.

Peripheral intravenous feeding can be used but if it is required for more than a week, a central vein access is necessary. With a central line the solutions can be of a higher concentration. Solutions with reduced protein and glucose concentrations are available and ideal for peripheral infusion if access to a central line is unavailable or the gastrointestinal tract route needs to be supplemented for a short period of time.

Taylor (1994) considers the success of total parenteral nutrition as being dependent on the choice of access site, with the subclavian route being preferable. The catheter should be for long-term use and is generally tunnelled and sutured in position to prevent skin and catheter trauma, with an occlusive dressing to cover the site. Once in position, the line is X-rayed to ensure correct positioning prior to the infusion commencing. As intravenous feeds bypass the intestinal tract, the gastric mucosa atrophies, making the tract more permeable to bacteria (Zainal 1995) and resulting in a higher risk of systemic infections and septicaemia.

The lack of oral fluids will quickly dry out the mouth and reduce saliva production, making it unpleasant for the patient. Regular mouth care is therefore essential for a patient on enteral or parenteral nutrition.

MULTIDISCIPLINARY APPROACH TO NUTRITION

Many professionals rightly expect the nursing team to coordinate the assessment and screening of patients. The nursing team are responsible for carrying out a nutritional assessment in the preadmission clinic or on admission to the ward, with repeated assessments as required. This reflects the nurses' unique role in nutritional care through being aware of what the patient is eating in hospital and any problems that arise.

As hospital meals do not always supply the vitamins and minerals required to meet the patients' needs, supplements need to be prescribed and used appropriately. These are designed to complement a patient's diet so need to be given at a time that does not compromise appetite at meal times. Keeping food supplements on the ward requires relevant storage conditions but they must be easily accessible when required by the nursing team.

Awareness of cultural differences in nutrition (Table 8.4) is vital to support the patient in the provision and choice of food. The involvement of the

Table 8.4 Cultural and religious dietary influences

	Avoid eating	Will eat
Very strict Hindus and Sikhs	Meat, poultry and eggs	Milk, yoghurt, butter, ghee, vegetarian cheese
Other Hindus	Beef and pork	Milk, yoghurt, butter, ghee, vegetarian cheese Possibly allowed eggs, chicken, lamb
Other Sikhs	Beef and pork	Milk, yoghurt, butter, ghee, vegetarian cheese Possibly allowed all cheese, poultry, lamb, fish, eggs
Muslims	Pork and non-Halal meats	Eggs, milk, yoghurt, fish, butter, ghee, vegetarian cheese, Halal meats Possibly allowed all cheese
Orthodox Jews	Shellfish, pork, game birds	Lamb, beef, poultry, fish with fins and scales
Vegetarians	Meat, poultry, fish	Dairy products, honey and plant products
Vegan	Animal foods or products, including milk and honey	All plant products

family can ensure that correct and preferred diets are maintained but the nurse has to remain aware of the nutritional implications of food provided by the family. Involving the patient and family in meeting the patient's nutritional needs will encourage the continued participation in recommended diets after the patient is discharged home.

A TEAM APPROACH

A specialist nurse or nutritional support nurse is ideally situated to support the ward team in implementing and monitoring the care of a patient with parenteral or enteral feeds as well as being involved in staff and patient education.

The orthopaedic nurse has to be aware of the nutritional needs of the patient, particularly the specific requirements related to musculoskeletal health, bone and wound healing, rehabilitation and how the patient will manage when discharged. This means nurses have to be actively involved in all aspects of nutritional assessment, support through supplements or enteral or parenteral feeds, physical support to eat and drink and evaluation of patients' nutritional intake.

Dieticians are trained to assess and provide appropriate nutritional support but are not resourced to carry out routine or continual assessments on all patients; they rely on referrals for identifying at-risk patients. The increased acceptance of direct referrals from nurses rather than through the medical team has reduced the time patients wait to be seen but may lead to the referral of inappropriate patients

if the nursing assessment and practice framework are inappropriate.

The dietician's role remains essential for assessing patients' nutritional status, identifying deficits and initiating appropriate diets or supplements. Their involvement at ward level benefits staff and patients through monitoring the ward's approach to patient assessment and individual care. In the long term this ensures the nursing team are clinically effective in the provision of nutritional care and the team as a whole are committed to the provision of a quality patient service.

The occupational therapist's role is assessing the patient's range of movement and mobility in relation to shopping for and preparing food, their ability to eat and the provision of advice or appropriate aids such as plateguards or long-handled cutlery for use in the hospital or home.

A speech therapist should be involved if the patient has problems in swallowing or chewing, for instance following a stroke, head or facial trauma, especially if it involves the jaw, mouth or tongue.

The involvement of a pharmacist on the ward on a daily basis can alert the team to the potential for any food or nutrient and drug incompatibilities. Being involved in the supply and monitoring of food supplements, enteral and parenteral diets gives the pharmacist a valuable support role for staff and patient education programmes.

The delivery, distribution and serving of food varies between hospitals, from cook-chill services with a limited serving period to individual ordering and timing of meals. Any compromise in the delivery, distribution or serving can affect the temperature, nutritional quality and presentation of the food.

All those involved in the catering, delivery and serving of meals are part of the patient care team. The serving of food by non-nursing staff has led to some practitioners viewing this role as unimportant rather than a valuable contribution to patient care and health. If nurses are responsible for coordinating nutritional care, they are by definition responsible for ensuring the patient receives the care they require and therefore need to be aware of what occurs during the meal-time period.

ENVIRONMENTAL INFLUENCES

The environment where patients eat is as important as the food. Stephen & Allison's (1997) audit of food waste showed that approximately 35% of food sent to orthopaedic patients was wasted, with a high number of meal trays being returned unused and 75% of patients eating less than the recommended daily intakes for energy. This reinforces the cost implications and the risk of patient malnutrition occurring.

Some of the reasons why patients are unable to eat while in hospital are listed in Box 8.2. Taking easily achievable steps can alleviate many of these problems, such as ensuring patients are comfortable and pain free prior to meal times and providing assistance so that food is served while it is hot and appetising.

Investigations and other patient activities such as physiotherapy should be avoided to allow patients to eat their meal hot, in a conducive atmosphere and at their own pace whenever possible. Oral hygiene, especially the chance to rinse the mouth and brush their teeth and dentures before and after food, makes the patient feel fresher and removes food particles that could cause oral problems.

NUTRITION AND THE ELDERLY

The elderly can be very vulnerable to malnutrition, so it is important to have appropriate assessment and screening processes in place (McLaren et al 1997, Tierney 1996).

Generally older patients are in hospital longer than a younger patient with the same illness. They may have a deficit in certain nutrients before admission and require specific consideration of their physical ability to eat and whether they have a smaller appetite or less desire to eat. It is important to offer a variety of sizes of portions, with supplementary meals and drinks.

EFFECTS OF AGEING

With older age there is a reduced energy requirement, slower metabolic rate and less energetic activity. Quinn (1997) confirms that while these reductions mean the individual needs less to maintain their body weight, they still require a high energy and protein intake with adequate micronutrients, to ensure they meet their physiological requirements.

The senses of taste, smell and thirst diminish with age, leading to a reduced desire to eat. This reduction in internal cues to hunger and thirst leads to reduced intake and higher risks of anorexia and dehydration. The presentation of food is used to encourage the visual senses which play a large role in persuading the patient to eat. The philosophy of 'little and often' can enable the elderly patient to cope with a larger volume or higher nutrient content than they are used to.

Poor dentition, gum disease and ill-fitting dentures affect the types of food chosen as well as increasing the risk of oral pain, oral infections or mouth ulcers. Reduced dexterity causes frustration, making the opening of a drink carton or cutting up food difficult, leading to avoidance of these activities and certain food options on a menu.

Elderly patients often drink less because they believe they will urinate less, especially if they find getting to the bathroom difficult at night. The importance of regular fluid intake must be reinforced and assistance, if required, should not be viewed as a problem or nuisance.

EVIDENCE FOR PRACTICE IN ELDERLY CARE

Lipski et al (1993) compared the nutritional status of long-stay elderly patients to individuals of a similar age, physical and mental health living at home. The findings are disturbing and highlight the issues of nutritional care in hospital. They showed that the energy requirements of long-stay patients are high despite reduced and even severely restricted mobility, yet they received only two-thirds of their dietary energy requirements. Long term, this reduces the patient's metabolic rate, causing loss of muscle tissue and impairing muscle function, reducing their physical activity further and creating a vicious cycle of events. The intakes of vitamin C and D, calcium and other minerals were low both for those living at home and the long-stay patients, but the latter were less likely to be on supplements. Overall, Lipski et al found that those living at home were nutritionally better off while the long-stay elderly patients were at greater risk of being nutritionally compromised.

Hallström et al's (2000) qualitative study of nine patients shows the effect on individuals when they are not allowed, not able or not wanting to eat. The cases described show the importance of all members of the nursing team understanding how to encourage and support diet and fluid intake, the role of the family and the need to challenge practices that lead to malnutrition.

Avenell & Handoll's (2001) Cochrane review of trials on nutritional interventions for older people with hip fractures supports the need for proactive measures to be taken by concluding that there is favourable, though not strong evidence for effective nutritional supplementation using oral protein and energy feeds in reducing postoperative complications and rehabilitation time.

Results such as these demonstrate the value of nutritional assessment, repeat assessments and the need to be aware of appropriate nutritional support and supplements for elderly patients.

CONCLUSION

All orthopaedic patients require a diet that promotes their musculoskeletal health. To ensure this, the nurse needs to understand the physiological processes and nutrition requirements for bone and wound healing, the energy required for rehabilitation and the potential causes of nutrition and fluid depletion that put a patient at risk.

The importance of raising awareness of nutritional needs with health professionals, patients and their families, along with the need to review practice where possible, cannot be overestimated. Nurses need to review their practice in the light of the evidence for the need to continually assess the nutritional status of patients at different stages in their care, how they are assessing patients, the actions taken as a result and the role of the healthcare team in providing a quality service. The nurse has a responsibility to inform, educate and empower the patient and their family in relation to healthy eating and the use of dietary supplements, with the aim of ensuring long-term compliance and appropriate lifestyle changes.

The specific needs of patients who are particularly vulnerable, through age, trauma or chronic illness, need to be appreciated and acted upon accordingly. To ensure this, the nurse must be involved in mealtime activities including the distribution of food, providing assistance where needed and collecting the food trays to ensure they know what has been consumed. This is not a waitress service, but a vital part of assessing whether patients' nutritional needs are being met.

Further reading

Allen DJ 1993 Adding food for thought; structuring nutritional support for elderly trauma patients. Professional Nurse 8(10): 632–637

Closs SJ 1993 Malnutrition: the key to pressure sores? Nursing Standard 8(4): 32–36

Collins CM 1996 Nutrition and wound healing. Care of the Critically Ill 12(3): 87–90

Dickerson J 1995 The problem of hospital induced malnutrition. Nursing Times 91(4): 44–45

Holmes S 1999 Nutritional support in hospital. Nursing Times Clinical Monographs No. 4. EMAP Healthcare, London

Reilly H 1996 Nutritional assessment. British Journal of Nursing 5(1): 18–24

Struthers F 1994 Identification of malnutrition; report on the identification of malnutrition within 5 surgical wards. Clinical Resource Audit Group Audit Symposium. Occasional Paper No. 66. The Scottish Office, Edinburgh

References

Avenell A, Handoll HHG 2001 Nutritional supplementation for hip fracture aftercare in the elderly. Cochrane Database for Systematic Reviews, issue 1. Update Software, Oxford

Bond S (ed) 1997 Eating matters. University of Newcastle upon Tyne, Centre for Health Service Research, Newcastle

Brown F 1997 Making eating better: having models and tools are not enough – it's using them and using them properly that counts! In: Bond S (ed) Eating matters. University of Newcastle upon Tyne, Centre for Health Service Research, Newcastle

Cumming RG, Klineberg RJ 1994 Aluminium in antacids and cooking pots and the risk of hip fractures in elderly people. Age and Ageing 23: 468–472

D'Eramo AL, Sedlak C, O'Bryan-Doheny M et al 1994 Nutritional aspects of the orthopaedic patient. Orthopaedic Nursing 13(4): 13–20

Department of Health (DoH) 2001 The essence of care: patient focused benchmarking for healthcare practitioners. Department of Health, London

Eastwood JB, Levin GE, Pazanias M et al 1990 Aluminium deposition in bone after contamination of drinking water supply. Lancet 336: 462–464

Freebody S 1998 Implementation of a nutritional assessment tool for patients undergoing surgery. Journal of Orthopaedic Nursing 2(1): 25–31

Greenfield SM, Webster GJ, Vicary FR 1997 Drinking before sedation: preoperative fasting should be the exception rather than the rule. British Medical Journal 314: 162

Grimley Evans J 1989 Ageing and nutrition; questions needing answers. Age and Ageing 18: 145–147

Hallström I, Gunnel E, Rooke L 2000 Pain and nutrition as experienced by patients with hip fracture. Journal of Clinical Nursing 9(4): 639–646

Handel C 1997 A review of the use and benefits of nutritional supplements in the wound healing of orthopaedic patients. Journal of Orthopaedic Nursing 1(4): 179–182

Holmes S 1996 The incidence of malnutrition in hospitalised patients. Nursing Times 92(12): 43–45

Jester R, Wlliams S 1998 Pre-operative fasting: putting research into practice. Nursing Standard 13(39): 33–35

King's Fund 1992 A positive approach to nutrition as treatment. King's Fund Centre, London

Lipski PS, Torrance A, Kelly PJ et al 1993 A study of nutritional deficits of long-stay geriatric patients. Age and Ageing 22: 244–255

McLaren S 1997 Patient case studies: 1 Florence Smith. In: Bond S (ed) Eating matters. University of Newcastle upon Tyne, Centre for Health Service Research, Newcastle

McLaren S, Holmes S, Green S et al 1997 The evidence about eating and nutritional needs. In: Bond S (ed) Eating matters. University of Newcastle upon Tyne, Centre for Health Service Research, Newcastle

Murphy S, Khaw KT, May H et al 1994 Milk consumption and bone mineral density in middle aged and elderly women. British Medical Journal 308: 939–941

Norton B 1996 Nutritional assessment. Nursing Times 92(26): 71–76

Porter KH, Johnson MA 1998 Dietary protein supplementation and recovery from femoral fracture. Nutrition Reviews 56(1): 337–340

Quinn C 1997 The nutritional screening initiative: meeting the nutritional needs of elders. Orthopaedic Nursing 16(6): 13–24

Royal College of Nursing (RCN) 1997 Orthopaedic clinical outcomes. Royal College of Nursing, London

Solanki T, Hyatt RH, Kemm JR et al 1995 Are elderly Asians in Britain at a high risk of vitamin D deficiency and osteomalacia? Age and Ageing 24: 103–107

Stephen A, Allison S 1997 Auditing dietary care: SIGMA, a study of food waste. In: Bond S (ed) Eating matters. University of Newcastle upon Tyne, Centre for Health Service Research, Newcastle

Sullivan DH, Nelson CL, Bopp MM et al 1998 Nightly enteral nutrition support of elderly hip fracture patients: a phase 1 trial. Journal of the American College of Nutrition 17(1): 155–161

Taylor M 1994 Total parenteral nutrition: part 1. Nursing Standard 8(23): 25–28

Tierney AJ 1996 Undernutrition and elderly hospital patients: a review. Journal of Advanced Nursing 23: 228–236

Wood DJ, Cooper C, Stevens J et al 1988 Bone mass and dementia in hip fracture patients from areas with different aluminium concentrations in water supplies. Age and Ageing 17: 415–419

Zainal G 1995 Nutritional demands. Nursing Times 91(38): 57–59

Chapter 9

Epidemiology influences

Julia D Kneale

INTRODUCTION

Musculoskeletal disorders cross the boundaries of age, culture and society. They arise from a wide variety of causes and affect the physical, psychological, social, cultural and economic lives of patients, their families and the society in which they live and work. The causes of ill health include the:

- patient's internal anatomy and physiology, for instance the development, repair and replacement of the skeletal system
- individual's behaviours such as making decisions about smoking, exercise or diet-related activities
- context in which people live and work, including their understanding of healthy lifestyles and ability to put them into practice, housing conditions or health and safety at work
- local, national or international structures that affect health, for instance the provision of primary care services, health screening and vaccination programmes.

To put these factors into context, consider a patient with osteoporosis. The effects on the patient's internal physiology relate to a changed skeletal structure, while their behaviours will include the level of exercise and calcium intake across their lifespan. The context in which they live could increase their chance of a fall, for example due to an uneven path, resulting in a Colles' fracture, and the health structures that could positively influence their health would include access to bone density screening and injury prevention advice.

The range and prevalence of musculoskeletal disorders and trauma are vast, with different causes being an individual, local, national or international issue. At a personal level issues such as safe moving and handling of heavy objects or putting healthy living advice into action can increase or decrease risks of injury, while at a local level the problems can relate to resource provision for healthcare, minor and major injury care or illness prevention. At a national level, the issues are likely to surround the financing of public healthcare, developing and implementing injury prevention measures where possible and identifying best practice that is economical to implement. At an international level, the same issues apply but on a larger scale. In addition, it becomes possible to identify trends that emerge across countries in relation to the occurrence and prevalence of disease, the benefits of treatments, the economic value of preventive measures and how all these impact on and affect world health issues. In many instances the diverse nature, unpredictability, size and severity of the conditions and injuries mean that prioritising care and resources is very complex.

This chapter illustrates some of these multifaceted aspects. It does not offer or emphasise solutions or how they should be tackled but identifies how epidemiology studies can influence musculoskeletal health and healthcare through their results. Due to the vast nature of this subject, a limited range of examples is used to illustrate the issues involved.

IDENTIFYING MUSCULOSKELETAL PROBLEMS

The apparently simple division of musculoskeletal problems into orthopaedic conditions and trauma injuries appears straightforward, but the relationship between the two occasionally shows cause and effect. For instance, a rugby player who has sustained a variety of knee injuries during his playing career (trauma injuries) is likely to develop osteoarthritis (an orthopaedic disorder) in later life. Alternatively, a child with osteogenesis imperfecta will have a high risk of fracture, with potentially several fractures at different stages of healing being present because of the orthopaedic condition. Hence, both cause and effect can occur sequentially or together.

Classification according to whether the damage is to the bone or soft tissues is less straightforward as a disorder that alters the position or function of a bone will affect the muscles, ligaments, blood or nerve supply to some degree.

Grouping conditions into anatomical regions, such as pelvic or shoulder problems, precludes conditions such as rheumatoid arthritis that affect multiple joints or bones.

An alternative is to study the distribution, effects and causes of the disorder or injury using an epidemiological viewpoint. While this is also an imperfect approach, viewing the specialty in this way can demonstrate issues of prevention, early detection and some, though not all, relationships between cause and effect.

AN EPIDEMIOLOGY APPROACH

Epidemiology involves looking for patterns that occur in health and illness within populations and the factors influencing those patterns. This approach offers a different view of health and disease by relating them to, for example, the environment and ways of living. Box 9.1 lists some of the issues studied in epidemiological research.

This approach enables the identification of those at risk of a disease or injury; any changes in the level of risk providing some evidence of the effectiveness of prevention or treatment strategies. It does not involve the development of intervention plans but collates information to inform the planning stage of care or the evaluation of patient outcomes. For instance, the number of injuries and deaths among car passengers highlighted the need for car designs to incorporate seatbelts. The initial optional use of seatbelts meant people were still being unnecessarily injured or

---

Box 9.1   Examples of issues investigated in epidemiological studies

- Social trends
- Public health trends
- Diet, nutrition
- Obesity
- Transport and road safety
- Accidents
- Lifestyle, sports and leisure
- Working environments
- Activity levels
- Exposure to chemical and hazardous materials
- Effect of housing and living conditions
- Effects of poverty, smoking, age and gender as health-related issues

killed. This has led to legislation in many countries resulting in a dramatic reduction in passenger and driver injury severity and deaths.

DEMOGRAPHY STUDIES

The monitoring of populations has occurred throughout history; examples are found in pre-Christian eras and within the Bible, while in Britain the first demographic study of the population led to the development of the Doomsday Book. These studies involved monitoring the size of a population, the principal function of demographic studies.

The demographic approach is relevant to studies of population groups and their health risks, particularly issues such as age ratios, where cultural groups live or the number of people in a household. Consequently demographic and epidemiological studies are related; for instance, the age ratios of a population will indicate potential changes in the future rates of osteoporosis and hip fracture among elderly patients.

HISTORY OF EPIDEMIOLOGY

It was not until the 19th century that measurements of the distribution of disease occurred with any accuracy. The first classic, frequently cited example was the work of John Snow who identified that the risks of cholera in London related to the drinking water supply. He located the houses where people had died from cholera during 1848–9 and 1853–4, noting an apparent association between these and the sources of drinking water they used. Using simple statistical comparisons, he identified that deaths and incidences of cholera were higher in areas supplied by the Southwark water company than in areas supplied by the Lambeth water company. From this, he developed a theory that linked cholera to its spread by contaminated water. This led to the cleaning of the water supplies and a reduction in incidences of cholera long before the identification of the organism responsible. He was unable to identify why everyone in one area did or did not get or die from cholera, as the links between illness, co-morbidity, immunity, susceptibility, physiological defences and other risk factors had not yet been established.

A more recent study by Doll & Hill (1964, cited by Beaglehole et al 1993) made the link between cigarette smoking and lung cancer. Although not all smokers get lung cancer and not all patients with lung cancer have been smokers, this important link led to the prevention campaigns we have today.

These examples demonstrate that for many conditions the causes are multifactorial, with some factors being a direct cause while others increase the risk of an event happening. An example would be children's limb injuries in cycling accidents: the speed at which they are cycling and the ground surface are direct causes but other factors increase the risk of injury such as a lack of protective clothing and inability to judge distance and speed.

AIMS OF EPIDEMIOLOGY

The key features of epidemiology are the identification or influence of various risk factors, the measurement of disease and its outcomes in relation to a population at risk. This can include determining the demographic make-up of the population.

The population can be a group that is healthy or sick, who have or are at risk of the disease or condition under investigation. The aim is to improve understanding of the cause, distribution or progression of the condition. Moon et al (2000) summarise the epidemiological approach as involving the following four factors.

- **Description**: identifies the incidences of a disease or injury and the relative frequency of occurrence within populations, for example falls in older people resulting in hip fracture or non-accidental injuries in children resulting in upper limb fractures. This leads to the discovery of changes or trends in the occurrence over time.
- **Explanation**: involves finding the causal factors and implications of an illness, for example the effect of calcium intake by adolescents and their risk of osteoporosis in adult life. In the case of infections, the mode of transmission of an infection such as tuberculosis within a homeless population group might be of interest.
- **Prediction**: estimates the number of cases likely to arise in the future, such as trends in primary bone tumours or predicting the potential effect on trauma admissions from an airport being developed or extended.
- **Control**: involves applying epidemiological knowledge to prevent new cases arising, for example whether driving speed restrictions reduce road traffic accident rates or the severity of injuries in a specific area. Other examples of control involve the eradication of disease, as with poliomyelitis, or

studying the effectiveness of drugs that improve function or the quality of life or prolong life.

EPIDEMIOLOGICAL RESEARCH

Conclusions based on the causes (aetiology) of disease often arise from comparison of:

- disease rates between groups
- those with different levels of risk, for example comparing why some older people are at greater risk of falling than others
- why those exposed to the same risks will or will not develop an illness or incur injuries, such as studies on the implementation of health and safety recommendations in the workplace.

The monitoring of health trends will show increasing, decreasing, changed or static distribution patterns. This identifies emerging short- or long-term trends and the effectiveness of interventions to reduce previous problems. Unfortunately, research is never that simple, as confounding factors intervene. The reasons for the reduction in major injury and death rates among car passengers and drivers include a combination of:

- seatbelt legislation
- reduced speeds in built-up areas
- the effect of speed cameras
- changes to the design and safety features of cars
- the training of paramedics in the care of the victim at the roadside and during transfer to hospital
- hospital improvements in resuscitation techniques, plus different treatment and rehabilitation methods.

Hence comparing death rates among car passengers per head of population between, say, 1954 and 2004 will not give clear data relating to the benefit of any of these factors. Consequently, changes over time are considered within the context and influences of the time periods concerned (Coggon et al 1993).

POTENTIAL BIAS

When drawing comparisons between cause and effect, the data need to be unbiased in order to identify at-risk groups.

If the data collection involves more than one person or more than one location, issues relating to the rigour, standardisation of the data collection process and the potential for biases to be created by one or more of the collectors or centres need to be considered in the design and implementation of the research. For instance, the rates of deep vein thrombosis (DVT) in patients after discharge from hospital could vary depending on how a hospital collects data relating to this. Differences could reflect whether the two events of surgery and thrombosis are linked, whether the patient is treated for the embolism in the same hospital, by the same orthopaedic team or by the haematology team. Here the research team must ensure these issues are accounted for; otherwise, it could incorrectly appear that one unit has a higher rate of DVT occurrence than another.

POPULATION GROUPS

Although ideally epidemiological data would be based on the whole target population, as with the majority of research it is based on a selection of this, the study sample (Coggon et al 1993), for example the number of patients attending one hospital with primary tumours who subsequently develop bone metastases. The representativeness of this sample group in terms of the generalisability of any findings could vary depending on the clinical area used. A hospital with a regional oncology unit is likely to see a wider range of primary tumours and more patients with bone metastases than a small hospital that normally refers patients on to a regional unit. The results from using either hospital could therefore have an inbuilt bias if not accounted for in the data analysis process.

Defining the study population depends on the topic concerned.

- **Geographical populations**: for example, those living in a specified area who attend a spinal assessment clinic.
- **Occupational populations**: such as children attending a specific sports facility or the employees of a factory.
- **Specific care facility populations**: including those on a community practitioner's register of clients, residents of a care home or attendees of a preadmission clinic.
- **Diagnostic populations**: for instance, patients with systemic lupus erythematosus (SLE).

In many cases a combination of these is of interest, for example a study reviewing the occurrence of

SLE in people of working age (20–60), living in a specific city and attending a specified rheumatology nurse-led clinic.

Equally, within these broad definitions inclusion and exclusion criteria normally apply such as gender, age, ethnicity, co-morbidity, mobility restriction or previous medical interventions.

MEASURING FREQUENCY

The measures of frequency of a condition depend on its incidence, prevalence and mortality rates.

Incidence

The incidence is the rate at which new cases occur in a population of previously unaffected individuals over a specified period of time (Coggon et al 1993). In studies of aetiology, the incidence is generally the most important factor.

Prevalence

The prevalence is the proportion of a population affected (cases) by a condition at a particular point in time. Prevalence is often easier to determine than incidence.

Generally, prevalence is more relevant for stable conditions than for acute disorders. As each new case arises, it enters the prevalence pool and the patient will remain in this category until they recover, are diagnosed as having a chronic condition or die.

Period prevalence is defined as the 'proportion of a population that are cases at any time within a stated period' (Coggon et al 1993, p9). The prevalence may fluctuate depending on other variables, making repeated or continuous assessments of prevalence relevant. An example is the prevalence of back pain amongst nurses which has changed over time, particularly following the introduction of lifting aids and non-lifting manual handling policies. Equally the number of nurses with back pain changes as individuals go through stages such as the acute phase, have repeated periods of acute pain, recover or move into a continuous chronic pain condition. The introduction of new moving and handling equipment, health and safety at work regulations and changes in the role of nurses are some of the additional variables affecting the prevalence of back pain cases over time.

Prevalence rather than incidence is used in relation to rarer diseases.

Mortality

Measures of mortality relate to the incidence of death from a disease or injury, for example the number of fatal pulmonary embolisms following hip replacement surgery. Mortality rates are measured using the cause of ill health, injury, age and gender. This allows comparisons over time to show whether preventive measures are beneficial.

Patterns of mortality can be misleading, as with the decline in mortality from spinal cord injury. If attributed to improved care by the paramedic and trauma teams, this ignores the reduction in incidence due to improved safety measures in sports and car safety. This illustrates the complexity and the need for accurate relationships between mortality and frequency to be related to all potential variables.

ACCIDENT DATA CONSISTENCY

The UK Measuring and Monitoring Injury Working Group (MMIWG 2002) recognised the need for a policy lead in prioritising the coordination of accident and injury prevention at local, regional and national levels. One problem in collating data on illness and injury is that the agencies involved collect information important to them but the type of information varies. They can have different definitions for the same terms and collect information using different data coding systems, making comparisons and analysis difficult. This is a problem both nationally and internationally.

Defining an accidental injury

Accidental injury is defined by the MMIWG (2002, p2) as an injury 'occurring as a result of an unplanned and unexpected event which occurs at a specific time from an external cause', for example a transport incident (by rail, road, air or water), falls or those caused by natural or environmental factors.

The terms used to define the severity of injuries include critical, major, serious, slight or minor but specific definitions of what these mean are not available and routinely used. A serious injury is defined by the Department of Health (1999) as one that requires an inpatient stay of longer than 3 days. However, many patients may be in hospital for 3 or more days due to preexisting conditions or other problems exacerbated by or as a consequence of the injury concerned. Consider a patient with a Colles' fracture. This is normally described as a minor accidental injury but if the patient's general health requires them to be in hospital for more than 3 days, is this now defined as a serious injury? How these terms are used in countries outside the UK may well differ again.

Accident rates

Data on injury rates and causes need to be meaningful, accurate and routinely collected and collated. Meaningful data can inform a population of their specific risk of injury or initiate an injury prevention scheme. At a local level, the number of injuries and deaths per year can be too small for the data to be of use for monitoring or evaluating prevention programmes for individual injury types. Hence, data relating to injury surveillance are normally collated at a regional or national level.

There is a lack of data relating to injury rates as defined by disability, ethnic groups and social class within local and regional areas. This again prevents identification of some causes of ill health and injury, as well as stopping local prevention schemes accurately targeting such groups, as their risk is unknown.

The Department of Health's (2002) current priority groups for monitoring and measuring injury are children and young adults of 0–24 years and the elderly of 65+ years (see Table 9.1). Table 9.2 illustrates the inequalities in death and serious injury by age and gender.

Reducing accidental injuries is a national and international issue. Table 9.3 shows some of the targets set for the reduction in injury rates within the UK by government departments.

EPIDEMIOLOGY AND ORTHOPAEDICS

The DoH estimates the cost to the NHS of treating accidental injuries and poisoning as being £2.2 billion per year (MMIWG 2002). This does not include the cost of rehabilitation, the cost to employers from lost working days or the cost to individuals in terms of the financial and physical effects.

FALLS AND HIP FRACTURE

The importance of looking at a population group at risk of an orthopaedic condition or injury is shown on the majority of trauma wards where the number of elderly people with a hip fracture could indicate that all people over 60 years have a very high risk of

Table 9.1 Measuring and monitoring injuries: priority areas (adapted from MMIWG 2002)

Priority area	Data collected on
Priority areas for immediate action	Young and older pedestrians
	Injuries to older people from falls and fractures
	Injuries to older car occupants
	Injuries to children from play and recreation
Priority areas for action over the period to 2002	Injuries to younger drivers and passengers
	Sports injuries to young adults
	Injuries at work
	Home and leisure injuries to working-age adults
Priority injury areas	Transport injuries: pedestrians, pedal cycle and car occupant injuries
	Sport, play and recreation-related injuries
	Falls and fractures
	Home and leisure injuries
	Work-related injuries
Priority populations	Children
	Young male adults
	Older people
	Socio-economically disadvantaged people

having a hip fracture. In reality, although many are at high risk, the level of risk varies with, for instance, their level of bone density, exercise and risk activity behaviours. Conclusions about risk and incidence rates cannot be made solely from clinical data as these would inevitably be based on the number of patients seen, not the total of those at risk within a population.

Hip fractures are one of the most studied orthopaedic conditions in relation to epidemiology because of the rates of occurrence and the multiple causes and factors related to this injury (Beaglehole et al 1993). As the number of older people as a proportion of the population is increasing, the number of patients with a hip fracture will likewise increase over time, leading to an increased need for acute and rehabilitation care facilities.

The elderly are at the greatest risk of falls. This is typified in Britain where approximately a third of the population over 65 years has a fall (Swift 2001) in any given year. It is women, especially those living alone, who are at greatest risk of having a fall compared to

Table 9.2 Health inequalities in injuries by age and gender (adapted from MMIWG 2002)

Data source	Type of injury	Inequality data
Based on 1999 data (from the ONS (Office for National Statistics) mortality figures)	All accidents	Death rate for those of 65+ years is 3 times the rate for all ages
	Falls	Death rate for those of 65+ years is over 5 times the rate for all ages
	Falls	Death rate for women of 65+ years is 1.5 times that for men
	All accidents	For those aged 15–24 and 25–64 years the death rate for men is over 3 times the rate for women
	All accidents	For all ages the death rate in men is 1.4 times that for women
Based on 1999–2000 data (from DoH)	All accidents	All-person serious injury rate for those of 65+ years is 4 times the rate for all ages
	Falls	All-person serious injury rate for those of 65+ years is 4.9 times the rate for all ages
	All accidents	For those aged 15–24 years the male rate is 2.6 times the female rate
	Falls	For those aged 15–24 years the male rate is 2.7 times the female rate
Based on 1999 data (from DETR (Department of Environment, Transport and the Regions))	For pedestrians	The casualty rate (killed or seriously injured) for those aged 0–15 years is 1.7 times the rate for all ages
	For pedestrians	The casualty rate (killed or seriously injured) for those aged 70+ years is 1.3 times the rate for all ages
	For all road users	The casualty rate (killed or seriously injured) for those aged 16–29 years is 1.8 times the rate for all ages
Based on England national estimates from 1998 data (from DTI (Department of Trade and Industry))	*Data by age*	
	All home accidents	A & E attendance rate for those aged 0–4 years is over 3 times the rate for all ages
	Falls at home	A & E attendance rate for those aged 0–4 years is over 3 times the rate for all ages
	All leisure accidents	A & E attendance rate for those aged 5–14 years is over 2.6 times the rate for all ages
	All home accidents	A & E attendance rate for those aged 75+ years is over 1.5 times the rate for all ages
	Falls at home	A & E attendance rate for those aged 75+ years is over 2.7 times the rate for all ages
	Data by gender	
	All home accidents	A & E attendance rate for boys aged 0–4 years is 1.3 times the rate for girls
	Falls at home	A & E attendance rate for boys aged 0–4 years is 1.3 times the rate for girls
	Falls (leisure activities)	A & E attendance rate for boys aged 5–14 years is 1.4 times the rate for girls
	All home accidents	A & E attendance rates for women aged 75+ is 1.7 times the male rate
	Falls at home	A & E attendance rates for women aged 75+ is 1.9 times the male rate
	All leisure activities	A & E attendance rates for women aged 65–74 is 1.7 times the male rate
	Falls (leisure activities)	A & E attendance rates for women aged 65–72 is 2.0 times the male rate
Based on 1999–2000 provisional data (from the Health and Safety Executive)		The commonest age for male employees to sustain non-fatal major injuries is 30–34 years, which accounted for 2890 injuries or 15% of injuries to all male employees
		The commonest age for female employees who sustained non-fatal major injuries is 50–54 years, accounting for 930 injuries or 15% of injuries to all female employees

men, with half of all women over 85 years having a fall in any one year (Swift 2001). Reduced bone density, typically seen in elderly women, increases their chance that a fall will cause a fracture. The relevance of osteoporosis prevention and hip fracture prevention strategies requires long-term studies that follow cohorts over time.

Not only do the majority of fractures associated with falls occur in the elderly but also the majority of deaths associated with falls are the consequence

Table 9.3   Targets set to reduce the rate of injuries (adapted from MMIWG 2002)

Publication	Target
Saving lives: our healthier nation (DoH 1999)	Accidental injury was 1 of 4 priority areas with targets to reduce by 2010: • death rates from accidents by at least a fifth • the rate of serious injury from accidents by at least one-tenth
Tomorrow's roads: safer for everyone (DETR 2000)	A national road safety strategy aiming by 2010 to achieve: • a 40% reduction in the number of people killed or seriously injured in road accidents • a 50% reduction in the number of children killed or seriously injured in road accidents • a 10% reduction in the slight casualty rate, expressed as the number of people slightly injured per 100 m vehicle kilometres
Health and Safety Commission (2001)	Targets for health and safety accidental injury include a reduction of: • 30% in the number of working days lost per 100 000 workers from work-related injury and ill health • 10% in the incidence rate of fatal and major injury accidents • 20% in the incidence rate of cases of work-related ill health
Department of Trade and Industry (MMIWG 2002)	Targets set for home accidents are: • a 20% reduction in home accidental deaths by 2007 • to maintain home accidental injuries at the 1999 levels despite adverse demographic changes

of hip fractures. Keene et al (1993) corroborated this as they identified a fractured femur as being associated with a 33% mortality rate per year.

Patients over 75 years admitted following an accident occupy a hospital bed for an average of 18 days (DTI 1997). Of these, patients with hip fractures account for the largest number of bed-days spent in hospital among orthopaedic patient groups. The potential increase in the annual incidence of hip fracture in England and Wales could rise to 96 000 by 2031, along with the increased need for extra bed-days and costs of care (Armstrong & Wallace 1994). This compares to 1985 when in England there were 43 230 fractures of the hip, with an average hospital stay of 29.8 days (OHE 1990). Despite the reduction in the length of hospital stay, hip fractures remain expensive to treat in terms of bed-days, surgery and rehabilitation.

These points illustrate some of the complexities for any study aiming to relate cause and effect within an orthopaedic population.

CLINICAL APPLICATION

Epidemiology research is quantitative in approach, focusing on the patterns that emerge about a disease or injury occurrence, determining the onset and the cause and effect relationships. Ideally, from the analysis, beneficial preventive strategies or treatment approaches can be determined for patient groups or an individual.

While the data may appear to be unrelated to orthopaedic nursing, it explores why patients appear in the accident and emergency or orthopaedic clinic departments. The subsequent care they receive and the outcomes for the individual, family and society are aspects that the orthopaedic nurse can influence. By being aware and acting upon the known risk factors and by understanding the implications for patients in the short or long term, the orthopaedic nurse can ensure an evidence-based care approach.

The fundamental difference between epidemiological research and clinical epidemiology is that the former looks at groups and the latter at how the risk factors affect specific individuals. The application of epidemiology to clinical practice is based on the interpretation and recommendations of the findings to the individual patient.

ENVIRONMENTAL FACTORS

The environment is perhaps one of the largest influences on orthopaedic epidemiology, especially in terms of trauma, as has already been seen with hip fractures. This would include the effects of psychological, biological, physical, chemical and accident factors (Beaglehole et al 1993).

The individual can identify or modify the effect of environmental factors by, for example, their nutritional status, physical condition, personality and body defences. Unfortunately, there are multiple effects of environmental factors on the cause and subsequent development of disease, making the identification of specific causes difficult to isolate. This often accounts for the differences between the findings of different epidemiological studies as they are using different population groups in different settings (Beaglehole et al 1993).

Community environment

This includes the surveillance and occurrence of disease or injury in real-world settings, such as spinal injuries from building site accidents. Also included in this group would be the benefits of community screening programmes, for example hip dysplasia screening in babies, and community-based causes such as the influence of alcohol and drugs on health.

In relation to transport as a cause of ill health and injury, the UK Department of Transport, Local Government and Regions (2001) estimated that in the year 2000, there were 233 729 road traffic accidents in Great Britain causing injury to at least one person (DTLGR 2001). The estimated value of preventing these accidents is £12 170 m (at year 2000 prices). Consequently, investigations into the causes of transport accidents and the resultant injuries are continuous and a major source of research interest in all countries.

Occupational environment

The Health and Safety Executive estimates that workplace injury and ill health cost employers £3300–6500 million per annum and impose costs to individuals from reduced income and additional expenditure of £7000 million (cited by MMIWG 2002). It further estimates that the total cost to society, including pain, grief and suffering plus additional individual and employer costs, is £14 500–18 100 million (based on 1995–6 prices).

The focus on the workplace as a cause of ill health includes the monitoring of levels of illness in a workforce and looking for causal links between occupational exposures and subsequent disease. This would include ergonomics and manual handling as causes of intervertebral disc injuries. Other factors influencing occupational causes of ill health are chemicals, including skin irritants, dust, shift work, noise, lighting, radiation, climate, stress and human relationships within the workplace.

Most studies of the workplace are based on fit male adults; they may not always be representative of other occupational or general population groups (Beaglehole et al 1993).

Home environment

The Department of Trade and Industry (DTI 2001) estimated that there are 2.8 million accidents in the home and 3.1 million leisure accidents (including sports) that result in injury. This reflects the injuries and accidents actually reported but many, especially minor injuries, go unreported. During 1999, accidents in the home environment cost 3974 people their lives (MMIWG 2002).

With the home environment being a dangerous place in relation to personal injury, the orthopaedic issues include injuries to children, adults falling down stairs or traumatic injury to a digit or limb by household or gardening equipment such as knives and chain saws. The cost to society of accidents in the home was estimated to be £25 000 million per year at 1994 prices (Hopkin & Simpson 1996).

The reasons for such injuries vary. The MMIWG recognises that obtaining data on injuries from sports, leisure and play is difficult but is required before the benefits of preventive initiatives are measured. Equally important are the data relating to the causes of injuries in children.

Stark et al's (2002) retrospective population-based study aimed to assess the links between deprivation and childhood fracture rates in Glasgow. They found that children living in deprived areas had a significantly higher fracture rate than those living in affluent areas. This supports Morrison et al's (1999) findings that showed higher mortality rates for children suffering injury who lived in deprived areas of Scotland. However, a similar study by Lyons et al (2000) in South Wales showed no such trends linking childhood fracture rates and deprivation. These differences reflect not just the difficulties in linking poverty and injury but also the problems encountered when comparing studies from different geographical areas, the difference in statistical approaches and the variations used in defining the term 'deprivation' (Stark et al 2002).

PREVENTION

General population

Research related to general population groups often looks at prevention; this would include identifying the risks in relation to falls in the elderly. The importance of looking at the causes of why people fall

> **Box 9.2   Risk factors for falls (adapted from Swift 2001)**
>
> - Impairment of gait, balance or mobility
> - Polypharmacy, especially drugs acting on the central nervous system and antihypertensives
> - Visual impairment
> - Impaired cognition
> - Depression
> - Postural hypotension
> - Associated medical history: stroke, Parkinson's disease, degenerative lower limb joint disease

> **Box 9.3   Risk factors relating to osteoporotic fractures (adapted from Swift 2001)**
>
> - Risk of falling
> - Radiographic evidence of osteopenia
> - Loss of height associated with osteopenic vertebral deformity
> - Previous fragility fracture
> - Prolonged corticosteroid treatment
> - Chronic disorders associated with osteopenia
> - History of premature menopause
> - History of maternal hip fracture
> - Low body mass index
> - Age and gender
> - Level of physical activity
> - Diet
> - Alcohol
> - Cigarette smoking

(Box 9.2), including the physiological, pathological and pharmacological factors, illustrates the need to incorporate these aspects into a multidimensional assessment and intervention approach in the care of older people (Swift 2001). Falls assessment and prevention clinics are aiming to address these issues.

High risk

Taking a selective prevention approach enables identification of, for example, those at high risk of repetitive strain injury (RSI) from work-related causes such as repeated use of computer keyboards. This would have implications for the design of the work environment, the cost to employers and individuals of time off work and the treatment approaches. The identification of RSI causes should then lead to the instigation of preventive measures for the individual and others.

Systemic changes

A clear example of systemic changes is the reduction in oestrogen levels in postmenopausal women. Oestrogen protects against bone loss, so the decrease in oestrogen level puts postmenopausal women at a significantly greater risk of vertebral body and hip fractures compared to premenopausal women (Box 9.3). This risk increases with age as the loss of bone density increases due to the continuous reduction in oestrogen levels. The increased proportion of older people in the population as a whole means this will continue to be a major issue as a cause of back pain and mobility problems in this population group.

A study by Coupland et al (1999) explored a means of reducing these risks, namely by the use of regular physical activity (stair climbing, brisk walking, with frequent walks of at least a mile) to increase bone density at the hip and in the whole body in postmenopausal women. Farahmand et al's (2000) study in Sweden supports this by concluding that recent physical activity is protective against hip fracture. This information should be built into patient advice for those identified as being at risk, as these physical activities are relatively straightforward for many middle-aged women.

SPECIFIC GROUPS

There is a potential multitude of studies; as discrete research studies, or part of larger studies. The areas addressed below are only a small range of examples; others would include epidemiology studies of genetic-related conditions, infections and immunity, paediatric conditions and trauma and oncology studies. Some of the following chapters pick up this theme and include specific epidemiology findings, trends or risk factors related to orthopaedic disorders and injury.

Degenerative conditions

With increased age, there is a gradual loss of muscular strength and stamina due to muscle cell atrophy. The accompanying loss of elastic fibres and collagen in muscle tissue, tendons and joint ligaments leads to reduced flexibility and increased stiffness. These natural degenerative changes have associated effects on the mobility of the individual. This does not have obvious implications for healthcare services until further problems arise, such as a fracture or the need for joint replacement surgery.

Such changes have a great effect on orthopaedic services as degenerative diseases affect the musculoskeletal system more than any other system, with osteoarthritis affecting most people over 75 years of age to some degree. With these physical changes come impaired mobility, chronic pain and an altered level of independence. This has implications for the long-term provision of healthcare, including joint replacement surgery, and ensuring individuals are able to return to their active lives and be independent in the community. However, some patients may require long-term community-based care to support their independent living or because they move to residential or nursing home facilities.

Postoperative thrombosis

The identification of health problems within specific patient groups includes the rates of postoperative complications such as venous thrombosis in patients following joint replacement surgery.

Edelsberg et al's (2001) review identifies the current risks after hip and knee arthroplasty, which appears to be about 2.5% for deep vein thrombosis and 1% for non-fatal pulmonary embolism in the 3 months following surgery. Although the risk of venous thrombosis has reduced over time, the cost of treating these events remains high. Edelsberg et al state that similar reliable results for the risk of embolism following hip fractures are lacking due to the complex factors related to the injury and the causes of embolism such as the time between injury and surgery and the patients' potentially poorer overall health.

Personal lifestyle

Research on the influences of an individual's lifestyle, their social setting and behaviours on the development of disease could involve investigating injuries from high-risk activities such as rally driving, the effects of major trauma resulting in disability, or why only some tennis players have repetitive injuries such as lateral epicondylitis.

IMPLICATIONS FOR NURSING

The cause of orthopaedic conditions, particularly trauma events, may not appear to relate to the role of the orthopaedic nurse.

The orthopaedic nurse may not be caring for an individual immediately following injury but in the secondary and tertiary phases of their care. Relevant activities will include raising the patient's awareness of how they can prevent a future event occurring, particularly in the case of sports and recreational activity-related trauma.

Patients admitted to the healthcare system with an orthopaedic condition will likewise receive care from orthopaedic nurses who need to be aware of the cause and progression of their condition.

All nurses are involved in the treatment and care of patients who have a secondary condition, for example wound and urinary tract infections. These secondary conditions are equally the subject of epidemiological studies as seen with the thrombosis risks.

With the increasingly important role of the nurse as a health promoter, every opportunity should be taken to educate patients in safety and the preventive aspects of health. This includes, where appropriate, raising awareness of the causes and progression of conditions and injuries.

Prevention as an aspect of care should not be undervalued. The prevention of ill health typically occurs at three levels.

- **Primary prevention** directed at healthy people, aiming to prevent ill health arising in the first place. This includes advice on exercise and diet to promote a healthy lifestyle, safety in sports activities and accident prevention measures.
- **Secondary prevention** aims at stopping acute ill health from moving to a chronic or irreversible stage and restores the person to their former state of health. The orthopaedic nurse's role here includes screening programmes such as nurse-led developmental dysplasic hip screening or the prevention of complications from a diagnosed condition or treatment, for example preventing healthcare-associated infections.
- **Tertiary prevention** enables patients and relatives to make the most of their potential for healthy living within the boundaries of their health problems. This is refelected in advice offered by nurse-led hospital-at-home, early-discharge schemes and nurse-led follow-up clinics.

Using the information provided by epidemiological studies to inform practice increases the toolkit all practitioners can access to ensure high-quality evidence-based care. The arenas for using these data to inform nursing practice are widening with the creation of more diverse nursing roles and the increased use of multidisciplinary approaches to practice problems. Nurses should therefore become more aware of the role of epidemiology in the identification of the causes and progression of ill health and use this information for the development of future nursing roles and practices.

Further reading

Beaglehole R, Bonita R, Kjellström T 1993 Basic epidemiology. World Health Organisation, Geneva

Coggon D, Rose G, Barker DJP 1993 Epidemiology for the uninitiated, 3rd edn. BMJ Books, London

Whitehead D 2000 The role of epidemiology in orthopaedic practice. Journal of Orthopaedic Nursing 4(1): 33–38

References

Armstrong A, Wallace WA 1994 The epidemiology of hip fracture and methods of prevention. Acta Orthopaedica Belgica 60 (suppl 1): 85–101

Beaglehole R, Bonita R, Kjellström T 1993 Basic epidemiology. World Health Organisation, Geneva

Coggon D, Rose G, Barker DJP 1993 Epidemiology for the uninitiated, 3rd edn. BMJ Books, London

Coupland CAC, Cliffe SJ, Bassey EJ et al 1999 Habitual physical activity and bone mineral density in post-menopausal women in England. International Journal of Epidemiology 28: 241–246

Department of Health (DoH) 1999 Saving lives; our healthier nation. Department of Health, London

Department of Health (DoH) 2002 Preventing injury – priorities for action. A report from the Accidental Injury Task Force to the Chief Medical Officer. Department of Health, London

Department of Trade and Industry (DTI) 1997 21st annual report home accident surveillance system. Accident data and safety research – home, garden and leisure. Department of Trade and Industry, London

Department of Trade and Industry (DTI) 2001 Working for a safer world. 23rd Annual report of the home and leisure accident surveillance system – 1999 data. DTI Consumer Affairs Directorate, London

Department of Transport, Local Government and the Regions (DTLGR) 2001 Road accidents Great Britain: the casualty report 2000. Stationery Office, London

Edelsberg J, Ollendorf D, Oster G 2001 Venous thromboembolism following major orthopaedic surgery: review of epidemiology and economics. American Journal of Health-System Pharmacy 58 (suppl 2): S4–13

Farahmand BY, Persson P-G, Michaëlsson K et al 2000 Physical activity and hip fracture: a population-based case-control study. International Journal of Epidemiology 29: 308–314

Hopkin JM, Simpson HF 1996 Valuation of home accidents: a comparative review of home and road accidents. Report 225. Transport Research Laboratory, Crowthorne

Keene GS, Parker MJ, Pryor GA 1993 Mortality and morbidity after hip fracture. British Medical Journal 307: 1248–1250

Lyons RA, Delahunty AM, Heaven M et al 2000 Incidence of childhood fractures in affluent and deprived areas: population based study. British Medical Journal 320: 149

Measuring and Monitoring Injury Working Group (MMIWG) 2002 Report to the Accidental Injury Task Force. Available online at: www.doh.gov.uk/accidents/pdfs/mmi.pdf

Moon G, Gould M et al 2000 Epidemiology: an introduction. Open University Press, Buckingham

Morrison A, Stone DH, Redpath A et al 1999 Trend analysis of socioeconomic differentials in deaths from injury in childhood in Scotland 1981–1995. British Medical Journal 318: 567–568

Office of Health Economics (OHE) 1990 Osteoporosis and risk of fracture. Office of Health Economics, London

Stark AD, Bennet GC, Stone DH et al 2002 Association between childhood fractures and poverty: population based study. British Medical Journal 324: 457

Swift CG 2001 Falls in later life and their consequences – implementing effective services. British Medical Journal 322: 855–857

Chapter 10

Process and prevention of infection

Dinah Gould, Julia D Kneale

INTRODUCTION

All patients are susceptible to infection from, for example, contamination of a trauma wound or healthcare-associated infection (HCAI). The risk of infection from surgery increases because of the long and complex nature of musculoskeletal procedures.

An HCAI complicates recovery, whether it is a skeletal infection or in another body system. If the infection affects an implant or weakens a bone, causing a pathological fracture, further surgery is often required. Orthopaedic and trauma nurses need to understand the causes of infection, how they develop and the principles of infection control to ensure the provision of high-quality care.

NORMAL DEFENCES

Before being able to prevent an infection occurring, an understanding of how the body normally defends itself from infection is needed. The natural barriers protecting the body include both the arrangement of tissues and bactericidal secretions:

- intact skin
- sebaceous secretions
- hairs and turbinal bones in the nose
- lysozyme in tears
- saliva in the mouth
- tonsils and adenoids
- cilia and mucus in the respiratory tract
- acid in the stomach
- normal intestinal flora and secretions
- flushing action of urine.

Disease and trauma can breech these defences and increase the risk of infection. The more invasive the trauma and the higher the number of invasive procedures required during treatment, the greater the risk of contamination of tissues that are normally free of microorganisms.

SKIN

Intact skin provides a mechanical barrier to invasion by microorganisms. The sebaceous glands excrete a mildly bactericidal secretion which, along with the normal skin flora, stops pathogenic bacteria from causing an infection. The normal skin flora is harmless unless it is able to penetrate the skin via a wound or injection site.

Staphylococcus aureus is carried asymptomatically on the skin of 10–30% of the general population but is carried more often by healthcare staff. The main sites of carriage are the nose, pharynx, forehead, fingers, toes and perineum. It commonly causes a wound infection or osteomyelitis when able to penetrate the tissues.

GASTROINTESTINAL TRACT

Many of the body's normal secretions are capable of destroying bacteria. The saliva contains lysozyme, an antimicrobial enzyme that removes the microorganisms mechanically by the flushing action of saliva production and swallowing. Patients with a dry mouth, due to dehydration or the effects of drugs, are at risk of oral infections occurring because of the lack of this lysozyme action.

The mucus secreted throughout the gastrointestinal tract acts as a mechanical barrier against infection, while secretions such as hydrochloric acid in the stomach and the bile in the duodenum destroy bacteria. If these secretions are suppressed, an enteric infection is likely to occur.

The normal flora of the large bowel can be destroyed by large doses of prophylactic antibiotics prescribed to protect the patient against a bone infection after surgery. The absence of the normal flora will allow pathogenic organisms, for example Gram-negative *Escherichia coli* (Box 10.1), especially resistant strains, to supervene. An additional consequence of this scenario is diarrhoea; if cross-infection occurs, an outbreak of infective diarrhoea among patients can occur.

Box 10.1   Pathogenic organisms

Gram–positive bacteria: many bacteria contain chemicals in their cell walls allowing them to take up the blue or purple colour of a laboratory dye, Gram's stain, that is widely used in identification and diagnosis of an infection, e.g. *Staphylococcus aureus*, streptococci, enterococcus, clostridia, *Mycobacterium tuberculosis*.

Gram–negative bacteria: these retain the red colour of the counterstain and are thus distinguishable, e.g. haemophilus, pseudomonas, salmonella, *Escherichia coli*. This group of bacteria is able to grow with or without the aid of oxygen and tend to thrive in warm moist environments such as sinks.

RESPIRATORY TRACT

The respiratory tract, except for the alveoli, is lined with ciliate mucus membrane. The coarse nasal hairs and the arrangement of the turbinal bones in the nasal cavity keep large particles out of the respiratory tract. Smaller and inhaled particles are trapped in the mucus and carried by the beating cilia up the respiratory tract to be either swallowed or expelled by coughing and sneezing. About 100 ml of mucus is secreted each day in a healthy person. The lymphoid tissues of the pharynx (tonsils and adenoids) provide additional protection against infection.

The effect of anaesthetic agents is to depress the protective actions of the cilia, putting postoperative patients at risk of a chest infection. Cigarette smoke is an irritant that also paralyses the cilia action and increases the secretion of mucus, which then stagnates in the respiratory tract. Therefore, patients are advised to reduce or stop smoking for several weeks prior to surgery to allow the cilia action to recover and reduce their risk of a chest infection.

GENITOURINARY TRACT

The genitourinary tract has several defences against infection.

For adult women the vagina has a protective pH of 4.5 from the resident population of lactobacilli that metabolise glycogen in the cervical secretions, forming lactic acid and thus an unfavourable environment for most bacteria. Vaginal infections are more common in young girls and postmenopausal women who lack the oestrogen necessary to maintain cervical secretions.

Two sexually transmitted diseases are occasionally encountered in orthopaedic practice. Gonorrhoea is responsible for septic arthritis and syphilis can cause progressive widespread damage to tissues and bones.

The tip of the urethra is colonised by the same microorganisms as the skin but the bladder is normally sterile. Catheterisation risks carrying bacteria into the bladder where the main defence is the flushing effect of emptying the bladder. As a result, urinary tract infections are common in catheterised patients. The risk of an infection increases with the length of time the catheter is in situ. The main points where microorganisms can invade the catheter system are:

- at the catheter tip at the time of insertion
- non-return valves do not completely prevent the backflow of bacteria to the bladder
- aspiration points on the drainage tube from where syringed urine samples are collected
- potential puncture holes in the collection bag
- if the outlet connection is contaminated when changing the drainage bag, by handling with contaminated hands, if it becomes disconnected or touches another surface, especially the floor.

A small number of patients each year develop an ascending urinary tract infection leading to renal infection and septicaemia. The Department of Health (DoH 2003a) guidelines for the prevention of infections associated with the insertion and maintenance of urinary and central venous catheters must be adhered to.

INVASIVE PROCEDURES

All invasive procedures carry the possibility of introducing microorganisms and the risk of infection occurring. Box 10.2 shows some of the portals of infection related to arterial and other intravenous lines. Similar points of entry are found with other procedures.

PATIENT FACTORS

In addition to the normal body defences, the patient may have other personal factors that increase their risk of an infection.

Box 10.2   Examples of portals of entry in intravenous infusion and similar lines

Intrinsic (present before use)
- Infusion fluid
- Crack or puncture holes in the fluid container
- Administration apparatus including the lines and connection points

Extrinsic (introduced during use)
- Contamination during insertion of the infusion line
- Contamination at the connection points, especially when the infusion fluid containers are changed
- During injections into and irrigation of the line
- Contamination of the infusion filters
- From the covering dressing

AGE

Very young and very old patients are particularly susceptible to infection as the immune system develops during childhood and declines in effectiveness with age. Consequently, a young adult patient with an open fracture that is managed well should not develop an infection, whereas an elderly patient with a closed fracture could develop an HCAI.

NUTRITION

A balanced diet that meets the physiological requirements will reduce patients' susceptibility to infection. The diet needs to be nutritionally appropriate with sufficient protein, calories, vitamins and minerals to ensure tissue growth and repair.

Patients who have a reduced nutritional intake due to their illness, dependence, fasting before and after surgery, nausea, pain or lack of appetite will be at risk of developing an infection. Even if a patient is able to eat in hospital, they may not be receiving an adequate nutritional intake. While at home, the patient may continue to have an inadequate intake because they are unable to shop, have no incentive to cook and prepare food or have difficulties in handling food and packaging.

Contamination of food, drinks and the equipment used for eating and drinking can easily occur during food preparation, presentation and consumption if hygiene standards are not adequate.

DEHYDRATION

Dehydration causes suppression of the body's normal defence mechanisms, leading to a dry mouth and respiratory tract, reduced gastrointestinal mucus and reduced urine production, resulting in loss of the effective urinary tract flushing mechanism. Nursing activities to counteract these effects, such as mouth care and treating the cause of dehydration to maintain homoeostasis, are essential to reduce the risk of infection.

IMMOBILITY

Not being mobile can result in urinary stasis, stasis of the cilia in the respiratory tract and pressure sores. Immobile patients are often less able to expectorate due to their position, especially if they are supine or unable to sit up for the greater part of the day.

Obese patients are at greater risk of developing a pressure ulcer, especially if they are immobile, as adipose tissue has a poor vascular supply, making healing slower. Sacral pressure ulcers are more likely to develop an infection as this area is more susceptible to contamination.

WARD ENVIRONMENT

Inappropriate cleaning of the ward and equipment, especially in the bathroom, toilets, commodes, washbowls, bedpans and urinals, increases the risk of cross-infection occurring as many are shared between patients.

The main factor in cross-infection remains the hands of healthcare staff, especially as the washing and drying of hands remains inadequate. The more a patient is touched by nursing, medical and other staff, the greater the risk of infection. Consequently a patient who is unwell or unable to care for themselves will require more physical contact during nursing, physiotherapy and medical care, but this will also increase their risk developing an HCAI.

ILLNESS AND DRUGS

The debilitating effects of illness and treatment regimes can compound the risk of infection.

- Radiotherapy and chemotherapy debilitate a patient already physiologically affected by cancer.
- The high levels of blood sugar and glycosuria occurring with diabetes mellitus may contribute to an infection, especially among elderly patients.
- Peripheral vascular disease changes the circulation to the limbs, commonly resulting in infections of the digits. Advice on foot care is therefore essential, especially for patients with diabetes as any infection can lead to necrosis, gangrene and the potential need for excision or amputation of the affected area.
- Even slight trauma will affect the microcirculation if the blood supply to the area is impaired. Healing is then slow and the area easily infected. The skin over the anterior tibia is one example, varicose ulcers commonly develop in this region because the skin layer is thin and poorly vascularised.
- The use of antibiotic therapy, will increase the risk of gastrointestinal infections as described above, thus unnecessary antibiotics are best avoided.
- The destruction of the normal mouth and vaginal flora increases the risk of a fungal infection, namely candida (thrush).
- Steroids, whether taken for an orthopaedic or other medical problem, suppress the normal inflammatory response that protects the body from infection, reducing the number of white cells and impairing phagocytosis.

Being aware of and identifying the potential causes and risks for a patient enables the healthcare team to take appropriate precautions.

INFECTION TRANSMISSION

Understanding how microorganisms are transmitted can enable the practitioner to take precautions. The principal methods of transmission are direct and indirect contact, through air-borne transmission, by food and water, and parenterally from one host to the next by infected body fluids, needles or other instruments. A few organisms, including HIV, can be transmitted from mother to baby via breast milk.

DIRECT CONTACT

The spread of infection by direct contact between people is particularly common in hospital, especially when very ill patients are receiving care from a number of different members of staff. This risk is minimised by individualised and team nursing approaches to care. Ensuring that practitioners are not involved in caring for highly susceptible patients and infectious patients on the same span of duty further reduces the risk of transmission by direct contact.

Hand washing remains the most significant action in infection control practice (DoH 2003).

INDIRECT CONTACT

Objects that carry microorganisms between people are referred to as fomites. This form of transmission occurs when equipment is not cleaned correctly. Bacteria require warmth, moisture and nutrients to grow and multiply. They therefore flourish in damp bedding and towels rather than on metallic surfaces. The prevention of infection relies on keeping all equipment clean and dry and removing all potential reservoirs of bacteria, such as flower vases and suction tubing.

AIR-BORNE SPREAD

When air-borne respiratory and salivary bacteria-laden droplets dry, they leave particles of dust which act as reservoirs of infection to be passed on to others. Early research by Duguid (1946) demonstrated that an average of 39 000 bacteria-containing droplets are released by a single unstifled sneeze, 710 from a cough and 36 during loud speech. The size of the droplets dictates how far they travel, with gravity causing larger droplets to fall sooner whereas smaller droplets will travel further, dry and the bacteria pass into the circulating air.

Typical infections in the community affecting the upper and lower respiratory tract are transmitted by air-borne droplets. The same effect is seen during surgery with wound infections being caused by the air-borne transmission of staphylococci from the nose and throat of the theatre staff. Minimising the number of people in the theatre, using ultra-clean air environments and laminar flow systems that allow rapid filtration of the air will reduce the risk of intraoperative air-borne contamination.

FAECAL–ORAL ROUTE

Faeces contain a large number of bacteria, which potentially contaminate the environment, food and water. Generally this occurs via inadequate personal hygiene. Microorganisms that form spores, for example *Clostridium perfringens*, are resistant to drying so remain infectious for long periods outside the body.

Outbreaks of food poisoning, often due to salmonella, occur in areas where food is prepared. This risk must be identified throughout hospital catering services. Food brought in by relatives may also be a source of infection transmission; this must be considered if a case of food poisoning occurs.

PARENTERAL SPREAD

Hepatitis B and C and HIV are the main infections spread by contaminated needles and body fluids. Although hepatitis B is more virulent, neither survives long outside the body. The risk of infection is higher for patients who have had a large number of different sexual contacts and for intravenous drug abusers. Good practice when handling and disposing of all sharps, blood samples and other body fluids is essential to protect both patients and healthcare personnel (May & Brewer 2001). All healthcare staff must be offered hepatitis B immunisation.

PATHOGENICITY

The ability of a microorganism to cause disease is referred to as pathogenicity. Most bacteria live harmlessly in the environment, in the soil and water, where they decompose animal and plant material. Some live on the skin and in the gastro-intestinal tract where they compete with foreign bacteria to prevent them multiplying and causing an infection. These beneficial bacteria are referred to as commensals.

Relatively few bacteria act as pathogens, causing disease. When they do, a sequence of events occurs:

- invasion of the tissues overwhelms the body's normal mechanical and bactericidal defences
- the pathogens evade the immune system defences
- multiplication of the pathogen
- destruction of the host tissues, often as a result of enzyme secretion
- release of toxins (potent poisons) that are responsible for the specific signs and symptoms of the infection.

The more virulent the pathogen, the greater the capacity it will have to invade tissues, destroy them and produce stronger toxins. *Staphylococcus aureus* owes its pathogenicity to an enzyme, coagulase, which converts the plasma protein fibrinogen to fibrin; this produces a fibrin mesh around the bacteria to protect them from phagocytosis. In contrast, *Staphylococcus epidermidis*, a commensal organism present in the normal skin flora, is unable to release coagulase so has a lower level of pathogenicity. It will develop as an active infection in severely debilitated patients with poor defence systems and is particularly associated with urinary tract and intravenous catheter infections.

Bacteria capable of causing a low-grade infection in severely debilitated patients are referred to as opportunists. They are a major source of infection because their growth requires moisture and simple environmental contamination, conditions present in many hospital situations.

The size of the infective dose of the pathogen is an important factor contributing to pathogenicity. Areas such as deep tissues of muscles, bones and joints are usually sterile and have a low resistance to bacteria; only a few organisms are therefore required to initiate a pathogenic sequence with devastating effects. In areas with better defence systems, such as the gastrointestinal tract, more organisms are required to initiate the pathogenic sequence.

The speed of bacteria multiplication will also affect pathogenicity. Under ideal conditions, bacilli such as *Escherichia coli* and pseudomonas can replicate approximately every 30 minutes. Urine left in a catheter bag is easily contaminated if left to multiply, a large infective dose can rapidly develop and then gain access to the bladder.

PHYSIOLOGICAL RESPONSES TO INFECTION

Pyrexia

Pyrexia is a systemic reaction of the body to an infection, provoked by microorganisms and their toxins. Body temperature is controlled by the hypothalamus, which regulates the temperature at about 37°C. This control is achieved by a process of negative feedback (Fig. 10.1).

Antigens are foreign substances that stimulate the immune system to respond by producing antibodies. An antigen can be bacterial cells, pollen grains or foreign cells from a tissue graft. When an infection occurs, antigens sited on the bacteria cell walls cause the normal temperature control to be reset at a higher temperature until they have been eliminated from the body. A higher temperature enhances the process of phagocytosis, the process by which the bacteria are engulfed by white cells (mainly neutrophils and macrophages) and are actively destroyed by the action of hydrolytic enzymes. The neutrophils release a protein that stimulates the pyrexia.

An increase in the body temperature will increase the metabolic rate, which in turn increases the speed of tissue repair and precipitates the immune response (Mackowiak 1994). For every 1°C rise above 37°C, the adult pulse rate will increase by approximately 20 beats per minute and the respiratory rate by seven breaths per minute. The body stores of glycogen become depleted and if the pyrexia is prolonged, a negative nitrogen balance will follow. The patient also feels lethargic or exhausted.

Pyrexia is not an infallible sign of infection. Elderly patients may not develop a pyrexia and the presence of confusion and restlessness in a previously lucid and cooperative patient may be the initial indicators of infection. As anaesthesia leaves some patients disorientated postoperatively, this initial sign can be missed.

Inflammation

Inflammation is the reaction of living tissues to injury. The response occurs chiefly through the activity of the vascular and connective tissues. There is no specific cause and the inflammation can relate to physical trauma (excessive heat, cold and radiation), chemicals or an infection. This is an important point as many nurses equate inflammation with an infection only. Following accidental trauma or surgery it is normal for damaged tissues to appear inflamed. The classic signs and symptoms of inflammation are:

- redness
- heat
- swelling
- pain
- loss of function.

At the microscopic level, these readily observable changes are explained by hyperaemia, exudation of plasma from the blood to the extracellular spaces and migration of white cells (Box 10.3) from the capillaries to the damaged area.

Hyperaemia.   This is the initial response, beginning within seconds of injury when the local area becomes momentarily white due to vasoconstriction.

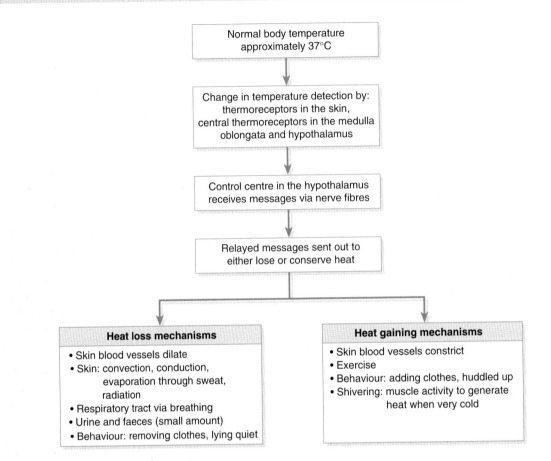

Figure 10.1   Temperature control.

Box 10.3   Neutrophils and macrophages

Neutrophils originate in the red bone marrow. They are continually replaced throughout life as they only survive 1–3 days. They are the first white cells to appear at the sites of acute inflammation. The number of neutrophils increases in an acute infection such as acute osteomyelitis.

Macrophages originate in the red bone marrow, enter the blood and migrate into the tissues. They are replaced throughout life but survive for weeks or months. They appear at the site of inflammation after the neutrophils but as they are larger, they have a greater capacity for phagocytosis. They are active in chronic infections such as tuberculosis.

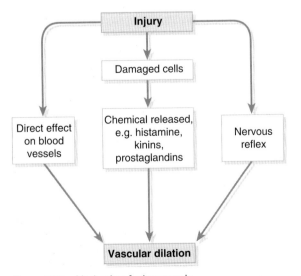

Figure 10.2   Mechanism for hyperaemia.

A dull red warm flush follows as the vessels dilate, increasing local blood supply. The mechanisms responsible for these changes interact, as shown in Figure 10.2.

Exudate. Chemicals released from the injured cells combined with damage to the endothelium of the capillaries increase their permeability, allowing plasma proteins to escape from the vessels into the surrounding extracellular space. Water follows by osmotic attraction, leading to oedema. Pressure from oedema on nerve endings and the action of chemicals such as prostaglandin and kinins released by the damaged cells explain the pain associated with inflammation.

Vasodilation and exudation are valuable defence mechanisms because they carry more white cells and antibodies to the damaged area to fight infection and more fibrinogen to produce blood clotting, thus stemming bleeding in the case of trauma injuries.

Migration. Vasodilation reduces the speed at which the blood is flowing in the capillaries immediately adjacent to the damaged area, causing neutrophils to congregate (marginate) close to the vessel walls. Chemicals released by the damaged cells attract neutrophils, which have the property of amoeboid movement. They are able to squeeze through narrow slits between the capillary endothelial cells and migrate towards the wounded area (see Fig. 10.3). Attraction by chemical substances is called chemotaxis. The ability to squeeze between the capillary cells is known as diapedesis. Once in the damaged area, the neutrophils begin, by phagocytosis, to engulf and digest bacteria and foreign debris contaminating the wound. Only bacteria to which host antibodies have become attached can be phagocytosed, showing how the specific immune system and non-specific inflammation cooperate to destroy an infection.

Antibodies are proteins produced by the body in response to foreign particles, including bacteria. The immune response is specific, as there are thousands of different antibodies, a different one produced in response to every different kind of foreign particle encountered by the tissues. During life, everyone is challenged by slightly different microorganisms, so everyone contains a unique spectrum of antibodies.

The neutrophils, which have a short lifespan, expire after successfully phagocytosing a given number of bacteria. They are later phagocytosed themselves by the much larger and longer-lived macrophages which arrive at the site of damage a day or so after the acute inflammatory response develops. Sometimes virulent bacteria resist attack by degradative enzymes within the neutrophil. Instead they multiply inside it, causing the neutrophil cell membrane to burst open, allowing the bacteria to escape again.

Sequels to acute inflammation

If the inflammatory response proceeds successfully it is followed by resolution, a return to normal conditions. This is possible under the following circumstances:

- minimal host cell death and damage
- rapid elimination of the causal agent
- local conditions favouring prompt removal of exudate and debris via the circulatory system.

Inflammation and resolution proceed more swiftly in tissues which are well vascularised than in those with poor circulation.

If bacteria and other contaminants are not readily removed, suppuration will follow. As dead neutrophils, dead bacteria and other debris accumulate they form pus and an abscess develops, 'pointing' towards an internal or external body surface under the influence of gravity. If the content of the abscess is discharged naturally or by a surgical incision, the pain and swelling will subside, the remaining cavity gradually heals and scar tissue forms.

An abscess deep in the tissues may be overlooked. Gradually a long tortuous track develops between the abscess and a body surface, resulting in the formation of a chronically discharging sinus, especially if contaminated material is retained. Sinuses are extremely difficult to heal and may require surgical intervention. Deep cavity wounds must be packed to prevent superficial healing over a potentially infected underlying layer.

WOUND HEALING

The process of wound healing involves two phases (Gould & Booker 2000) (Fig. 10.3).

1 **Proliferation**: during which tissue regeneration occurs involving four processes:
   - an acute inflammatory reaction continuing for about 3 days
   - collagen synthesis, involving the regeneration of tissues lost through trauma
   - angiogenesis, repair of the blood vessels
   - epithelialisation, the replacement of the skin covering the wound.

2 **Maturation**: the process by which the tissues become stronger. This phase can last from 21 days to 2 years (Collier 1996).

Not all cells share this property of regeneration. The ability of cells to repair following trauma

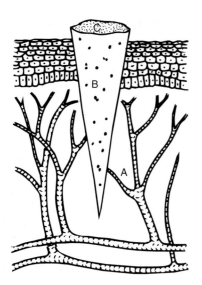

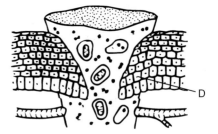

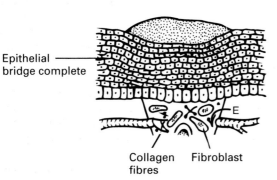

Epithelial
bridge complete

Collagen   Fibroblast
fibres

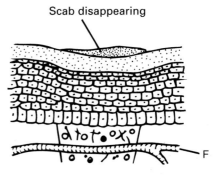

Scab disappearing

Organized new tissue

Inflammatory phase (0–3 days): injured capillary network (A) fills wound with blood to form clot (B), scab forms as a mechanical barrier (C). Damaged tissues release histamine, which causes vasodilation. Additional blood supply brings macrophages and neutrophils. Epitheliasation begins (D) below the scab, epithelial bridge is completed about 3 days post injury.

Proliferation phase (3–24 days): granulation tissue develops from the collagen fibres produced by the fibroblasts and capillary growh stimulated by low oxygen levels, with capillary loops (E) growing into the clot area. Angiogenesis completed when new capillary network is formed (F). Scab will gradually disappear.

Destructive phase (2–5 days): neutrophils and macrophages remove dead tissue and stimulate multiplication of fibroblasts.

Maturation phase (21 days to 2 years): collagen fibres continue to develop and are reorganised to increase the scar tissue strength.

Figure 10.3   Healing by primary intention.

depends on their ability to regenerate and undergo mitosis, a phenomenon known as totipotency. Generally the more highly differentiated (specialised) a tissue has become, the less totipotency is retained by the cells.

● The epithelium and fibroblasts found in connective tissue form a population of labile cells that

retain the ability to regenerate throughout the person's lifetime. The epithelial cells found on the skin and lining of the gastrointestinal tract are in areas where trauma is most likely to occur so they are capable of continually replacing themselves.

● The cells of many internal organs such as the liver and kidney are described as being stable. They do not normally undergo mitosis but can do so in response to damage. Some regeneration following trauma is therefore possible.

- Permanent cells are unable to multiply after their growth phase is complete in early life. Nerve and muscle cells fall into this category. They are unable to regenerate so healing of these tissues is by granulation but there is a degree of permanent loss of function. This has implications for the prognosis of patients with major muscular and nerve injuries.

Bone is classified as connective tissue with osteocytes lying in a non-cellular matrix reinforced with mineral salts. After a fracture, there is an inflammatory reaction comparable to that of soft tissue healing followed by regeneration and healing, generally without loss of function.

Thus a combination of healing processes are involved at the same time with different tissues and organs healing at different rates.

HEALING BY PRIMARY INTENTION

This occurs in clean, incised wounds with good apposition of the tissue margins. Typical examples are cuts and surgical incisions (Fig. 10.3).

Towards the end of the inflammatory response, macrophages in the wound attract fibroblast cells. Fibroblasts are connective tissue cells that produce collagen, the protein that provides the strength in the skin, fascia, tendons and ligaments. In a healing wound, collagen forms granulation (scar) tissue. In surgical wounds, collagen synthesis becomes optimal between the 5th and 7th postoperative days, forming a network of collagen fibres that supports granulation tissue in the cleft of the wound, holding the two edges together. Although collagen provides tensile strength, the damaged tissues never quite regain their original strength.

Collagen formation depends on an adequate supply of nutrients and oxygen but in an infected wound, collagen is competing with bacteria for these, thus delaying healing. The infection further disrupts healing because any pathogenic bacteria will release the enzyme collagenase, which digests the collagen.

Fibroblast activity is stimulated in an acidic environment, rich in lactate and vitamin C. This environment is found deep within the tissues where viable cells are metabolising and releasing lactic acid. The collagen formation therefore begins deep inside

the wound, then extends outwards and upwards as the wound heals.

Wounding severs the local capillaries which then need to undergo repair by angiogenesis at the same time as collagen synthesis. The new capillary growth, stimulated by low oxygen levels, starts at the healthy margins of the wound and later invades the area of regeneration. The new tissue is highly vascular, causing it to appear pink, but these new vessels are easily traumatised, especially by the unnecessary removal of dressings.

While it is forming, the surface of the wound is reepithelialised, a process beginning less than 24 hours after the clean wound is made and completed within 2–3 days. The healthy epithelial tissues at the edge of the wound multiply and form an epithelial bridge (Fig. 10.3) across the wound that is impermeable to bacteria. Often at this stage, the dressing applied in theatre is removed to allow for inspection of the healing tissues. The scab over the epithelial bridge provides an effective mechanical protection against infection, which should not be removed, yet the dressing inspection may damage or remove this protective scab. The process of reepithelialisation proceeds more readily in a moist environment, yet many nursing and medical practitioners remain convinced that a wound should remain scab free and dry. Once reepithelialisation is complete, the scab naturally begins to slough away without any intervention.

As the inflammation subsides, the wound begins to mature, losing its red, raised appearance as the collagen fibres gradually realign, lacing themselves together in a strong, three-dimensional weave. Maturation is accompanied by decreasing vascularity and shrinking of the fibroblasts as they become quiescent. The scar eventually becomes white and less pronounced. Patients often worry about the appearance of the wound and should be advised of these changes before they leave hospital.

HEALING BY SECONDARY INTENTION

Healing by secondary intention proceeds more slowly. This mechanism of healing occurs in open wounds where there has been loss of tissue, necrosis or infection. Burns, ischaemic and varicose ulcers and pressure sores fall into this category.

The wound is subject to recurring episodes of inflammation, fibroblast activity, excess collagen formation and renewed damage. After tissue

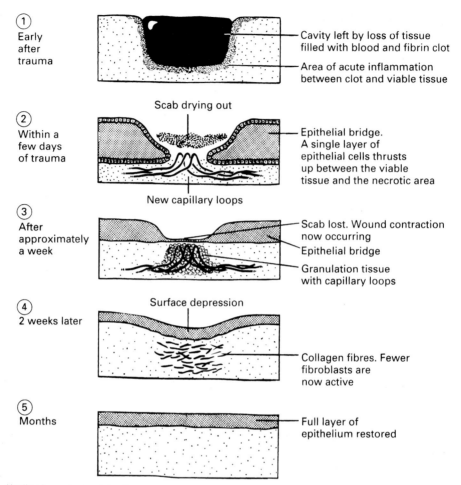

① Early after trauma — Cavity left by loss of tissue filled with blood and fibrin clot / Area of acute inflammation between clot and viable tissue

Scab drying out

② Within a few days of trauma — Epithelial bridge. A single layer of epithelial cells thrusts up between the viable tissue and the necrotic area

New capillary loops

③ After approximately a week — Scab lost. Wound contraction now occurring / Epithelial bridge / Granulation tissue with capillary loops

Surface depression

④ 2 weeks later — Collagen fibres. Fewer fibroblasts are now active

⑤ Months — Full layer of epithelium restored

Figure 10.4 Healing by secondary intention.

destruction, the wound cavity fills with blood and fibrin (Fig. 10.4). Acute inflammation commences at this junction, with viable cells remaining at the base and around the edge of the cavity. Within a few days, the scab covering the wound dries and new epithelial cells thrust their way upwards between the surface debris and underlying tissue. Capillary loops grow into the new epithelium, bringing macrophages and fibroblasts. In time, the cavity fills with granulation tissue and the scab is shed. Epithelium covers the surface of the wound completely within about 2 weeks, although this depends on the size of the wound. There can be excessive and inappropriate collagen deposition and pronounced scarring. Any infection will exacerbate this situation and prolong the healing time.

The maturation phase can take up to one year, with the fibres realigning themselves to provide strength; the area will become less vascular and the fibroblasts begin to shrink as the collagen gains strength (Gould 2001).

CONTAMINATED WOUNDS

Trauma patients can have heavily contaminated wounds (Box 10.4), especially if an open fracture is contaminated by dirt from the road, clothing or chemicals (Cooper & Lawrence 1996). For many pathogenic microorganisms, a large infective dose of bacteria (10^5 colony-forming units) is necessary before infection supervenes in a healthy adult (Gould 2001). Host defence mechanisms can usually cope with smaller doses; hence, many bacteria present in contaminated wounds are destroyed. However, the local defence mechanism is overwhelmed when large amounts of necrotic tissue are present, for example following an open fracture.

Box 10.4   Wound classification

Clean wounds: no evidence of inflammation, no lapse in aseptic technique during surgery and no entry into the respiratory or gastrointestinal tract.

Clean contaminated wounds: those generated by surgical procedures which involve entry into the respiratory tract or gastrointestinal tract, but in which no significant spillage has occurred.

Contaminated wounds: those in which there is evidence of acute inflammation without the formation of pus. An otherwise clean operation in which there has been a major breach of aseptic technique and recent traumatic wounds is considered to be contaminated.

Dirty wounds: those in which pus or a perforated internal organ is encountered. Traumatic wounds not of recent origin, especially if a discharging sinus is present, are also placed in this category.

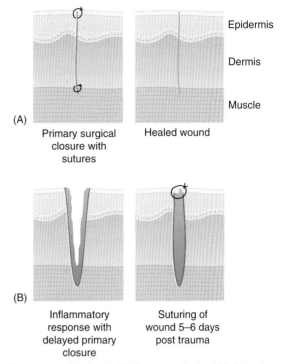

Figure 10.5   Healing by (A) direct suturing and (B) delayed primary closure.

This provides an ideal medium for bacterial growth, especially the species responsible for tetanus (*Clostridium tetani*) and gas gangrene (*Clostridium perfringens*). In these circumstances as few as 15 bacteria may be sufficient to cause an infection in joints and bones. Surgical debridement under general anaesthesia and appropriate antibiotics are required, often for several weeks or more.

Minor wounds heal spontaneously but in the case of more severe trauma, surgical intervention is essential to speed tissue repair, minimise deformity and avoid infection. The method of wound closure will depend on the amount of tissue lost. Direct suturing of the wound edges is appropriate for clean wounds and for contaminated wounds where thorough debridement has been possible (Fig. 10.5A).

Delayed primary closure is the method of choice for heavily contaminated and dirty wounds (Fig. 10.5B). As damaged tissues reach the height of their immune response within 4–5 days of injury, suturing is delayed until then, as the natural resistance to infection will be at its maximum. Initially, the wound is covered with a sterile, non-adherent dressing. When wound closure ultimately takes place, the minimum amount of suture material is employed. Sutures operate as foreign bodies, greatly decreasing the threshold necessary for any remaining bacteria to cause an infection. It has been estimated that the presence of one silk suture reduces the threshold for a clinical infection by a factor of 10 000.

Patients for whom a policy of delayed primary closure has been decided will require a great deal of support to allay the psychological fear of being left 'not intact' or 'cut open' and to relieve any anxiety that they are being neglected. Physical nursing care is crucial to prevent urinary stasis, pressure sore formation and respiratory tract infections through the patient's reluctance to move. Pain control is vital for any patient with a trauma injury as pain can be exacerbated by fear and anxiety.

SURGICAL WOUND INFECTIONS

A number of factors influence the development of infections in surgical wounds. The longer a patient is in hospital, the greater the chance that they will develop an infection, especially from contamination with multiresistant organisms. The use of preadmission clinics has been advantageous in reducing the length of time a patient is in hospital prior to planned surgery. Equally, the transfer of patients into intermediate care settings and early discharge schemes reduces the length of stay for both planned orthopaedic surgery and trauma patients. These developments in orthopaedic care should therefore have a positive influence on infection rates. Other factors influencing infection rates include:

- the patient's age, as older people are at higher risk
- their general health, especially diabetes and cancer
- the position of the wound
- of particular importance in orthopaedic surgery, the degree of contamination and the number of bacteria able to access the open tissues during surgery.

Theatre environment

Although complete elimination of surgical site infections is not possible, the sharing of good practices and information on incidence and surveillance initiatives, can influence behaviours and reduce the incidence (Schneeberger et al 2000).

Staphylococci are a typical example of bacteria transmitted in the theatre environment. They are shed in large numbers from the nose, throat, perineum and on skin scales. A single skin scale may carry 100 individual bacteria, presenting a threat when the deep tissues are exposed. Contamination may occur via the air-borne bacteria or contact with bacteria originating from elsewhere on the patient or the theatre team.

In the early 1960s John Charnley was responsible for the development of a mechanically satisfactory hip joint prosthesis but success was marred by a high rate of sepsis, often exceeding 10% in some centres. Infections sometimes developed months after surgery, representing a disaster for the patient who became less able to function than they were prior to the original surgery. Charnley concluded that the implanted prosthesis must be particularly susceptible to infection, requiring only a small airborne inoculum for sepsis to develop. Between 1960 and 1970 he refined a system of theatre ventilation and clothing that reduced contamination of the ambient air in a theatre suite to less than 1%. Even without prophylactic antibiotics, the rate of infection fell to less than 1%.

Cotton is not suitable for theatre clothing as bacteria can escape through its loose weave. Charnley advocated the use of special non-woven fabric (Ventile) used in conjunction with a total body exhaust gown and helmet. Air is removed from the helmet and the upward flow helps to keep the individual cool. Bacteria are dispersed beneath the gown so the system is fully effective only if there is a unidirectional ultraclean air flow within the theatre. Many theatre staff find the total body exhaust system hot and claustrophobic and the exhaust hose restricts movement. More recent developments in operating theatre design have superseded this system but will only be deemed effective if the infection rate remains at or below 1%.

Filtered air systems reduce the air-borne bacteria count but must be started before the operating list commences and checked regularly to ensure they are working correctly. The air flow is from clean to dirty areas of the suite by maintaining a higher level of pressure in the operating room than in other areas such as the sluice. In high-risk areas such as orthopaedic theatres, high-speed laminar flow systems are effective in removing airborne particles swiftly from the patient's vicinity. The air flows at approximately 30 m per minute, passing through a bank of filters before being extracted through the opposite wall or floor. Down-flow systems appear to be more effective than cross-flow systems but both are rendered less effective by excessive movement of personnel and large obstacles within the theatre, making it essential that only essential personnel are in the area and equipment is stored elsewhere. Guidelines for monitoring airflow and microbiological levels in operating departments are available (Humphreys & Taylor 2002, Stacey and Humphreys 2002) to ensure evidence-based infection control practices and procedures are developed and implemented at a local level.

Anaesthetic equipment must be thoroughly cleaned and decontaminated after use, as the warm, moist tubing can harbour bacteria, especially Gram-negative bacilli. Appropriate infection control policies relating to anaesthetic equipment and its decontamination are essential (king and Cooke 2001).

The risk of infection increases with the length of the surgical procedure so the length of procedures is kept to a minimum.

Mask and gloves

The efficiency of masks in reducing the airborne bacterial count is variable. If the mask is made of a thin material, usually paper, or is ill fitting because it is small and stiff, the effectiveness can be as little as 50%. Loss of efficiency occurs through small particles escaping round the sides. Most of the cheaper brands fall into this category. Effective masks are manufactured from one thick layer of fabric or laminated material, they are soft, pleated and fit the facial contours. However, a systematic review by Lipp & Edwards (2003) found limited results in trials evaluating the wearing of disposable surgical facemasks by the surgical team to prevent postoperative wound infections. They suggest there is a lack of significant evidence to demonstrate whether wearing masks affects the infection rates for patients having clean surgical procedures.

Although there is evidence to suggest that the wearing of theatre masks has little effect, orthopaedic procedures carry such high risks of infection and consequences that they must be worn.

The bacteria carried on the hands are reduced by the use of skin disinfection. The bacteria present from environmental contamination are removed this way while those remaining tend to be resident flora, sheltered in the sweat glands. Gloves are therefore essential during surgery to prevent these organisms gaining access to the wound. As gloves are easily punctured during surgery, double gloving has been adopted by many surgeons with a variety of techniques, including the use of a glove liner between the two pairs, indicator gloves and cloth gloves (Tanner & Parkinson 2003).

Wound position

The site of a wound is closely related to the degree of contamination and infection. A well-vascularised wound is capable of a more efficient inflammatory response and is more likely to heal while remaining free of infection. Hence, a sacral pressure sore carries a very high risk of infection, especially if the damage is deep in the tissues as dressings are very difficult to hold in position. Leg wounds have a high incidence of infection, often from bacteria that are faecal in origin, suggesting that the legs should be regarded as a potentially contaminated site during preoperative preparation.

Preoperative care

Except in an emergency, most patients will be encouraged to have a bath or shower prior to surgery. The use of antiseptic skin preparation at this point has been debated. Shaving the skin is known to increase the risk of sepsis as it damages the epithelial cells, increasing the rate of growth and multiplication of bacteria. Shaving at the last minute in theatre reduces the risk of infection. Most orthopaedic surgeons appear to be against shaving unless essential due to the increased risk of infection.

WOUND MANAGEMENT

The purpose of wound cleaning is to remove heavy contamination from the area. This is achieved either prior to going to theatre, especially if delayed primary closure is to be used, or during surgery. The use of a stream of fluid under hydrostatic pressure may dislodge the contaminants but may also damage tissue defences, so intermittent irrigation is therefore recommended.

The surgical technique and handling of tissues during surgery can contribute to the infection rate. The beneficial effects of the inflammatory process depend on a good blood supply but can be impaired by rough tissue handling, tissue compression and inappropriate diathermy use. The use of monofilamentous suture material is recommended as braided threads are linked with infections because microorganisms can invade through the thread weave.

Following orthopaedic surgery, seepage of serous and serosanguinous fluid through the wound occurs unless removed via a closed suction drain. Wound drains inserted following surgery are designed to remove excess accumulation of fluid but they also serve as a focus of infection. Two drains are often used, to remove fluid from deep in the wound and from the superficial tissues, with the drain inserted through a separate stab wound rather than the incision site to reduce the risk of infection. There has been some debate about the relevance of the routine use of drains following orthopaedic surgery. However, the systematic review by Parker & Roberts (2003) suggests that there is currently no conclusive proof from randomised trials to support or refute the use of suction drains for these patients. They recommend that further randomised trials are required to identify significant outcomes.

The implications of infections arising in the pre-, intra- and postoperative period need to be understood as many infections commence during exposure of the tissues but the effects are not evident until much later. Nurses have a responsibility to ensure that any concerns about infection risks are highlighted to the medical, theatre and infection control staff. The care of postoperative and chronic wounds is the responsibility of the nursing staff. The wide range of dressing materials and apparently conflicting advice on the cleaning and management of these means that the support of specialist infection control and tissue viability nurses is vital, especially when a protracted wound infection or delayed healing is involved.

Implications for management

Outside a very narrow pH range, living tissues lose their metabolic function because the enzyme activity is disrupted. Alterations in pH rapidly have a deleterious effect on reepithelialisation and phagocytosis, which is important when choosing which wound cleaning agent to use.

An adequate oxygen supply is essential for tissue healing. Hyperbaric oxygen enhances the rate of epithelial migration by increasing the oxygen tension in the blood supply to the wound. A high level of oxygen will kill anaerobic bacteria such as clostridia, which cause gangrene.

Rapidly dividing cells depend on a good blood supply to provide nutrients and remove the toxic waste materials resulting from metabolism. External topical nutrients are generally not beneficial as they provide an excellent culture for bacteria. There are several exceptions to this, although they must be used with care.

- The high sugar content in honey, when applied to a wound, has a hydroscopic action, drawing fluid out of the bacterial cells to destroy them.
- Papaya contains an enzyme, papain, which operates as a debriding agent because of its proteolytic action.

Such nutrient applications are only to be used within commercially produced products to ensure they are safe and their use supported by current evidence of effectiveness.

Choice of dressing

There is a critical balance between optimal wound humidity and the amount of fluid present. A wound that is allowed to dry will develop a hard, impermeable scab, impairing the migration of the epithelial bridge. Research in the 1960s and 1970s demonstrated that occlusion beneath a dressing designed to retain moisture promoted reepithelialisation, angiogenesis and granulation. Polyurethane and hydrocolloid dressings fall into this category.

Concerns arise about excessive exudate under polyurethane dressings. This exudate is bactericidal, containing large numbers of active neutrophils. Providing the edges of the dressing are not lifted from the skin, no bacteria can get in from the outside. With some dressings, excess exudate can be aspirated via a sterile needle and syringe but care must be taken not to tear the dressing in the process.

Thermal insulation is required to maintain the wound at body core temperature. The rate of cell multiplication doubles in wounds maintained at a steady 37°C, compared to the ambient temperature of the skin surface. At lower temperatures, cell division is reduced and white cells, which are particularly sensitive to low temperatures, may fail to undergo phagocytosis. The wound can take up to 3 hours to return to its previous level. Lengthy dressing changes and unnecessary inspection of the wound site are therefore discouraged.

To provide optimum protection, a dressing must absorb excess exudate (unless aspiration is possible), prevent contamination of the wound and surrounding environment and not adhere to the healing tissues. However, exudate must not be absorbed in excess otherwise the wound surface begins to slough and if the dressing surface becomes moist, bacteria can gain access from outside the wound. Passage in the opposite direction is also possible, with bacteria in a wound becoming a source of cross-infection. Adherence to the wound bed is a problem, especially if there is little exudate once healing is under way. Serous exudate dries on the undersurface of the dressing and when this is removed the scab and new tissues are torn away, adding to the patient's discomfort, provoking inflammation and delaying healing. Gauze is a particular problem because the loose weave allows bacteria to pass through, it adheres to the wound bed, the fibres can become isolated and act as a focus of infection, and if left in place too long, capillary loops grow into the gauze, causing fresh trauma when removed. Non-adherent dressings are therefore more appropriate.

It is no longer acceptable for the same dressing to be used for every wound or every patient. The choice of a wound dressing has to be based on the type of wound, the method of healing and the potential environment created by the dressing of choice. The development of a wide variety of dressings has led to confusion over which are best in a given circumstance. Research into different dressings and their relative advantage for each type of wound is ongoing and will continue as new dressings come on to the market. To reduce the confusion some clinical areas stock, or are only able to access, a small range of dressings. This restrictive approach often means that less commonly used dressings have to be prescribed and accessed through the pharmacy department.

When a patient is discharged from hospital, it is essential that the resources of the community nursing team be considered, as their range of dressings is often smaller. If a specific dressing has proven to have a positive effect and should be continued, the community team must be contacted in advance and the patient sent home with a supply of dressings.

Chronic wounds

A holistic approach is needed to assess the cause of delayed healing. Reviewing the patient's diet, level of mobility, position in bed and pain management are just as important as reviewing the wound cleaning agent and dressings. Accurate documentation of wound care is essential to provide feedback on the healing or deterioration of the wound. Links between the stage of healing, types of dressings used and the general health of the patient may give practitioners a clue as to the cause of delayed healing and indicate positive actions.

Chronic wounds will not heal within the same time period as surgical wounds, hence changing a dressing will not lead to reepithelialisation within 2–3 days. It is here that the art and science of nursing meet with the nurse's clinical judgement, knowledge of the patient's history and understanding of the scientific properties of the dressings complementing each other.

If a wound is not healing by primary or secondary intention, the patient can become despondent. It is essential that the nursing team remains positive and supportive to avoid feelings of neglect, especially in the case of a pressure sore, the breakdown of a large wound or if an infection develops. Encouraging the patient to take an active role in their care may increase their motivation, including teaching them how to dress the wound if this is appropriate.

ANTIBIOTIC THERAPY

In the 1950s large outbreaks of staphylococcal cross-infection led to the closure of many hospital wards. From these events many infection control policies developed. During the 1980s, it became evident that staphylococci were developing resistance to a wide range of antibiotics. Strict policies on the use of broad-spectrum and prophylactic antibiotics have since been instigated to reduce the risk of bacteria developing resistance to all antibiotics. By reserving some drugs, they can act as a valuable reserve for patients with a multiresistant infection.

Patients undergoing orthopaedic surgery are placed at high risk of developing a bone infection,

making the use of prophylactic antibiotic therapy justifiable, but it should not be used indiscriminately. The aim is to protect the patient from bacteria known to represent a specific threat. The review by Gillespie & Walenkamp (2003) supports the use of prophylactic antibiotics for patients having surgery for proximal femoral and other closed long bone fractures. They found a single dose significantly reduced deep wound infections, superficial wound infections, urinary tract and respiratory tract infections.

Gram-negative bacilli (*E. coli*, proteus, klebsiella, pseudomonas) are spread by contact. They have been found in deep-seated orthopaedic wounds and are responsible for problematic HCAIs, especially of the urinary tract. Few antibiotics are effective against these, supporting the need for the strict implementation of prophylactic antibiotic treatment.

The following good practice guidelines are identified in the use of antibiotics:

- not to be given for trivial reasons
- use preventive measures rather than prophylactic antibiotics wherever possible
- prophylactic use to be reserved for high-risk patients and only if their use is cost effective compared to the patient acquiring an infection
- appropriate specimens to be taken as soon as an infection is suspected
- use antibiotics only if clinically indicated
- avoid broad-spectrum antibiotics, use drugs based on specificity results
- give the correct dose, for the appropriate length of time and stop only at the end of a course or if no clinical response is seen.

Wound swabs taken to identify the microorganisms involved and their sensitivity to antibiotic therapy must be collected carefully to prevent contamination from the normal flora on the skin. Samples of wound exudate should be aspirated as a swab sample is at risk of drying out prior to reaching the laboratory (Gould 2001).

HEALTHCARE–ASSOCIATED INFECTION

Although patients are admitted with bacteria acquired in the community that put them at risk of developing an infection, many infections develop after admission to hospital. These infections are notorious for complicating the course of an illness and delaying recovery. The causes of these infections and the costs they incur have raised many issues that orthopaedic nurses need to be aware of.

HCAIs cannot be prevented completely but they must be detected and dealt with appropriately (NAO 2000). This includes the need for surveillance and feedback of clinical staff, improvements in education and training on infection control practices and auditing of compliance with local and national infection control guidelines.

The DoH (2003b) has identified the current healthcare issues for the UK, these include:

- infections that occur during care and treatment are common and potentially life threatening
- effective evidence-based measures are not consistently implemented
- more infections are difficult to treat because of the increase in antibiotic resistance
- multiresistant strains are a particular threat, especially MRSA, vancomycin-resistant enterococci and penicillin-resistance *Streptococcus pneumoniae*.

To address this, the DoH (2003b) advocate a cultural change in the health service that will ensure: strong leadership with the commitment of managers and clinical leaders at local and national level, high-quality information for the public, patients and clinical teams, and the identification of evidence-based interventions the interventions identified include making HCAIs an indicator of quality and safety in patient care, and ensuring rigorous and consistent implementation of effective measures to reduce the rates and risks of HCAI. The suggested strategies include clear infection control guidelines, clean hospital environments, good hygiene practice, strict antibiotic prescribing policies and isolating infected patients in side-rooms or cubicles.

To support these initiatives, the DoH (2003b) has identified seven action areas that are around the themes of:

- active surveillance and investigation
- reducing the infection risk from catheters, tubes, cannulae, instruments and other devices
- reducing reservoirs of infection
- high standards of hygiene in clinical practice
- management and organisation
- research and development.

These interventions, strategies and actions, will only be effective if implemented and enacted by all practitioners. Orthopaedic nurses must be aware of how these are to be addressed in their own clinical area and work with the Infection Control Team to ensure practice is based on current best evidence.

COSTS

HCAIs are enormously costly to any healthcare provider because of the increase in bed occupancy, antibiotics, nursing time and resources required to manage infections, especially if isolation is required.

These infections carry significant personal costs for the patient and their family, including physical and psychological suffering in addition to those imposed by their original orthopaedic problem or trauma. An extended length of treatment and lasting disability can arise from the infection and consequent surgery that affect the patient's employment, social and financial status. The prolonged length of care can impose on the extended family and friends involved in supporting the patient, possibly causing personal and relationship effects for all concerned.

The longer the hospital stay, the more difficult the period of rehabilitation and adaptation is likely to be.

A comprehensive study of HCAI in the UK by Plowman et al (2001) identifies their incidence and economic burden. They found an incidence rate of 7.8% of patients developing one or more HCAI, the highest incidence of these being urinary tract infections. This supports Emmerson et al's (1996) prevalence study, which found 9% of patients developed an infection, the commonest sites being: blood 6%, wound 9%, lung 22% and the urinary tract 23%. The DoH (2003b) suggests that 80% of urinary tract infections are traceable to catheters.

Plowman et al (2001) found that those developing an infection remained in hospital longer and incurred costs of almost three times that of treating uninfected patients. For orthopaedic patients, the additional costs were 2.6 that of uninfected patients and required patients to be in hospital an additional 12.3 days longer on average. Although not all HCAIs are preventable, Plowman et al suggest that even a 15% reduction can bring significant benefits to the individual and the health service in terms of cost savings.

MULTIRESISTANT INFECTIONS

The threat of antibiotic resistance is an increasing global issue, with more microorganisms developing resistance to one or more drugs. The indiscriminate use of antibiotics increases the risk of bacteria acquiring a multiresistant status. The natural speed of multiplication of bacteria means that genetic changes occur over a short time period. Drug resistance will therefore quickly become a problem once resistance has been established.

A range of bacteria have now adapted and cause problems in treating patients with infections (Glover 2000):

- methicillin-resistant *Staphylococcus aureus*
- vancomycin-resistant enterococcus
- penicillin-resistant pneumococcus
- multiresistant *Pseudomonas aeruginosa*
- multiresistant *Mycobacterium tuberculosis*.

Methicillin–resistant *staphylococcus aureus*

Methicillin-resistant *Staphylococcus aureus* (MRSA) is carried by an estimated 30–50% of the general population (Gould & Booker 2000). It only becomes a problem when transmitted to a person at high risk of developing an infection, especially if there is a break in their skin. In high-risk areas, precautions are taken both to prevent carriers from developing an infection and to protect other patients, including nursing the patient in isolation and ensuring they are last on the day's operating list. Orthopaedic patients are generally classed as high risk because of the potentially serious consequences of MRSA infections following trauma and surgery, especially following the insertion of a prosthesis or other metal implants (Schierholz & Beuth 2001). A prevalence study of MRSA colonisation amongst surgical and orthopaedic patients admitted to a Welsh hospital (Samad et al 2001), found a rate of 5.3%, of which 65% were nasal carriers. They found the main risk factors to be gender (male), age (over 70 years), previous hospital admission and being a nursing home resident. They suggest that all patients fitting some or all of this profile be screened for MRSA prior to admission for surgery. Ideally, patients with positive results should then be treated and only admitted once a negative result is obtained or prophylaxis against MRSA infection be used in the case of trauma or other patients whose admission cannot be delayed.

Wilcox et al (2001) report on the benefits of using perioperative prophylaxis, using nasal mupirocin to prevent MRSA surgical site infections in orthopaedic patients. The marked decrease in infections found had benefits in terms of savings in bed days and the savings in treatment costs with a noticeable 23% reduction in vancomycin being reported. This suggests that mupirocin can reduce the incidence of MRSA surgical site infections, a particularly relevant implication for patients having prosthesis or fixation surgery. It also supports Samad et al's (2001) preference to treat known carriers prior to surgery.

MRSA is treated by the use of glycopeptides, for example vancomycin and teicoplanin. The main precaution in preventing the spread of MRSA remains hand washing, along with the use of protective clothing, especially gloves, and the safe disposal of linen, conforming to hospital policies on handling and laundering linen (British Society of Antimicrobial Chemotherapy 1998).

PREVENTING INFECTION

Many sources of infection threaten the patient in hospital:

- exogenous infections originate from the environment and other people (Fig. 10.6)
- endogenous infections arise from the transfer of bacteria to a more susceptible site on the same person, as with wound infections.

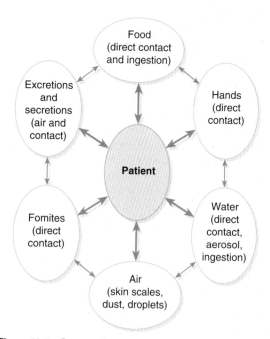

Figure 10.6   Sources of exogenous infection.

The nursing team must assume all patients and staff are carriers and take appropriate strategies to prevent cross-infection (Lee-Smith 1999). Many of the precautions taken in the operating theatre to prevent endogenous infections are costly but on the ward, many preventive measures are relatively simple and cost effective. The principal method of preventing infection remains adherence to universal precautions (Box 10.5).

The infection control team will provide relevant policies and procedures based on current research evidence. Nursing teams are responsible for ensuring these are implemented (Lee-Smith 1999). Regular audits of practices and ward hygiene levels are essential to monitor adherence to and the impact of such policies and procedures (McCulloch 1998). The publication of positive results and reductions in the rate of hospital-acquired infections can reassure the public that their health will not be compromised.

Hand washing

This is the single most inexpensive and highly effective form of infection control. Yet many healthcare staff fail to wash their hands at appropriate times, do not use a correct technique and do not challenge other members of the multidisciplinary team who do not follow infection control policies (Lee-Smith 1999).

Education, feedback and reinforcement (Swoboda 2004), improved facilities (Cochrane 2003) including making alcohol-based hand rinse gels available and the positive effect of good role models, have all been shown to increase compliance with successful hand hygiene practice (Arroluga et al 2004). Everyone, including patients and visitors, needs to understand the importance of good hand hygiene in preventing the spread of infection, Nurses and other healthcare practitioners must recognise their responsibility and accountability to maintain and continually reinforce good practices.

As a general guide, hands should be washed (RCN 2000):

- before and after handling patients
- after handling any soiled item, body fluids or items contaminated with body fluids
- after removing protective clothing
- before any aseptic procedure and handling invasive devices
- before handling food
- immediately hands have been visibly soiled.

Adequate hand washing involves thoroughly lathering all the surfaces, taking care not to neglect the tips of the fingers and webs between fingers, palm and thumb, which are often overlooked. Rings should be removed before hand washing, as bacteria tend to collect beneath them. These need to include the appropriate location and size of sinks, which are free of clutter and, where appropriate, the use of posters to encourage the correct guidelines to be followed (Cochrane 2003). Nail brushes must be for single use only and either disposed of or sterilised after use (Larson 1995). Wall-mounted disposable

---

Box 10.5   Universal precautions (HMSO 1995, RCN 2000, Scotter and Davis 1999)

- Prevent puncture wounds, cuts and abrasions in the presence of blood and body fluids
- Protect all breaks in exposed skin by means of waterproof dressing and/or gloves
- Avoid the use of and exposure to sharps when possible, but if unavoidable, take particular care in handling and disposing of them
- Protect the eyes and mouth by means of a visor, goggles or safety spectacles and a mask when splashing is a possibility
- Avoid contamination of the person or clothing by use of waterproof/water-resistant protective clothing, plastic apron, gloves, etc.
- Wear rubber boots or plastic disposable overshoes when the floor or ground is likely to be contaminated
- Use good basic hygiene practices including hand washing and avoiding hand to mouth/eye contact
- Control surface contamination by blood and body fluids by containment and appropriate decontamination procedures
- Maintain cleanliness of the ward environment, patient-related equipment and soft furnishing
- Store equipment clean and dry
- Never reuse disposable equipment
- Dispose of all contaminated waste safely
- Maintain an appropriate staff–patient ratio
- Avoid overcrowding of wards
- Avoid unnecessary transferring of patients between wards
- Isolate patients with a known or suspected infection

towels are preferable to avoid recontamination but hard paper towels can cause abrasions of the skin (Gilmour & Hughes 1997). Foot-operated pedal bins are ideal to avoid recontaminating the hands by opening a bin lid. All members of the healthcare team can expect to have basic hygiene resources provided in their workplace (Gilmour & Hughes 1997).

Alcohol-based hand rubs are increasingly popular but are only effective if the solution comes into direct contact with the entire surface of the hand and allowed to evaporate effectively. Hilburn et al (2003) found an alcohol hand wash to be effective in their study, demonstrating a significant reduction in HCAIs on an orthopaedic unit, compared to previous practices using soap-based products. This supports previous studies by Voss and Widmer (1997), Boyce et al (2000) and Pittet et al (2000). The waterless, alcohol-based solutions containing ethanol or isopropanol are effective in reducing the number of viable pathogens found on the hands (Hilburn et al 2003), including MRSA (MacDonald et al 2004). These products are proving to be quick to use and convenient, with both pocket and wall-mounted dispensers being available.

MacDonald et al (2004) used an alcohol gel as part of a study on giving clinical staff feedback on the effectiveness of good hand hygiene, using changes in hospital-acquired MRSA rates as an indicator of effectiveness. Positive benefits were seen in the drop in infection rates and a change in the culture on the medical, surgical and orthopaedic wards involved, cost savings were identified from comparisons of the cost of the gel compared to the potential costs of treating patients with teicoplanin had they acquired an MRSA infection.

Cimiotti et al (2003) compared skin reactions to alcohol and chlorhexidine products, they found fewer skin reactions occurring with a shorter duration when the alcohol products were used. In comparison, the chlorhexidine products appeared to cause longer term reactions that got progressively worse with continued use of the product.

The hands, like the rest of the skin, are covered by transient flora picked up and shed on skin scales during daily activities and permanent flora carried deep in the sweat gland ducts. Hand washing can remove the transient flora but will never eradicate the permanent flora. Gloves must be worn when potentially contaminated items are handled and to prolong the effects of hand disinfection when the risk of infection is high, as when catheterising

a patient. If the gloves are removed carelessly or punctured, recontamination of the hands will occur.

Cleaning the environment

Any items within the healthcare environment (structure, fixtures, fittings, furnishing) can be contaminated with potentially infectious material. When a new hospital is commissioned or an area refurbished, care must be taken to minimise the risks of future infections occurring through the choice of building design, the environment and equipment.

Decontamination is achieved at four levels that are progressively more effective at reducing the threat of infection but are increasingly costly to achieve:

1 cleaning
2 disinfection
3 sterilisation
4 incineration.

The method chosen depends on cost effectiveness and feasibility. When considering prevention of infection, attention must be given to the sources of microorganisms, including opportunists, and the method of their dissemination.

Knowing that bacteria thrive in moist, nutrient-rich environments is sufficient to deduce that clean, dry conditions should prevail in clinical areas. Good ventilation will help disperse air-borne bacteria and the ultraviolet in sunlight can destroy microorganisms. Particular care must be taken in situations of high contamination and infection risk, especially where there are:

- spillages or organic waste material that is not cleaned up properly, e.g. blood, vomit, faeces, urine
- materials that have been in contact with an infected site, e.g. dressings, sharps, excretions, secretions, specimens
- patients with a virulent infection, e.g. multiresistant staphylococci, or a communicable disease, e.g. tuberculosis
- clinical waste
- any equipment that appears wet or soiled, e.g. baths, mops, medical equipment
- raw food in the hospital or ward kitchen, especially meat and fish.

Cleaning

Although cleaning is not usually part of a nurse's role, it is their responsibility to ensure the care environment is clean. Nurses must therefore understand the principles of decontamination and monitor the performance of those involved in carrying it out so that inadequacies can be reported. Hospital policies and procedures on cleaning and infection control must be followed at all times.

Nurses remain responsible for cleaning medical equipment and in high-risk areas, such as theatres and intensive care units, are required to assist with routine cleaning. Wherever possible, equipment should be stored clean and dry. Potential reservoirs of infection, especially in sluice areas, should be prevented from occurring.

Individual patient equipment, especially for hygiene and personal care, must be cleaned well to prevent cross-infection. Medical and pressure area care equipment must be cleaned appropriately to prevent them acting as fomites.

Disinfection

This is the destruction of vegetative microorganisms that will, for instance, destroy bacteria but not their spores. Disinfection is achieved chemically and by heat. The relevant health and safety procedures must be followed when using these to ensure the correct levels of heat or concentration of the chemicals. The correct storage of chemicals is essential.

Sterilisation

Sterilisation is the destruction of all microorganisms present, including spores, by the use of autoclaving, chemical sterilisation and radiation. This is a costly process that should not be used indiscriminately.

Disposal

The disposal of clinical waste and used materials can lead to contamination of the environment and hospital personnel if not carried out correctly. Simple actions are easily overlooked, such as cleaning the inside of waste bins after a disposable bag has burst, leading to contamination of the outside of the next bag and the staff removing it. Socially

acceptable standards and the use of hospital health and safety based policies ensuring the safe disposal of waste are essential. This includes the safe disposal of sharps, all of which should be treated as if contaminated.

Isolation procedures

Isolation procedures are on occasion essential to contain a source of infection but should not be undertaken lightly. Being in a single room, especially when on enforced bedrest, can result in boredom and loneliness. Any stigma associated with having an infection is made worse by the staff and visitors having to wear protective clothing.

A rational approach to isolation is based on the:

- causative organism
- reason for the precautions to be taken
- mode of transmission
- items likely to be contaminated
- appropriate methods of decontamination.

The most important aspect of successful prevention of infection is staff education, identifying the gaps in knowledge and knowing where to find more specialised help, including infection control staff, policies and the microbiology team.

CONCLUSION

The consequences of developing an infection are varied, including wound, chest or urinary tract infection and the development of osteomyelitis. Each carries further risks of extended length of hospital stay, increased cost of treatment, delayed bone and wound healing and the possible need for further surgery. To reduce these risks, orthopaedic and trauma teams need to be aware of how infections occur and thus how important preventive measures are.

Further reading

Gammon J 1998 A review of the development of isolation precautions. British Journal of Nursing 7(6): 307–310

Parker LJ 1999 Managing and maintaining a safe environment in the hospital setting. British Journal of Nursing 8(16): 1053–1066

Roitt IM 1997 Essential immunology, 9th edn. Blackwell, Oxford

Wilson J 2001 Infection control in clinical practice, 2nd edn. Baillière Tindall, Edinburgh

References

Arroliga AC, Budev MM, Gordon SM 2004 Do as we say, not as we do: healthcare workers and hand hygiene. Critical Care Medicine 32(2):592–593

Boyce JM, Kellelhers S, Vallande N 2000 Skin irritation and dryness associated with two hand hygiene regimens: soap and water handwashing versus hand antisepsis with an alcoholic hand gel. Infection Control Hospital Epidemiology 21: 442–448

British Society of Antimicrobial Chemotherapy 1998 Combined working party report: revised guidelines for the control of methicillin resistant *Staphylococcus aureus* infection in hospitals. Journal of Hospital Infection 39: 253–290

Cimiotte JP, Marmur ES, Nesin M et al 2003 Adverse reactions associated with an alcohol-based hand antiseptic among nurses in a neonatal intensive care unit. American Journal of Infection Control 31(1): 43–48

Cochrane J 2003 Infection control audit of hand hygiene facilities. Nursing Standard 17(18): 33–38

Collier M 1996 The principles of optimum wound management. Nursing Standard 10(43): 47–54

Cooper T, Lawrence JC 1996 The prevalence of bacteria and implications for infection control. Journal of Wound Care 5(6): 291–295

Department of Health (DoH) 2003a Hospital acquired infection: the EPIC project. Developing national evidence-based guidelines for preventing healthcare associated infections. Available online at: www.doh.gov.uk/hai/epic.htm

Department of Health (DoH) 2003b Winning ways: working together to reduce health care associated infection in England. DoH, London

Duguid JP 1946 The size and duration of air carriage of respiratory droplets and droplet nuclei. Journal of Hygiene 44: 471–479

Emmerson AM, Enstone JE, Griffen M et al 1996 The second national prevalence survey of infection in hospital: overview of the results. Journal of Hospital Infection 32(3): 175–190

Gillespie WJ, Walenkamp G 2003 Antibiotic prophylaxis for surgery for proximal femoral and other closed long bone fractures (Cochrane Review). Cochrane Library Issue 4. John Wiley, Chichester

Gilmour J, Hughes R 1997 Handwashing: still a neglected practice in the clinical area. British Journal of Nursing 6(22): 1278–1284

Glover TL 2000 How drug-resistant microorganisms affect nursing. Orthopaedic Nursing 19(2): 19–25

Gould D 2001 Clean surgical wounds: prevention of infection. Nursing Standard 15(49): 45–52

Gould D, Booker C 2000 Applied microbiology for nurses. Macmillan, London

Hilburn JMT, Hammond BS, Fendler EJ et al 2003 Use of alcohol hand sanitizer as an infection control strategy in an acute care facility. American Journal of Infection Control 31(2): 109–116

HMSO 1995 Protection against blood-borne infections in the workplace: HIV and hepatitis. HMSO, London

Humphreys H, Taylor EW 2002 Operating theatre ventilation standards and the risk of postoperative infection. Journal of Hospital Infection 50: 85–90

King TA, Cooke RPD 2001 Developing an infection control policy for anaesthetic equipment. Journal of Hospital Infection 47: 257–261

Larson EL and the Association for Professional in Infection Control and Epidemiology 1992–1993 and 1994 APIC practice guidelines committee: APIC guidelines for handwashing and hand antisepsis in health care settings. American Journal of Infection Control 23: 251–269

Lee-Smith J 1999 Can the orthopaedic team reduce the risk of infection? Journal of Orthopaedic Nursing 3(2): 95–98

Lipp A, Edwards P 2003 Disposable surgical face masks for preventing surgical wound infection in clean surgery (Cochrane Review). Cochrane Library Issue 4. John Wiley, Chichester

MacDonald A, Dinah F, Mackenzie D et al 2004 Performance feedback of hand hygiene, using alcohol gel as the skin decontaminant, reduces the number of inpatients newly affected by MRSA and antibiotic costs. Journal of Hospital Infection 56: 56–63.

Mackowiak PA 1994 Fever: blessing or cure? A unifying hypothesis. Annals of Internal Medicine 120: 1037–1040

May D, Brewer S 2001 Sharps injury: prevention and management. Nursing Standard 15(32): 45–52

McCulloch J 1998 Hospital-acquired infection. Nursing Standard 13(3): 33–35

National Audit Office 2000 The management and control of hospital acquired infection in acute NHS trusts in England. National Audit Office, London

Parker MJ, Roberts C 2003 Closed suction surgical wound drainage after orthopaedic surgery (Cochrane Review). Cochrane Library Issue 4. John Wiley, Chichester

Pittet D, Hugonnets S, Harbarth P et al 2000 Effectiveness of a hospital-wide programme to improve compliance with hand hygiene. Lancet 356: 1307–1317

Plowman R, Graves N, Griffin MAS et al 2001 The rate and cost of hospital-acquired infections occurring in patients admitted to selected specialities of a district general hospital in England and the national burden imposed. Journal of Hospital Infection 47: 198–209

Royal College of Nursing (RCN) 2000 Working well initiative: methicillin resistant *Staphylococcus aureus*, guidance for nurses. Royal College of Nursing, London

Samad A, Banerjee D, Carbans N et al 2002 Prevalence of Methicillin-resistant *Staphylococcus aureus* colonization in surgical patients, or admission to a Welsh hospital. Journal of Hospital Infection 49: 87–93

Schneeberger PM, Smits MHW, Zick REF et al 2002 Surveillance as a starting point to reduce surgical site infection rates in elective orthopaedic surgery. Journal of Hospital Infection 51: 179–184

Scotter J, Davis PS 1999 The importance of preventing infection. Journal of Orthopaedic Nursing 1 (suppl): 22–27

Stacey A, Humphreys H 2000 A UK historical perspective on operating theatre ventilation. Journal of Hospital Infection 52: 77–80

Swoboda S, Earsing E, Strauss K et al 2004 Electronic monitoring and voice prompts improve hand hygiene and decrease nosocomial infections in an intermediate care unit. Critical Care Medicine 32(2): 358–363

Tanner J, Parkinson H 2003 Double gloving to reduce surgical cross infection (Cochrane Review). Cochrane Library Issue 4. John Wiley, Chichester

Voss A, Widmer AF 1997 No time for hand washing? Handwashing versus alcohol rub: can we afford 100% compliance? Infection Control Hospital Epidemiology 18: 205–208

Wilcox MH, Hall J, Pike H et al 2003 Use of perioperative mupirocin to prevent methicillin-resistant *Staphylococcus aureus* (MRSA) orthopaedic surgical site infections. Journal of Hospital Infections 54: 194–201

Chapter 11

Orthopaedic infections

John Burden, Julia D Kneale

INTRODUCTION

The last 100 years have seen dramatic changes in the presentation and epidemiology of infections involving the musculoskeletal system. The high infection rates seen following trauma, gangrene and tetanus, along with life-threatening infections in other body systems, have all reduced. A similar reduction in tuberculosis was also seen, although this trend has been changing with a gradual increase in recent years. The use of prophylactic antibiotics has reduced the rates of osteomyelitis after surgery, although antibiotic resistance has created new problems in the therapeutic management of patients with infections. This same period has seen a dramatic rise in the use of metallic implants for joint replacement surgery and fracture fixation, bringing challenges for preventing infection and patient management when an infection has occurred.

This chapter reviews specific nursing and medical implications of musculoskeletal infections. Any bone infection increases the risk of non-union of fractures or further pathological fractures from severe bone destruction and necrosis of bone tissue. The prevention of infections and their early detection is therefore essential. The increased length of hospital stay or the need for repeat hospital admissions and surgery increase the costs of care dramatically for the patient and healthcare providers.

As the recommendations and developments of antibiotic therapies are under constant review and development, specific drug regimes are not included here. Readers are advised to refer to their local pharmacology departments for current advice and support in relation to these.

Box 11.1   Indicators of increased infection risk

- Electrolyte imbalance and poor nutrition
- Medical conditions including anaemia, diabetes, cancer, alcoholism and patients who are immunocompromised
- Presence of MRSA
- Other infection foci, for example a urinary tract or chest infection
- Poor skin integrity from trauma, pressure sores, blisters or other skin lesions
- Presence of a foreign body
- Treatment therapies including steroid therapy and the stress of surgery
- Repeat surgical interventions required
- Age, with children and older people being more at risk

RISKS AND INDICATORS

Every patient is at risk of developing an infection, particularly following trauma or surgery; some patients, though, are at more risk than others. This risk increases with age and the length of stay in hospital. Older patients, who are more likely to have additional risk indicators (Box 11.1), are most affected.

The initial indicators of a musculoskeletal infection generally include discomfort, pain, pyrexia, a raised skin temperature over the area, along with the patient feeling generally unwell. These symptoms may be present without any external indicators of an infection such as redness around the area, the presence of exudate on a dressing or wound breakdown.

FRACTURE RISKS

Planned orthopaedic surgery and closed trauma injuries carry an infection risk but the presence of open trauma carries the highest risk, which increases with the severity of the injuries and the extent of contamination from the environment or clothing at the time of injury.

X-rays taken to monitor healing will not show the initial stages of an infection. Consequently conservative fracture treatment, especially of minor trauma injuries, can result in an infection becoming severe before it is recognised.

The infection risk increases if open surgery and internal fixation are required. The risks are balanced against the benefits of surgical stabilisation. Where possible, these issues are discussed with the patient prior to progressing with a treatment plan.

If an infection occurs after fracture fixation, removal of the metalwork is generally advisable, with the fracture site being supported and stabilised in traction, a cast, splint or with an external fixator if the wires can be placed away from the site of infection. The risk of a pin-track infection needs to be balanced against the benefits of using skeletal traction or an external fixator, either as a primary treatment method or when changing the method of stabilisation because of infection. Clear protocols for recording and auditing pin-track infections are essential to identify when these occur (Lee-Smith et al 2001, Ward 1997).

The incidence of pin-track infection is difficult to establish because it is recorded in different ways, for example by the number of patients with a pin-track infection or the number of infected pin tracks compared to the number of pins a patient has. Equally, the degree of infection recorded varies from a mild reaction to a severe infection requiring removal of the pin. These differences are not always identifiable in reports on pin-track infections unless there are clear definitions of how the infections were counted and how the degree of infection was measured.

INFECTION UNDER A CAST

The presence of an infection is often indicated when a patient complains of itching, heat or discomfort under their cast, when there are unexplained stains on the cast or it has an unpleasant odour. Equally, delayed or non-union of a fracture should alert the team to the possibility of an undetected infection.

Depending on the extent and site of infection, either the cast or a section of it is removed to inspect the area for a wound or bone infection. The bone will need continuing support to promote healing, typically by the use of a backslab, splint or traction.

PROSTHESIS RISKS

To reduce the risk of cross-infection, patients, particularly those having joint replacement surgery, should never be nursed in a room with a patient who has a chest or urinary infection, abscess or open skeletal infection.

A prompt diagnosis is essential to reduce the risk of bone destruction, particularly around an implant, which could lead to further disability. Redness, heat and swelling are often the initial indicators of an infection around an implant but as these are the natural indicators of an inflammatory response to surgery, a delay in diagnosing an infection can occur.

Late-onset infections, especially around a prosthesis, occurring 3 or more months post surgery are indicated by the return of pain around the joint, reduced movement and X-ray evidence, along with the systemic signs of an infection. Salvaging an infected joint is difficult. The prosthesis is removed and a temporary spacer is generally inserted until the infection clears. Intravenous antibiotics are essential to clear the infection and this therapy can continue at home with appropriate patient education and support. The successful replacement of the prosthesis is not guaranteed, as it will depend on the amount of bone removed and quality of the remaining bone.

SURGICAL RISKS

The intraoperative period is a prime point on the patient's journey for the introduction of infection. Although not all risks can be reduced prior to surgery, the nursing and medical teams need to be aware of them and act accordingly. Such actions include:

- treating known infections prior to surgery, especially respiratory and urinary tract infections
- consider testing all samples taken pre-, intra- and postoperatively for multiresistant organisms, especially MRSA
- prescribing prophylactic antibiotics for high-risk patients and procedures, for example trauma patients with open fractures and patients having metal implants
- maintaining high standards of intraoperative asepsis during procedures, including appropriate clean air exchange systems
- elevating the limb post surgery where appropriate
- avoiding catheterisation unless essential. If required, appropriate antibiotic cover is provided
- the early introduction of exercises to reduce oedema.

ACUTE OSTEOMYELITIS

The most common causative organism resulting in osteomyelitis is *Staphylococcus aureus*, especially where the infection is spread via the bloodstream following a bacteraemic event. Other organisms implicated, especially in infections affecting debilitated elderly patients, are streptococci, pseudomonas and *Escherichia coli*.

Organisms generally reach the focus of infection by one of three routes:

1 direct inoculation at the time of surgery or trauma incident
2 haematogenous spread from a core point of infection such as an abscess or chest infection
3 local spread from an infected wound, especially from burns and other soft tissue trauma.

Once bacteria have gained access to the bone, they often accumulate in the metaphyseal region where they proliferate and trigger an initial infection response. If untreated, the build-up of pressure in the bone causes the infected material to migrate to the cortex, separating the periosteum from the underlying bone to form a subperiosteal abscess (Fig. 11.1). The white cells cannot remove the infected material, resulting in the accumulation of infected and ischaemic tissue, with the eventual necrosis of the underlying bone (sequestrum). The infection can then track to the skin via a sinus. If the area infected is near a joint, the infection may track into the joint and cause septic arthritis. This risk is greatest at the hip, knee, shoulder, elbow and wrist joints (Dandy & Edwards 2003).

If initial treatment is either unsuccessful or is not initiated, the sequestrum becomes isolated, the periosteum develops new bone around it and leaves a reservoir of infection within. This scenario indicates the presence of chronic osteomyelitis, the bone is weakened and there is an increased risk of a pathological fracture.

PRESENTATION AND DIAGNOSIS

A detailed history may reveal recent trauma affecting the bone or an infection elsewhere in the body. The patient is normally admitted for a definitive diagnosis, antibiotic therapy and, if required, surgical intervention.

As osteomyelitis is a local infection with systemic effects, patients may present with the classic

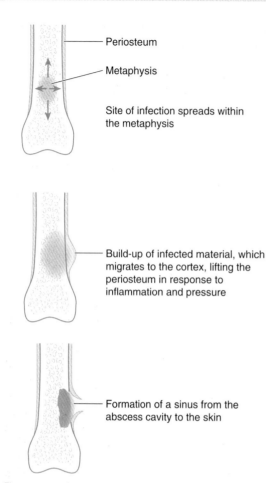

- Periosteum
- Metaphysis

Site of infection spreads within the metaphysis

Build-up of infected material, which migrates to the cortex, lifting the periosteum in response to inflammation and pressure

Formation of a sinus from the abscess cavity to the skin

Figure 11.1   Acute osteomyelitis.

Box 11.2   Classic symptoms seen in acute osteomyelitis

Local symptoms:	Pain over the site of infection
	Heat
	Redness over the affected area
	Joint effusion
Systemic symptoms:	Increase in body temperature
	Headache
	Sore throat
	Nausea
	Sweating
	Malaise

PATIENT MANAGEMENT

The goals of care are to return the patient to their normal lifestyle, free of infection and with as much normal mobility and limb function as possible. Although most cases do not recur, patients on steroid therapy, those who smoke, are nutritionally compromised or diabetic have a reduced healing potential, causing delays in their bone healing. The principal nursing issues relate to pain management, antibiotic therapy and understanding of the surgical management options. Mobility and nutrition are of equal relevance; these are addressed in Chapters 5 and 8.

Pain management

Patients remain concerned about their progress and long-term health throughout their period of treatment. To help alleviate some of the anxiety experienced, involving the patient and their family or carer in planning and assisting with care where possible is encouraged. The symptoms that cause the most anxiety are generally discomfort and pain.

Elevating and supporting the affected bone will reduce the discomfort and pain experienced. The use of traction, splints and casts needs to be considered, especially when a limb is affected. Using a removable splint or cast will allow regular inspection of the area and assist in wound care without causing unnecessary discomfort for the patient. The use of inhalation analgesia and preemptive analgesia prior to wound care will provide additional patient comfort.

Using a validated pain assessment score to reflect accurately the changes in a patient's level of pain over time is essential. The choice of analgesia will

symptoms of infection and a local infection reaction (see Box 11.2).

Laboratory investigations are crucial in determining the causative organisms. Blood cultures, wound swabs or needle biopsy samples are taken for culture and sensitivity prior to the administration of antibiotics. Sinus track swabs need to be taken with care to prevent contamination with normal skin flora. An infection is indicated by increased white blood cell (WBC) count, erythrocyte sedimentation rate (ESR) and C-reactive protein (CRP). The diagnosis is confirmed once an organism is isolated.

A plain X-ray will exclude other causes for the symptoms and demonstrate the presence of a pathological fracture. Computed tomography (CT) can identify cortical abnormalities, abscesses, sinus tracks and sequestrum. Magnetic resonance imaging (MRI) is useful in the detection of soft tissue and bone marrow involvement.

depend on the patient's own pain assessment. Aspirin and paracetamol are valuable as they have both analgesic and antipyretic properties. If the pain is more severe, the use of opiate analgesia is beneficial, either orally or via a patient-controlled analgesia system.

The involvement of the hospital acute pain team will ensure appropriate analgesics are given as the patient's pain and condition change.

Antibiotic therapy

Antibiotic therapy is started once blood or wound cultures have been obtained. A broad-spectrum antibiotic is prescribed until the sensitivity results are known and the ideal antibiotic identified. Intravenous antibiotics are given initially to establish an effective therapeutic blood level. Regular measurement of the serum concentration of the antibiotic is undertaken to ensure an adequate therapeutic level of the drug.

The most commonly used antibiotics for *Staphylococcus aureus* infections are cloxacillin, cefazolin and clindomycin. Benzylpenicillin is used against streptococcus infections. Patient compliance with the antibiotic regime is essential, as the antibiotics are continued from 4 weeks to several months. Regular antiemetics are needed for some patients experiencing nausea as a side effect of the drugs. The correct administration of antibiotics is important to prevent the development of antibiotic resistance. The patient generally remains in hospital until the efficacy of the therapeutic regime is established. The long-term antibiotic therapy is generally changed to oral administration, once the infection is controlled. Intravenous antibiotic therapy is continued in the community with the involvement and support of the community nursing team or by patients who are taught to self-administer their antibiotics.

Monitoring drug efficacy is essential for deciding whether to continue on a particular regime and determining the length of treatment required, especially following discharge from hospital. Radiological studies, bone scans, reduced CRP and a fall in the ESR levels are used to measure the response to treatment.

Patients can suffer adverse reactions to the prescribed antibiotics. These should be reported and changes made to the drug regime if the reactions are unacceptable or severe. Immunosuppressed and elderly patients are at risk of resistant infections developing in the oral cavity, genitourinary tract,

gastrointestinal tract and vaginal mucous membranes following antibiotic therapy.

While the patient is pyrexic, other nursing actions can help alleviate their discomfort, for example using fan therapy and cool, light clothing or bedding. Intravenous fluids and increasing oral fluid intake will correct any fluid loss from the pyrexia, prevent dehydration and correct an electrolyte imbalance.

A gradual reduction in the body temperature until a predetermined norm has been reached is ideal; 4-hourly monitoring of the body temperature will indicate such changes.

Surgical management

Surgical intervention is indicated if the antibiotic therapy is ineffective or the pressure of infected material requires decompression to release it from the medulla or subperiosteal abscess (Lew & Waldvogel 1997).

The surgical management of an infected bone or joint generally involves the removal of infected and necrotic material followed by the promotion of normal soft tissue and bone healing. Tissue and exudate samples are taken to confirm the causative organism and antibiotic sensitivities. Surgery can involve extensive debridement to control the infection, irrigation of the area, skeletal fixation, bone grafting or limb salvage involving external fixation and bone transportation.

Repeated debridement is required if the infection is extensive. The wound is left open to allow for removal of the exudate, wound drainage and regular dressing changes. Wound closure is carried out once the area is clean and healthy, and granulation tissue is evident.

Increasing the concentration of antibiotics in the area is beneficial but poor tissue circulation will reduce the antibiotic concentration. Acrylic beads or bone cement impregnated with an antibiotic, normally gentamicin, are the principal methods used to overcome this (Klemm 1993).

If a joint is infected, an open or arthroscopic exploration, with debridement and irrigation of the joint, is required. A sample of exudate is obtained for culture prior to antibiotics being commenced.

In the worst scenario, an infection can lead to extensive bone destruction, non-union of a fracture and chronic osteomyelitis. Excision or amputation may be the only recourse to prevent the infection spreading and resulting in septicaemia.

CHRONIC OSTEOMYELITIS

The onset of chronic osteomyelitis may be insidious, taking months or even years to develop. It is diagnosed when there is a relapse of a previously treated or untreated infection, if clinical signs persist after 10 days and there is an associated bone necrosis (Lew & Waldvogel 1997).

The presence of a Brodie's abscess on X-ray increases the risk of repeat infections. The abscess forms when an infected area is partly overcome by the body's defences, leaving a pocket of infected material dormant within an abscess lined by cortical bone.

The high risk of bone and soft tissue destruction requiring extensive surgery and long-term therapy indicates the need for patients to be referred to specialist centres for treatment.

MANAGEMENT OF CHRONIC OSTEOMYELITIS

Isolating the causative organism is essential. This is usually *Staphylococcus aureus*, although streptococci, pneumococci and *Mycobacterium tuberculosis* can be responsible.

The presence of a deep-seated infection and sequestrum indicates the need for surgical debridement.

The same antibiotics are indicated as for acute osteomyelitis with a combination of drugs generally being used to prevent the development of antibiotic resistance. An alternative to using antibiotic-impregnated beads to concentrate antibiotics in the affected area is the Lautenbach irrigation method. This involves instilling antibiotics through irrigation tubes to the site of the infection every 4 hours. The antibiotic remains in the bone cavity until drained out prior to the next instillation of antibiotics. The irrigation is continued for 3–6 weeks, making this a prolonged but effective procedure (Sims et al 2001).

Once all the necrotic bone and tissue are removed and the infection is under control, the need for further interventions to aid bone healing is assessed. Extensive reconstructive surgery using bone transportation to bridge the bone gap is often required, leading to prolonged and repeated hospital admissions. The patient may need to continue antibiotic therapy for a year or more until bone healing is completed.

Occasionally, reconstructive surgery is not possible, does not provide a functional joint or fails to produce expected benefits. Amputation of part or all of the limb is then considered as a positive treatment option, especially if mobility and function can be regained with or without an orthosis.

Nursing management

Caring for a patient with chronic osteomyelitis poses a challenge for the nursing team. The patient can have a lengthy hospital stay, repeat admissions or require an extensive period of care at home. They can be faced with changes in their body image from the surgery, scarring or amputation of the affected limb. The debilitating effects of infection and continued antibiotic therapy are also a problem for many patients.

The pain experienced will become chronic in nature, requiring different approaches to pain management to enable the patient to cope with the potentially long-term condition and possible disability.

Patients experience anxiety and powerlessness related to the uncertainty over their limb viability and the long-term nature of their condition. The multidisciplinary team needs to create a positive climate, encouraging the patient to participate in decisions made about their care. With appropriate support and information, the patient can understand the disease process, treatment options and objectives, leading to increased compliance with their care. This promotes a positive outlook and helps the patient to make plans for the future.

The potential for long-term disability needs to be considered, as it will be the cause of increased anxiety for the patient in relation to their education, employment or financial status. Appropriate professional support or the involvement of the school or employer can reduce the anxiety experienced and enables the patient to regain a sense of control over their situation.

TUBERCULOSIS

The cause of skeletal tuberculosis is *Mycobacterium tuberculosis*, often called the tubercle bacillus, which causes infection in cattle, birds, reptiles and fish, although spread of the infection from animals other than cattle is rare. Bovine tuberculosis was once a common source of human disease spread via unpasteurised milk. All cattle are now tested and milk is rendered tuberculosis free by pasteurisation. The main spread of infection from one person to another is by air-borne cross-infection. The tuberculosis bacterium is one of a group of organisms that includes *Mycobacterium leprae*, the causative organism in Hansen disease (leprosy).

The incidence of tuberculosis infections dramatically reduced during the last century from improved living conditions and the use of early and aggressive drug therapies. In some areas, though, the rate is gradually increasing again due to changes in socioeconomic conditions.

- A significant number of tubercular infections occur in people immunosuppressed due to infection with HIV because this virus attacks the T-lymphocytes and bone marrow, the body's main defence against the tubercle bacillus.
- The increased incidence is linked to the movement of people who are not protected through vaccination, especially the increase in travel to, and immigration from, countries where the pathogens are endemic.
- An increase in homelessness, the role of alcohol consumption and poor diet amongst vagrant populations and their close proximity in hostel accommodation cause a rapid rate of cross-infection.
- Patients not completing their course of treatment can lead to a rebound infection later from dormant bacilli.

This resurgence has produced resistant strains. These are particularly prevalent among patients previously treated for the disease, those infected with the human immunodeficiency virus (HIV) and intravenous drug abusers.

In Britain the majority of children are vaccinated with the BCG vaccine (Bacille-Calmette-Guerin) at 10–13 years but in spite of this, a significant number of infections occur each year amongst children.

A primary infection usually occurs in the lower two-thirds of the lungs and may then spread to the skeletal system. An endogenous or secondary infection can occur many months or years after the original infection because of inadequate treatment or poor patient compliance with drug therapy.

The mycobacteria are slow to develop and multiply, requiring treatment to be prolonged. Inadequate or incomplete treatment can result in a relapse of infection and the emergence of multidrug-resistant strains. As the pathogens are more likely to develop resistance to an antibiotic if only one is given, combination therapies of two or three drugs are used.

SKELETAL TUBERCULOSIS

Along with the increased incidence of tuberculosis has come a rise in the number of patients with bone and joint tuberculosis. About half of all cases of skeletal infections occur in the vertebral column. The thoracic and cervical vertebrae are the most commonly affected sites.

Skeletal manifestations of tuberculosis can occur at any age, with the very young and the very old being at particular risk.

PATHOLOGICAL CHANGES

Tubercle bacilli reach the bone metaphysis through the bloodstream, secondary to an active or inactive primary lesion usually in the respiratory tract. The infection causes bone destruction, which starts centrally and produces the classic cavity seen on X-rays.

If a sinus develops between the skin and the infected bone, the infection is termed 'open'. At this point other patients are at risk as the bacteria can be expelled through the sinus.

Tuberculosis of the vertebral column causes a cavity in the vertebral body which then collapses, causing a wedge fracture. This vertebral collapse can be the first sign of an infection. The infection has the potential to cross the disc spaces, causing destruction of the anterior vertebral margin, and spreads to adjacent vertebrae. A kyphosis can then develop as further wedge fractures occur. The sharp angle of the spinal curve from several wedge fractures is referred to as a sharp gibbus.

Paraplegia can occur from the pressure created by the infection within the vertebral body. If the pressure is too great, it causes compression of the spinal cord or compromises the vascular supply to the spinal cord, especially in the area of the gibbus.

PRESENTATION AND DIAGNOSIS

The clinical features will reflect the nature of the disease process and the areas involved. Symptoms are usually slow to develop with minimal local redness and warmth over the area initially. Some patients experience muscle spasms. If the spine is affected the pain is often localised and there may be evidence of a kyphosis and neurological involvement. Typically pain in the affected bone or joint is worse at night and a low-grade fever is often more evident at night. If the lungs are involved, a persistent non-productive cough is often present.

The diagnosis is confirmed following a thorough clinical history, laboratory and radiological findings (Box 11.3).

Box 11.3 Investigations for skeletal tuberculosis

- Blood specimens: ESR and CRP are elevated and WBC shows a mild increase in lymphocytes
- Early morning specimens of sputum and urine may show evidence of the bacilli
- Mantoux or Heaf skin test: purified protein derivative of tuberculin is injected intradermally using single syringe for Mantoux or multipuncture gun for the Heaf test. A positive result indicates the person has been infected in the past and has some cell-mediated immunity. A strongly positive result indicates either earlier BCG vaccination or active tuberculosis
- Chest X-ray: evidence of pulmonary infection
- Skeletal X-rays: show bone destruction, diffuse rarefaction around the site of infection, vertebral body collapse, wedge fractures
- MRI: shows extent of soft tissue involvement
- CT: of limited value as differentiation between an infection and other soft tissue changes such as a tumour or trauma is difficult

PATIENT MANAGEMENT

A holistic nursing care approach involving the multidisciplinary team will address the patient's psychosocial and physical care needs in hospital and for continued care at home.

Long-term hospitalisation and treatment can affect patients' education, employment, financial status and relationships. These implications can be as important to the patient as the physical changes imposed by their skeletal infection.

Identifying the organism is essential but as this takes time, drug therapy is started once the specimens have been collected. The mainstay of medical treatment remains antituberculous chemotherapy managed in two phases: the initial phase involving at least three drugs, then a continuing phase using two drugs. In the initial phase a combination of drugs include isoniazid, rifampicin, pyrazinamide and ethambutol, given for 2 months (Table 11.1). Isoniazid and rifampicin are then continued for a further 4 months.

Streptomycin, once the mainstay of drug treatment for tuberculosis, is rarely used in Britain except in cases of drug resistance. It is one of a group of drugs

Table 11.1 Antitubercular drug therapies

Drug	Side effects	Nursing responsibilities
Isoniazid – highly effective but resistant bacteria strains now found	Peripheral neuropathy	Note any changes in sensation to hands and feet
Rifampicin – very potent	Accelerates metabolism of corticosteroids, phenytoin, anticoagulants and oestrogen. Reduces effectiveness of oral oestrogen contraceptive pill. Causes red–orange discolouration of urine and other body fluids. Liver failure	Patients must be warned about the possible effects and possible staining of clothes from body fluids
Pyrazinamide – given only in initial phase but not to pregnant women	Liver and gastrointestinal disturbances and gout	Patient education regarding possible side effects
Ethambutol – used in initial phase. Reserved to treat resistant strains and atypical mycobacteria	Visual disturbances including colour blindness and restriction of the visual field	Patient education regarding the potential visual effects
Streptomycin	Nephrotoxic, ototoxic, skin rashes, anaphylaxis	Given by intramuscular injection, as it is not absorbed from the gut. Is a skin irritant hence when preparing and administering streptomycin, gloves and, if there is danger of aerosol spray, a facemask are advised. Observe patient for vertigo, buzzing in the ears and loss of hearing

known as amino glycosides that are toxic and nephrotoxic.

Multidrug-resistant tuberculosis is becoming a problem in some countries. This is the result of inadequate medical treatment and patients' non-compliance with treatment. Full recovery from skeletal tuberculosis may take up to 2 years and chemotherapy will be required for a large part of that time. The prevention of further multidrug resistance is of prime importance. The nurse must ensure the patient understands the length of the treatment period involved and the dangers of non-compliance with their therapeutic regime, including their own secondary infection risk and the risk to others. Successful supervision and monitoring of drug therapy is achieved by the orthopaedic team working together with the help, if available, of a specialist tuberculosis team, the infection control unit and the community team.

Despite antibiotic treatment and draining of any sinus that forms, some patients will require surgical interventions, for example joint arthrodesis and fusion of the vertebrae to prevent further skeletal collapse. Joint replacement, to provide a functional joint, is not carried out in the infectious phase but later once the disease is quiescent.

SEPTIC ARTHRITIS

Organisms invading a joint cavity create an infection referred to as infective, pyogenic, suppurative or septic arthritis. The most common causative organism is *Staphylococcus aureus*. *Escherichia coli* and streptococci infections affect infants and the elderly, while gonorrhoea infections affect sexually active teenagers and young adults (ARC 2004a). Acute septic arthritis is an urgent condition as permanent joint damage is likely to occur unless prompt action is taken.

The classic symptoms of septic arthritis are joint pain, swelling, redness and heat. An elevated WBC count is generally conclusive. Unfortunately, many other conditions mimic these symptoms such as gout, Reiter's syndrome, rheumatic joint disease and Lyme disease. These must be ruled out before treatment is commenced. Reiter's syndrome is seen as a late sequel to septic arthritis that also involves urethritis and conjunctivitis.

The infecting organism can enter the joint cavity by:

- the local spread of osteomyelitis from an adjacent bone

- direct inoculation from a penetrating joint injury
- as a complication of open joint surgery
- haematologous spread from a distant focus of infection, typically a respiratory tract infection.

In most instances, an infection involving a joint cavity represents a failure of the body's defence mechanisms, since many such infections are the result of haematologous spread. Once the organism has gained entry, the synovial membrane is damaged first and the joint becomes distended. If unchecked, the infection can quickly damage the joint capsule, articular cartilage and the subchondral bone. Abscesses can develop within the subchondral bone and synovium.

In children with septic arthritis of the hip, pressure on the femoral head, articular cartilage and within the joint space causes necrosis of the femoral head; this can be confused with Legg–Calvé–Perthes disease (Salzbach 1999).

PRESENTATION AND DIAGNOSIS

A rapid assessment of the patient's clinical condition will indicate an acute joint infection. A detailed medical history can uncover another preexisting infection or recent surgery to the joint.

The significant indicators are a red, hot, swollen joint that is painful to touch. As the infection can destroy the articular cartilage, the patient will hold the joint in a position of ease, usually flexed, abducted or externally rotated. If the infection is not identified and treated, the joint can fuse in this position.

Relevant haematology investigations (WBC, ESR, CRP, blood cultures) are completed before a wide-spectrum antibiotic is given. Aspiration and culture of synovial fluid from the affected joint will identify the organism involved and antibiotic sensitivity.

Radiographic investigations have a role in confirming the diagnosis, although significant changes are evident on joint X-rays only after destruction of the articular cartilage and underlying bone has occurred. CT and MRI scans will identify the presence of an abscess and the degree of bone destruction.

PATIENT MANAGEMENT

Patients, especially children, experiencing pain, are not able to tolerate active or passive movements of the joint and are unable to bear weight if a lower limb joint is involved.

Thorough drainage of the joint coupled with the administration of the appropriate antibiotics are the mainstay of treatment. Drainage of the joint is achieved by needle aspiration, arthroscopic irrigation or an open surgical approach. A wide-spectrum antibiotic, such as cloxacillin, is administered initially. This is changed if necessary once the antibiotic sensitivity is known and continued for a 2–3-week course. Vancomycin tends to be reserved for use with antibiotic-resistant strains of staphylococcus.

If not treated successfully, skeletal changes, including pathological dislocation and arthritic changes, occur. Long-term changes in mobility and joint function arise from reduced range of movement and leg length discrepancies, especially when the hip joint is affected (Salzbach 1999).

OTHER JOINT INFECTIONS

There are many causes of infective arthritis, including fungal, viral and bacterial infections. Most practitioners will rarely see these infections but for patients they can result in severe joint changes.

INFECTIVE ARTHRITIS

Infective arthritis can also be caused by a variety of fungi of which *Candida albicans* is one example. This infection is commonly seen in children, patients with a long-term indwelling catheters and immunosuppressed adults. As the organism is difficult to isolate, the diagnosis is made on clinical examination only. A progressive synovitis damages the joint, causing discomfort and pain. Treatment involves antifungal drugs and occasionally surgical interventions to correct severe joint changes.

Occasionally viruses such as hepatitis B, herpes simplex or rubella are responsible for acute infective arthritis. The infection is usually monoarticular, affecting a large weight-bearing joint. In most patients the disease is self-limiting.

REACTIVE ARTHRITIS (REITER'S SYNDROME)

Reactive arthritis generally follows a bacterial or viral infection; however, in some cases no causative organism is found.

The clinical features can include urethritis, conjunctivitis, and polyarthritis affecting the weight-bearing joints and skin rash over the hands and feet

and inflammation of the genitalia. Other causes of these symptoms must be excluded before treatment is commenced.

Bedrest is recommended during the acute phase of the disease with gradual mobilisation once the symptoms resolve. Other aspects of the condition are treated symptomatically, for example:

- urinary tract infections are treated with doxycycline or erythromycin
- antiinflammatory drugs, (NSAIOs) and analgesia are used for arthritic symptoms
- if conjunctivitis is present, the patient is referred to an ophthalmologist for appropriate treatment.
- It is usually short lived, lasting about 6 months, and normally disappears with minimal residual symptoms (ARC 2004b).

LYME DISEASE

Lyme disease, which has a musculoskeletal component, was first described as a distinct entity in 1975 when an epidemic of a disease resembling juvenile rheumatoid arthritis occurred at Old Lyme, Connecticut, in America. Since then Lyme disease has been reported widely in America but is not often seen in Britain.

This inflammatory disorder of the joints is caused by the spirochete *Borrelia burgdorferi* which is spread by the bite of the *Ixodid* tick. The ticks settle in warm, moist body areas, particularly the popliteal surface, axilla or groin.

Three distinct stages of the disease are recognised: early localised changes, early systemic changes and late Lyme disease. The musculoskeletal manifestations occur in the second and third stages. Typically the knee and other large joints are affected by joint pain, swelling and intermittent episodes of arthritis which get progressively longer and mimic rheumatoid arthritic changes. Other associated symptoms such as fever and malaise may occur. The disease is recurrent and may be acute or chronic.

Diagnosis is confirmed by clinical examination supported by WBC count, synovial biopsy and antibody titres. Gram's stain and culture are often negative.

Treatment by antibiotic therapy is usually effective; penicillin is recommended for children and tetracycline for adults. In monoarthritis where antibiotic therapy has failed, a synovectomy can relieve the symptoms. Isolating the patient is not required, as the infection is not passed from person to person.

INFECTIONS OF THE HAND

An infection in the tendon sheaths and fingers will affect the smooth movements of the hand and wrist (Dandy & Edwards 2003). The lack of space between the structures of the hand results in any infection being very painful. Initial treatment involves cleaning the area, elevation of the arm and antibiotic therapy. The treatment aims to avoid the development of adhesions that will further impede movements.

Paronychia, an infection of the nail, starts in the skinfold and spreads to the subungual space, causing pressure under the nail. If there is severe pain, the edge of the nail can be lifted or part of the nail removed to release the exudate and pressure. A regional block or general anaesthesia is used, as a ring block risks spreading the infection (Dandy & Edwards 2003).

Penetrating injuries can result in one of three scenarios (Dandy & Edwards 2003).

1 **Pulp space infections of the fingertips**: these can require an oblique or transverse incision along the side of the finger to relieve the pressure.
2 **Infection of the finger tendon sheath**: these are very painful and result in the finger being held in flexion. The patient is admitted for intravenous antibiotics but if no response is seen, the sheath is opened and irrigated.
3 **Infections of the thenar and hypothenar fascia sheath**: although these are less painful, movements are still restricted. Surgery is indicated if there is no response to intravenous antibiotics.

CLOSTRIDIAL INFECTION

This is a variable group of anaerobic bacteria. Some are present as normal gastrointestinal flora whereas others, such as *Clostridium difficile*, cause diarrhoea. The two conditions associated with trauma are tetanus and gangrene.

Cases of tetanus are rare because of immunisation. The *Clostridium tetani* bacteria enter the body from infected material during penetrating trauma. They have an incubation period of 3–21 days (Worf 2003) which means that a patient with a minor injury may have returned home prior to symptoms developing. The bacteria release potent toxins that affect the motor nerves, causing spasm and muscle stiffness, typically seen in lockjaw. If untreated, muscle rigidity will lead to respiratory distress, asphyxia, exhaustion and death. Treatment is by tetanus immune globulin to neutralise the toxins, diazepam to counteract muscle spasm and metronidazole as the antibiotic of choice (Worf 2003). To minimise the risk of infection, all trauma patients must be checked to ensure they have tetanus toxoid protection, even if the injury is relatively minor.

The gangrene scenario occurs when there is extensive tissue damage to internal organs from a road traffic accident, severe compound fractures, an interrupted blood supply or contamination of the wound by water, soil or a foreign body. *Clostridium perfringens* multiplies in the necrotic tissues, releasing proteolytic enzymes that attack the muscle and healthy tissues in the area. Septicaemia develops if the infection spreads via the systemic circulation. Treatment is by removal of the necrotic tissue and relevant antibiotic therapy.

CONCLUSION

All patients admitted for surgery or following trauma are at risk of developing an acute or chronic infection of the skeletal system.

The pattern of infections has changed during the last century. Poliomyelitis has disappeared as a major cause of musculoskeletal disability in Britain. In comparison, tuberculosis, once a fatal infection, almost disappeared as a skeletal infection problem but is now returning due to changes in society.

Osteomyelitis and joint infections remain difficult to treat, especially when antibiotic-resistant organisms are involved. Any delay in identifying an infection, the causative organisms and instigating treatment can lead to prolonged periods of hospital care, antibiotic therapy and bone loss requiring extensive surgery. The resultant infection and skeletal changes can have serious and costly implications for patients and the healthcare team.

Prevention remains the best protection from infection and the healthcare team are all responsible for minimising the risk of infection throughout the patient's care.

References

Arthritis Research Campaign (ARC) 2004a Infection and arthritis: rheumatic disease: Topical reviews. Available online at: www.arc.org.uk/about_arth/med_reports/series4/tr

Arthritis Research Campaign (ARC) 2004b Reactive arthritis: an information booklet. Available online at: www.arc.org.uk/about_arth/booklet

Dandy DJ, Edwards DJ 2003 Essential orthopaedics and trauma, 4th edn. Churchill Livingstone, Edinburgh

Klemm KW 1993 Antibiotic bead chains. Clinical Orthopaedics and Related Research 295: 63–67

Lee-Smith J, Santy J, Davis P et al 2001 Pin site management. Towards a consensus: Part 1. Journal of Orthopaedic Nursing 5(1): 37–42

Lew DP, Waldvogel FA 1997 Current concepts: osteomyelitis. New England Journal of Medicine 336(14): 999–1007

Salzbach R 1999 Paediatric septic arthritis. AORN Journal 70(6): 986, 988, 991–992, 994–998, 1000, 1002–1004, 1006, 1009–1010

Sims M, Trent J-C, Lake S 2001 The Lautenbach method for chronic osteomyelitis: nursing roles, responsibilities and challenges. Journal of Orthopaedic Nursing 5(4): 198–205

Ward P 1997 A one-hospital study to determine the reaction, prevalence and infection risk indicators for skeletal pin sites. Journal of Orthopaedic Nursing 1(4): 173–178

Worf N 2003 Tetanus – still a problem. Registered Nurse 63(6): 44–49

Chapter 12

Patient admission: planned and emergency

Seamus O'Brien, Jennifer Cody

INTRODUCTION

Preoperative assessment clinics were established with the aim of reducing the number of surgical delays and cancellations. They ensure the better use of resources and that patients are admitted fitter for their surgery and in a less anxious state. Patients are given clear information on their condition and treatment, with time to absorb and reflect on this, having had the opportunity to discuss their surgery and care.

Trauma patients do not have this advantage. When admitted, the impact of the trauma may not yet be realised or patients are stressed by the events, concerned for the health of other injured patients, the reactions of their family and possible effects on their personal or family life. The nursing focus on admitting the patient has, of necessity, to concentrate on the physiological status, assessment and management of the injuries. Therefore, practitioners' actions may not reflect the patient's concerns at the time of admission.

Both trauma and elective surgery patients have similar requirements when admitted and these similarities and some of the differences are addressed in this chapter. The need for immediate assessment of physiological status is met either in a preassessment clinic or by the primary and secondary survey of a trauma patient; in both situations, pathology-based assessments for monitoring physiological boundaries are needed. Specific issues arising for diabetic patients and those with rheumatoid arthritis are discussed here. General issues surrounding the use of health outcome measures and the need for discharge planning to commence on or before admission to improve patient care are addressed.

ELECTIVE PATIENT ASSESSMENT

Traditionally patients were admitted to hospital up to 2 days before surgery to enable routine laboratory tests, radiography and medical assessments to take place. Treatment of any medical problems identified at this time was not always possible before the patient was admitted for their surgery. This resulted in delays or cancellations of surgery, inconveniencing patients, wasted limited resources, increased waiting times for admission for surgery and the education needs of patients were inadequately addressed. The increased costs to healthcare providers and the emotional distress for patients and relatives were unacceptable.

Preoperative assessment clinics were introduced to meet these challenges, maximising the use of available resources such as theatre times and hospital bed occupancy and to improve the patients' experience of surgery. The clinics vary, with some providing a multidisciplinary approach (Sutcliffe & Potter 2002) while others are solely medically focused (Baines 2000, Davies 2000, Hocking & Shaikh 2000). An increasing number of these clinics are totally nurse led (Lucas 1998) and there is evidence to suggest that these work well (Haines & Viellion 1990, Read & Graves 1994, Whiteley et al 1997).

With the increase in life expectancy, there is more elective orthopaedic surgery being carried out on older patients with more demanding and challenging health problems. This makes the preoperative evaluation of their health by the surgeon, anaesthetic and nursing staff beneficial. The addition of physiotherapy and occupational therapists to the assessment team further enhances the patient's care at this stage.

The preoperative assessment clinic provides the opportunity to:

- carry out a full general and disease-specific medical history
- carry out a thorough physical examination
- assess the patient's health status and fitness for surgery
- order and carry out any necessary investigations, usually guided by clinical protocols, with sufficient time for the return and interpretation of results and the opportunity to delay or cancel their admission if required.

PREADMISSION ASSESSMENT CLINICS

The reporting of successful preoperative assessment clinics in America, Australia and the UK (Kirkpatrick 1984, Sutcliffe & Potter 2002) has encouraged units to develop nurse-led clinics. However, information for guiding the development of such a service and the management of clinics is limited in the UK literature (Murray et al 1995, Read & Graves 1994, Richardson & Maynard 1995).

The advent of hip and knee clinics in some areas for patients awaiting joint replacement surgery has led to patients experiencing improved mobility prior to their attendance at the preadmission clinic. These clinics enable the patient to meet the preadmission team early, their mobility and general health can be assessed and patients feel supported during the period of time they are awaiting admission for surgery (Haines & Viellion 1990).

WHEN TO ASSESS

Generally, the preadmission clinic facilitates the investigations and nursing interventions that lead to positive patient outcomes, through the establishment of clinical and outcome measurement baselines, the promotion of realistic patient expectations and the provision of patient support and education. Together these enhance the quality of care.

The assessment takes place in several stages and by different healthcare personnel, depending on how the individual clinics are organised.

Prior to attending for assessment, patients should be phoned at home to conduct an initial health screen covering such issues as dental status, skin status and latest health monitoring. The aim is to introduce the patient to the assessment team and to ensure the patient still wants and needs the surgery. This call can prevent patients being found unfit at the assessment and avoid their unnecessary attendance at the clinic.

Standardised approaches and algorithms for the management of the assessment process are increasingly commonplace (Beaty 1999). These have been developed to standardise processes and improve the quality of healthcare by identifying best practice, concepts familiar to most orthopaedic nurses.

Attendance at preoperative assessment clinics takes place 2–6 weeks before surgery. The information obtained during the assessment allows the establishment of potential and actual patient problems and a care management strategy. This allows the healthcare team to anticipate and prepare for postoperative problems unique to the individual.

Aims of assessment

The aims of specific clinics will vary depending on the healthcare staff involved in the assessment process. It is an ideal opportunity to identify problems within the care delivery process and to find imaginative solutions to these.

Patients should be encouraged to bring a relative, named carer or friend with them. As Raleigh et al (1990) found, relatives and friends also benefit from preoperative education and are then better able to aid the patient's recovery. In addition, the nurse can discuss with them the discharge plans and postdischarge needs to avoid delays for social reasons at the time of discharge.

The following are the general aims of most clinics and have been demonstrated to be successful in addressing these aspects of care (Asimakopoulos et al 1998, Messer 1998).

- To identify previously unrecognised medical problems, allowing time for the correction and treatment of these. This reduces delays and cancellations of surgery, decreasing the health service costs and improving the effective use of theatre time and hospital beds.
- To identify treatable co-morbid conditions and patients who pose a high anaesthetic risk (Box 12.1), with the aim of reducing perioperative morbidity and optimising patients' preoperative condition.
- To identify co-morbid conditions that are not reversible and may impact on the surgical outcome.
- To ensure the patient and relatives are involved in planning for the patient's discharge and postdischarge care needs, thereby reducing the overall length of hospital stay.
- To enhance the quality of patients' perioperative experiences, ensuring happier, less anxious, better informed and fitter patients. Relatives should be similarly well informed and prepared for all aspects of the surgery and postdischarge care.
- To reinforce teaching and ensure realistic expectations, by providing literature and videos that relate to the specific procedures as well as general information regarding anaesthesia and postoperative care.
- To establish standardised baseline measures of healthcare outcomes that are generic and disease specific.

NURSING ROLES IN ASSESSMENT

One of the principal driving forces in the UK for the development of nurse-led assessment has been the changes in junior hospital doctors' roles and clinical hours (Calman 1993, NHS Management Executive 1991).

Following a programme of relevant and often intense training, orthopaedic nurses are now developing and using the skills necessary to undertake a wide range of preoperative assessment (Kinley et al 2001, Lucas 2002). In most orthopaedic units, nurses are now undertaking patient assessments that were previously the domain of their medical colleagues, even in the absence of formal evaluations of the effectiveness of nurses performing such roles (Richardson & Maynard 1995).

CONSENT FOR TREATMENT

Legal issues around consent for examination and treatment (Adam 2001, DoH 2002a) have led to changes in the way in which patients are asked to give their consent to treatment, care or research, in order to ensure that the process is properly focused on the rights of individual patients. The importance of patient-focused consent for procedures also emerged as a key theme in the Bristol Royal Infirmary Inquiry Report (Kennedy 2001).

Each hospital has consequently reviewed its procedures for consent and this has in some cases included the need to gain written consent for procedures formerly deemed acceptable without, such as a blood transfusion or nerve blocks used within a surgical procedure. This consent may be obtained

---

Box 12.1   Anaesthetic high-risk patients

Past history of anaesthetic problems
Unstable diabetes
Medical problems that are not being treated,
    e.g. hypertension
Severe obesity
Current history of alcohol abuse
Symptomatic emphysema
Certain allergies, e.g. to drugs
Difficult airway
Undiagnosed aortic stenosis
Previously unidentified heart murmurs
Unstable ischaemic heart disease
Abnormal urea and electrolyte levels

within the preadmission clinic visit or patients are given the information in the clinic and the surgeon and anaesthetist gain the written consent on the patient's admission.

ANAESTHETIC ASSESSMENT

The anaesthetist confirms the patient's general health state and assesses problems specifically concerning the choice of anaesthetic and their fitness for surgery. For this reason, some clinics have this assessment built into the patient's clinic visit rather than on the day of their admission for surgery.

PHYSIOTHERAPY ASSESSMENT

Rehabilitation for any orthopaedic surgery starts long before the operation date itself. At the preoperative assessment clinic, physiotherapists will give patients exercises to maintain the muscle strength and ranges of movement in the joint following surgery. The patient's walking pattern is corrected if necessary, with walking aids provided and their use demonstrated as required. The provision of information leaflets prepares patients for their operation, increasing the chances of them having a quick recovery. When patients are admitted for their operation, they are seen by the ward physiotherapist to check for any more recent problems, they review their walking ability, answer questions and remind them of the exercises to be done while they are recovering in the 24–48 hours after the operation.

Following the operation, the physiotherapist may be involved in assessing the patient's breathing, providing chest physiotherapy and assessing muscle strength. The preplanned exercises, such as taking a few deep breaths every hour and moving their feet up and down at the ankle 20 times every hour to encourage the circulation in the limbs, are encouraged by both the physiotherapist and nurses.

Once the patient is able to get up and start walking, the physiotherapist is involved in the constant reassessment of the patient's mobility. Patients are shown how to get out of bed safely, initially standing by the side of the bed to ensure they do not experience any nausea or dizziness from the change in position. Once ready, patients are taught to use their walking frame, crutches or stick with a good walking gait where possible.

Patients are then encouraged to concentrate on improving their mobility skills, supported by the physiotherapy and nursing teams until they are walking independently, able to care for themselves as required to be discharged safely.

The surgeon, the treatment and the physiotherapist's judgement of the patient's physical ability dictate the amount of weight a patient can put through their affected leg.

General advice on the need to be active and suggestions of sensible activities can be given for both preoperative fitness and for increasing postdischarge fitness levels. These may include using a static bicycle, swimming, walking, bowls and dancing, depending on the physical status of the patient and their abilities. Activities to be avoided may include high-impact sports such as jogging, tennis, squash, downhill skiing, extreme walking, football, rugby and basketball until full fitness is achieved by the increased use of graduated exercises.

OCCUPATIONAL THERAPY ASSESSMENT

The occupational therapist is an integral part of the team and their involvement in the preadmission phase is increasing with the use of preadmission home visits and assessments. During a home visit the patient's safety in the home is assessed along with a complete evaluation of the impact of the disease on the patient's activities in the home, at work, the effects on hobbies and recreational activities.

Aspects of personal care are addressed as required such as hygiene, grooming, eating, drinking, dressing, getting in and out of bed, driving, cleaning, cooking, shopping, working and the patient's sex life. The therapist also conducts a physical examination concentrating on range-of-motion and the observation of any disabilities that might hinder performance. The need for any living aids or assistive devices, including raised toilet seats, dressing aids or stair rails, is assessed. These are put in place, preferably prior to the patient's admission or in time for their discharge from hospital.

FALLS PREVENTION

The patient's risk of falling needs to be determined while in the clinic. This is based on their previous and current medical status, the number of medications the patient is on, the type of medications, their environment and other associated factors, for example the decreased visual ability and balance of elderly people (DoH 2002b). This evaluation needs to be reviewed after surgery and on discharge. Tips for accident prevention can be given, such as having good lighting at home, avoiding rugs or thick carpets and having a clear route with sufficient lighting from the bed to the bathroom.

PATIENT EDUCATION

Although it has been documented that patients have difficulty retaining information given preoperatively (Lepczyk et al 1990), there is also evidence that it improves patient's awareness of their treatment and has a positive impact on postoperative behaviour, indicated by the recall of information given (Haines & Viellion 1990). Providing such education and information can reduce anxiety levels significantly. It is generally the nurse who will be involved in information giving, covering areas such as all the potential complications, what to expect, what to do if the patient experiences problems after discharge from hospital and contact numbers for staff.

Patients are given information about their admission, education about what to expect pre- and postoperatively and advice on pain management, including information on the possible use of epidural and patient-controlled analgesia. Booklets and handouts supporting and reinforcing what is said allow patients to consider the information later (Lucas 1998, 2002, Pi-Chu et al 1997).

ORTHOPAEDIC TRAUMA PATIENTS

Orthopaedic patients in the accident and emergency department constitute a sizeable proportion of the workload. Although a general practitioner could treat many of the injuries, some are life or limb threatening, especially for the elderly and children. The A & E nurse must be conversant with a variety of presenting conditions and must know what effects the condition may have on the patient if an intervention is not implemented within an acceptable time.

The A & E nurse's role is not an easy one as all the patients who present to the department are reliant on the skills and knowledge of the nurse to prioritise their problems, instigate investigations and interventions before a doctor has actually seen them. It is with this skill and knowledge that the nurse ensures that the orthopaedic patient is treated in a timely, appropriate and safe environment.

Over 15 million people attend A & E departments in the UK every year and this number is increasing (Robertson-Steel 1998). Each department sees and treats a variety of conditions in any one day, with the management of limb injuries appearing to account for the majority of their caseload. Presentation of such injuries differs, from the patient involved in a road traffic accident having suffered multiple trauma to the patient who walks in having tripped and sprained an ankle. The diverse nature of the injuries and illnesses, plus the unpredictable workload, requires nurses to think on their feet, make spontaneous decisions and master many expanded roles. Consequently, the nurse needs a considerable knowledge of a large range of medical problems.

TRAUMA NURSE ASSESSMENT SKILLS

Since the introduction in the UK of the Patient's Charter (DoH 1997), A & E departments have been required to carry out an initial assessment on all patients who come through the door. This is to evaluate and prioritise the care and needs of patients to ensure that those who require urgent treatment and intervention get it.

The assessment process is a combination of both knowledge and intuition grounded in experience and formal training. It is dependent on the hospital's policies and protocols, plus the skills, experience and confidence of each individual nurse. The assessment itself requires the nurse to make a judgement on the basis of objective and subjective data and to have the depth of knowledge and expertise to perform the assessment safely. Communication and interpersonal skills provide the basis for collaboration between the nurse and patient to ensure that all relevant information is gathered, enabling the nurse to make an informed judgement regarding the priority of the patient's condition. Accurate initial assessment in the form of history taking and observation is key to effective emergency care.

To make an accurate assessment, it is important to be an astute observer. Even the patient who walks through the door will have an assessment of his airway carried out. Although the nurse will do this subconsciously, she will soon notice if the breathing is compromised! The remainder of the assessment is concerned with taking a detailed history either from the patient, if able, or from an accompanying person. This includes when the injury occurred, how and what the mechanism of injury was.

Observation of the patient is vital, especially observation of the affected limb, its position, any marks and the neurological and vascular competence.

After the assessment, the nurse allocates the patient to a priority group. This is not standardised throughout the UK, although the Manchester Triage System (Manchester Triage Group 1997) has been adopted by many A & E departments and has gone a long way in ensuring that A & E departments are using the same format to prioritise patients. By doing so, accurate comparisons between departments are possible.

The Manchester Triage System was devised, as its name suggests, in Manchester by a group of like-minded professionals who considered it important to ensure that whatever their level of experience, the nurse carries out the assessment using the same format and subsequently arrives at the same priority as all other assessment nurses. Five coloured priority ratings are used.

- Red is life threatening; the patient must be seen immediately.
- Orange is very urgent; the patient must be seen within 10 minutes.
- Yellow is urgent, meaning the patient will be seen within 1 hour.
- Green is not urgent which means that intervention will take place within 2 hours.
- Blue is allocated to patients who could be seen in the primary care setting. These patients could wait as long as 4 hours for examination by the doctor.

Accurate and full documentation of the nurse's assessment is essential for several reasons, the most important of which is the possibility of it being called on in court. However, internally, the nurse may have to give an explanation as to why that particular patient was given a specific priority rating or to jog the memory when requested to provide a statement for management purposes. Audit is an essential part of A & E practice so the nursing records play an important part in aiding examination and comparison of documentation with protocols and policies.

All patients in the A & E department are seen in order of the priority given to them by the assessment nurse which can literally mean life or death for the patient if not carried out methodically and accurately. It can also ensure that procedures are instigated which expedite fast tracking for those whose conditions warrant quick intervention.

ORTHOPAEDIC TRAUMA PATIENT GROUPS

Fractured neck of femur

The elderly, because of failing faculties and other degenerative changes, are more prone to accidents that can be far more serious than in a younger person, particularly as they may have major rehabilitation and social problems. One of the commonest injuries from an elderly person falling is a fractured neck of femur, the majority of which occur in those over 65. With the increasing elderly population, it is estimated that the number of hip fractures will double by the year 2040 (Zuckermann et al 1991). The causative injury mechanism is usually minimal, such as a low-impact fall or stumble, but the consequences are far reaching for the individual concerned.

Meeting the needs of people who have a fractured neck of femur can present significant challenges in A & E departments. Long waiting times can affect the general state of health of frail elderly patients, which may result in longer hospital stays and poorer outcomes. Older people are particularly susceptible to dehydration and pressure ulcers. A good department will recognise that the person with this injury needs early intervention and requires early admission to a hospital bed. A policy to instigate fast tracking is generally used to ensure this.

A typical history is that the patient tripped and fell, was unable to get up again unaided and subsequently was unable to take weight on the injured limb. However, even being jostled in a crowd on the street or a bus can lead to a fall and a fracture. In about 95% of cases there is marked displacement. The presentation of external rotation, sometimes as much as 90%, along with leg shortening, makes it easy for the assessment nurse to make the diagnosis. Any movement of the hip causes severe pain. Once the nurse has carried out the assessment and after any underlying medical history is known and rules out any contraindications, fast tracking may begin.

A good A & E department will develop fast-tracking procedures for various illnesses and injuries and one such policy should be developed for this patient group. Using the guidelines, the A & E nurse will insert a large-bore Venflon and connect it to an intravenous infusion. Blood samples are taken for investigation and analgesia administered for the pain. An ECG is done and an X-ray requested of the injured hip and the chest. Many A & E nurses are now able to carry out these roles, which has led to patients being transferred onto a bed in a ward without having seen a doctor at all.

Close liaison with the trauma ward ensures the rapid allocation of a bed. Whilst the patient is in the imaging department, the orthopaedic surgeon is informed to expect the patient and once the nurse has confirmed the fracture, transfer to the ward is expedited. In these days of full wards, if a bed is not available on an orthopaedic ward the patient is allocated a bed elsewhere or, failing that, the patient must be transferred onto a bed in the A & E department. Ideally, the fast tracking from arrival in the department to admission to the ward should not take longer than 1 hour.

The patient who has suffered from an impacted abduction fracture will not present with the obvious signs for fast tracking, as there is no detectable shortening or rotational deformity. Indeed, the patient may have been able to walk short distances or may not have sought medical help for a few days. Most policies and protocols allowing nurses to request X-rays specify that there must be an obvious fracture or dislocation. In this case, the priority for intervention will be lower and the patient will need a detailed examination by the doctor.

The A & E fast-tracking policy should be audited on a regular basis to ensure not only that it is being adhered to but to identify any learning needs, which may be required by the nurses.

Supracondylar fracture of the humerus

One of the commonest and important fractures in children, occurring mostly in the 3–11 year age group, is a supracondylar fracture of the humerus (Davis et al 2000) (Fig. 12.1). It is therefore of the utmost importance that the assessment nurse can identify this injury and take the necessary action to expedite rapid intervention. This has a 'very urgent' priority due to the risk of injury to the brachial artery and the median nerve.

The history is that of a fall onto the outstretched arm, often involving falling from a height. Any displacement is regarded as dangerous, the distal fragment normally being displaced and tilted backwards. Identification and observation of the limb is crucial. Attention is paid to the circulation, colour, sensation and temperature of the forearm and hand; these and the presence of a radial pulse are documented every 15 minutes.

A record is made of the last time the child had any food or drink. The arm is placed in a broad arm sling and then, following examination by the doctor, the patient is transferred to theatre for fracture reduction under anaesthetic as soon as possible.

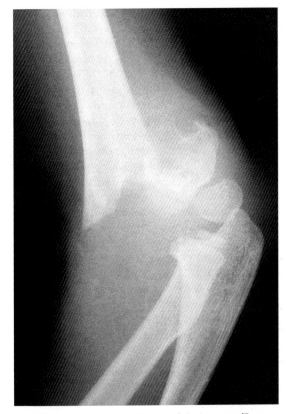

Figure 12.1   Supracondylar fracture of the humerus. (From Dandy & Edwards 2003.)

After reduction, the arm is immobilised in plaster with the elbow flexed. Again, a careful watch is kept on the circulation to ensure that complications do not occur.

Fracture–dislocations of the ankle

Along with the radius, injury to the ankle is one of the most common presentations in the A & E department. Fractures of the malleolus with or without dislocation can occur in three different ways:

1. abduction or lateral rotation force, or the combination of both
2. adduction force
3. vertical compression force.

Fracture dislocation of the ankle joint with neurovascular compromise is treated as an emergency. It is identified by the gross deformity of the ankle joint and the excruciating pain experienced by the patient. The pedal pulse is not present, the foot is cold to the touch and blanching of the toenails proves negative.

If manipulation is not undertaken almost immediately the patient may lose their foot. It is not uncommon for the nurse to interrupt the examination of another patient to ensure that the doctor reduces the dislocation and restores the circulation to the foot.

The reduction is done very quickly, using Entonox as the analgesia of choice. The nurse provides the traction required while the doctor undertakes a rapid manipulation of the joint. An X-ray has not been taken at this point; such is the emergency that at this stage it is deemed unnecessary. Once the limb has been immobilised in Plaster of Paris, analgesia will be administered and an X-ray requested of the reduced ankle. The patient will remain nil by mouth until the ankle can be stabilised in theatre.

A nurse must always be aware that compartment syndrome (Ashworth & Patel 1998) involving the muscles in the calf may develop within hours as a complication of a fracture dislocation of the ankle. It is a condition that must be diagnosed and treated promptly as it can compromise the integrity of the limb. The presenting signs and symptoms are very severe pain, neurological dysfunction, occasionally oedema and muscles that are stiff on palpation. Acute muscle necrosis will develop if the condition is left untreated. Often the clinical signs and symptoms are sufficient to warrant the diagnosis. When acute compartment syndrome is suspected an orthopaedic surgeon must be alerted immediately as decompression surgery will be required to prevent permanent loss of function.

ASSESSING FRACTURES AND DISLOCATIONS

It is important for the assessment nurse to identify obvious fractures or dislocations so that an appropriate priority can be assigned to the patient's injury. In the assessment bay the nurse will record the:

- pulses distal to the injury
- colour and temperature of the limb
- capillary refill
- neurological status of the area and distal to the site of injury.

First aid must be implemented to ensure that the patient is comfortable while waiting. This will include:

- removal of any rings or bracelets
- control of bleeding
- application of dry dressing
- application of a sling

- administration of mild analgesia if appropriate
- identification of tetanus status and allergies.

With the expanding role of A & E nurses, many are able, within agreed protocols, to request an X-ray of the injured limb and in the case of minor or uncomplicated injuries, are able to treat the patient, discharging or referring them on as appropriate. This decreases the number of patients waiting for examination by the doctor and provides a more efficient service.

Nurse X-ray requests

A & E departments are very busy places and unfortunately, for some groups of patients, long waiting times do occur. One such group is those who have suffered isolated limb injuries.

The traditional model for patients having suffered an isolated limb injury is for them to be assessed by the nurse who places them in a priority category, usually not a very high one. The patients are then required to sit in the waiting room until the doctor examines them and decides whether an X-ray is required. Studies have found that this process occurs in 90% of cases (Davies 1994) and results in the patient queuing to see the assessment nurse and then the doctor, queuing for an X-ray and queuing again to see the doctor for a discussion about the results and recommended treatment. These patients have two consultations and three waits in various areas.

Allowing triage nurses to request X-rays can decrease delays for patients (Davies 1994, Parris et al 1997) and lead to a more efficient service. Results of one study suggests that waiting times for patients can be reduced by an average of 45 minutes (Kelly et al 1995) while other studies suggest that time saving for patients can range between 8 and 60 minutes (Davies 1994, Macleod & Freeland 1992). The document *Reforming emergency care* (DoH 2001) sets targets for A & E departments, one of which was that by April 2002, 75% of patients must be seen and discharged within 4 hours of registration. Departments have therefore instigated new initiatives to reduce patients' waiting times such as X-ray requesting by nurses.

Many A & E departments have already trained their nurses in the role of X-ray requesting. This education includes sessions on radiation protection and examination of limbs. The patients who benefit from this initiative are those with limb or digit injuries as the protocols must be very succinct in nature and usually stipulate that there must be an obvious fracture or dislocation.

At the assessment the nurse will take the history as usual and carry out any first aid required, including the administration of analgesia. An X-ray form is then completed and the patient goes to the imaging department. The radiology department is involved in the nurse training because the department must gain their consent and cooperation before the initiative can commence.

Many radiology departments request that the nurse details a good history of the injury on the X-ray request form so that the radiographer can decide which views are required. When patients return to the A & E department with their X-ray they wait for their first examination by the doctor. If the X-ray proves to be positive a higher priority will be assigned to the patient. Some A & E departments have gone one step further and trained their nurses to read the X-ray and prescribe the treatment. In most cases these are emergency nurse practitioners and again it is those patients with limb injuries, such as sprains, strains and uncomplicated fractures, who benefit from their experience.

MANAGEMENT OF THE MULTIPLY INJURED PATIENT

Multiple trauma has become known as the neglected disease. Trauma kills more people between the ages of 15 and 24 than any other causes combined and is the leading cause of death and disability for all groups up to the age of 40.

The arrival of a multiply injured patient is potentially one of the most difficult situations that can confront the A & E nurse and if they do not take a firm, confident hold of the situation at the beginning, chaos and confusion can result. The nurses know that many of the deaths resulting from major trauma are from conditions amenable to appropriate and timely life-saving interventions. A plan of action, usually involving the trauma team, is put into action to identify and prioritise the life-threatening problems and set in motion the interventions required. A reduction in deaths can occur if the patient is appropriately assessed and life-saving interventions are initiated in the A & E resuscitation room.

The team approach, involving doctors and nurses, has evolved as one of the most effective and prevalent means to ensure the delivery of high-quality, comprehensive trauma care.

Multiple trauma patient assessment

Certain mechanisms of trauma result in predictable injuries. Consequently, the history of the event, taken from the patient or a witness, may reveal information leading to the identification and treatment of injuries commonly associated with the specific injury seen. Table 12.1 shows some commonly seen injuries and their mechanisms of occurrence. Many of these are musculoskeletal in nature; nevertheless, the priority they are given is secondary to other problems experienced by the patient and must be dealt with first by the trauma team. The trauma team must adopt a systematic approach so that life-saving interventions can be instituted.

Primary survey

Once the patient arrives in the trauma room the primary survey is commenced. This is a rapid assessment of the patient's injuries, vital signs and body functions and the initiation of life-saving treatment. This process constitutes the ABCs of trauma care and identifies life-threatening conditions (Scollon et al 1997).

Table 12.1 Expected injury in relation to mechanism of trauma

Mechanism of injury	Anticipated injuries
Pedestrian hit by car	Fractures of the femur, tibia and fibula on the side of the impact (adult)
Pedestrian hit by large vehicle or dragged under vehicle	Pelvic fractures
Unrestrained front-seat passenger (frontal impact)	Posterior dislocation of acetabulum, fractures of femur and/or patella
Unrestrained driver	Head, chest, abdomen and pelvis injuries
Back-seat passenger in vehicle without head restraint (rear impact)	Hyper-extension of neck with associated high cervical fractures
Fall injuries landing on feet	Compression fractures of lower vertebral spine and fractures of calcaneus

A. Airway maintenance with cervical spine control
B. Breathing and ventilation
C. Circulation with haemorrhage control
D. Disability: neurological signs
E. Exposure and environment control: completely undress the patient, but prevent hypothermia

During the primary survey, life-threatening conditions are identified and management is begun simultaneously. All the members of the trauma team will know what specific role they will be taking which enables many of the life-saving interventions to be instigated at the same time.

Secondary survey

The secondary survey does not begin until the primary survey (ABCs) is complete. If resuscitation is initiated, the primary survey status is reassessed. An unstable patient may not progress onto the secondary

---

Box 12.2   Assessment of the extremities

Circulatory status assessment is:
- Inspection of colour, skin temperature and symmetry
- Palpation of distal pulses

Sensory function assessment is:
- Testing of gross sensory function by touching various parts of the injured extremity, especially fingertips and toes
- Comparison with the uninjured extremity

Motor function assessment is:
- Inspection for spontaneous motor function of injured and uninjured extremities
- Testing the presence and symmetry of motor strength and range of motion

Soft tissue injuries require inspection for:
- Lacerations
- Abrasions and contusions
- Avulsions
- Puncture wounds
- Impaled objects
- Ecchymosis
- Oedema
- Angulations
- Deformity
- Open wounds in proximity to a deformity
- Palpation for crepitus

---

survey before leaving the department for emergency surgery or to the intensive care unit for ventilation, if they are severely cardiopulmonary compromised.

It is not until the secondary survey that limb fractures are identified and stabilised. The secondary survey is a head-to-toe evaluation of the patient including vital signs. Each area of the body is completely examined. A complete evaluation may require repeated examinations of the patient. The extremities are inspected for contusion or deformity. Palpation of the bones, examination for tenderness, crepitation or abnormal movement all aid in the identification of fractures.

Significant extremity injuries may exist without fractures; for instance, ligament ruptures produce joint instability. In contrast, pitfalls may occur from not diagnosing fractures because the team concentrates on a vascular compromise or when digital fractures are missed on patients with more severe injuries that take priority.

Any splints that have been applied pre-hospital are not removed if they do not interfere with the assessment. The extremities are assessed for circulatory, sensory and motor functions plus soft tissue injuries (see Box 12.2).

If there is time, any extremity injury is treated conservatively until the patient's more severe injuries have been treated and the patient is stable. However, on occasions when the patient must be rushed to theatre, these injuries will be treated at a later date when the patient is not in a critical condition.

DIABETIC PATIENT ASSESSMENT

About 1.4 million people in the UK have been diagnosed with diabetes, a number set to double by 2010. Another million probably have the condition but are unaware of it. Type 1 diabetes is a state of insulin deficiency associated with ketoacidosis, commonly seen in the young, normally requiring insulin-based management. Type 2 diabetes is a resistance of endogenous insulin or the disturbance of the glucose–insulin coupling: it is not associated with ketoacidosis. Type 2 diabetes is managed by diet, oral hypoglycaemic medication, insulin or a combination of all three.

Diabetes can cause cardiac complications, with both symptomatic and asymptomatic cardiac disease seen in patients over 50 years. A preoperative electrocardiogram (ECG) is therefore required for all diabetic patients. The incidence of silent ischaemia is higher in diabetic patients so other forms of cardiac testing may be relevant for individual patients.

Diabetic patients should be screened for changes in serum electrolytes, creatinine, proteinurea and hypertension.

GLUCOSE AND INSULIN MANAGEMENT

It is important that preoperative assessments detect any cases of previously undiagnosed diabetes. Treatment can then be commenced prior to admission for surgery.

The goal of glucose management is to keep the blood glucose levels at or below 240 mg/dl or an equivalent based on local practice guidelines, while avoiding perioperative hypoglycaemia below 80 mg/dl. This decreases the rate of glycosuria, reduces the risk of dehydration and, from some studies, has shown to improve wound healing (Beaty 1999).

The management of diabetic patients must be planned in advance of surgery to allay their anxiety and ensure prevention of potential intra- and postoperative complications.

Patients on oral medication or insulin should stop this on the day of surgery. The blood glucose is checked in the morning, then every 4–6 hours pre-, intra- and postoperatively or as per local guidelines. Insulin can be administered on a sliding scale for any blood glucose level over 240 mg/dl. An intravenous infusion of 5% dextrose is administered to prevent ketosis. The patient recommences their oral hypoglycaemic medication on the morning after surgery if they are tolerating food.

PATIENTS WITH RHEUMATOID ARTHRITIS

Patients with rheumatoid arthritis often require total joint replacement and other orthopaedic surgery. This form of arthritis is associated with anatomical and physiological changes including cervical spine disease, anaemia, pulmonary and cardiac involvement, all of which must be assessed for.

Studies have shown that 30–40% of patients with rheumatoid arthritis admitted to hospital have radiological evidence of cervical spine subluxation (Beaty 1999). This generally involves the first and second cervical vertebrae. Subluxation of the C1–C2 joint during endotracheal intubation may compromise the respiratory centre in the medulla. A careful history of C1 and C2 nerve root pain and cervical spine X-rays are vital.

The patient with rheumatoid arthritis is at risk of associated lung disease that can restrict their vital capacity and cardiac problems such as pericarditis, myocarditis, valve and conduction deficits. A full medical history, physical examination and ECG are important.

If the patient has been on corticosteroids within the previous 9 months, they will require steroid prophylaxis based on local protocols. Liaison with the rheumatology team will enable appropriate care and administration of steroid therapy and disease-modifying antirheumatic drug therapies.

SPECIFIC INVESTIGATIONS

RADIOLOGY ASSESSMENT

The regular use of chest X-rays dates from the prevalence of tuberculosis and screening for lung cancers. However, the cost of chest X-rays for every patient is considerable, so they are ordered on the basis of local protocols.

Chest X-ray abnormalities are very common, being present in 20–60% of people over 50 years of age. The influence of a preoperative abnormality on the surgical plan and patient outcome is relatively small. An example of the recommendations for chest X-ray screening can be seen in Box 12.3. Patients who have been X-rayed within the previous 6 months only need it repeating if there are other clinical indicators found on physical examination of their history. Chronic obstructive airways disease and changes consistent with heart disease may influence patient management decisions but the patient's medical history and physical examination are likely to be more important in assessing cardiopulmonary function than a chest X-ray.

Box 12.3   Guidelines for the use of selective preoperative chest X-rays

Thoracic procedure involved
Age over 65 years
History of cardiovascular disease
History of pulmonary disease
Current smoker of more than 20 per day or smoker for over 50 years
History of prior malignancy

The decision to order a skeletal X-ray is easy if there is an obvious skeletal injury. This is not always the case, leading to decisions on whether to X-ray or not being based on Nicholson & Driscoll's (1995) criteria relating to the presence of one or more indicators.

- Moderate or severe pain, especially on movement or weight bearing
- Tenderness on palpation
- Deformity or instability
- Bruising or severe swelling
- Crepitus
- Suspected muscle, tendon, blood vessel or nerve injury
- Suspected foreign body.

The interpretation of X-rays is formally by the radiologist report but increasingly nurses need to be able to interpret X-rays (Kneale 2000) in order to instigate treatment or before planning the next stages of care. For instance, an emergency nurse practitioner in A & E will interpret limb X-rays to identify and treat uncomplicated digit fractures, fracture clinic staff need to identify the progression of fracture healing and the position of a fracture prior to reapplying a cast, while ward nurses need the same skills for identifying joint or skeletal integrity post treatment or surgery to decide whether they can safely mobilise a patient.

LABORATORY INVESTIGATIONS

The importance of routine laboratory testing for elective surgery patients is debatable. Screening to uncover hidden disease is logical and the selective use of routine examinations can supplement other physical and subjective examinations, providing a complete preoperative assessment. The findings of abnormalities may not have an impact on the treatment decision and overall surgical outcomes.

For trauma patients the use of laboratory-based assessments will depend on the nature and cause of the injury, the time available prior to surgery and the physical status of the patient.

Most units have selective testing using unit or national guidelines or protocols based on age, gender and co-morbid conditions. The use of these must be balanced against the potential omission of a necessary investigation. Therefore there is a need to continuously update such guidelines.

Haematology assessment

The full blood count is important, as many patients are on long-term medications, including non-steroidal antiinflammatory drugs, which can predispose the patient to iron deficiency anaemia secondary to gastric erosions and bleeding. The rate of preoperative anaemia varies. Anaemia of less than 8 g haemoglobin will increase the patient's surgical risk. As some orthopaedic procedures are associated with significant blood loss, a baseline value is vital.

Severe abnormalities in WBC counts are uncommon, possibly indicating the need to investigate further for an infection if high or leukaemia if low.

A drop in the platelet count will need investigation as this can impact on clotting times. Encountering an unexpected thrombocytopenia requiring platelet transfusion is uncommon, necessitating a haematology referral. Bleeding time assessments have little use in predicting postoperative haemorrhage except in patients taking aspirin or non-steroidal antiinflammatory drugs. Preoperative prothrombin time and partial thromboplastin are reserved for patients with a personal or family history of a haematology disorder or hepatic disease or who are currently on anticoagulant therapy. A patient with end-stage renal disease can develop platelet dysfunction, which is best evaluated by a bleeding time.

A serum chemistry level will assess renal function, hepatic enzyme abnormalities, serum glucose and electrolyte levels. These enable screening for asymptomatic disease for problems such as hypokalemia, which can be detected and treated prior to surgery.

PULMONARY ASSESSMENT

Pulmonary complications following surgery are a significant cause of surgical morbidity, the main causes being atelectasis, aspiration, infection, pulmonary oedema and pulmonary embolism. Patients with restrictive lung disease or problems due to neuromuscular disorders or position, such as being supine for long periods, are at particular risk.

Surgery can be carried out on patients with chronic obstructive airways disease and asthma with minimal risk when they are free of bronchospasm. Standard steroid and bronchdilator therapies are generally used for at least 2 weeks prior to surgery to ensure stability of pulmonary function. These are continued throughout the postoperative period.

Patients should be encouraged to stop smoking for several weeks preoperatively and for at least 6 weeks post surgery, due to the increased risk of infection among smokers.

Antibiotics should be used if there is any evidence of a chest infection and supported by physiotherapy advice, along with the use of spirometers, coughing and deep breathing exercises. Along with early mobilisation to reduce the risk of a chest infection, these can be encouraged by both physiotherapists and nurses.

CARDIOLOGY ASSESSMENT

Preoperative risks of myocardial infarction (MI) and congestive heart failure based on the patient's history and examinations are of clear importance. An abnormal ECG will require investigation. A high percentage of patients over 45 years may have an abnormal ECG reading on routine assessment with the incidence increasing with age (McKee & Scott 1987, Turnbull & Buck 1987).

Detecting a silent infarction on ECG readings alone is difficult but a recent history of infarction will greatly increase the risk of peri- and postoperative cardiac problems. The use of set criteria for identifying risks of perioperative cardiac complications is recommended (Detsky et al 1986, Goldman 1983).

Patients with a history of MI or pulmonary oedema within the previous 6 months, aortic stenosis or multiple risk factors are at greatest risk. Stable angina, controlled hypertension, left ventricular failure or non-specific ST wave changes on the ECG do not appear to increase cardiovascular risks. It is important to be aware that history alone is insufficient to establish cardiac risk, as many elderly patients with joint disorders do not exercise enough to cause angina.

Any heart murmurs need to be further investigated with an echocardiogram.

Congestive heart failure can be due to cardiac or non-cardiac disorders such as an MI, aortic or mitral valve disease, arrhythmias, hypertension, anaemia or haemochromatosis. Patients with poor exercise capacity and severe impairment of left ventricular function with an ejection fraction of less than 25% are at increased risk of congestive heart failure. In all cases the underlying disease and cardiac function should be treated prior to surgery.

Aortic and mitral stenosis are associated with increased preoperative myocardial ischaemia and pulmonary oedema.

Patients with mechanical valves need to be heparinised preoperatively and their warfarin stopped 3–5 days prior to surgery. These patients must have antibiotic prophylaxis if they have a urinary catheter to reduce the risk of their developing a valve infection.

Patients with atrial fibrillation with controlled ventricular rates are reported to pose no significant problems (Beaty 1999). The team must be concerned about the cause of atrial fibrillation and whether it poses a surgical risk for the individual patient. It is commonly seen in elderly patients after surgery, generally due to underlying heart conditions.

Postoperative tachycardia is often multifactorial due, for example, to anaemia, hypovolaemia, pain or anxiety. Electrolytes, haemoglobin, haematocrit levels and an ECG are required to rule out or detect other causes.

Assessment for hypertension

The key to the assessment of hypertension is to have protocols with acceptable parameters, agreed by the anaesthetic and surgical teams, that take into account the rise in blood pressure from preoperative anxiety. It is important to check the blood pressure in both arms, as required by the British Hypertension Guidelines (Ramsay et al 1999a, b).

If the blood pressure is elevated it should be rechecked later when the patient has had an opportunity to rest. If the result remains higher than the agreed threshold, referral of the patient to the general practitioner for monitoring and stabilisation is required, prior to reassessment at the clinic 3–4 months later.

RENAL AND HEPATIC FUNCTION ASSESSMENT

Urinalysis

Urinalysis will indicate the presence of glycosuria and proteinuria, important in patients with a known renal dysfunction and for identifying patients with an unsuspected urinary tract infection. Treating asymptomatic infections preoperatively is beneficial in reducing the risk of a secondary infection around a surgical implant, especially in joint replacement surgery (Lawrence & Kroenke 1988). The insertion of a catheter prior to surgery can lead to transient bacteraemia, resulting in such an infection.

Renal function risks

The elderly are more prone to renal complications due to multiple co-morbidities, their medication and age-related decline in the glomerular filtration rate.

Acute renal failure occurring in the acute postoperative phase, within 24 hours of surgery, is often the result of hypovolaemia, hypotension or unrecognised preoperative volume depletion. Late postoperative renal failure is usually due to fluid volume depletion from poor oral intake with inadequate intravenous fluid support.

Patients with chronic renal insufficiency and end-stage renal disease have a higher risk of postoperative complications, for example dehydration, hyperkalaemia or fluid overload, which, if prepared for, can be avoided.

Liver function assessment

Asymptomatic abnormalities in liver function tests are common in preoperative assessments, following anaesthesia and after surgery. Liver disease such as viral hepatitis, alcohol hepatitis or cirrhosis can lead to significant changes in liver function, transient hepatic decompression, poor wound healing and excessive bleeding. Each case will need to be investigated and handled according to the results.

Patients with a history of hepatic or renal impairment may require alterations to the type and dose of anaesthesia and medications used, especially analgesics.

PATIENT OUTCOME MEASURES

The aims of orthopaedic surgery are to:

- prevent death following trauma
- restore function, especially mobility
- prevent future decline in function as seen in paediatric patients
- relieve pain, as achieved by joint replacement surgery.

Orthopaedic evaluations in the past have focused primarily on impairment measures such as range of movement or radiographic outcomes. Impairment measures have the advantage of being objective and easily measured by the surgeon. Their main disadvantage is that they may have little relevance to the reason why the patient had the surgery or the patient's evaluation of the outcome. Impairment measures are therefore relevant but do not provide a complete picture.

Some of these measures involve preoperative evaluations to compare later to postoperative or postdischarge scores, allowing demonstration of improved patient outcome such as mobility or walking gait. The addition of patient-based subjective outcome assessments based on health status, quality of life and satisfaction with care is needed. Patient satisfaction is important as it evaluates directly the patient's experience of their treatment. These measures are addressed in more detail in Chapter 2.

HEALTH ASSESSMENTS

Measures of health status are classified as generic or disease specific. Generic instruments, for example the SF-36 assessment tool (Ware et al 1994), measure a broad perspective of health status including physical function, role limitations imposed by physical and emotional health, vitality, mental health, social functioning, bodily pain and general health. The problem with generic instruments is that they may not focus on the concerns relevant to the patient or disease.

Disease- or condition-specific instruments such as the Oxford Hip and Knee Score (Dawson et al 1996) or the Harris Hip Score (Harris 1969) address the shortcomings of generic tools by focusing on the problems arising from the conditions relevant to the surgeons and patient. As a result, they will show greater sensitivity and responsiveness to change in measurements before and after treatment.

PATIENT SATISFACTION

Patient satisfaction outcome measures have emerged as important components in healthcare evaluation, reflecting the culture of patient-focused and -led healthcare services. In response to this, several standardised measurement tools, generic and disease specific, have been developed. Most are used preoperatively to establish a baseline and repeated at 3 months, 1 year and at least 5 yearly thereafter.

MENTAL HEALTH STATUS

Delirium and confusional states are common in the posttrauma and postoperative periods. Elderly patients and those with several medical problems are more susceptible to confusion. Preoperative baseline assessments of mental health such as mini mental health status scores (Folstein et al 1975) are important, especially for patients at risk.

Postoperative confusion increases the risk for postoperative complications, aspiration, higher mortality rates, longer length of stay and aggressive behaviours, leading to increased risks of falling or other injury. The management and treatment of patients with confusion must be directed at any underlying disorder or cause such as ensuring the patient is hydrated or stopping medications.

CONCLUSION

Simply transferring responsibility for patient assessments from the medical to nursing staff is not appropriate. Where orthopaedic nurses are taking on assessment roles of trauma and elective surgery patients, they must do so only if confident, competent and with the appropriate knowledge and skills. Some centres believe this requires education to Master's degree level, while in others in-house training is given. Whichever route is used, the nurse remains responsible for acting within their code of practice and legal guidelines for nursing actions (NMC 2002), it being their own professional responsibility not to take on actions they are ill equipped to perform. Having developed these skills, the nurse can have wider career opportunities as a nurse practitioner or other specialist nurse roles.

Most elective orthopaedic units have a preassessment clinic service. The aim is to better utilise existing facilities by reducing the number of cancellations and to prioritise the preparation of patients for surgery. These aims are achieved by improved patient education and establishing prior to their admission to hospital the patient's realistic expectations of their surgery, rehabilitation and longer-term outcomes.

Multiprofessional, one-stop clinics allow routine investigations to be carried out and for the patient to be seen by the medical, nursing, physiotherapy and occupational therapy staff.

The advent of hip and knee clinics or clubs has allowed peer patient support to develop. The group education session can include a video of the pre-, intra- and postsurgery care. If necessary, the GP is contacted about any problems identified. If the admission date has to be cancelled, the opportunity will be available for another patient to be brought into hospital for their planned surgery. Since introducing such clinics, patients' length of stay in hospital has reduced.

The successful preoperative assessment of the elderly elective patient is dependent on understanding why they differ from younger patients and how much of the difference is due to ageing, disease and residual damage from past ill health. The information gathered about the patient informs the surgical team of whether or not the patient is likely to tolerate, or survive, their operation.

The trauma nurse needs to have an insight into the assessment of patients admitted as an emergency. Although ward nurses are not involved in the ABCs of major trauma patients, they need to have an understanding of the process to ensure the secondary survey can be continued on the ward once the patient is admitted.

This chapter has shown the significance of these admission issues and how some continue as repeated assessment throughout the patient's stay.

References

Adam S 2001 Good practice in consent: achieving the NHS Plan commitment to patient-centred consent practice. Health Service Circular HSC 2001/023. Department of Health, London

Ashworth MJ, Patel N 1998 Compartment syndrome following ankle fracture-dislocation: a case report. Journal of Orthopaedic Trauma 12(1): 67–68

Asimakopoulos G, Harrison R, Magnussen PA 1998 Pre-admission clinic in an orthopaedic department: evaluation over a 6-month period. Journal of the Royal College of Surgeons of Edinburgh 43: 178–181

Baines DB 2000 Pre-anaesthesia assessment clinics [comment, letter]. Anaesthesia 55: 813

Beaty JH 1999 Orthopaedic knowledge update (home study syllabus). American Academy of Orthopedic Surgeons, Rosemont, Illinois

Calman K 1993 Hospital doctors: training for the future. Report of the working group on specialist medical training. Department of Health, London

Dandy DJ, Edwards DJ 2003 Essential orthopaedics and trauma, 4th edn. Churchill Livingstone, Edinburgh

Davies J 1994 X-ray vision of shorter queues. Nursing Times 90(21): 52–54

Davies JR 2000 Pre-anaesthesia assessment clinics [comment, letter]. Anaesthesia 55: 812–813

Davis RT, Gorczyca JT, Pugh K 2000 Supracondylar humerus fractures in children. Clinical Orthopaedics 376: 49–55

Dawson J, Fitzpatrick R, Murry D et al 1996 The problem of 'noise' in monitoring patient-based outcomes: generic disease-specific and site-specific instruments for total hip replacement. Journal of Health Policy and Research 1: 224–231

Department of Health (DoH) 1997 The patient's charter. Department of Health, London

Department of Health (DoH) 2001 Reforming emergency care. Department of Health, London

Department of Health (DoH) 2002a Consent: reference guide to consent for examination or treatment. Available online at: www.doh.gov.uk/consent/refguide.htm

Department of Health (DoH) 2002b National service framework for older people. Available online at: www.doh.gov.uk/nsf/olderpeople

Detsky AS, Abrams HB, McLaughlin JR et al 1986 Predicting cardiac complications in patients undergoing non-cardiac surgery. Journal of General Internal Medicine 1: 211–219

Folstein MF, Folstein SE, McHugh PR 1975 A practical method for grading the cognitive state of patients for the clinician. Journal of Psychiatric Research 12: 189–198

Goldman L 1983 Cardiac risks and complications of non-cardiac surgery. Annals of Internal Medicine 98: 504–513

Haines N, Viellion G 1990 A successful combination: preadmission testing and preoperative education. Orthopaedic Nursing 9(2): 53–57

Harris WH 1969 Traumatic arthritis of the hip after dislocation and acetabular fractures: treated by mould arthroplasty: an end-result study using a new method of result evaluation. Journal of Bone Joint Surgery 51A: 737

Hocking G, Shaikh L 2000 Anaesthetic pre-assessment clinics to identify patients at risk [comment, letter]. Anaesthesia 55: 812

Kelly A-M, McCarthy S, Richardson S et al 1995 Triage nurse initiated x-rays for limb injuries are accurate and efficient. Emergency Medicine 7: 81–84

Kennedy I 2001 Learning from Bristol: the report of the public inquiry into children's heart surgery at the Bristol Royal Infirmary 1984–1995. Stationery Office, London

Kinley H, Czoski-Murray C, George S et al 2001 Extended scope of nursing practice: a multicentre randomised trial of appropriately trained nurses and pre-registration house officers in preoperative assessment in elective general surgery. Health Technology and Assessment 39(5): 20

Kirkpatrick S 1984 Ambulatory surgery nurse practitioners step in to keep pace with growing day surgery. AORN Journal 40: 826–827

Kneale JD 2000 Radiological investigations. Journal of Orthopaedic Nursing 4(3): 138–143

Lawrence VA, Kroenke K 1988 The unproven utility of preoperative urinalysis. Archives of Internal Medicine 148: 1370

Lepczyk M, Raleigh EH, Rowley C 1990 Timing of preoperative patient teaching. Journal of Advanced Nursing 15: 300–306

Lucas B 1998 Orthopaedic patients' experiences and perceptions of pre-admission assessment clinics. Journal of Orthopaedic Nursing 2(4): 202–208

Lucas B 2002 Developing the role of the nurse in the orthopaedic outpatient and pre-admission assessment settings: a change management project. Journal of Orthopaedic Nursing 6(3): 153–160

Macleod AJ, Freeland P 1992 Should nurses be allowed to request x-rays in an accident and emergency department? Archives of Emergency Medicine 9: 19–22

Manchester Triage Group 1997 Emergency triage. BMJ Publishing, London

McKee RF, Scott EM 1987 The value of routine preoperative investigations. Annals of the Royal College of Surgeons of England 69: 160

Messer B 1998 Total joint replacement pre-admission programs. Orthopaedic Nursing 17(suppl 2): 31–33

Murray C, Read S, McCabe C 1995 Reduction in junior doctors' hours: the nursing contribution (phase 2): a methodological study. University of Sheffield, Sheffield

Nicholson DA, Driscoll PA 1995 ABC of emergency radiology. BMJ Books, London

NHS Management Executive 1991 Junior doctors: the new deal. NHSME, London

Nursing and Midwifery Council (NMC) 2002 Code of professional conduct. Nursing and Midwifery Council, London

Parris W, McCarthy S, Kelly A-M et al 1997 Do triage nurse initiated x-rays reduce patient transit time? Accident and Emergency Nursing 5: 14–15

Pi-Chu L, Li-Chan L, Jin-Jen L 1997 Comparing the effectiveness of different educational programs for patients with total knee arthroplasty. Orthopaedic Nursing 16(5): 43–49

Raleigh EH, Lepczyk M, Rowley C 1990 Significant others benefit from pre-operative education. Journal of Advanced Nursing 15: 941–945

Ramsay LE, Williams B, Johnston DG et al 1999a Guidelines for management of hypertension: report of the third working party of the British Hypertension Society. Journal of Human Hypertension 13: 569–592

Ramsay LE, Williams B, Johnston GD et al 1999b British Hypertension Society guidelines for hypertension management: summary. British Medical Journal 319: 630–635

Read S, Graves K 1994 Reduction of junior doctors' hours in Trent Region: the nursing contribution. Sheffield Trent RHA/NHS Executive Trent, Sheffield

Richardson G, Maynard A 1995 Fewer doctors? More nurses? A review of the knowledge base of doctor–nurse substitution. Discussion paper 135. Centre for Health Economics, University of York

Robertson-Steel IRS 1998 Providing primary care in the accident & emergency department. British Medical Journal 316: 409–410

Scollon D, Graham CA, McGowan J et al 1997 Resus 111: advanced trauma life support. British Journal of Hospital Medicine 58(94): 162–165

Sutcliffe A, Potter A 2002 Multidisciplinary pre-admission clinics for orthopaedic patients. Nursing Standard 16(21): 39–42

Turnbull JM, Buck C 1987 The value of preoperative screening investigations in otherwise healthy individuals. Archives of Internal Medicine 147: 1101

Ware JE, Kosinski M, Keller SD 1994 SF-36 physical and mental health summary scales: a user's manual. New England Medical Centre, Boston

Whiteley MS, Wilmott D, Galland RB 1997 A specialist nurse can replace pre-registration house officers in the surgical pre-admission clinic. Annals of the Royal College of Surgeons of England 79(suppl): 257–260

Zuckermann J, Sakales S, Fabian D et al 1991 Hip fractures in geriatric patients. Clinical Orthopaedics and Related Research 274(1): 213–225

Chapter 13

Joint and limb problems in children and adolescents

Julia Judd, Liz Wright

INTRODUCTION

Paediatric orthopaedics is a growing specialty and today subspecialties have evolved within it (Salter 1997). These are due to orthopaedic surgeons taking a specific interest in different areas of paediatric disorders. The majority of these disorders can be categorised as congenital, developmental, genetic, traumatic, infectious, inflammatory, metabolic or neoplastic (Gamble 1998).

Children are unique and require specialist nursing care. Their bones grow and mature at different rates. They are physically smaller, with a growing skeleton and are vulnerable to accidental injury. To nurse a child, the healthcare professional needs to be aware of their developmental stage, level of cognitive comprehension and how the social environment can affect the child's health and recovery.

This chapter will discuss:

- the effect on the infant, child and adolescent in relation to common joint and limb problems and their associated causes; developmental dysplasia of the hip, Perthes' disease, slipped upper femoral epiphysis and congenital foot deformities
- musculoskeletal trauma in children, which focuses on growth-plate injuries, skeletal trauma in child abuse, the treatment and nursing management of some typical childhood fractures, home traction and the role of the multidisciplinary team in discharge planning.

The remit of this chapter does not allow for full discussion of the care of the child with special needs.

DEVELOPMENTAL DYSPLASIA OF THE HIP

The condition where the hip is dislocated at birth used to be called congenital dislocation of the hip or CDH but is now referred to as developmental dysplasia of the hip (DDH). The new name recognises that hip conditions can develop after birth, up to 1 year of age. It also reflects that children presenting with acetabular dysplasia (a shallow or misshapen hip socket) are treated under the same regime as those with a truly dislocated hip. The incidence of DDH is approximately two per thousand live births (Broughton 1997).

HIP SCREENING

It is recommended that a paediatrician clinically assesses all babies for a potential hip problem soon after birth. For those infants whose hip stability is of concern or where there is a family history of DDH, an ultrasound of their hips should be performed within 2–6 weeks of birth.

A period of 2 weeks is left between identifying a potential problem and undertaking diagnostic hip screening. This allows excretion of the mother's labour hormones from the infant's body. The reason for this is an unproven theory that suggests relaxin, produced by the mother during labour, is transferred to the infant and causes temporary ligamentous laxity (Forst et al 1997, Vogel et al 1998). This hormone remains in the infant's body for a short period, making the joints more lax and increasing the possibility of a false-positive result when the paediatrician assesses the hips.

Hip screening involves obtaining a medical history and undertaking clinical assessment of the baby, followed by an ultrasound scan of the hips. X-rays at this stage are of very limited value as the hip joint of the young infant does not show up because it is cartilaginous. X-rays are taken when the head of the femur begins to ossify, with the ossific nucleus becoming evident around 6 months of age. Ultrasound scans have the advantage of being dynamic, allowing movement of the hip joint to be observed, and there are no radiation risks.

There are three potential outcomes.

1 The hip is normal and the child is discharged.
2 The child is diagnosed as having acetabular dysplasia.
3 A diagnosis of a dislocated or subluxing hip is made.

For all but the first outcome, the management is the same. The baby should be treated as soon as possible in a Pavlik harness following confirmation of the diagnosis by ultrasonography.

Some centres place the baby in double nappies to encourage hip abduction. This is only useful as a temporary measure following a paediatrician assessment and a diagnosis of suspected hip dislocation.

THE PAVLIK HARNESS

The Pavlik harness is a soft harness composed of shoulder and leg straps (Fig. 13.1). The harness holds the child's hips in a position of flexed abduction. This locates the head of the femur concentrically within the acetabulum. The child's naturally rapid growth and the stimulus of the positioned head of femur promotes acetabular growth to form a containing socket shape. The treatment is concluded when the socket has been restored, the dislocated or dysplastic hip resolved and the ossific nucleus is present within the femoral head (Fig. 13.2).

The Pavlik harness treatment continues for approximately 26 weeks. Throughout this time the child has weekly harness checks and ultrasound scans. The harness is worn continuously for the first 6 weeks. The amount of time that the child spends in the harness each day is then gradually reduced until it is being worn at night only. This continues until the ossific nucleus develops. Successful treatment is confirmed by ultrasound scans showing that the acetabulum is developing in response to the correctly positioned head of femur.

This effective and non-invasive treatment for DDH is reported to be successful in 95% of cases (Taylor & Clarke 1997), minimising the likelihood of surgical intervention. However, the 26-week management of a child in a harness, predominantly by the parents, requires careful instruction on the practicalities of daily care and continuous support. Following application of the harness, the parents are shown how to clean the harness and how to care for their baby's hygiene needs, change the nappy and vest. Preferable types of clothes are advised and the use of car seats and baby seating devices are discussed. The use of baby bouncers and baby walkers is not recommended for the baby with an underdeveloped hip.

Some parents find it difficult to comprehend that their happy, healthy-looking newborn baby has a medical condition that warrants this treatment. Showing the scan to the parents, explaining the

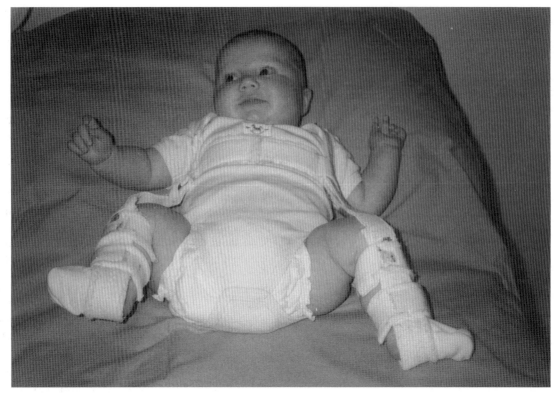

Figure 13.1   Child in Pavlik harness.

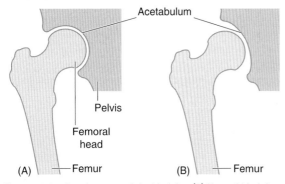

Figure 13.2   Development of the hip joint. (A) Normal hip joint. (B) Femoral head in a dysplastic acetabulum.

evidence and the poor prognosis if not treated can help to overcome their apprehension. Careful explanation of the principle of treatment is supported with information leaflets, which describe the care of their baby in detail.

SURGICAL PROGRAMME

For the small percentage of hips that do not respond to treatment with the Pavlik harness, a surgical programme is undertaken. This is also the treatment of choice for children who present and are diagnosed late, as the Pavlik harness is not effective in children over 3 months because its success depends on the rapid growth of the infant.

Surgery is performed when the ossific nucleus has developed. This occurs between 6 and 15 months of age. The principle of the surgery is to seat the femoral head within the acetabulum, stimulating it to grow into a socket (Malvitz & Weinstein 1994).

A closed or open hip reduction can be used to treat children from the time the ossific nucleus is present up to approximately 3 years of age. Each child's case is considered individually.

Preoperative gallows traction

Prior to surgery the child is admitted into hospital for a 1-week period of gallows traction (Fig. 13.3). The traction aims to gently stretch the soft tissue attachments around the hip joint, the blood vessels and nerves. This increases suppleness for the surgery and reduces the risk of complications from vascular impairment (Gage & Winter 1973). Avascular that children being nursed on gallows traction have a greater predisposition to chest infections and otitis media, so special attention should be paid to these risks.

Surgical options for DDH

The traction is removed after 1 week and the child is bathed prior to surgery. This cleans the skin and allows for the gentle removal of the adhesive traction. It is important at this stage not to traumatise the skin. The surgeon may consider delaying the surgery if the skin is sore or there are any lesions present, as this would increase the risk of infection and because the skin is unfit for encasing in plaster.

Whilst waiting for surgery, free of traction, the child should be discouraged from weight bearing as this counteracts the aim of the traction.

Parents should be encouraged to escort their child to the anaesthetic room as it reduces their anxiety (Glasper & Powell 2000). The operative management for the closed or open reduction of the hip involves four key stages.

1 An arthrogram is performed, injecting dye into the hip joint to enable viewing under an image intensifier. This has two functions: it allows the whole hip joint to be viewed, including the cartilaginous aspects that do not show on X-ray, and it is dynamic, allowing the joint function to be assessed.

2 An adductor tenotomy allows release of the tendon, promoting the mobility of the femoral head.

3 A closed reduction of the hip is attempted, with the surgeon aiming to manipulate the femoral head into the acetabulum without surgically opening the joint capsule. A successful closed reduction is confirmed by the image intensifier view. The child will be placed in a hip spica plaster to maintain the position (Fig. 13.4).

4 If a closed reduction is not achieved, then an open reduction is performed (Weinstein & Ponseti 1979). This involves surgically opening the joint capsule and removing the labrum from the acetabulum. Often true hip dislocation causes the soft tissue labrum to fill the empty acetabular space and mechanically obstruct the head of femur from being concentrically reduced by manipulation only. Following an open reduction, the hip joint is immobilised in a hip spica plaster (Fig. 13.4).

If the child is over the age of 2, a femoral shortening is incorporated with the open reduction (Galpin et al 1989) by surgically cutting through the proximal

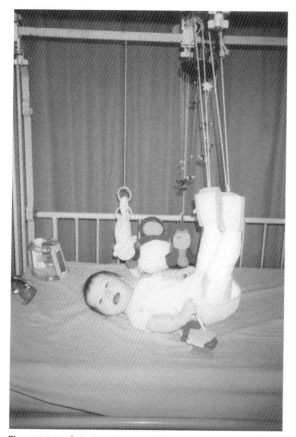

Figure 13.3   Baby in gallows traction.

necrosis of the femoral head is the main complication risk following the surgery.

For the child weighing over 10–16 kg Pugh's traction should be used (Davis & Barr 1999, Fish et al 1991), as gallows traction in this group of children is thought to predispose to avascular necrosis itself.

A child in gallows traction requires all the care associated with a person immobilised on traction. Particular attention must be paid to the integrity of the child's skin. A small piece of adhesive tape taken from the skin traction set should be used as a patch test to assess for any potential skin allergies. Non-adhesive traction is recommended if the test is positive, indicating an allergic reaction.

Once applied, the child's legs are evenly tied or weighted to prevent back pain. It should be possible to place a flat hand between the child's buttocks and the mattress. The outer bandages of the traction should be removed daily and the skin checked for blistering or sores. Neurovascular observations must be maintained. It is the authors' observation

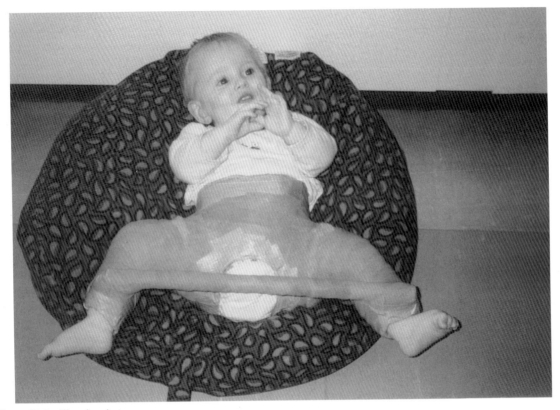

Figure 13.4 Hip spica plaster.

femur on the affected side, removing a part of the femur and using a plate to secure the two bone ends. This shortens the femur and reduces the stretch of the attached femoral nerves and blood vessels, thus reducing the complication of avascular necrosis of the femoral head post surgery.

For children of 4 years and over, a pelvic osteotomy is performed. This is also indicated in the child whose hip joint fails to respond to a closed or open reduction. An osteotomy involves surgically cutting and realigning the pelvis to provide better cover over the head of femur and create a deeper acetabulum. There are many different surgical approaches that can be used, with a Salter innominate pelvic osteotomy being preferred in many centres (Salter 1961). The osteotomy is performed just above the acetabulum and filled with a wedge-shaped bone graft taken from the iliac crest. This alters the angle of the acetabulum to facilitate covering of the femoral head and deepening the cup. The osteotomy site and the bone graft are stabilised with two surgical pins. The child is immobilised in a hip spica cast for 6 weeks and then

readmitted to hospital for removal of the spica and pins under general anaesthetic.

Children who exhibit persistent DDH may require a varus femoral derotational osteotomy (Kasser et al 1985). This involves surgically cutting through the proximal femur and rotating the femoral head so that it sits more concentrically within the acetabulum. This surgery is sometimes undertaken alongside other operations. The child is nursed in a hip spica plaster for approximately 6 weeks postoperatively.

Postoperative management and hip spica care

The postoperative management of these children is multifaceted. It involves regular observations of the cardiovascular system and neurovascular observations of the limbs encased in plaster. Observing for indications of infection and effective pain control are essential. There will be specific patient management issues pertaining to the type of pain control selected, with preference given to the use of an epidural or morphine infusion when appropriate.

Box 13.1   Developmental dysplasia of the hip plaster programme

Closed reduction	Open reduction
Hip spica for 6 weeks	Hip spica for 6 weeks
Repeat hip spica for 6 weeks	Broomstick plaster for 6 weeks
Broomstick plaster for 6 weeks	Night splints for 6 weeks
Night splints for 6 weeks	

The duration of the plaster programme is dependent on the type of surgery undertaken (Box 13.1). The minimum time in plaster is 6 weeks and the maximum is 24 weeks. Each plaster is on for 6 weeks and then changed as required under general anaesthetic on a day surgery basis.

The extent of the plaster programme has a major impact on the lives of the child and family. The 'normal-looking' mobile child who entered the hospital is now rendered immobile, in a fixed position with a very visible plaster. This makes achieving all the activities of daily living a challenge. It is of paramount importance that the child and family have a full understanding of the treatment programme and are willing to comply with it. If family compliance is not gained or appropriate plaster care not continued, the plaster may have to be removed, resulting in the operative correction of the hip being lost.

Caring for a child in a hip spica plaster has three key elements: skin care, mobility and psychosocial care. As soon as the child returns from theatre the plaster should be protected from soiling. Initially this is achieved by inserting strips of thin plastic sheet around the groin area of the plaster and allowing the urine to be collected in a receptacle placed underneath the child or placing a nappy over the plaster. Nursing the child on a raised wooden block supported with pillows for the first 24 hours postoperatively can facilitate this. The block allows ventilation and therefore drying of the plaster, utilises gravity to drain excrement away from the hip spica and permits a receptacle to be placed under the child. When the postoperative swelling in the groin area has subsided then a nappy can be tucked up into the plaster and the protective plastic inserts removed.

Once dry, the hip spica cast can be further protected with a layer of fibreglass plaster. The groin area of the hip spica is protected with waterproof tape that can be changed if necessary. The child cannot be bathed whilst in plaster; hygiene is maintained by thorough cleansing of the area whilst not getting the hip spica wet.

Parental involvement in the child's care should commence immediately on the child's return from theatre. It is essential the family are taught to care for their child appropriately, that they understand the importance of the care and their confidence in caring for their child gradually develops.

It is equally important that carers feel comfortable lifting and turning their child. The risk of developing a pressure ulcer is as relevant at the end of the plaster programme as it is at the beginning. The child in a hip spica is considerably heavier and the parents should be taught to lift correctly so as to avoid incurring a back injury.

The role of the occupational therapist cannot be over-stated with regard to promoting the child's mobility at home. Issues such as provision of an appropriate wheelchair or buggy, car seats, hoists and seating apparatus are essential for the family to be able to meet the child's daily needs.

Some older children may not be able to fit through a conventional doorway, so it may be more appropriate for them to be cared for in hospital for the whole treatment period.

Discharge from hospital needs to be planned prior to the operation and involves all members of the multidisciplinary team.

It is advantageous for the older child's psychosocial well-being if they can return to school. Medically there is no reason for the child not to do so and it has untold benefits. The child can socialise with their peers and the family has a little respite from the ongoing care needs, not to mention maintaining the child's educational development.

In the authors' centre the programme of care is explained in detail prior to the commencement of treatment. This is backed up by written information and the paediatric orthopaedic nurse practitioner provides ongoing family support. Informing and empowering the family in their child's treatment is essential to the success of the programme of care.

PERTHES DISEASE

Perthes disease is also known as Legg–Calvé–Perthes disease after the three orthopaedic consultants who identified it.

> **Box 13.2   Stages of Perthes skeletal changes (from Herring 1998)**
>
> | | |
> |---|---|
> | Stage 1 | The blood supply is interrupted or fails; the femoral head begins to degenerate; on X-ray it appears dense with some irregularity of the head being noted |
> | Stage 2 | The degeneration continues and the necrosed bone becomes fragmented or appears to have "crumbled away" |
> | Stage 3 | The healing stage: the blood supply returns and the femoral head starts to regenerate |
> | Stage 4 | The residual stage: when the femoral head has redeveloped, possibly misshapen |

Perthes is a condition in which the femoral head becomes necrosed due to an interruption in its blood supply. It commonly occurs in boys aged 4–10 years. These children are often skeletally immature, small for their chronological age and of thin build. Generally the younger the child is at the time of diagnosis, the better the prognosis. The cause of the condition is unknown, although it has been suggested that it may be related to children with abnormalities of thrombolysis (Glueck et al 1996). The disease commonly has a 2-year duration and moves through four stages (Herring 1998) as outlined in Box 13.2.

Treatment for children with this condition is dependent on the severity of the necrosis and their symptoms. Many children are referred to the hospital with a history of intermittent hip pain and a limp. As well as a medical history and clinical examination, anteroposterior and frog lateral hip X-rays are obtained as a routine diagnostic measure to identify an early Perthes disease. Often sequential hip X-rays are needed before a diagnosis can be made, as the hip changes are insidious. The child's bone age is calculated via a hand X-ray to determine the child's skeletal maturity and compared with their chronological age. The disease prognosis is more closely related to the child's skeletal age; the younger the child is at the time of diagnosis, the more optimistic the outcome.

CLASSIFICATION

There are two classification systems used to grade the hip affected by Perthes disease: the Catterall and Herring classifications. Catterall (1971) grades

the hip into one of four groups, dependent on the amount of necrosis and collapse of the femoral head identified on X-ray.

- Group I has up to 25% femoral head involvement.
- Group II has up to 50% femoral head involvement.
- Group III has up to 75% femoral head involvement.
- Group IV has 100% femoral head involvement.

Herring et al (1992) grade Perthes disease in three groups, A–C, according to the amount of flattening of the femoral head as seen on X-ray. This is calculated by assessing the height of the femoral head or lateral pillar involvement.

MANAGEMENT

If Perthes disease is diagnosed then the child may enter one of three treatment routes.

Observation

Following diagnosis the child attends outpatient clinics and the course of the disease is mapped using X-rays. The child continues normal activities of daily living.

Conservative treatment

The child may experience intermittent episodes of severe hip spasm, preventing the hip joint being put through a full range of movement and bearing weight.

During these episodes the child is admitted to hospital for a short period on Pugh's traction to rest the joint and relieve muscle spasm. Non-steroidal antiinflammatory drugs can be prescribed at this time. Once the episode has settled the child can return to normal activities.

Sporting activity sometimes initiates pain and the child may choose to reduce these. However, swimming is strongly recommended as it mobilises the joint, whilst being non-weight bearing and not stressing the infarcted area.

Surgery and abduction braces

The third option includes children with a severe Perthes lesion. This is the fragmentation stage where there is significant femoral head involvement of greater than 50% (Catterall 1971).

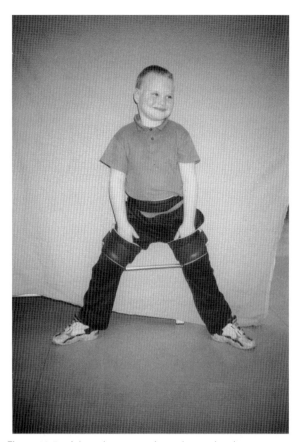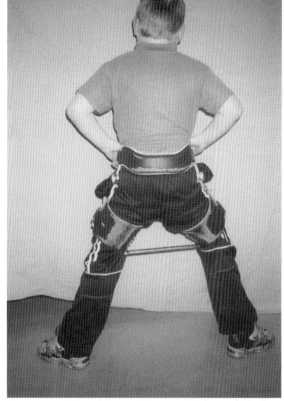

Figure 13.5   Atlanta brace, anterior and posterior views.

These children may need to undergo surgery or wear an abduction splint, the aim being to locate the femoral head concentrically in the acetabulum. When the healing stage commences the regeneration of the femoral head is influenced by the shape and proximity of the acetabulum, encouraging regrowth to its natural shape. If this is not achieved and a misshapen femoral head is evident, the residual stage is reached and a diminished range of hip movement may result.

There are different types of abduction splints available. In some centres hip abduction is achieved by applying broomstick plasters. Other units use a specific splint such as an Atlanta brace (Fig. 13.5); this is worn for 23 hours per day for approximately 1–1½ years. The child can walk in this type of splint and continues their normal life activities. Again it needs to be emphasised that the effectiveness of this treatment relies on the understanding and compliance of the patient and family. Whilst splint-based treatment is known to work, there is medical debate as to whether or not it is more or less beneficial to the child than surgery (McAndrews & Weinstein 1983).

The aim of surgery is to contain the femoral head concentrically within the acetabulum and to promote optimum healing. There are several operations that can achieve this, including pelvic and femoral osteotomies as previously discussed. Generally children who undergo this surgery are nursed post-operatively either in a hip spica plaster or on Pugh's traction.

SLIPPED UPPER FEMORAL EPIPHYSIS

Slipped upper femoral epiphysis is a condition in which the head of the femur slips off the physis or growth plate (Fig. 13.6). It occurs mainly in boys aged 9–16 years and less frequently in girls aged 8–15 years. Children with this condition are often obese and usually present with pain in the hip and

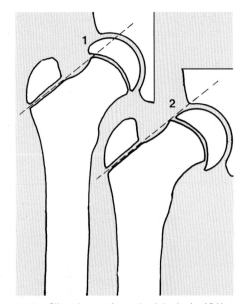

Figure 13.6 Slipped upper femoral epiphysis. An AP X-ray view of both hips allows comparison. In the normal hip (1) a tangent line to the neck should cut through the epiphysis. In a slip (2) this is no longer the case. (From MacRae & Esser 2002.)

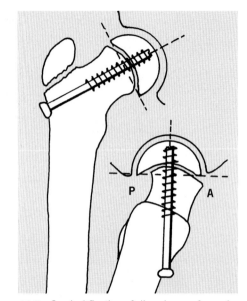

Figure 13.7 Surgical fixation of slipped upper femoral epiphysis. In stable cases fixation is by a single percutaneous cannulated screw inserted so the screw lies in the centre of the head, perpendicular to the epiphysis and without penetrating the femoral head. (From MacRae & Esser 2002.)

possibly a limp. It is not uncommon for the child to complain of referred pain in the thigh or knee.

The exact cause of slipped upper femoral epiphysis is not known. Many episodes are idiopathic in origin but there is a school of thought that overloading of the growth plate at the hip joint due to obesity contributes to the mechanical failure of the physis (Staheli 1992).

The onset of symptoms can be sudden or insidious. Traumatic slipped upper femoral epiphysis is possible but rare. It is classified by the duration of symptoms: less than 2 weeks is classified as acute, greater than 2 weeks is classified as chronic. The term acute-on-chronic is used to describe someone with chronic pain who experiences a sudden onset of severe pain. Pre-slip is a classification for a child with X-ray appearances of slipped upper femoral epiphysis but without symptoms (Canale 1998).

MANAGEMENT

The principle of treatment is to prevent the slip from worsening, until the physis naturally fuses and the issue is resolved. Attempting to manipulate the femoral head into alignment runs the risk of initiating avascular necrosis. Consequently this is usually achieved by surgically pinning the femoral

epiphysis, securing it in the slipped position (Fig. 13.7). If the child experiences an acute slip with severe pain then Pugh's traction is applied to relieve hip spasm and reduce the injury prior to surgery (Nattrass 1997).

The main elements of caring for a young person with this condition are those associated with any immobilised patient in bed. However, special attention should be paid to the child's pain, psychosocial care of the adolescent and if obese, then the opportunity for health promotion should be utilised. It is not uncommon for this group of patients to have been teased at school; the nurse should be aware of this and the effect it may have on the child's emotional state.

The child is allowed to mobilise non-weight bearing on crutches, usually 48 hours postoperatively, when comfortable. Normal weight bearing is resumed at the surgeon's discretion and determined by the original severity of the slip. The child's progress is monitored by regular follow-up appointments. They are generally asked to refrain from sports for approximately 3 months. If the initial condition is unilateral there is a high probability that the femoral epiphysis on the unaffected side will slip. The child and family should be informed of this and the symptoms to be aware of.

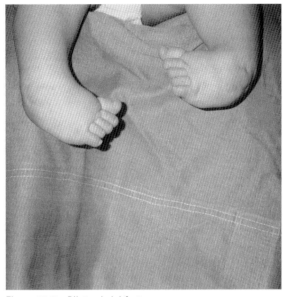

Figure 13.8 Bilateral clubfeet.

CONGENITAL FOOT DEFORMITIES

CONGENITAL TALIPES EQUINO VARUS

Congenital talipes equino varus or clubfoot (Fig. 13.8) is one of the most common congenital deformities, occurring in approximately 1:1000 live births, twice as often in boys and with 50% being bilateral (Bender 1998).

The condition is either idiopathic or associated with other disorders, for example neuromuscular diseases, chromosomal abnormalities or linked with a syndrome. For this reason, all babies born with clubfoot should undergo a thorough musculoskeletal assessment. Although the cause of clubfoot is undetermined, research suggests different causative theories such as fetal developmental arrest, genetic familial links, teratogenic factors and intrauterine moulding (Herring 2002).

Central to the foot deformity is the abnormal shape of the talus, with the relationships of all other connecting bones being abnormal (Norris & Carroll 1998). The position of the foot and ankle is altered.

- The ankle is in a position of equinus; the heel is high, causing the foot to point downwards.
- The heel is in varus; turned inward.
- The forefoot is in adduction, turned inward towards the heel.

The deformity varies from mild, postural and easily correctable to a severe fixed form. It should be stressed to the parents at an early stage of management that a clubfoot will remain smaller in size and may be underdeveloped.

Whichever treatment plan is decided upon, the aims are the same: to achieve a plantargrade, functional and pain-free foot or feet (Bender 1998), enabling the child to participate with their peers in all activities.

Conservative management

The initial treatment for all babies born with clubfoot is stretching of the tight soft tissues, to achieve as much flexibility of the foot as possible.

The orthopaedic surgeon assesses the foot and may use a classification system (Dimeglio et al 1995) to grade the severity of the deformity (Uglow & Clarke 2000). This allows for uniformity of care and a baseline for measurement of final outcome. There are regional variations to the management of clubfoot; however, the initial management involves a combination of soft tissue stretching with serial plaster casts replaced on alternate weeks.

Ponseti method. The Ponseti method of non-operative treatment has recently been introduced in this country (Ponseti 1996). The clubfoot is corrected by simultaneous serial casting addressing each of the components of the deformity separately: the cavus, varus and adductus. The plaster is applied above the knee to prevent the cast slipping and although temporarily upsetting to the baby, the parents should be reassured that they will quickly become accustomed to it. The plasters are changed weekly, correcting the deformity gradually. Some centres allow the parent to soak plasters off in the bath the night before the clinic appointment. Following 5–6 manipulations and cast applications, an Achilles tenotomy is performed to correct the equinus deformity prior to a final cast worn for 3 weeks. On removal of the cast, a splint is worn consisting of boots attached at each end of a bar (a variation of the Denis Browne splint) with the feet placed in external rotation. The affected foot is placed at 70° external rotation with the unaffected foot at 40°. The boots and bar need to be worn by the baby for 3 months full time and at night only for a further 2–4 years to prevent a relapse of the condition.

A child that presents with a severe, stiff deformity may require surgical correction.

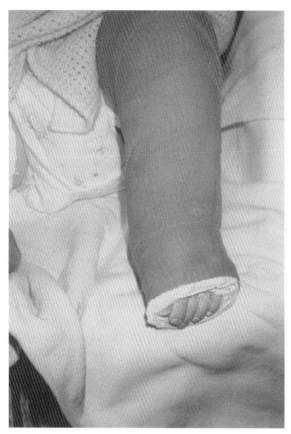

Figure 13.9   Fibreglass cast for clubfoot.

Surgical correction

Surgery varies according to the age of the child and the nature of the residual deformity. One approach is a two-stage procedure performed at 9 months of age before the child is walking. Operating in two stages has been shown to reduce the incidence of wound infection (Bender 1998, Uglow & Clarke 2000).

- First-stage surgery involves a plantar medial release of the soft tissues to bring the front of the foot round to face forwards.
- Second-stage surgery is performed 2 weeks later with a posterolateral procedure to lengthen the Achilles tendon to bring the heel down.

The complete surgical process is best explained to the parents using pictorial resources and information leaflets. It is important they have a full understanding of the whole care pathway.

Above-knee plasters are used for a total of 3 months with a change of plaster under anaesthetic at 6 weeks. It often requires reinforcement with

additional fibreglass during this period due to general wear and tear from the surprising amount of activity of the child (Fig. 13.9). For the final part of this surgical pathway, the child wears night splints and orthotic boots until approximately 2 years of age.

Surgery for clubfoot may differ not only in its timing but also in technique. The Ilizarov frame is used in some centres for primary correction in the young baby followed by serial plasters. This choice of treatment needs to be carefully considered with the parents, ensuring they comprehend fully the impact it will have in caring for their child.

RELAPSED CLUBFOOT

Clubfoot is an extremely difficult deformity to correct. From birth, the severity of the deformity can be assessed and the more components of the foot that are stiff, the more likelihood of relapse and further surgery being required. Recurrent deformity may occur in 20% of cases (Bradish & Noor 2000). Surgery can take the form of either repeated soft tissue corrections, a tendon transfer using the tibialis anterior tendon, or bony surgery involving a lateral column shortening or osteotomies. Plaster immobilisation is required, the duration of which is determined by the surgeon. For a child aged over 3 years, the plasters are usually below the knee, making it easier for management, especially with toileting and seating.

Ilizarov frame

An alternative to the above treatment methods is to use the Ilizarov circular frame (Fig. 13.10) which gradually corrects the deformities, the position being maintained by subsequent plaster immobilisation and a tendon transfer (Bradish & Noor 2000). The family and child need verbal, written and pictorial information to facilitate an informed decision and to ensure patient compliance (Santy 2000).

The acceptance of the frame by the child and family, especially its appearance, is paramount for a successful outcome. The team of nurses, doctors, physiotherapist, occupational therapist and community nurses all have important roles to play, providing the necessary network of support.

Recent reports indicate that the child under 5 years has a better outcome than an older child whose feet, whilst having a reasonable position, tend to be stiff. It could be argued that for the adolescent a cosmetic result is important; however, there might be a loss of function.

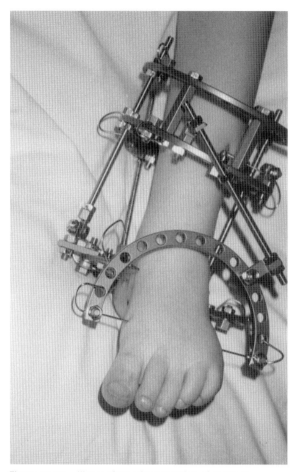

Figure 13.10   Ilizarov frame for correction of clubfoot.

Management of the Ilizarov frame requires complete understanding and the compliance of both the child and family. This is achieved by giving them information and involving them in discussion of the management of the pin sites, the potential complication of pin infection, the risk of pain due to pin loosening, how to prevent soft tissue contractures and how to enable the child to be mobile.

Pin-site care needs to be evidence based. Consensus of opinion to date (Lee-Smith et al 2001) amalgamated by orthopaedic nurses suggests cleaning daily with normal saline or, at home, cooled boiled water, using new non-shredding gauze or non-shredding cotton wool buds for each pin (Sims & Saleh 2000) (Fig. 13.11). Scabs or crusts should be removed to allow free drainage of fluid and dressings applied only if there is exudate (Sims & Saleh 2000).

The child and parents are taught how to perform the daily adjustments to the frame, using a turn chart, which can be personalised by the child.

Parents soon become adept at adapting clothing, using Velcro fastenings or trousers with side openings. A cloth covering can be made to go over the frame to protect it and prevent it catching.

Whilst a young child may accept the appearance of the frame, the adolescent is more likely to have concerns about their body image (Shelley 1993) and the impact on their lifestyle. As Burr stated (1993, p10), "Adolescence is an important time for gaining independence and developing self control". Giving them control of their circumstances with education and support will enhance the opportunity for compliance and successful outcome. A survey of service provision for adolescents in hospital in the early 1990s highlighted the need for staff support in caring for the adolescent. The addition of a psychologist and youth worker to the team benefits the staff and the adolescent undergoing treatment such as Ilizarov frame correction (Charles & Russell-Johnson 1995).

NURSING INTERVENTIONS IN CLUBFOOT MANAGEMENT

Need for support

The implications of clubfoot for the parents mean they require early emotional support from the nursing team, with information and education on the meaning of the diagnosis and treatment plan. This is backed up with pictorial leaflets and ideally, a contact telephone number.

Treatment needs to start at birth, outlining the programme of care and involving the parents to establish a partnership in setting objectives (Mount 1993), educating them and instilling the importance of their commitment to the planned care. Early on in the management, parents should be made aware that the treatment aims to give the child a foot which functions normally, allows wearing of shop-bought shoes and is pain free. The foot may be one or two sizes smaller than the normal foot with less calf muscle bulk.

Involving the parents

Initially parents are taught stretching exercises for the affected foot or feet, with encouragement to supplement this with continual playing with their child's foot.

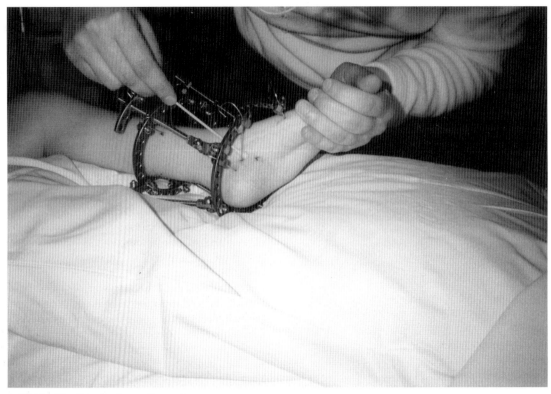

Figure 13.11 Cleaning pin sites on Ilizarov frame.

Following application of a cast, clear verbal and written instructions should be given to the parents on how to care for their child's plaster. This includes basic neurovascular observations of colour, warmth, movement and pain. Parents need to feel confident in handling their child with the knowledge they can contact the nursing team with any problems.

Postoperative observations

For the child who has undergone a surgical correction, the foot should be elevated on pillows for the first 48 hours to reduce swelling. Routine plaster care is performed with careful monitoring of toe movement, pain on passive extension of the toes, colour and capillary refill time. Any blood ooze through the plaster should be marked and monitored.

Parents are encouraged to participate in their child's management by observing for toe movement and ensuring they keep the leg(s) elevated. Plasters are reinforced with synthetic fibreglass, usually the day after surgery.

Pain management

Effective analgesia is essential. A nerve block given perioperatively can last for 4 hours, providing effective pain relief. Further analgesia may be required in opioid form for the first 24 hours, followed with an oral preparation such as paracetamol or junior ibuprofen, which the parents can continue at home.

The baby is normally discharged from hospital 1–2 days after surgery, providing they are comfortable and the neurovascular observations are satisfactory. Support at home can be arranged through the baby's health visitor or the children's community nurse.

Adapting to circumstances

The impact on the family of an older child undergoing further procedures differs from the care provided for the 9 month old. For the preschool or school-age child, immobilisation requires provision of a suitable buggy or child's wheelchair. Often a compromise is reached regarding the period of time for non-weight bearing, as children in this age group will continue to mobilise if pain free. In most cases the child is able to continue schooling, with staff support.

Neurovascular observations

Whether immobilised in a plaster or external fixator, neurovascular observations are closely monitored to detect signs of possible compartment syndrome (Altizer 2002). The affected limb is compared to the untreated limb to assess and record changes in the colour, capillary refill time, the presence of distal pulses, the degree of swelling, movement and noting the presence of any pain on passive and active movement (Grippen Bryant 1998).

Adapting to immobility

The patient undergoing correction of a foot deformity will be immobilised for a period of time. An adolescent may perceive this as enforced immobility. Through explanation and achievable goals, the nurse can help them adjust to their limitations. Discussion on coping strategies when discharged from hospital will highlight potential problems early.

The adolescent will require help with daily living activities. Their respect and dignity need to be ensured; this is an area that will need discussion between the parent and child.

Other problems causing concern at home and leading to families needing reassurance can be addressed by telephone contact with the nurse practitioner or ward team, or by liaison with the community nurse.

OTHER FOOT CONDITIONS

Parents often seek medical advice with regard to a perceived problem with their child's feet or toes. Referrals for orthopaedic assessment of minor deformities such as metatarsus adductus, pes planus (flat feet), curly or overriding toes are commonly prompted by discussion with relatives or shoe fitters.

Treatment is rarely required but diagnosis of these physiological conditions should exclude possible associated conditions such as hip dysplasia. Most cases of metatarsus adductus, thought to arise from intrauterine positioning, spontaneously resolve (Drennan 1998). Flat feet are the norm in children until the arch develops at the age of 6 (Kerr Graham 1997a). Treatment for curly and overriding toes is not a requisite unless problematic; that is, they are painful or causing pressure ulcers (Meehan 1998).

It is essential that anxious parents have a true understanding of the nature of these presentations. Reassurance is achieved following a thorough examination and explanation, with the knowledge that usually an element of time is all that is needed for natural resolution.

CHILDHOOD TRAUMA

Few children go through their childhood without sustaining an injury of some description; 10–15% of these injuries are skeletal, of which 15% are physeal injuries (Fothergill et al 1998).

Certain social indicators increase the incidence of limb fractures. Childhood crazes such as skateboarding, in-line skating and mini scooters are responsible for many admissions to hospital.

The peak incidence of fractures in children can be seasonal, increasing during school holidays and good weather.

Fractures in children differ from those in adults, due to the increased density and porosity of their bones. The thick periosteum helps to support the fracture and contributes to quicker healing.

In children an injury involving the immature growth plate, especially of a long bone, has long-term implications. These epiphyseal fractures are graded using the Salter Harris classification system, with type 1 being unlikely to affect growth outcome, to the rare type 5 which will result in growth arrest of the affected bone (Snyder 1998). Problems of this nature may not be noted until many months after injury when a leg length discrepancy becomes apparent.

SKELETAL TRAUMA IN CHILD ABUSE

When a child presents to the emergency department with a fracture it is important to establish the position, type and mechanism of the injury. This will not only facilitate a treatment plan but should allow the nurse to correlate the history with the injury sustained.

Discrepancies in the pattern of injury, presentation time in the emergency department, inconsistent medical history and fractures in the child under 1 year of age should alert the nurse to the possibility of child abuse. Other causes such as bone dysplasias must be excluded before this diagnosis is reached.

As 30% of children suspected of being abused have fractures (Pieper 1994), it is important to perform a skeletal survey which will establish the presence of previously healed fractures. When a cause for concern is raised, advice on action should be sought from the hospital's lead professionals in this area, such as a designated clinical nurse specialist and the Social Services (Stower 1999).

UPPER LIMB FRACTURES

Forearm fractures are commonly treated via closed reduction and plaster immobilisation. An unstable fracture may require internal fixation, using wires, plates or a flexible intramedullary nail.

Healing and consolidation are more rapid in children compared to adults, and their bones have the ability to remodel, allowing for a non-exact anatomical reduction. Four to six weeks is an average time for a forearm fracture to become consolidated. If wires are inserted these are removed at 4 weeks, followed by a further 2 weeks in a plaster cast. The child should refrain from sports activity for at least 4 weeks following removal of the cast.

Supracondylar fractures

Supracondylar fractures occur at the distal end of the humerus. The severity of the injury is generally described using the Gartland classification, varying from a Grade 1 to Grade 3 (Kerr Graham 1997b). A Grade 1 is treated with a simple backslab plaster and immobilised for 3 weeks, whilst a completely displaced Grade 3 fracture requires percutaneous pinning for 3 weeks. An open reduction is necessary if the fracture is unstable (Hart & Kester 1999).

These fractures carry a high risk of complications. The close proximity of the nerves and blood vessels around the elbow makes them susceptible to associated damage at the time of injury or during reduction of the fracture.

FEMORAL SHAFT FRACTURES

Paediatric femoral shaft fractures are a common injury in children, with most being attributable to accidental trauma. The male to female ratio is 2.5:1, with peaks in children under the age of 5 and in the mid-teenage years (Hakala & Blanco 2000). The aetiology varies; in younger children falls are the main cause, with high-energy trauma such as a road traffic accident being the more usual cause of injury in older children.

Treatment methods are designed to achieve fracture alignment whilst relieving pain and achieving good functional outcomes. Considerations taken into account by the orthopaedic team include the age of the child, the position and type of fracture plus any associated injuries, for example a head injury (Hakala & Blanco 2000). The orthopaedic assessment of these children is secondary to the initial management of life-threatening problems. Once the patient is stabilised, the orthopaedic injuries can be managed.

TREATMENT OPTIONS OF A FRACTURED FEMUR

Pavlik harness

For a child under 3 months of age, a Pavlik harness is used (see Fig. 13.1). Padding to the posterior strap gives additional support to the fracture. The harness is used for approximately 3 weeks and discontinued after a satisfactory radiological review. Healing of a fractured femur in this age group is extremely rapid.

Gallows traction

Gallows traction can be used for children from 3 to 18 months of age (see Fig. 13.3). This is weight dependent, with a suggested maximum weight of the child being 16 kg (Davis & Barr 1999). Adhesive extension tapes applied to both legs are secured with bandages. The cords are either attached to an overhead beam of the cot, or a pulley and weight system can be used. This raises the child's hips so they are flexed at 90° and the sacrum is lifted off the bed to enable a flat hand to pass underneath. The child's own body weight provides countertraction (Davis & Barr 1999). This age group can also be managed in a hip spica cast (see Fig. 13.4).

Depending on the position and type of fracture and to some extent surgeon preference, the older child may be treated in a variety of ways.

Hip spica cast

The child may be placed immediately in a spica, or after a week in gallows or Thomas splint traction. This supports the early callus formation and prevents an angulation deformity. Before this method is used, the family need to be consulted and advised on the implications for caring for their child at home. The child is discharged to be cared for in the home environment with support services available. See the previous section under DDH for the care of a child in a hip spica.

Fixed and balanced traction

From an average of 2 years of age and up, femoral fractures may be treated conservatively via fixed or balanced traction, using either skin or skeletal traction. The type depends on the anticipated length of time in traction and the amount of weight required to reduce the fracture (Nichol 1995).

There have been a variety of traction types devised by orthopaedic surgeons over the years. Thomas splint traction can be applied in either fixed or balanced form. Hamilton Russell traction may be used as a balanced framework with a sling to support the knee. Alternatively the fracture may be treated simply with "straight pull" traction with only a pillow under the knee.

Application of Thomas splint traction

The need to apply a Thomas splint does not occur daily in the life of an orthopaedic nurse. In the authors' centre a photographic diary of the traction bed with every stage of splint application has made an ideal resource pack for staff, ensuring correct traction application.

The splint can be applied in the emergency department by the nurse practitioner or ward staff. This facilitates postapplication radiological review prior to transferring the child to the ward. An explanation of the treatment is given to the child and parents whose anxiety levels are high at this early stage of management. It is important to reiterate this when they are able to focus more clearly on the future implications.

Of primary importance is the administration of appropriate analgesia prior to the application of the splint. Parents find themselves at a loss and feel ineffective in their ability to comfort their child in pain. The early assessment and treatment of the child's pain lessens the traumatic experience for both child and parent. Ketamine, a strong analgesic and dissociative anaesthetic, is ideal as it has a rapid onset and lasts approximately 20 minutes (Glickman 1995). It is often used with a femoral nerve block as an effective analgesic combination.

The child's unaffected leg is measured, with extra length added to allow for foot plantarflexion. When measuring around the circumference of the top of the leg, an allowance is made to accommodate for swelling of the fractured limb. This space between the skin and the ring will enable hygiene and ring care to be carried out, preventing pressure ulcers developing (Mellet 1998).

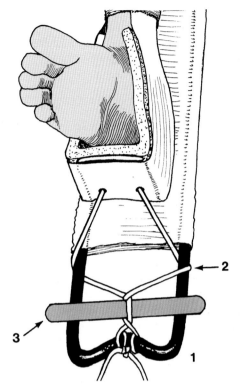

Figure 13.12   Thomas splint. The traction is completed by tying the cords to the end of the splint (1). Passing the cord under the corresponding bar will help control lateral rotation (2). A Chinese windlass using a spatula is used to take up the slack (3). (From MacRae & Esser 2002.)

Applying the traction takes two people. An assistant applies manual traction while supporting the leg and ankle, pulling the fracture into alignment, and correct the leg length, ensuring the foot pulses remain present. An adhesive extension tape is applied to the affected leg, making sure the medial and lateral malleoli are well padded. This is secured with bandaging, ensuring the patella remains free; this will protect the peroneal artery and allow checks on correct alignment with the foot. The affected leg rests on the covered and padded splint with the ring fitting in the groin resting posteriorly against the ischial tuberosity. The extension tapes are either secured to the splint end with a windlass in position, known as fixed traction (Fig. 13.12), or the cord is attached with the prescribed weight and placed over a pulley system to hang free.

The fractured limb is now immobilised. En route to the ward an X-ray is taken to confirm satisfactory alignment. Once on the ward, the splint can be suspended using traction cord, weights and pulleys to enable the child to move freely around the bed. For balanced traction the bed end is elevated to achieve the required countertraction of the child's body weight (Davis & Barr 1999).

Home traction

In today's healthcare economic climate there is a shift to reduce the period of hospitalisation. The trend for use of traction is on the decline due to changes in orthopaedic management and pressure caused by the impact on nursing services and bed shortages.

If a hip spica cast is inappropriate, the option to care for the child on traction at home with the support of the community nursing team is explored. As the child generally requires from 6 to 10 weeks in traction, depending on their age and fracture healing, this option needs to be carefully planned with the family and the multidisciplinary team. Protocols and guidelines for the child's management at home and how potential problems should be managed need to be established in advance and well understood by both the primary and secondary care teams.

Specifically designed home traction kits are available for use with either a hospital bed or the child's own bed. These children are best cared for in or close to the main living area, allowing them to remain interactive and involved in family life. The child's and other family members' needs should be taken into account. On the positive side, there is the bonus of the child being in their own environment and a reduction in travelling costs for the parents.

Elastic intramedullary nailing

This minimalist surgical approach involves the insertion of flexible long nails the diameter of which corresponds to the child's age (Fig. 13.13). Wires are placed to ensure stabilisation and reduction of the fracture. This method when used for femoral fractures is recommended in the 6–14 year age group (Hakala & Blanco 2000). The nails are removed approximately 9 months following insertion (Hakala & Blanco 2000), although this is not required if the patient is asymptomatic.

External fixation

This method is used for all age groups, commonly being used with open or comminuted fractures with associated soft tissue damage. It facilitates early

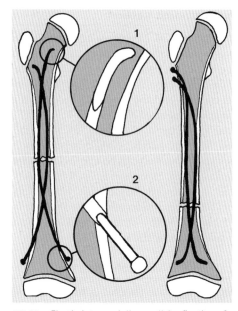

Figure 13.13 Elastic Intramedullary nail for fixation of a fracture femur. The flexible pins bend to fit and have flattened ends (1) to engage in the cancellous bone and control rotation. The other protruding end (2) is atraumatic.

mobilisation and discharge from hospital. Either a monolateral frame or a circular frame (Ilizarov frame) is used. The former is attached via pins inserted proximally and distally to the fracture. The circular frame is composed of a number of wires fixed to the bone and attached to a series of rings or half rings. For the care of pin sites, see under Congenital talipes equino varus (p 253).

SPECIFIC NURSING CARE ISSUES FOLLOWING TRAUMA

There are many aspects to be considered in the total care of a child following a fracture. Routine care such as an appropriate fluid regime, analgesia and observations are recorded as part of the postoperative procedure. Specific care includes neurovascular observations, care of the plaster cast, care of the traction or fixator and the overall care of the immobilised child.

Neurovascular observations

A skilled nurse is able to distinguish the relevance of certain findings when carrying out neurovascular observations, with the aim of detecting early signs of compartment syndrome. As Love (1998, p160) states, "Nurse-led pain assessment could make all the difference between recovery or loss of limb…". However, the young child can be difficult to assess and is therefore at risk (McQueen et al 2000). An understanding of the child's normal cognitive level and how they express pain is useful information acquired from the parents. Observations of colour, temperature of the extremity, sensation, distal pulses and movement (Pieper 1994) are recorded hourly initially and collated with observations of temperature, pulse and respiratory rates to form a true picture.

An increase in pressure within the compartment will give rise to the first signs of compartment syndrome (Ross 1991). The problem can arise following trauma, surgery and immobilisation (Tucker 1998). The discriminating signs of compartment syndrome are: pain out of proportion to the injury or surgery, pain on passive stretching of the digits of the affected limb, parasthesia, tense skin and possibly an absent or weak pulse. It should be noted that distal pulses can remain normal even with a high intracompartmental pressure (Whitesides 1978 & McQueen 1993, cited by Love 1998). Prompt action to address the problem is necessary to prevent tissue death occurring. Simple repositioning of the limb or splitting a tight plaster cast, including the padding, can help prevent or resolve the early signs of compartment syndrome. Once established, a fasciotomy to release the fascia surrounding the muscle is essential (Ross 1991).

Care of child's plaster

Many children undergo plaster application in the emergency department and are then discharged home. This makes teaching about caring for the plaster cast and observing for the prevention of potential complications essential through verbal instruction supported with a written information card.

Whether at home or on the ward, the child's limb is elevated to reduce swelling within the plaster. If there is a forearm fracture, the arm is elevated in a roller towel or similar apparatus. For supracondylar fractures the arm may be more comfortable rested on two or three pillows. A lower limb in plaster is elevated either on pillows or on a Braun frame.

Care is necessary in handling a newly applied plaster so as not to cause an indentation that could lead to pressure on the enclosed limb.

The child is taught how to exercise the joints not encased in plaster to prevent potential joint stiffness.

Care of traction and the immobilised child

The acceptance of being on traction can be a major issue for the child or adolescent. Teaching the child and family about the traction helps to relieve anxieties and will reassure them. The aspects of care discussed should include moving the child, handling and positioning, dietary needs, personal hygiene, plus problems and anxieties related to elimination. Simple explanations in the use of the urinal bottle and bedpan can alleviate misunderstanding and fear and the child is reassured that their privacy and dignity will be maintained.

The nurse should make constant observations of the traction apparatus, checking that:

- clamps are secure and the pulleys run freely
- traction cords are secure and not frayed
- weights hang freely
- countertraction is maintained.

If the child is on Thomas splint traction, the skin integrity under the ring must be checked regularly, ideally by performing 1–2 hourly ring care. If the child is involved in this aspect of care, the nurse needs to ensure they are doing it correctly. Any bandaging is checked to make sure it is neither too tight nor too loose. Complaints of itching can highlight blister formation under the skin extensions and should be investigated.

A nutritious diet is essential for bone healing and the prevention of constipation. The child on traction is apt to be treated with sweets and snacks; these are best in moderation.

The behaviour of hospitalised children may regress (Pieper 1994), often demonstrated by boredom. This can be relieved through play for the young child, enlisting the services of the hospital play specialist. The child's education via the hospital school helps continuation of normality.

A team approach to care

From admission, the care of the child involves the whole multidisciplinary team working in partnership with the family. The aim is for optimum care both in hospital and on discharge back to the community.

The nurse practitioner or the nurses on the ward are able to coordinate the team of staff, enabling a smooth pathway of care through the hospital and back to the community setting. The nurse needs to consider the impact on the family of the child's injury and how it is to be managed once at home.

Early intervention from both the physiotherapist and the occupational therapist as part of the total package of care will assist the facilitation of a safe discharge. Restoring and maintaining normal joint and limb function through teaching a range of exercises is paramount to achieving mobility. Mobility aids such as buggies, wheelchairs and hoists require teaching on their safe use; this is vital for a well-managed and informative hospital discharge.

Parents are involved throughout and instructed on further care of their child and future potential complications. Names and contact numbers of the nurse practitioner and other personnel involved in the child's care are made available to the parents for follow-up support and advice (Pieper 1994). The community nurse and health visitor are informed early of the planned discharge date, allowing time for identified problems to be addressed.

Schooling is another area to be explored; either a home tutor or assistance made available in the school can be arranged.

THE CHILD WITH A PAINFUL LIMP

The child who presents with a history of hip, thigh or knee pain and is possibly non-weight bearing, requires careful consideration and management to achieve a prompt diagnosis and correct treatment.

Irritable hip, also known as transient synovitis of the hip, is an acute condition that resolves quickly with rest. Children may present with a limp and pain in the knee or hip with a non-specific medical history. Passive movements of the hip are restricted but all other investigations are normal. A diagnosis of irritable hip can only be made on exclusion of other possible causes (Taylor & Clarke 1995) by performing a series of investigations (Box 13.3).

If the investigative results are normal and the child is apyrexial but has reduced mobility in the hip, they are treated on bedrest with or without Pugh's traction to relieve any muscle spasm. Taylor & Clarke (1995) suggest that two abnormal findings out of the following indicate the necessity for admission to hospital and intravenous antibiotic therapy to treat sepsis:

- ESR greater or equal to 20 mm per hour
- severe hip pain or spasm
- local tenderness
- pyrexia.

Box 13.3 Initial investigations for the child with a painful hip

Blood investigations	Radiological examination
Full blood count	AP of hips and pelvis
Erythrocyte sedimentation rate	Frog lateral hips and pelvis
C-reactive protein	

Blood culture analysis is required for sensitive intravenous antibiotic treatment but a broad-spectrum antibiotic can be given whilst awaiting the definitive result.

An incorrect or delayed diagnosis with no recognition of the signs and symptoms of septic arthritis or osteomyelitis can have a detrimental effect on the child's growing bones. Early detection with aspiration of the joint and aggressive intravenous treatment of the infection will significantly encourage a positive outcome.

CONCLUSION

It has not been possible to consider the whole of the vast spectrum of joint and limb problems within this chapter. However, important issues have been discussed. Paramount to effective treatment and management is the well-being of the child and the support given to the family.

In past years children with orthopaedic disorders were kept in hospital for months or even years. Today with advancing treatments, technology and recognition of changing socio-economic factors, discharging the child with appropriate support can be advantageous to both the child and family. However, this is not always the case and each situation needs to be assessed individually with consideration of the home environment, available community support, hospital back-up, the 24-hour parental care required and their coping mechanisms, before home care is arranged.

Paediatric orthopaedic nursing continues to evolve to meet these challenges with new posts developing to enhance care. Nurse practitioners are in a position to coordinate, advise and plan care for the individual child. A team approach, whether the child is nursed in the hospital or community environment, will ensure uniformity of care with the child and family's needs being met.

References

Altizer L 2002 Neurovascular assessment. Orthopaedic Nursing 20(4): 48–50

Bender LH 1998 Congenital and developmental disorders. In: Maher AB, Salmond SW, Pellino TA (eds) Orthopaedic nursing, 2nd edn. WB Saunders, Philadelphia

Bradish CF, Noor S 2000 The Ilizarov method in the management of relapsed club feet. Journal of Bone and Joint Surgery 82B(3): 387–391

Broughton NS 1997 Developmental dysplasia of the hip. In: Broughton NS (ed) A textbook of paediatric orthopaedics. WB Saunders, London

Burr S 1993 Adolescents and the ward environment. Paediatric Nursing 5(1): 10–13

Canale ST 1998 Slipped capital femoral epiphysis. In: Staheli LT (ed) Pediatric orthopaedic secrets. Hanley & Belfus, Philadelphia

Catterall A 1971 The natural history of Perthes disease. Journal of Bone and Joint Surgery 53B: 37–53

Charles M, Russell-Johnson H 1995 Campaigning for adolescent care. Paediatric Nursing 17(10): 6–7

Davis P, Barr L 1999 Principles of traction. Journal of Orthopaedic Nursing 3(4): 222–227

Dimeglio A, Bensahel H, Souchet P et al 1995 Classification of clubfoot. Journal of Pediatric Orthopaedics 4(2)B: 129–136

Drennan JC 1998 Metatarsus adductus. In: Staheli LT (ed) Pediatric orthopaedic secrets. Hanley & Belfus, Philadelphia

Fish DN, Herzenberg JE, Hensinger RN 1991 Current practice in the use of prereduction traction for congenital dislocation of the hip. Journal of Pediatric Orthopaedics 11: 149–153

Forst J, Forst C, Heller KD 1997 Pathogenic relevance of the pregnancy hormone relaxin to inborn hip instability. Archives of Orthopaedic and Trauma Surgery 116(4): 209–212

Fothergill J, Fox N, Jewkes F et al (Advanced Life Support Group, Working Group) 1998 Advanced paediatric life support: the practical approach, 2nd edn. BMJ Publishing Group, London

Gage JR, Winter RB 1973 Avascular necrosis of the capital femoral epiphysis as a complication of closed reduction of congenital dislocation of the hip. Journal of Bone and Joint Surgery 54A: 373–388

Galpin RD, Roach JW, Wenger DR et al 1989 One stage treatment of congenital dislocated hip in older children, including femoral shortening. Journal of Bone and Joint Surgery 7A: 734–741

Gamble JG 1998 Etiology of orthopaedic disorders. In: Staheli LT (ed) Pediatric orthopaedic secrets. Hanley & Belfus, Philadelphia

Glasper EA, Powell C 2000 First do no harm: parental exclusion from anaesthetic rooms. Paediatric Nursing 12(4): 14–17

Glickman A 1995 Ketamine: the dissociative anesthetic and the development of a policy for its safe administration in the pediatric emergency department. Journal of Emergency Nursing 21(2): 116–124

Glueck CJ, Crawford A, Roy D et al 1996 Association of antithrombotic deficiencies and hypofibrinolysis with Legg–Perthes disease. Journal of Bone and Joint Surgery 78A: 3–13

Grippen Bryant G 1998 Modalities for immobilisation. In: Maher AB, Salmond SW, Pellino TA (eds) Orthopaedic nursing, 2nd edn. WB Saunders, Philadelphia

Hakala BE, Blanco JS 2000 Pediatric femoral shaft fractures. Medscape Orthopaedics and Sports Medicine 4:1. Available online at: www.medscape.com/medscape/ OrthoSportsMed/journal

Hart KM, Kester K 1999 Supracondylar fractures in children. Orthopaedic Nursing 18(3): 23–27

Herring JA 1998 Legg–Calvé–Perthes disease. In: Staheli LT (ed) Pediatric orthopaedic secrets. Hanley & Belfus, Philadelphia

Herring JA (ed) 2002 Tachdjian's pediatric orthopaedics, 3rd edn. WB Saunders, Philadelphia

Herring JA, Neustadt JB, Williams JJ et al 1992 The lateral pillar classification of Legg–Calvé–Perthes disease. Journal of Pediatric Orthopaedics 12: 143–150

Kasser JR, Bowen JR, MacEwan GD 1985 Varus derotational osteotomy in treatment of persistent congenital dislocation of the hip. Journal of Bone and Joint Surgery 67A: 195–202

Kerr Graham H 1997a Normal variants: intoeing, bow legs and flat feet. In: Broughton NS (ed) A text book of paediatric orthopaedics. WB Saunders, London

Kerr Graham H 1997b Upper limb trauma. In: Broughton NS (ed) A text book of paediatric orthopaedics. WB Saunders, London

Lee-Smith J, Santy J, Davis P et al 2001 Pin site management: towards a consensus Part One. Journal of Orthopaedic Nursing 5(1): 37–42

Love C 1998 A discussion and analysis of nurse-led pain assessment for the early detection of compartment syndrome. Journal of Orthopaedic Nursing 2(3): 160–167

MacRae R, Esser M 2002 Practical fracture treatment, 4th edn. Churchill Livingstone, Edinburgh

Malvitz TA, Weinstein SL 1994 Closed reduction for functional and radiographic results after an average of thirty years. Journal of Bone and Joint Surgery 76A: 1777–1792

McAndrews MP, Weinstein SL 1983 A long term follow-up of Perthes disease treated with spica casts. Journal of Pediatric Orthopaedics 3: 160–165

McQueen MM, Gaston P, Court-Brown CM 2000 Acute compartment syndrome: who is at risk? Journal of Bone and Joint Surgery 82B(2): 200–203

Meehan PL 1998 Toe deformities. In: Staheli LT (ed) Pediatric orthopaedic secrets. Hanley & Belfus, Philadelphia

Mellett S 1998 Care of the orthopaedic patient with traction. Nursing Times 94(22): 52–54

Mount M 1993 Self-care to home care: the way forward. Paediatric Nursing 5(5): 20–23

Nattrass GR 1997 Slipped upper femoral epiphysis. In: Broughton NS (ed) A text book of paediatric orthopaedics. WB Saunders, London

Nichol D 1995 Understanding the principles of traction. Nursing Standard 9(46): 25–28

Norris C, Carroll MD 1998 Clubfoot. In: Staheli LT (ed) Pediatric orthopaedic secrets. Hanley & Belfus, Philadelphia

Pieper P 1994 Pediatric trauma. Nursing Clinics of North America 29(4): 563–584

Ponseti IV 1996 Congenital clubfoot: fundamentals of treatment. Oxford University Press, Oxford

Ross D 1991 Acute compartment syndrome. Orthopaedic Nursing 10(2): 33–38

Salter RB 1961 Innominate osteotomy in the treatment of congenital dislocated hip. Journal of Bone and Joint Surgery 43B: 518–539

Salter RB 1997 Foreword. In: Broughton NS (ed) A text book of paediatric orthopaedics. WB Saunders, London

Santy J 2000 Nursing the patient with an external fixator. Nursing Standard 14(31): 47–52

Shelley H 1993 Adolescent needs in hospital. Paediatric Nursing 5(9): 16–18

Sims M, Saleh M 2000 External fixation – the incidence of pin site infection: a prospective audit. Journal of Orthopaedic Nursing 4(2): 59–63

Snyder P 1998 Fractures. In: Maher AB, Salmond SW, Pellino TA (eds) Orthopaedic nursing, 2nd edn. WB Saunders, Philadelphia

Staheli LT 1992 Fundamentals of pediatric orthopaedics. Raven Press, New York

Stower S 1999 Principles and practice of child protection. Paediatric Nursing 11(7): 35–42

Taylor GR, Clarke NM 1995 Recurrent irritable hip in childhood. Journal of Bone and Joint Surgery 77B(5): 748–751

Taylor GR, Clarke NM 1997 Monitoring the treatment of developmental dysplasia of the hip with the Pavlik harness: the role of ultrasound. Journal of Bone and Joint Surgery 79B: 719–723

Tucker KR 1998 Compartment syndrome: the orthopaedic nurse's vital role. Journal of Orthopaedic Nursing 2(1): 33–36

Uglow MG, Clarke NMP 2000 Relapse in staged surgery for congenital talipes equinovarus. Journal of Bone and Joint Surgery 82B(5): 739–743

Vogel I, Andersson JE, Uldbjerg N 1998 Serum relaxin in the newborn is not a marker of neonatal hip instability. Journal of Pediatric Orthopaedics 18(4): 535–537

Weinstein SL, Ponseti IV 1979 Congenital dislocated hip: open reduction through a medial approach. Journal of Bone and Joint Surgery 61A: 119–124

Chapter 14

Care of patients with bone tumours

Chris Henry

INTRODUCTION

Bone tumours are a challenge to orthopaedic nurses because they may be rare, difficult to diagnose, life threatening and require a combination of treatments involving chemotherapy, radical surgery and radiotherapy. This requires nurses to develop an extended knowledge of oncology and counselling, be able to communicate difficult information, relate to issues around terminal illness and collaborate effectively with multi-agencies, community teams and other treatment centres.

Bone tumours are benign or malignant, primary or secondary, slow growing or aggressive. Characteristically, benign tumours grow moderately slowly, are well differentiated, are only locally invasive and generally do not metastasise; however, certain types can develop malignant changes over a period of time. Conversely, primary malignant bone tumours are rare, they are locally invasive and metastasise (Gray 1994). Most primary bone tumours are classified according to the cell type from which they originate (Table 14.1), although the origin of some tumours is uncertain. The presentation of both types can be similar.

Age is an important factor as some tumours peak at certain stages of growth.

- Primary malignant bone tumours rarely occur before the age of 5 years.
- It is uncommon for giant cell tumours to establish before the epiphyseal closure (O'Sullivan & Saxton 1997).
- The incidence of osteosarcoma peaks in teenage years.
- Chondrosarcoma is a disease of the mature skeleton.

Table 14.1 A classification of bone tumours

Tissue of origin	Benign tumour	Malignant tumour
Bone	Osteoid osteoma	Osteosarcoma
	Osteoblastoma	
	Aneurysmal bone cyst	
Cartilage	Osteochondroma	Chondrosarcoma
	Chondroma	
	Enchondroma	
Fibrous	Fibroma	Fibrosarcoma
Marrow		Myeloma
Uncertain	Giant cell tumour	Ewing's sarcoma
	Benign fibrous	Malignant fibrous
	histiocytoma	histiocytoma

This chapter offers a broad explanation of the different types of tumours, their management and relevant nursing care issues. Secondary bone tumours occur as the metastatic deposits from primary tumours in the breast, prostate, lung, thyroid and kidney. These are not connected with primary bone cancer so are dealt with separately at the end of the chapter.

CLINICAL PRESENTATION

The patient may have a history of trauma, often relating to a sporting injury which, although not the cause, can reveal the presence of a tumour. If the pain is assumed to be from soft tissue damage, this can delay the start of investigations and treatment.

The patient can present with a variety of symptoms, the commonest for patients seeking advice being pain or discomfort. This is caused by the rapid expansion of the tumour within the bone, which stretches the surrounding tissues. If close to a joint, it eventually causes pressure on the nerves and blood vessels. Screening for a pathological fracture is necessary. A history of night pain and pain not relieved by rest is indicative of a malignant tumour. Initially, non-steroidal antiinflammatory drugs (NSAIDs) are effective in the management of pain from a tumour but if the pain becomes severe, morphine tends to be the most effective drug to use.

Swelling will be present in varying degrees. The first indication of a tumour can be a swelling away from a joint with little pain. The area is usually hard, radiates heat if the tumour is malignant and is tender if palpated. If the swelling is large, dilated blood vessels are visible on the skin surface.

Limb movement is limited by pain and swelling, especially if a joint is involved. If a lower limb is affected the patient can be reluctant to bear weight. Sporting activities are usually curtailed voluntarily before treatment is sought.

Altered neurology can be present, especially if the tumour is in the spine or pelvis, causing pressure on adjacent nerves. In these cases a change in bowel and bladder function can occur.

Patients may experience a nighttime pyrexia with complaints of night sweats. A recent decrease in appetite and associated weight loss are reported if there is a delay in referral and identifying the presence of a tumour.

INVESTIGATIONS

Investigations to establish the type and extent of the tumour are generally undertaken on an outpatient basis or during a short hospital admission. If a malignancy is suspected, especially in a young person, inpatient investigations allow a more informative approach and offer support to all the family.

The nurse can play a key role in helping patients to express their feelings of anger, fear and resentment that their lives may be at risk. Encouraging participative decision making in their future management and treatments, together with accurate information, can help to reduce the feelings of isolation and loss of control (Ross Bell 1994). Ineffective coping is common at this stage due to fear of the unknown before a confirmed diagnosis is made. This can cause extreme anxiety and confusion for the patient and family while awaiting the final results and reduces their ability to assimilate information.

Blood tests may show an elevated serum alkaline phosphatase level due to increased osteoblastic activity, especially in patients with metastatic disease (Mertens & Bramwell 1994). In certain tumours the erythrocyte sedimentation rate (ESR), white cell count and serum lactic dehydrogenase (LDH) are raised. Serum LDH is used as a prognostic factor, showing a reduction if there has been a response to drugs and elevation if the tumour has recurred (Sailsbury & Byers 1994).

IMAGING

Plain X-rays are the first imaging technique used. These will show the site, approximate size and outline of the tumour, significant changes to the periosteum, hollow cavities in the bone, new bony activity and the presence of any pathological fractures.

A magnetic resonance imaging (MRI) scan should be taken before any disturbance is made to the tumour, such as a biopsy. This non-invasive technique utilises a magnetic field to produce a two- or three-dimensional image (Fig. 14.1). It provides detailed information about the inside of the bone, the joints and soft tissues, making it a valuable tool in assessing the extent of the tumour spread (Apley & Soloman 1993). A repeat MRI scan during treatment will demonstrate the response to treatment. As the scan will also show the association between the tumour and the local nerves and blood vessels, it is valuable in planning surgery as it shows the extent of the clearance margins required at the time of resection. The scanning process may take up to 1 hour, often with the patient lying in a supine position in the tunnel; this can be claustrophobic, uncomfortable and noisy. Patients should be assessed prior to scanning to ensure they have adequate analgesia cover.

Computed tomography (CT) scans provide multiple cross-sectional views of tumour involvement in bone, soft tissues and neurovascular structures. This is of particular value in demonstrating interosseous tumours in the spine and pelvis (Ross Bell 1994). CT scans of the lungs are taken when the tumour is suspected to be malignant as the lungs are the primary source for bone metastases. This will require careful explanation if the patient is to be prepared for this outcome.

Radionuclide bone scanning will detect or exclude other tumours in the skeleton. The scan is taken of the whole skeleton about 3 hours after an intravenous injection of a radionuclide such as technetium-99m. This will detect metabolically active areas, known as 'hot spots' (Fig. 14.2). Hot spots indicate the presence of malignant tumours, fractures, bone infection, arthritis and bony metastases (Ross Bell 1994). They will also show normal bony activity around the growth plates in young people. These differences need to be understood by the healthcare team and explained carefully to the patient and family.

BIOPSY

A biopsy is an essential part of the investigative process. The aim is to provide a representative sample of the tumour for both histopathology and

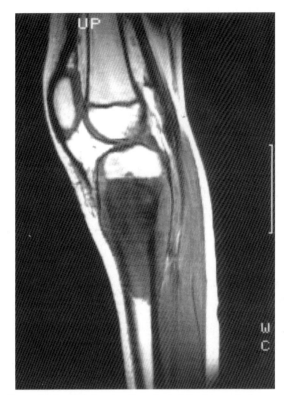

Figure 14.1 MRI showing the extent of the tumour in the proximal tibia.

microbiology. Differences of opinion exist over the optimum method but it is generally agreed that it should be performed at a specialist centre. Grimer & Sneath (1990) found that complications were 10 times more likely to occur if biopsies were not carried out at a specialist tumour centre. Carrying out the biopsy at such centres allows planning of the biopsy site and the route of access to be part of the definitive surgical management because the biopsy scar may have to be included in the subsequent surgical excision of the tumour (Apley & Soloman 1993, O'Sullivan & Saxton 1997). Cannon & Dyson (1987) showed that where the biopsy site could not be excised, 38% of tumours recurred.

Needle, excision and open biopsies are commonly practised. Needle biopsy, the least invasive method, involves a core of tissue being withdrawn through a needle, often under CT or ultrasound guidance. If a soft tissue sample is taken, a local anaesthetic may be adequate but if a bone sample is needed, this is more painful, requiring a general anaesthetic, especially if the tumour is already causing distress. Stoker et al (1991) reviewed 208 needle biopsy procedures and concluded that

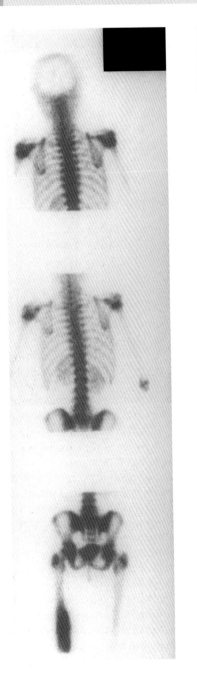
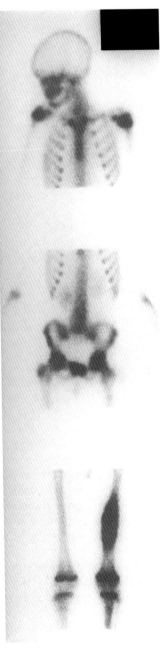

Figure 14.2 Bone scan, anterior and posterior views, showing marked increased uptake of isotope in the mid-shaft of the left femur. No other area of abnormal skeleton activity indicated.

when experienced practitioners carried out the procedure, it was safe and accurate with a correct diagnosis reached in 97% of cases, the potential for limb-sparing surgery was increased and there were fewer disturbances to a viable tumour, reducing the risk of local and systemic spread.

Excisional biopsies are reserved for benign lesions where the tumour is completely removed.

Open biopsies involve removing a section of the tumour under a general anaesthetic.

Waiting for the results of the biopsy is a very anxious time for the patient and family; this can vary from 2 days to 2 weeks. Soft tissue samples are quicker to diagnose than those taken from bone as they need to undergo a process of decalcification before the slides can be prepared (Ross Bell 1994).

The bone is weakened following biopsy, increasing the risk of a pathological fracture. If the lower limb is involved, the patient may need to use crutches and avoid full weight bearing.

BENIGN TUMOURS OF BONE

OSTEOID OSTEOMA

An osteoid osteoma is a small painful tumour composed of newly formed bone. It occurs in patients under 30 years of age, more commonly in men than women (ratio of 3:1), with 50% developing in the femur and tibia. Those occurring in the spine may cause a painful scoliosis (Apley & Soloman 1993). Patients can experience quite severe pain that is worse at night; aspirin-based drugs usually provide relief.

A small radiolucent area, called the nidus, may show on X-ray. A thin-slice CT scan may show the nidus more clearly, strongly suggesting the diagnosis and allowing accurate location of the tumour in the bone. A radio-isotope bone scan will show an area of increased uptake.

These tumours may eventually resolve without any intervention, but the degree of pain experienced makes this an unlikely method of management. The standard treatment has been surgical excision of the nidus, which must be complete to prevent recurrence. However, although the lesion may be small, an extensive operation may be needed to remove it. As these lesions tend to occur in weight-bearing bones, it is sometimes necessary to use bone grafting and internal fixation to prevent the risk of fracture, especially if a large amount of cortical bone is excised (Rosenthal et al 1998).

In recent years, conservative approaches to treatment have been developed and successfully used in selected cases. They involve CT-guided percutaneous techniques, performed under a general anaesthetic, to destroy or remove the nidus. These procedures are minimally invasive and include percutaneous resection or the thermal destruction of the nidus using laser photocoagulation or radiofrequency ablation (Linder et al 2001). The advantages of these for patients are a fast reduction in tumour pain within 48 hours, just an overnight stay in hospital and the immediate resumption of all activities. Rosenthal et al (1998) were unable to show any significant differences, with regard to rate of recurrence, between patients undergoing a surgical procedure and those managed by percutaneous ablation.

OSTEOBLASTOMA

These tumours are similar to an osteoid osteoma but are larger. The surgical management differs because the whole lesion must be excised completely, otherwise it may recur (O'Sullivan & Saxton 1997). These tumours may be aggressive but do not metastasise. About 50% occur in the spine, incurring a higher risk of complications from spinal cord involvement with motor or sensory changes, possibly leading to a fatal outcome (Gray 1994).

OSTEOCHONDROMA

This is the commonest benign bone tumour, sometimes called an exostosis, which usually starts growing in adolescence. It develops from an outgrowth of normal cartilage, close to a growth plate, and becomes ossified (O'Sullivan & Saxton 1997). The growth continues on a stalk until skeletal maturity, giving a cauliflower appearance. Any enlargement of the tumour after its growth period has ended may indicate malignant transformation to chondrosarcoma. There can be single or multiple tumours, usually sited in the metaphysis of long bones. Multiple lesions develop as part of a familial disorder known as diaphyseal aclasis, causing bony deformity (Apley & Soloman 1993).

Surgical treatment is undertaken if the tumour is impairing the function of the adjacent muscles, tendons, nerves and joints. Wide excision will be required as there is a high rate of recurrence in inadequately resected tumours (Williams & Cole 1991).

CHONDROMA

A chondroma is a benign tumour arising from the cartilaginous elements of growing bone. When a chondroma arises as a single lesion in the small bones of the hand and foot it is called a cystic chondroma; those arising elsewhere are known as an enchondroma (Duthie & Bentley 1983). Multiple enchondromata, commonly known as Ollier's disease, affect the metaphysis of long bones, arising in the cartilage cells remaining from incomplete ossification.

Operative treatment is indicated if these tumours are rapidly growing, cause discomfort or loss of function. Surgical excision or curettage with bone grafting is usually effective. They can recur after incomplete removal; this risk is higher with tumours

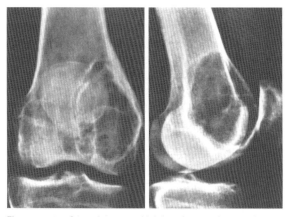

Figure 14.3 Osteoclastoma which has destroyed most of one femoral condyle; it extends close up to the joint surface. (From Adams & Hamblen 1990.)

of the long bones and if the patient is over the age of 35 years (Duthie & Bentley 1983).

GIANT CELL TUMOUR (OSTEOCLASTOMA)

This common benign tumour, seen in young men after fusion of the epiphysis, is of unknown origin. The typical sites are the distal end of the femur and proximal tibia, with the tumour starting in the metaphysis and extending into the epiphysis, maintaining an outer thin shell of cortex (Duckworth 1995). Giant cell tumours are composed of large numbers of giant cells, which give a 'soap-bubble' appearance on X-ray (Fig. 14.3). They are soft, friable tumours, presenting as pain near a joint, with a swelling or pathological fracture. Apley & Soloman (1994) describe the term 'benign' as misleading when applied to these tumours as one-third will be benign, one-third locally invasive and one-third will metastasise.

Surgical treatment is by excision of some bones such as the fibula and clavicle. In other areas, curettage and grafting may be adequate but for an aggressive or recurrent lesion, endoprosthetic replacement is required to ensure complete excision.

ANEURYSMAL BONE CYST

This tumour occurs mainly in teenagers and is rarely seen in patients over the age of 30 years; 50% arise in the metaphysis of long bones and 30% in the spine (O'Sullivan & Saxton 1997). The cyst that develops contains cavities filled with blood, which on X-ray may resemble a giant cell tumour. However, no other benign lesion spreads into the

adjacent bones in the same way. Although benign, this lesion varies between being active and highly aggressive, requiring full investigation to clarify the level of development (Gray 1994).

Patients present with pain and swelling in varying degrees. Treatment is by curettage, occasionally with bone grafting. There is a risk of recurrence after surgery if a wide excision is required. If the tumour grows in the spine, where resection is difficult, radiotherapy may be effective.

MALIGNANT TUMOURS OF BONE

Primary bone cancers are classified as high or low grade; they all have the potential to metastasise, usually to the lung. Low-grade tumours tend to have a slower rate of growth, invade locally and are slower to metastasise. If inadequately resected, they will recur and are at risk of transforming into a high-grade type (Enneking & Conrad 1988). High-grade tumours are rapidly growing, aggressive and destructive lesions, with a high incidence of metastases.

OSTEOSARCOMA

Osteosarcoma is the commonest primary bone cancer to occur in young people up to the age of 30 years and is slightly more common in boys and men than in girls and women, with a ratio of 1.5:1 (Souhami & Tobias 1986). There is a peak incidence around 14 years of age and it appears to be more likely to occur in young people who will be taller than average for their age. It also occurs in adults with Paget's disease, indicating a link with increased bone activity (Schwartz et al 1993). It accounts for 3–4% of childhood malignancies with about 150 new cases diagnosed in Britain each year (Souhami & Tobias 1986).

There are five main types of osteosarcoma: osteoblastic, chondroblastic, fibroblastic, mixed and telangiectatic (O'Sullivan & Saxton 1997). The tumour arises in the metaphysis of the bone where growth is more active. The majority are seen in the lower limb, particularly in the distal femur (Figs 14.4, 14.5) and proximal tibia, with other common sites being the proximal humerus, proximal femur and pelvis.

Approximately 10–20% of patients have lung metastases at the time of diagnosis (Lewis 1996); this significantly affects their prognosis. Although pain is a frequent complaint, a study by Grimer & Sneath

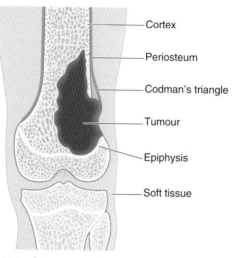

Figure 14.4   Osteosarcoma in the distal femur. (Adapted from Gibson & Evans with permission from Whurr Publishers.)

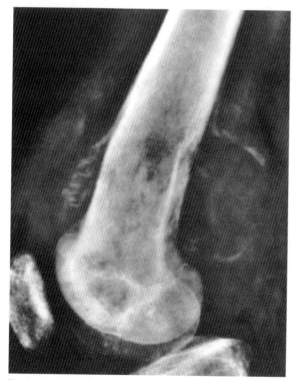

Figure 14.5   Osteosarcoma of the lower end of the femur, the most common site of these tumours. The tumour has destroyed much of the lower end of the femur and has burst through the cortex into the soft tissues. (From Adams & Hamblen 1990 with permission.)

(1990) demonstrated that, on average, it was 6 weeks before a patient with osteosarcoma contacted their general practitioner for advice and a further 7 weeks before a diagnosis was made.

Aetiology

Patients with hereditary retinoblastoma have an increased risk of developing an osteosarcoma as a secondary tumour, indicating a genetic predisposition to this disease (Jurgens et al 1992). The incidence is also higher in irradiated bones. Osteosarcoma is one of the tumours identified in Li-Fraumeni cancer families, where there may be the early onset of breast cancer in mothers and close relatives due to a P53 germline mutation (Porter et al 1992).

Historically, osteosarcoma of the jaw was commonly found in workers painting luminous watch dials due to the ingestion of radium when they moistened the paintbrushes in their mouths (Ross Bell 1994, Souhami & Tobias 1986).

Radiographic features

The plain X-ray films may show destruction of the cortex and some periosteal reaction. A wedge of new bone develops at the angle where the periosteum is pushed away from the bone, called a Codman's triangle (Figs 14.5, 14.6). There may also be the 'sunray' appearance of new bone tumour (Gray 1994) (Fig. 14.6).

Management

The optimum treatment for osteosarcoma is a combination of chemotherapy and radical surgery, either limb sparing or amputation. This approach has advanced the management of osteosarcoma over the last 30 years, with survival rates of about 55% for tumours without metastases at the time of presentation. A good response to chemotherapy is an important prognostic factor; if 90% tumour necrosis is achieved at the time of resection, the patient's survival is significantly improved (O'Sullivan & Saxon 1997). Trial chemotherapy protocols using a combination of drugs are constantly reviewed both nationally and internationally to seek the optimum treatment.

Grimer (1996) found that local recurrence of osteosarcoma was more likely to arise after limb-sparing surgery if the patient had a poor response to chemotherapy. He suggests that the effect of chemotherapy is more significant than the extent of surgical margins in preventing this.

Osteosarcoma is not very sensitive to radiotherapy. Its use is therefore limited but is indicated at the end of treatment to irradiate the soft tissues where the tumour has only been marginally resected. If this is around the joint of an endoprosthetic implant, adhesions may occur which can limit function.

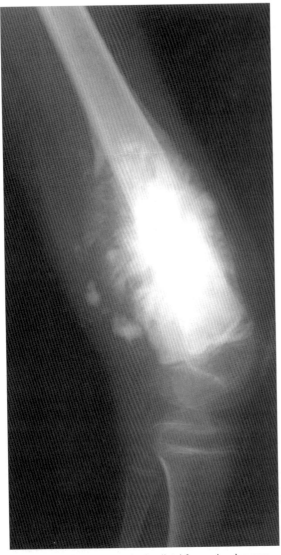

Figure 14.6   Osteosarcoma in the distal femur showing new bone formation and elevated periosteum.

EWING'S SARCOMA

Ewing's sarcoma is the fourth commonest primary malignant bone tumour and the second commonest in young people, 75% occurring in patients under the age of 20 years, with a male to female ratio of 3:2 (O'Sullivan & Saxton 1997). The majority of patients are white, with a very low incidence in the black Afro-Caribbean population.

This aggressive, small, round, blue cell tumour is of uncertain origin. It arises in the diaphysis or shaft of the bone (Fig. 14.7). Although it may occur in any

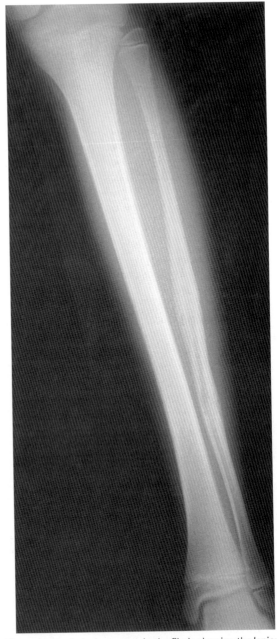

Figure 14.7   Ewing's sarcoma in the fibula showing the 'onion layers' of periosteal reaction.

bone, it is more common in the femur, tibia, fibula, humerus and pelvis. It usually spreads into the soft tissue area more rapidly and more extensively than an osteosarcoma (Pringle 1987). Approximately 25% of patients have lung metastases at the time of diagnosis and the tumour can infiltrate the bone marrow, which is routinely aspirated before treatment is commenced.

Patients with a Ewing's sarcoma may present with a pyrexia, often occurring at night along with night sweats. A raised ESR and white cell count (WCC) are probably due to the necrotic nature of the tumour (Duckworth 1995). The clinical features can resemble osteomyelitis.

The tumour pain generally increases in intensity at a slower rate than with an osteosarcoma. This may be the reason for delays in diagnosis. Grimer & Sneath (1990) found that patients waited an average of 21 weeks before consulting a doctor, with a further wait of 31 weeks before a diagnosis was made.

A number of significant factors relate to a poorer outcome.

- The site of the tumour: those in the pelvis and sacrum have the worst prognosis, followed by those in the proximal end of long bones.
- Lung metastases present at the time of diagnosis.
- A large soft tissue component involved.
- A high serum lactic dehydrogenase (LDH), which is related to the size and activity of the tumour.
- A high leukocyte count, which appears to be linked to an increased risk of tumour recurrence (Schwartz et al 1993).

Aetiology

Cytogenic studies have shown a translocation of chromosome 22 in patients with Ewing's sarcoma; this is also seen in patients with a neural tumour. Peripheral primitive neuroectodermal tumours (PNET) are now included in the Ewing's sarcoma group, demonstrating a translocation of chromosome 11; these are currently managed in the same way. This cytogenic abnormality is supported by the increased risk of these patients developing osteosarcoma in irradiated areas (Schwartz et al 1993). No hereditary link has been demonstrated.

Radiographic features

The plain X-rays frequently show a large soft tissue swelling and a destructive lesion with a moth-eaten appearance without any new bone formation. There may be a periosteal reaction aptly described as 'onion layers'. This is caused by layers of new tumour bone forming under the periosteum, and being destroyed, leaving only the shells parallel to the shaft of the bone (Duthie & Bentley 1983).

Management

Ewing's sarcoma is very sensitive to chemotherapy and radiotherapy. A combination of multi-agent chemotherapy, surgery and the later option of radiotherapy has improved the outlook for young people if they have no metastatic disease, with a 5-year survival rate of 50–55% (Schwartz et al 1993).

Autologous bone marrow transplantation with stem cell rescue, following high-dose chemotherapy, is currently part of the European chemotherapy protocol being used in clinical trials for patients deemed to have a poor prognosis. As randomisation in this trial does not generally occur until after surgery, it is important that practitioners are aware that all patients undergoing surgery for Ewing's sarcoma will require irradiated blood to protect against the later possible complication of graft versus host disease if transplantation is required.

CHONDROSARCOMA

Chondrosarcoma is the second commonest primary malignant bone tumour. It occurs in the mature skeleton with a peak incidence in patients of 40–60 years of age. These tumours are derived from cartilage cells, with large areas of cartilage becoming ossified (Piasecki 1987). There are two forms (O'Sullivan & Saxton 1997):

1 the central form arising within the bone from an enchondroma and
2 the peripheral form arising on the surface of the bone from an osteochondroma.

The tumours occur more frequently in the pelvis and proximal ends of long bones (Duckworth 1995) (Fig. 14.8). They are slower growing than other malignant tumours, metastasise later and as the swelling gradually increases in size, pain becomes a persistent feature. These tumours appear to grow more rapidly in younger adults.

Low-grade chondrosarcoma tumours are well differentiated, tend to be locally invasive and unlikely to metastasise. The high-grade tumours, known as dedifferentiated chondrosarcoma, are poorly differentiated with a high incidence of lung metastases. A low-grade tumour that recurs has the potential to change to a higher grade.

Plain X-rays show a destructive bone lesion containing flecks of calcification, possibly invading the soft tissues (Duthie & Bentley 1983).

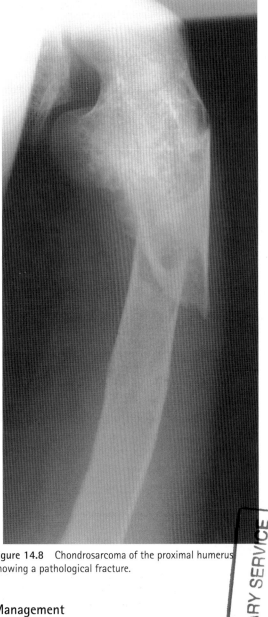

Figure 14.8   Chondrosarcoma of the proximal humerus showing a pathological fracture.

Management

The optimum treatment is complete excision of the tumour together with any associated soft tissues. This may necessitate endoprosthetic replacement or amputation to obtain adequate clearance margins to prevent recurrence.

Unfortunately, chondrosarcomas are resistant to both radiotherapy and chemotherapy, although these treatments may have some part to play in the management of high-grade tumours following surgical excision and in containing unresectable tumours. A study by Capanna et al (1988) showed that out of 46 patients treated for dedifferentiated chondrosarcoma by radical surgical excision alone, only three patients survived more than 2 years.

MULTIPLE MYELOMA

A myeloma is a malignant tumour of the plasma cells of the bone marrow. It may arise as a single lesion, a plasmacytoma, but more commonly, multiple lesions are present, occurring wherever there is red bone marrow.

Patients are generally over the age of 45 years and present with symptoms of bone pain, tenderness, weakness and anaemia due to the bone marrow destruction. Pathological fractures occur, especially in the spine due to vertebral body collapse. Patients who have widespread disease may show signs of renal failure.

Plasma cells normally produce protein antibodies; as a result, in multiple myeloma large quantities of protein can be detected in the blood and urine. The investigations commonly include (Apley & Soloman 1993):

- urinalysis, with over half the cases showing Bence-Jones protein
- electrophoresis of the plasma and urine proteins
- blood tests which may show hypercalcaemia and a significantly raised ESR
- a sternal marrow puncture to identify typical myeloma cells.

Radiographic features

Plain X-rays are similar to those of metastatic disease showing a reduction in bone density. A typical X-ray feature shows multiple 'punched-out' areas in the bones with no surrounding new bone formation; these are best seen in the skull. In addition, as myeloma is one of the commonest causes of secondary osteoporosis and vertebral compression fractures in patients over the age of 45 years, these features will be visible on X-ray.

Management

There is no curative treatment for multiple myeloma. Radiotherapy and chemotherapy may relieve the pain and pressure, possibly prolonging survival. Pathological fractures are treated symptomatically with internal fixation but the bone will be crumbly, often requiring the support of bone cement to ensure a good fixation (Apley & Soloman 1993).

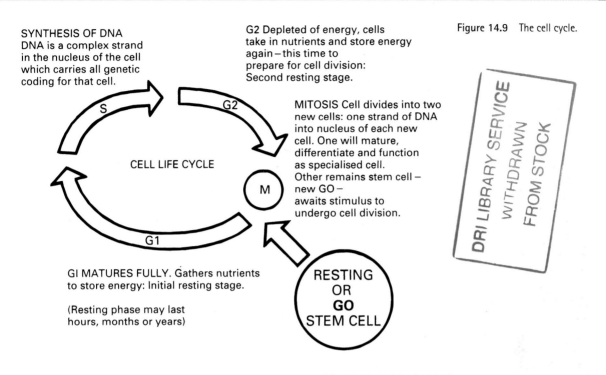

SYNTHESIS OF DNA
DNA is a complex strand
in the nucleus of the cell
which carries all genetic
coding for that cell.

G2 Depleted of energy, cells
take in nutrients and store energy
again – this time to
prepare for cell division:
Second resting stage.

Figure **14.9** The cell cycle.

CELL LIFE CYCLE

MITOSIS Cell divides into two
new cells: one strand of DNA
into nucleus of each new
cell. One will mature,
differentiate and function
as specialised cell.
Other remains stem cell –
new GO –
awaits stimulus to
undergo cell division.

GI MATURES FULLY. Gathers nutrients
to store energy: Initial resting stage.

(Resting phase may last
hours, months or years)

RESTING
OR
GO
STEM CELL

CHEMOTHERAPY FOR PRIMARY BONE TUMOURS

RATIONALE

Chemotherapy is given to:

- reduce the tumour size and its associated oedema, potentiating limb-sparing surgery
- kill the tumour cells making the tumour necrotic
- eradicate micrometastases (Ross Bell 1994).

The data from clinical trials (Mertens & Bramwell 1994) demonstrate that the use of adjuvant chemotherapy has improved long-term survival in patients with osteosarcoma and Ewing's sarcoma. Chemotherapy is commenced immediately after the diagnosis is confirmed to allow time for the manufacture of an endoprosthesis (Jurgens et al 1992). When the tumour is resected after the first few cycles of chemotherapy, it is possible to study the effects of chemotherapy on the tumour cells. A good response is said to be when 90% or more of the tumour cells have been killed, leaving only a small percentage of viable tumour (Jurgens et al 1992). If less than 90% of the tumour has been killed, it may be considered appropriate to adjust the combination of cytotoxic drugs to enhance tumour necrosis.

COMBINATION CHEMOTHERAPY

All primary bone tumours are treated with a combination of cytotoxic drugs, which act on different phases of the cell cycle (Fig. 14.9). The cell cycle is the process by which all immature stem cells have the ability to reproduce themselves. The reasons for combining selected drugs are to:

- have maximum impact on the tumour cells in a shorter course of treatment
- reduce drug resistance
- lessen the toxic side effects of the drugs (Brown 1987).

Protocols for the administration of cytotoxic drugs allow a short period of rest between cycles. This reduces the accumulation of side effects from these drugs, allowing normal tissue time to recover (Williams & Cole 1991).

CLINICAL TRIALS

Despite major advances in the use of cytotoxic drugs to treat primary bone cancers, only 50–60% of patients with osteosarcoma and Ewing's sarcoma are long-term survivors. There are controversies around which drugs are most effective, which is the best combination and the optimum dose intensity.

Clinical trials are an important part of the research studies to evaluate past and present effectiveness and aim to improve future survival rates.

Patients may be worried about the concept of being randomised into a trial, especially if there is a time discrepancy between the regimens. They need to understand that although it is a trial, all the drugs they will receive are effective in treating their condition. They need support when making the decision to enter a trial, including reassurance about their safety and emphasising that there is no obligation to take part in any trial.

SIDE EFFECTS OF CHEMOTHERAPY

Cytotoxic drugs have a non-specific effect on all rapidly dividing cells. Their side effects arise from their action on normal cells that rapidly divide, especially those in the bone marrow, gastrointestinal tract, hair follicles and reproductive cells (Brown 1987).

Bone marrow suppression will limit the amount and frequency of the dose given as leukocytes, erythrocytes and thrombocytes are affected. The nadir or crisis is when blood cells have fallen to their lowest level, usually 7–10 days after treatment. At this point patients are at risk from infection, anaemia and bleeding. Cell counts must recover before further chemotherapy or surgery, creating the delay between treatment regimes.

Nausea and vomiting cause patients a great deal of distress, together with a loss of appetite, stomatitis, bowel disturbances and an associated weight loss. Antiemetics that control the chemoreceptor trigger in the brain show a good effect that can be enhanced by the addition of a corticosteroid such as dexamethasone. Sedation, relaxation and distraction therapies are also used to help to control the nausea. Oral hygiene is very important to lessen the effects of stomatitis, often caused by a candida infection.

Partial or total alopecia will occur in all patients having chemotherapy for primary bone cancer. It is one of the most obvious and distressing side effects, although the hair will grow back at the end of treatment. Eyebrows, eyelashes and pubic hair may also be lost. The patient's self-image is substantially altered at this time; the use of a wig, bandanas, hats, scarves and caps help to lessen the impact. Scalp-cooling devices, which cause vasoconstriction, are of limited success.

Infertility is a later side effect of chemotherapy; as prepubertal children generally tolerate higher doses of drugs, they may be more at risk (Jurgens

et al 1992). The option of sperm banking should be discussed with men before treatment commences and, where appropriate, boys may need to be assessed for sexual maturity when exploring this option. Many patients have successfully become parents following chemotherapy but they need to understand that this is not advisable immediately following treatment. Unfortunately, there is no provision for the storage of ova prior to chemotherapy due to the time required for this.

Other long-term side effects of chemotherapy include cardiomyopathy, high-frequency hearing loss, peripheral neuropathy, liver damage, impaired renal function and the possibility of a secondary malignancy.

Nursing interventions can help to educate the patient and family about the goals of chemotherapy, possible side effects and how these will be managed. They need emotional support throughout the arduous treatment with patients' self-esteem being helped by allowing them to retain some control within the restrictions of the treatment plan.

SURGICAL PERSPECTIVES

The goal of surgery is to remove the tumour completely with sufficient surgical margins to prevent local recurrence (Grimer 1996). This is either by limb-sparing surgery or amputation. Several factors influence the choice such as the age of the patient, the location of the tumour and the expected functional result postoperatively. Very young children may be considered unsuitable for limb-sparing surgery if the limb will not be able to grow sufficiently in length as they get older. Amputation is the only surgery possible if the tumour encases major nerves and blood vessels, such as the neurovascular bundle behind the knee. Major reconstruction following an extensive resection may offer very limited function, making the alternative of an amputation a practical solution.

Surgery normally takes place after several cycles of chemotherapy. Chemotherapy is beneficial in limb-sparing surgery by reducing the size and soft tissue component of the tumour, facilitating its eradication (Gray 1994). As there is very little time between recovery from bone marrow suppression and surgery, a growth factor called the granulocyte colony-stimulating factor (GCSF) may be required. This may be given preoperatively to stimulate the stem cells into producing white cells at a faster rate, thus preventing surgery being delayed due to neutropenia. A platelet transfusion may be required immediately before surgery if the count is low. Chemotherapy is generally resumed 2–3 weeks postoperatively.

Psychologically, the transition from chemotherapy to surgery is difficult for patients. They have had little time to feel well, having had many hospital admissions and reduced time with their families. Although they are pleased to have their tumour removed, many express concern about how well their pain will be controlled and how the loss of function will cause them to be more dependent on others. Patients also have to face further chemotherapy as soon as their wound is healed. An empathic and flexible nursing approach is essential to fully support these patients.

LIMB-SPARING SURGERY

This surgery has been available for over 15 years, allowing the effectiveness of the procedures to be evaluated (Grimer 1996). Rougraff et al's (1994) retrospective study of the outcome of treatment for non-metastatic osteosarcoma in patients compared a limb-sparing procedure to amputation. It showed that although there was a slight risk of local recurrence in those having the limb-sparing surgery, there was no difference in long-term survival.

The most commonly used replacements for excised tumour bone are allografts and endoprostheses. Allografts have been associated with a higher incidence of complications including infection, non-union and fracture (Roberts et al 1991). Excision of the scapula, fibula and pubic rami are relatively uncomplicated procedures if no other bone is involved. Conversely, tumours in the pelvis require complex surgery and were deemed inoperable until recent years. A hemipelvectomy and replacement is performed either by an autograft, using struts from the patient's fibula, or by an endoprosthesis in cases involving the acetabulum. Complications may include infection, nerve palsy and skin necrosis (Piasecki 1992).

Endoprostheses are custom-made metal implants, commonly used to replace tumours in the femur, tibia and humerus (Figs 14.10–14.12). They may include the associated joints for adequate clearance margins and can be designed to extend to accommodate limb growth in skeletally immature patients. To ensure close limb symmetry, measurement X-rays of the existing limbs are taken and incorporated

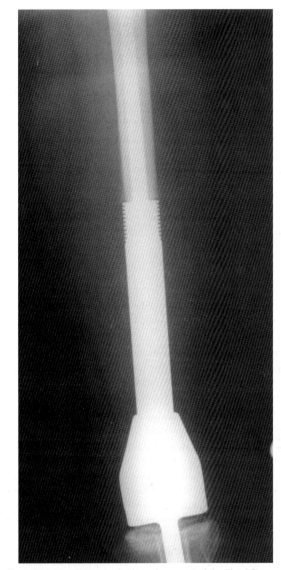

Figure 14.10 Endoprosthetic replacement of the distal femur showing grooved collar.

into the prosthetic design. It is important the patient understands the extent of the proposed surgery, how much bone is to be replaced and the expected functional results, especially if nerves and muscles are to be excised (Ross Bell 1994). It can be very helpful to have replica prostheses for demonstration purposes.

Reconstructive surgery is considered for tumours in the diaphysis when they are away from the growth plate. As the majority of the fibula is expendable, it is used in pelvic surgery and to replace any bone removed from the mid-shaft of the tibia.

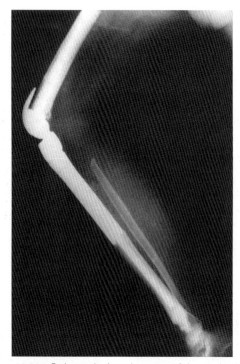

Figure 14.11 Endoprosthetic replacement of the proximal tibia (lateral view) with distal femoral component and excision of head of fibula.

POSTOPERATIVE ISSUES

Pain management

Epidural analgesia is very effective in the management of postoperative pain following pelvic and lower limb surgery, especially after amputation as it appears to delay the awareness of painful phantom limb sensations. Patients need to be aware of the possible temporary side effects, especially urinary retention and altered sensation. Changes in sensation make it difficult to assess the patient's neurovascular status accurately.

The use of patient-controlled analgesia for upper limb surgery gives patients a degree of choice and control over their pain relief (Kaufmann Rauen & Ho 1989). It is the analgesic method favoured by teenagers.

Pain that becomes difficult to control may indicate excessive swelling beneath the pressure bandages, particularly following surgery around the knee. The bandages should be released to relieve the pain and prevent pressure necrosis of the wound over the knee where the vascular status is easily compromised.

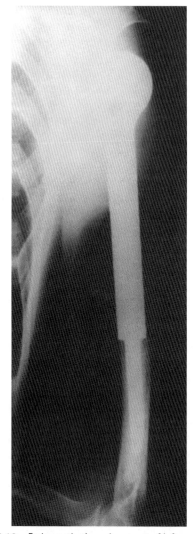

Figure 14.12 Endoprosthetic replacement of left proximal humerus.

Skin integrity

Skin integrity is compromised due to the large surgical incisions used in both limb-sparing surgery and amputation, devascularisation of the skin edges and immobility and impaired sensation (Hockenberry & Lane 1988). Impaired sensation is caused by nerve involvement in the tumour or at the time of surgery and the epidural analgesia.

Nursing interventions include the prevention of pressure ulcers, the early detection of skin necrosis and infection, plus encouraging an adequate nutritional intake to promote healing and maintenance of good skin condition (Ross Bell 1994). A lower limb should be placed so that the heel is free from the bed, the leg straight and the foot in a neutral position.

Wound drainage

Effective wound drainage will reduce the risk of haematoma formation, especially around the knee, which may delay the recovery of function. Research by Willett et al (1988) in routine hip replacement surgery showed there is minimal wound drainage after 24 hours. In comparison, wound drainage following endoprosthetic surgery involving the knee was double that in hip surgery at 24 hours and up to 10 times greater at 48 and 72 hours (unpublished audit, Royal National Orthopaedic Hospital 1994). Hence, the removal of wound drains in limb-sparing surgery is assessed on an individual rather than routine basis.

Mobility and function

Swelling, pain and muscle excision will reduce function initially.

Opiate analgesia is usually required to maximise the benefit from physiotherapy regimes. Patients who have been undergoing chemotherapy can find it difficult to gain motivation to practise their exercises because they are easily fatigued. Goal setting with young people is often an effective way to help them as they are able to monitor their own progress.

Patients who have had an endoprosthetic replacement for a proximal femoral tumour, necessitating the removal of the hip joint, will be at risk from dislocation (Ross Bell 1994). They may require a hip orthosis when actively mobilising until they regain adequate muscle control.

Patients who have had lower leg surgery require temporary splinting to protect the prosthetic knee joint until the quadriceps muscle is powerful enough to control the movement.

Long-term function is affected if a nerve has had to be sacrificed to gain adequate clearance of the tumour; for example, if the peroneal nerve has been compromised during surgery to the proximal tibia or fibula, a drop foot orthosis is required.

Collaborative discharge planning involving the patient, family and the multidisciplinary team will identify any deficits in the tasks of daily living, coordinate essential aids for independent management and ensure that the patient is safely rehabilitated before discharge home. Links should also be made, where appropriate, with the community team and oncology centre if further chemotherapy is planned.

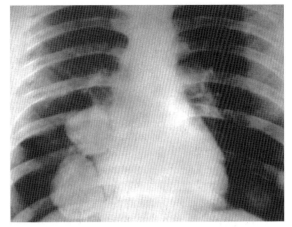

Figure 14.13   Chest metastases in a case of osteosarcoma of the tibia. (From Adams & Hamblen 1990.)

METASTATIC DISEASE FROM PRIMARY BONE TUMOURS

The lungs are the primary focus for metastatic spread from malignant bone tumours (Fig. 14.13). If lung metastases are present at the time of diagnosis, selective chemotherapy treatment protocols are used. If they develop during or after treatment, patients generally have a poor prognosis (Jurgens et al 1992), although there is evidence that a small number of patients may be successfully treated (Lewis 1996).

The management of lung metastases after the completion of treatment is complex and decisions have to be made about whether additional chemotherapy is given before resection or just surgery alone (Lewis 1996). Favourable factors for prognosis following resection are where:

- metastases are present in one lung only
- there are less than six metastatic lesions
- the lesions appear after chemotherapy has stopped
- they are entirely resected (Souhami & Tobias 1986).

In some cases, the metastases follow a fairly indolent course and are contained by several episodes of surgery to the lungs.

Bony metastases can be present at diagnosis or develop later, in which case the prognosis is extremely poor. Surgical resection may be indicated although bone pain from these metastases is usually treated by radiotherapy at the end of treatment.

PSYCHOSOCIAL PERSPECTIVES

A diagnosis of cancer causes a major disruption to the lives of patients and their families. It is especially hard for young people to understand why it should happen to them (Maguire 1996). Intense anxiety and pain result in sleep disturbances, patients may become depressed and marital or parental relationships become strained. Teenagers who have started to become independent will regress and become more dependent on their parents.

At the time of diagnosis patients may be overwhelmed with support but as treatment progresses this can lessen, possibly resulting in feelings of isolation (Ross Bell 1994), especially as the period of treatment ends. Penson (1991) identified the main fears in patients with cancer:

- fear of the unknown and uncertainty about survival
- fear of dependence and a feeling of loss of control and helplessness
- fear of rejection and isolation, together with a feeling of not belonging or contributing
- fear of disfigurement with the inevitable changes in body image.

The orthopaedic nurse is in a special position to help patients discuss these fears and find ways to lessen and overcome them. The fear of dependence and loss of control is helped by encouraging patient participation in the planning and implementation of their care, by honest communication and by supporting informed choice.

Alterations in body image result from both chemotherapy and surgery. The hair and weight loss from chemotherapy are reversible but the surgical interventions will cause permanent changes. Scarring, limb length discrepancy, altered function and an artificial joint will require many adjustments but patients who have lost a limb through amputation will need the most support. Strategies to promote acceptance should be practical and positive, with the focus on cure rather than loss (Ross Bell 1994). The advantages of amputation versus limb sparing should be openly discussed as patients experience conflict between preserving their body image and the consideration of more vigorous surgery (Grimer 1996).

A quality of life study on patients with osteosarcoma did not show a significant difference between those who had an amputation and those who had limb-sparing surgery (Postma et al 1992). Both groups felt equal lowering of their quality of life, mostly from physical complaints for patients who had limb-sparing surgery, while lower self-esteem and social isolation were experienced by patients following amputation.

Peer identification is of particular importance to teenagers and is one of their developmental tasks (Nirenberg 1985). During the cancer experience, this is hampered by changes to their appearance, making them feel self-conscious, having to use walking aids and restrictions on their sporting activities, all of which can threaten their acceptance by peers. School and college education is often disrupted, reintegration can be difficult in terms of the work missed and peer relationships, especially as their hair will not be fully grown for about 6 months and they may not be able to play sports, which can be isolating. Some young people report feeling more mature than their peers after the trauma of diagnosis and treatment, consequently old friendships are less close.

Problems may occur for adults wishing to return to work following treatment. They carry the stigma of a cancer diagnosis and they may be considered an employment risk, even if free from disease (Ross Bell 1994). The treatments require up to 9 months absence or greatly reduced time at work, causing considerable reduction in income. Even when patients are entitled to disability benefits whilst on treatment, these may take many months to process, making the support from a social worker essential.

FUTURE TRENDS

More effective chemotherapy regimens are constantly being researched, with the focus on drug combinations and dose intensity. The availability of haematological growth factors to reduce the severity of neutropenia has been valuable. However, the overall survival rate for malignant primary bone tumours has not significantly altered over the last decade. Current research in cell biology and the molecular genetics of sarcomas, identifying genetic mutations in DNA and the translocation of chromosomes, may significantly influence future management.

Endoprosthetic designs are continuously improved. The introduction of a grooved collar (see Fig. 14.10), coated with hydroxyapatite (HA), to the ends of proximal and distal femoral prostheses has advanced technology towards reducing the incidence of aseptic loosening, the most common cause

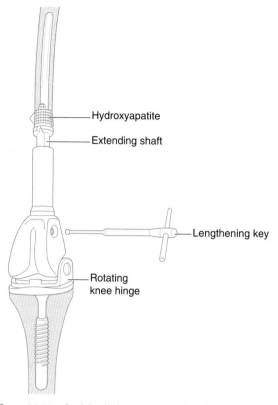

Figure 14.14   A minimally invasive extending distal femoral prosthesis. (Adapted from Gibson & Evans 1999 with permission from Whurr Publishers.)

of endoprosthetic failure in younger patients (Unwin et al 1995). The HA coating encourages bony ingrowth at the end of the prosthesis, it is non-toxic and is biologically compatible with bone.

Limb-sparing surgery in skeletally immature patients involves the use of an extendable prosthesis (Fig. 14.14), which requires lengthening until growth is complete. Although lengthening is a minimally invasive procedure, a general anaesthetic is needed and will be repeated several times. An exciting, pioneering development in the United Kingdom, by Stanmore Implants, is an extendable prosthesis that is lengthened in the outpatients department by applying a magnetic field. Several of these prostheses have successfully been inserted into young people with osteosarcoma, after resection of their tumours, to replace the distal part of the femur and knee. The femoral component of the prosthesis contains a magnetically driven gearbox, which is activated by placing the limb through a hole in a box, called a mobile limb extender. When switched on, this box creates a spinning magnetic field which, in turn, causes a magnet inside the gearbox to spin rapidly, turning a screw which lengthens the prosthesis. The prosthesis lengthens 1 mm in 4 minutes. Typically, the prosthesis is lengthened by 4 mm on each occasion, taking only 16 minutes. There is no discomfort, no loss of function and the limb can be lengthened to keep pace with the patient's normal rate of growth. An X-ray is taken after each session to check the increased length. Current research is now in progress to produce a smaller gearbox to enable this method to be used with prostheses in smaller limb bones such as the tibia and humerus.

Until recently, a hindquarter amputation, one of the most mutilating forms of ablative surgery, was the only surgical choice for the local control of a large pelvic tumour. A pioneering operation called a 'femoral swing' procedure has successfully provided an alternative in a few cases, where control rather than cure is the goal. This major surgery is used on patients requiring a total hemipelvectomy. The proximal femur is excised and replaces the hemipelvis; the head of the femur replaces the pubic ramus, with the cut proximal femur providing the ileum. The greater trochanter is then fashioned to accept a proximal femoral prosthesis, complete with acetabulum. The visible results and functional outcome of the surgery are very acceptable to the patient. The nursing challenges include wound healing, maintenance of optimum position, preserving skin integrity and pain control.

Various reconstructive techniques are being developed to excise tumours in the lower limb while preserving knee function and, if possible, the epiphyseal growth plate. This involves an endoprosthesis with specially designed fixation plates or bone transportation to relocate a free fragment of bone by using an external fixator and distraction to fill the gap left by the removal of a tumour (Hart 1994). Bone transportation is of particular value in tumours of the proximal tibia.

SUMMARY OF BONE TUMOUR CARE

Neoadjuvant chemotherapy, advances in limb-sparing surgery and the management of pulmonary metastases all contribute to the drive forward to improve the survival rates for patients with primary malignant bone tumours. The orthopaedic oncology patient provides a challenge requiring a collaborative approach involving the surgical, oncology, nursing, physiotherapy, occupational therapy, social work, psychological and community healthcare teams.

Nursing interventions involve:

- understanding the different illness pathway of the orthopaedic oncology patient
- giving effective and accurate information
- supporting a strategy for discussion, coping and dealing with the distress of a life-threatening illness
- presenting an empathic, positive approach, promoting independence and autonomy
- encouraging a positive attitude to self-esteem and body-related issues
- promoting a flexible, patient-participative approach to care, incorporating an understanding of the particular needs of the oncology patient, especially in relation to fatigue, immunosuppression and the trauma of the chemotherapy experience.

Before surgery, orthopaedic oncology patients have had to face a sudden cancer diagnosis, the immediate commencement of chemotherapy with its associated debilitating side effects, attending different centres for treatments and a complete disruption to their existing lives. Patients are often admitted for surgery within a very tight schedule between doses of chemotherapy, with little time for recovery in between. Orthopaedic nurses need to understand this pathway, listen to patients' experiences and avoid comparisons to the general orthopaedic patient.

A comprehensive, holistic approach, utilising all the available expertise and support, ensures the patient receives the optimum treatment for primary bone cancer, with a smooth transition between treatments and an outcome of maximum function without compromising long-term survival.

METASTATIC BONE DISEASE

Metastatic bone disease is very different from primary bone tumours in its development, management and nursing care.

Secondary deposits of tumours commonly occur in bone. Approximately 30–70% of all new cancers develop skeletal metastases. Of these, 80% result from carcinomas of the breast, prostate and lung, with those of the kidney and thyroid to a lesser degree (Dupuy & Goldberg 2001).

The commonest sites for bone metastases are the femur, humerus and acetabulum. The lesions are termed osteolytic, osteoblastic or mixed. Osteolytic lesions tend to destroy bone and need to be larger than 1 cm to be visible on a plain X-ray. Bone metastases from breast cancer are usually osteolytic and more likely to cause a pathological fracture. Osteoblastic metastatic lesions are formed from excessive bony growth by the tumour and these are more likely to be secondary deposits from prostate cancer (Tillman 1999).

Metastases can occur in bone in three ways (Piasecki 1987):

1 directly from the primary tumour to an adjacent bone
2 direct venous spread through the vertebral and pelvic veins
3 arterial spread after passing through the right cardiopulmonary circulation.

Tumour cells can pass directly into the vertebral circulation without first travelling to the lungs, which is why prostate cancer often results in spine metastases.

A bone scan will establish the extent of the disease. Plain X-rays, MRI scans and CT scans of the chest are helpful in planning further management. Blood tests used include bone chemistry, as in extensive cases hypercalcaemia may be present. If the primary disease site is known, a biopsy is not always required.

Patients usually present with a dull aching pain, which gradually increases in intensity during the day and can be severe enough at night to disturb sleep. Patients can also find that weight bearing aggravates their pain. The metastatic tumour cells infiltrate and proliferate in the bone marrow; this stimulates bone absorption, which in turn stimulates new bone formation. This process causes pain from the proliferation of bone cells, local tissue necrosis, inflammation and increased prostaglandin synthesis. Pressure on the periosteum or adjacent nerves causes both local and radiating pain (Coward & Wilkie 2000). The sudden onset of severe pain may indicate a pathological fracture, which may be the first sign of metastatic disease.

Metastatic bone disease means that the cancer is advanced or that initial cancer treatment has failed. It leaves the patient frightened, anxious and uncertain whether their cancer can be controlled. These emotions affect their strategy to cope with the pain. Coward & Wilkie (2000) found the pain from metastatic bone disease affected patients' work, leisure activities, family relationships and independence. They complained that the pain was constant, wore them out and reminded them that the cancer was there. Patients were reluctant to take analgesia for a variety of reasons. Some felt that the pain was a warning to protect the area and stop them doing too much when uncomfortable, while others had a fear of addiction to the analgesia or hated the side effects of the drugs. This study also showed that patients have a reluctance to admit to having pain; for some this was to avoid disappointing others who would view this as a sign of their condition getting worse. Another reason patients give for refusing opioid analgesia, not mentioned in the study, is the belief that it will shorten their life. Some parents are also reluctant for their children's pain to be relieved by opioids for the same reason.

TREATMENT OPTIONS

The aim of treatment, which is usually palliative, is to improve quality of life by controlling the disease, relieving pain and preserving mobility. Treatment options include analgesia, chemotherapy, hormone therapy, radiotherapy, radiofrequency ablation, surgery and bisphosphonates. The decisions about patient management will depend on the location and extent of the bony metastases, the degree of morbidity and general health of the patient.

As metastatic bone pain can be intense, a combination of analgesia, including NSAIDs and opiates, is often required. Careful pain assessment is needed, as some patients are reluctant to admit the extent of their pain. In many cases, analgesia alone will not be adequate and side effects may interfere with the patient's quality of life.

A less aggressive regimen of chemotherapy may be appropriate when first-line chemotherapy has failed. This can be given concurrently with radiotherapy as a palliative form of treatment. Hormone treatment can be an effective form of palliation for patients with bone metastases from breast and prostate cancers. Again, an acceptable balance between efficacy, side effects and quality of life is essential, with the patient being fully informed and involved in all palliative treatment decisions.

For some patients, local radiotherapy to symptomatic lesions is very effective as it kills the local tumour and the inflammatory cells causing the pain. This form of radiotherapy is quick, with few side effects, and although studies have shown that a relapse after an initial response is common (Dupuy & Goldberg 2001), most patients benefit from retreatment (Saarto et al 2002). If the metastases are more widespread, radio-isotopes can provide a more effective pain management option. Radiotherapy is used effectively to prevent pathological fractures in the spine and long bones, and for the treatment of spinal cord compression, a serious complication of metastatic bone disease (Saarto et al 2002).

Radiofrequency ablation is a new local treatment for bone metastases aimed at improving patients' quality of life. The tumour cells are killed immediately by the single percutaneous image-guided procedure using thermal energy, giving rapid pain relief. Studies are currently in progress to demonstrate the efficacy of this treatment and, in the future, will compare the results with treatment by local radiotherapy (Dupuy & Goldberg 2001).

The surgical management of metastatic bone disease aims to relieve pain and restore function. Surgery can provide a prophylactic stabilisation of the metastatic bone where there is a risk of a fracture, the fixation of a pathological fracture and the decompression of the spinal cord and/or stabilisation of the spine (Tillman 1999). The surgery should allow the patient to mobilise quickly and the fixation should last the patient's lifetime. If there is a risk of a pathological fracture, for example when 50% of the cortex of a long bone is destroyed, prophylactic internal fixation is required; this may be followed by treatment with radiotherapy. If a pathological fracture has occurred in the diaphysis of the bone, intermedullary nailing with locking screws is usually the treatment of choice. Fractures in the epiphysis, commonly around the hip, are treated with an endoprosthesis, as are metaphyseal lesions. Any major bone defects are filled, where appropriate, with methylmethacrylate cement.

Bisphosphonates, commonly used in the treatment of osteoporosis, have an increasing role in the management of metastatic bone disease. In vitro studies have shown that the nitrogen-containing bisphosphonates, such as pamidronate and zoledronic acid, have an antitumour activity (Coleman 2002). Although bisphosphonate therapy is palliative for patients with bone metastases, there is evidence to suggest that it can delay or prevent the bone lesions, cause existing lesions to regress and, in certain cases, help to improve survival (Coleman 2002).

Bisphosphonates interfere with the blood supply and growth factors necessary for the secondary tumour to continue invading the bone, establishing a less favourable environment in which the cells can multiply. They can slow down the process of bone resorption from osteoclast activity, thereby reducing or preventing the osteopenia from bone metastases. This action appears to inhibit the growth of the tumour cells in the bone (Coleman 2002). There is also some evidence to show that bisphosphonates can provide some pain relief for patients with bone metastases but should not be used as first-line therapy for this purpose (Wong & Wiffen 2003).

Metastatic bone disease causes debilitating pain, reduced mobility, loss of independence and a further reduced quality of life in patients whose life expectancy is already severely compromised. It is important, therefore, to have a coordinated team approach to their treatment and management involving a dedicated orthopaedic surgeon, oncologist, radiologist, radiotherapist and metabolic consultant, to ensure an individualised plan of treatment for the patient; this is most likely to be achieved at specialist centres. Included in this plan must be the support of the palliative care team, not only to monitor symptom control but to provide essential psychosocial support for the patient and their family as they struggle to cope with the practical and emotional difficulties of the inevitability of end-stage disease.

References

Adams JC, Hamblen DL 1990 Outline of orthopaedics, 11th edn. Churchill Livingstone, Edinburgh

Apley A, Soloman L 1993 Apley's system of orthopaedics and fractures, 7th edn. Butterworth Heineman, Oxford

Apley A, Soloman L 1994 Concise system of orthopaedics and fractures, 2nd edn. Butterworth Heinemann, Oxford

Brown J 1987 Chemotherapy. In: Groenwald S (ed) Cancer nursing: principles and practice. James and Bartlett, Boston

Cannon S, Dyson P 1987 Relationship of the site of open biopsy of malignant tumours to local recurrence following resection and prosthetic replacement. Journal of Bone and Joint Surgery 69B: 492

Capanna R, Bertoni F, Bettelli G et al 1988 Dedifferentiated chondrosarcoma. Journal of Bone and Joint Surgery 70A(1): 60–69

Coleman R 2002 Future directions in the treatment and prevention of bone metastases. American Journal of Clinical Oncology 25(6) (suppl 1): S32–38

Coward D, Wilkie D 2000 Metastatic bone pain: meanings associated with self-report and self-management decision making. Cancer Nursing 23(2): 101–108

Duckworth T 1995 Neoplastic conditions – primary neoplasms. In: Lecture notes on orthopaedics and fractures, 3rd edn. Blackwell Science, Oxford

Dupuy D, Goldberg N 2001 Image-guided radiofrequency tumour ablation: challenges and opportunities – part II. Journal of Vascular and Interventional Radiology 12(10): 1135–1148

Duthie R, Bentley G 1983 Tumours of the musculoskeletal system. In: Mercer's orthopaedic surgery, 8th edn. Edward Arnold, London

Enneking W, Conrad E 1988 Common bone tumours. Clinical Symposia 41(3): 2–32

Gibson F, Evans M 1999 Paediatric oncology – acute nursing care. Whurr, London

Gray D 1994 Bone tumours. In: Benson M, Fixen J, MacNicol M (eds) Children's orthopaedics and fractures. Churchill Livingstone, Edinburgh

Grimer R 1996 Costs and benefits of limb salvage surgery for osteosarcoma. In: Selby P, Bailey C (eds) Cancer and the adolescent. BMJ Books, London

Grimer R, Sneath R 1990 Editorial. Journal of Bone and Joint Surgery 72B(5): 754–756

Hart K 1994 Using the Ilizarov external fixator in bone transport. Orthopaedic Nursing 13(1): 35–40

Hockenberry M, Lane B 1988 Limb salvage procedures in children with osteosarcoma. Cancer Nursing 11(1): 2–8

Jurgens H, Winkler K, Gobel U 1992 Bone tumours. In: Plowman P, Pinkerton C (eds) Paediatric oncology: clinical practice and controversies. Chapman and Hall Medical, London

Kaufmann Rauen K, Ho M 1989 Children's use of patient controlled analgesia after spinal surgery. Paediatric Nursing 15(6): 589–637

Lewis I 1996 Medical management of bone tumours. In: Selby P, Bailey C (eds) Cancer and the adolescent. BMJ Books, London

Linder N, Ozaki T, Roedl R et al 2001 Percutaneous radiofrequency ablation in osteoid osteoma. Journal of Bone and Joint Surgery 83B(3): 391–396

Maguire P 1996 Psychological and psychiatric morbidity. In: Selby P, Bailey C (eds) Cancer and the adolescent. BMJ Books, London

Mertens W, Bramwell V 1994 Osteosarcoma and other tumours of bone. Current Opinion in Oncology 6(4): 384–390

Nirenberg A 1985 The adolescent with osteogenic sarcoma. Orthopaedic Nursing 4(50): 11–15

O'Sullivan M, Saxton V 1997 Bone and soft tissue tumours. In: Broughton N (ed) A textbook of paediatric orthopaedics from Royal Children's Hospital, Melbourne. WB Saunders, London

Penson J 1991 Psychological needs of people with cancer. Senior Nurse 11(3): 37–41

Piasecki P 1987 Bone malignancies. In: Groenwald S (ed) Cancer nursing: principles and practice. Jones and Bartlett, Boston

Piasecki P 1992 Update in orthopaedic oncology. Orthopaedic Nursing 11(6): 36–43

Porter D, Holden S, Steel C et al 1992 A significant proportion of patients with osteosarcoma may belong to Li-Fraumeni cancer families. Journal of Bone and Joint Surgery 74B(6): 883–886

Postma A, Kingma A, De Ruiter J et al 1992 Quality of life in bone tumour patients comparing limb salvage and amputation of the lower extremity. Journal of Surgical Oncology 51: 47–51

Pringle J 1987 Pathology of bone tumours. In: Souhami R (ed) Clinical oncology. Baillière Tindall, London

Roberts P, Chan D, Grimer R et al 1991 Prosthetic replacement of the distal femur for primary bone tumours. Journal of Bone and Joint Surgery 73B(5): 762–769

Rosenthal D, Hornicek F, Wolfe M et al 1998 Percutaneous radiofrequency coagulation of osteoid osteoma compared with operative treatment. Journal of Bone and Joint Surgery 76A(5): 649–656

Ross Bell N 1994 Neoplasms of the musculoskeletal system. In: Maher A, Salmond S, Pellino T (eds) Orthopaedic nursing. WB Saunders, Philadelphia

Rougraff B, Simon M, Kneisl J et al 1994 Limb salvage compared with amputation for osteosarcoma of the distal end of femur. Journal of Bone and Joint Surgery 76A(5): 649–656

Saarto T, Janes R, Tenhunen M et al 2002 Palliative radiotherapy in the treatment of skeletal metastases. European Journal of Pain 6(5): 323–330

Sailsbury J, Byers P 1994 Osteoblastic and cartilaginous neoplasms. In: Sailsbury J, Woods C, Byers P (eds) Diseases of bones and joints. Chapman and Hall Medical, London

Schwartz C, Constine L, Putman T et al 1993 Paediatric solid tumours. In: Rubin P (ed) Clinical oncology: a multidisciplinary approach for physician and students, 7th edn. WB Saunders, Philadelphia

Souhami R, Tobias J 1986 Bone and soft tissue sarcoma. In: Cancer and its management. Blackwell, Oxford

Stoker D, Cobb J, Pringle J 1991 Needle biopsy of musculoskeletal lesions. Journal of Bone and Joint Surgery 73B(3): 498–500

Tillman R 1999 The role of the orthopaedic surgeon in metastatic disease of the appendicular skeleton. Journal of Bone and Joint Surgery 81B: 1–2

Unwin P, Walker P, Blunn G 1995 A radiographic and retrieval study, comparing porous collared and hydroxyapatite coated segmental femoral replacements. Transactions of Orthopaedics 20: 747

Willett K, Simmons C, Bentley G 1988 The effect of suction drains after total hip replacement. Journal of Bone and Joint Surgery 70B(4): 607–710

Williams P, Cole W 1991 Bone tumours. In: Orthopaedic management in childhood, 2nd edn. Chapman and Hall Medical, London

Wong R, Wiffen P 2003 Bisphosphonates for the relief of pain secondary to bone metastases (Cochrane Review). The Cochrane Library Issue 1. Update Software, Oxford: 1–2

Chapter 15

Care of patients with rheumatoid arthritis

Naomi Flasher, Sharon Church

INTRODUCTION

Rheumatoid arthritis is the most commonly referred to rheumatic disease but the physiological changes, affects on the individual and management of the disease are less well known to practitioners outside rheumatology teams.

This chapter describes the current understanding of this complex, variable disease and its impact on all aspects of the individual's life. The effect of the disease process necessitates a multidisciplinary team approach to patient management and support at all stages of the disease process. The principles and aims of care are highlighted throughout the text, along with the interventions and outcomes.

HISTORICAL PERSPECTIVE

Arthritis and gout have been referred to in the writings of physicians since the first century AD. Throughout the centuries, artists have visually recorded what appear to be people with inflammatory arthritides, indicating the condition was known to a variety of cultures.

Paleopathology, the study of human disease using mummified or skeletal remains, has enabled diseases to be placed in a chronological order of occurrence along a timeline. The subtle differences between different rheumatic diseases make their individual identification on such a timeline difficult. This is not helped by documentary evidence, which makes historical diagnoses inaccurate when compared to current understanding of rheumatological disease and medical knowledge.

In the 17th century, diseases began to be classified according to accurate observation. These have evolved into the current diagnostic criteria for rheumatoid arthritis (RA), osteoarthritis, ankylosing spondylitis and systemic lupus erythematosus.

The major milestones in the pathway of RA include the science and progress in radiological imaging, developments in haematology, biochemistry and serological testing, plus the advent of drugs such as aspirin, steroids and more recently disease-modifying antirheumatic drugs (DMARDs).

The current management of care is generally based in specialist rheumatology units, with many national and international centres of excellence delivering patient care and being involved in research into RA and other rheumatological diseases. The British Society of Rheumatology currently recommends one consultant rheumatologist per 80 000 of the population.

Patients with RA are found in almost every healthcare setting, including community clinics, nursing and residential homes, nurse-led wards and acute hospital wards of every specialty. Orthopaedic wards are generally involved in the care of patients seeking preventive or corrective surgery or procedures requiring practitioners from both specialisms to work together for the benefit of effective and evidence-based patient care.

The expansion of rheumatology nursing roles has resulted from developments in the medical specialism and the reduction in the number of hospital beds for rheumatology patients. The latter is due to changes in patient care from hospital to community-based care, from prolonged bedrest or restorative cures such as spa treatments to more preventive and proactive therapies. The expansion of specialist nursing roles in rheumatology has led to developments in nursing practice based on the philosophy of rheumatology nursing (RCN 2001), involving the need to:

- enter into a therapeutic relationship with the patient to address physical, psychological, social and sexual needs within a multidisciplinary context
- enable the patient to achieve a state of adaptation
- empower, support and guide the patient and their family through care episodes
- provide effective research-based practice.

EPIDEMIOLOGY

As the underlying cause of rheumatoid arthritis remains unknown, a clear definition of the disease is difficult. However, it can be described as a bilateral, symmetrical, chronic inflammatory polyarthritis, predominantly affecting the synovium, with systemic involvement.

Rheumatoid arthritis is a relatively common disease with a worldwide distribution; most recent studies into its prevalence have estimated an overall rate of about 1%. This equates to about 1.5 million people in the UK (Hickling & Golding 1984). It is more common in women than men, with a ratio of 3:1 (Kragg 1989). There is a prevalence in those aged 20–70 years, with the peak age of onset being 45–65 years. The prevalence of RA increases with age in both women and men, although there is evidence to suggest it is more common in men than women of 75 years and over (Symmons et al 1994).

The approximate annual incidence rate in the UK has varied considerably between different studies since the 1950s, reflecting the difficulty in data collection. In view of this the Norfolk Arthritis Register was established to rigorously assess the incidence of rheumatic disease. Based on notification by general practitioners, the annual rate of new diagnoses in the UK in 1990 was 36 per 100 000 for women and 14 per 100 000 for men (Symmons et al 1994).

AETIOLOGY

The explicit cause of RA remains unknown, despite intensive worldwide research that continues in the attempt to clarify the underlying cause of the disease. What is clear is that the aetiology is multifactorial. The identification of the causes is important for improving the efficacy of treatments and for identifying the triggering mechanisms and factors that appear to affect the prognosis and disease presentation. Many hypotheses are being tested but the dominant theory relates to the immune system.

IMMUNOLOGY

The evidence for an immune system dysfunction in RA, although complex, is persuasive (Isenberg & Morrow 1995, William 1998). The two main features are:

1 rheumatoid factor in the synovial fluid or blood serum, indicating a seropositive patient
2 increased activity of the immune system cells within the synovial membrane.

It is the disruption of this autoimmune response which currently forms the basis of drug therapies used to suppress the disease activity.

Although no microbial agents have been identified as a direct causative factor in RA, it is considered that infectious agents trigger the disease in a genetically susceptible person. A presenting antigen, bacterial or viral, initiates the autoimmune response and the production of rheumatoid factor, but a repeat antigen event would not appear to be required for disease progression (Denman 1995).

GENETIC

Genetic factors play a key role in the development and presentation of RA. Studies have shown that those with a family history are three times more likely to develop the disease than those without. The identification of the human leukocyte antigens (HLA) DW4 and DR4 has provided evidence into the genetic contribution as people testing positive to these HLA tissue types are genetically predisposed to RA with an increased probability of developing the disease.

HORMONAL

Hormonal status may contribute to the presentation of RA. It is well recognised that pregnancy reduces rheumatoid disease activity (Nicholas & Panayi 1988) and that both the oral contraceptive pill (Spector et al 1991) and hormone replacement therapy (Carette et al 1989) are protective factors in genetically predisposed women.

RA is more prevalent in women after the menarche and before the menopause, making it paradoxical that female hormones appear to play a key role in reducing the severity of the symptoms and disease progression.

DIET

Although there is a lack of good evidence implicating food types as a cause of RA, Darlington et al (1990) support the conclusion that diet may temporarily exacerbate symptoms in a minority of patients.

The volume of anecdotal evidence relating to diet and arthritis has led to numerous publications. There are a large number of patients who will try most non-toxic treatments, including diets, in the hope of a remission or cure. These patients are a particularly vulnerable group, open to a barrage of confusing and conflicting information and advice. Patients should be advised to discuss any supplements to their diets and if using an exclusion diet, careful monitoring is needed to ensure vital nutrients are not lost.

Generally a healthy, balanced diet, low in fats and sugars, is advised. If a patient is overweight, losing weight will significantly reduce the pressure on the lower limb joints, thereby reducing pain.

Patients who frequently associate diet with their symptoms may find the booklet *Diet and arthritis* (Arthritis Research Campaign 1998) a useful starting point.

OTHER FACTORS

As yet no direct link between the environment or lifestyle and RA has been identified. However, these, along with psychological, emotional and educational factors, may play a part in the way the disease presents and progresses.

Dieppe et al (1985) describe how emotional stress and anxiety can often precipitate deterioration of the disease progression; this unpredictability often impacts on the individual, family and their socio-economic status (Williams 1986).

A significant number of people link a deterioration with particular weather conditions. Small-scale studies have shown joint stiffness correlates with humidity (Rasker et al 1986) and that pain scores are higher in warm, wet weather (Patberg et al 1985). However, there is insufficient evidence to suggest that climate is implicated in the course or prognosis of the disease.

PATHOLOGY

Pathological changes in rheumatoid arthritis are primarily concerned with synovial tissues. Figure 15.1 illustrates a typical synovial joint. The synovium is usually two cell layers of synoviocytes overlying connective tissue. The primary function of this membrane is the secretion of viscous, lubricating synovial fluid that surrounds the joint. This synovium layer is also present in bursae and tendon sheaths.

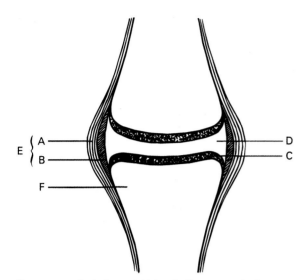

Figure 15.1 Typical synovial joint. A: fibrous capsule. B: synovial membrane. C: articular hyaline cartilage. D: joint cavity filled with synovial fluid. E: joint capsule. F: articulating bone. (From Gunn 1992.)

The pathological changes in RA progress through three phases (Fig. 15.2).

● **Phase 1 Cellular changes**. The synovial membrane becomes highly vascular, along with proliferation of synoviocytes and fibroblasts. Thickening of the synovial membrane and oedema occur as lymphocytes and plasma cells aggregate to form follicles. The follicles synthesise rheumatoid factor and inflammatory prostaglandins and these then react with immunoglobulins, leading to the formation of immune complexes within the joint.

● **Phase 2 Inflammatory response**. As the disease progresses into the second phase, the immune complex activates complement. Complement is a protein that aids the body's defences against invading antigens by attracting neutrophils into the synovial fluid. The immune complexes are phagocytosed by the neutrophils; during this process, the chemical mediators of the inflammatory process are released.

● **Phase 3 Destructive phase**. As the inflammatory response perpetuates, the disease enters the destructive phase. The high concentration of lysosomal enzymes in the synovial fluid start the irreversible damage to the hyaline cartilage. Fibrin accumulation on the synovial surface forms a vascular granulative tissue known as the pannus. The pannus eventually invades the articular surface adjacent to the synovium, secreting prostaglandins and proteases that erode the already damaged cartilage at the margins. Eventually large areas of the cartilage are destroyed and erosion of the bone commences.

Chronic synovitis and joint effusions cause distension of the joint capsule, leading to weak and lax ligaments. This, in combination with the damage to the joint and weakening of the supporting muscles, leads to joint instability. This instability results in the joint deformities typical of rheumatoid arthritis.

DIAGNOSIS

A diagnosis of RA can be made when a patient presents with a clinical picture within the diagnostic criteria of the American Rheumatism Association (Arnett et al 1988) (Table 15.1). The onset of RA can be:

● insidious, dated by the patient to the nearest month
● subacute, dated by the patient to the nearest week
● acute, dated by the patient to the specific day or even hour
● palindromic, whereby acute irregular episodes of joint pain and swelling occur for about 2 or 3 days.

Studies by Jacoby et al (1973) and Lawrence (1965) found that an insidious onset is the most common, occurring in approximately 80% of cases. An insidious onset with a symmetrical presentation is associated with a more progressive disease with severe outcomes, whilst a sudden onset with an asymmetrical presentation appears to have a more favourable course of disease progression and outcomes.

The most common sites of onset involvement are shown in Figure 15.3. Symmetrical polyarthritis, distributed peripherally, is predominant, occurring in 75% of cases. Asymmetrical or monoarticular onset, usually in the knees or wrists (Edmonds & Hughes 1985), occurs in the other 25% of cases. Patients will complain of a general feeling of ill health and malaise, which may have preceded the joint symptoms by several months. Pain, in and around the joints, with marked early morning stiffness and weakness impairing function are of major concern. The involvement of muscles, tendons, tendon sheaths and bursae may or may not be present. The majority of patients will have a variable disease course over many years with episodes of exacerbation and remission.

CLINICAL FEATURES

The symptoms and signs of articular inflammation, often accompanied by extraarticular and

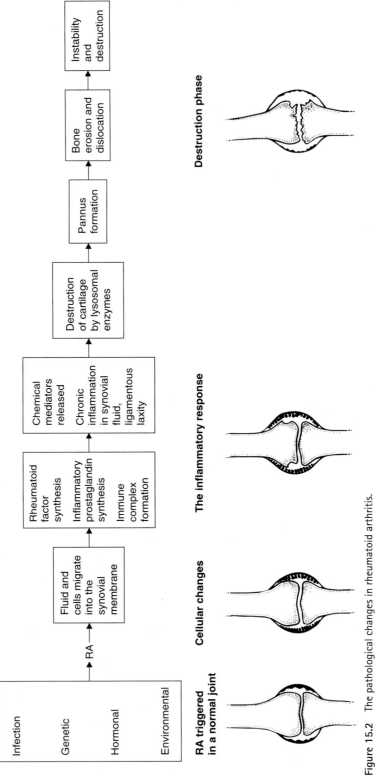

Figure 15.2   The pathological changes in rheumatoid arthritis.

Table 15.1   The revised American College of Rheumatology criteria for classification of rheumatoid arthritis (Arnett et al 1988). To satisfy the diagnosis of rheumatoid arthritis, at least four of the seven following criteria must be present: the first four must all be present for a minimum duration of 6 weeks

Criterion	Definition
1 Morning stiffness	Morning stiffness within and around the joint for a duration of greater than 6 weeks
2 Arthritis of three or more joint areas	At least three painful joints with simultaneous soft tissue swelling or effusion; bony overgrowth alone is not of criterion significance
3 Arthritis of the hand joint area	At least one hand joint swollen (as criterion 2): wrist, MCP or PIP for a duration greater than 6 weeks
4 Symmetrical arthritis	Simultaneous involvement of the same joint areas (as defined in criterion 2) on both sides of the body Bilateral involvement of the PIP, MCP or MTP joints without absolute symmetry is acceptable
5 Rheumatoid nodules	Subcutaneous nodules over bony prominences, extensor surfaces or in juxtaarticular regions
6 Serum rheumatoid factor	Demonstration of abnormal amounts of serum rheumatoid factor, by any method, that has been positive in less than 5% of normal control subjects
7 Radiographic changes	Typical radiographic rheumatoid changes as seen on postero-anterior hand and wrist films, which must include erosions and definite periarticular bony decalcification

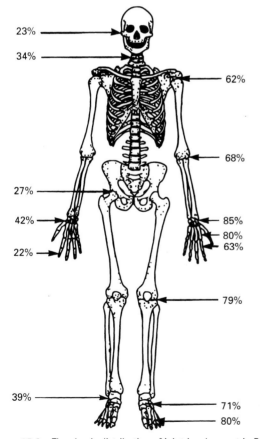

Figure 15.3   The classic distribution of joint involvement in RA. (From Dieppe et al 1985.)

constitutional factors, typify the onset of RA. The additional emotional effects of RA vary between patients and over time.

ARTICULAR FEATURES

Joint stiffness is generalised, being most severe following periods of inactivity. Early morning stiffness is common, ranging from 30 minutes to several hours in duration. The stiffness typically affects the small joints of the hands, feet and neck, with larger joints being involved as the disease progresses.

Patients experience pain deep within the joints at rest and during movement. The pain results from the inflammatory process and increased pressure within the joint pressing on the nerve endings. Damage to the joint mechanics causes pain predominantly during movement or weight bearing later in the disease process.

Tenderness on or around the joint is commonly experienced following a knock or bump that under normal circumstances would go unnoticed.

Warm joints are the result of the inflammatory process and increased vascularity of the synovium. It is important to note that red, hot joints are not a normal feature of RA; if this occurs, the possibility of an infection in or around the joint must be investigated.

Swelling is common at the wrists and knees but is most noticeable at the metacarpophalangeal (MCP)

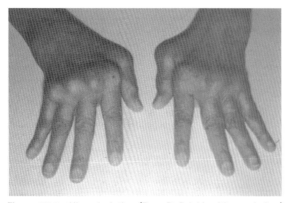

Figure 15.4   Ulnar deviation. (From Dr R Jubb with permission.)

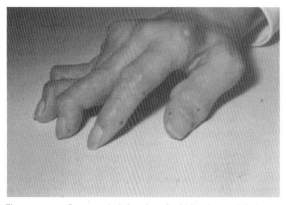

Figure 15.5   Swan neck deformity of middle, ring and little fingers. (From Dr R Jubb with permission.)

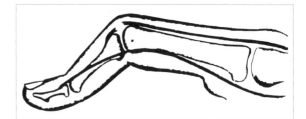

Figure 15.6   Boutonnière deformity. (From Kane 1981.)

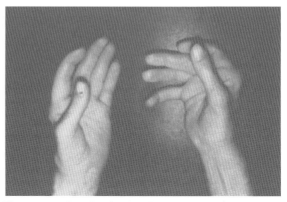

Figure 15.7   Early Z deformity of the left thumb. (From Dr R Jubb with permission.)

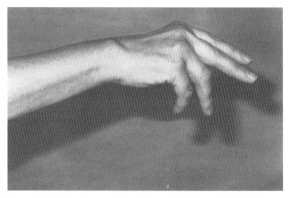

Figure 15.8   Rupture of the extensor tendons of the fourth and fifth fingers. (From Dr R Jubb with permission.)

and proximal interphalangeal (PIP) joints. Swelling is associated with synovial thickening as well as an effusion.

In the early disease phase, functional impairment predominantly presents as a reduced range of movement from pain, swelling and stiffness, along with a noticeable loss of power and grip strength in the hands. The functional impairment in later disease tends to correlate with the extent of ligament laxity and joint damage. Deformities of the hand typically seen in RA include ulnar deviation of the digits at the MCP joints, often accompanied by radial deviation at the wrists, swan neck and Boutonnière deformities of the fingers and Z-deformity of the thumb (Figs 15.4–15.7).

Although in the early phases these deformities can be passively corrected, in later disease the loss of hand function is more extensive, for example,

rupture of the extensor tendons (Fig. 15.8), preventing the patient from making a fist. Carpal tunnel syndrome, where there is compression of the medial nerve as it passes through the wrist, causing pain and numbness in the index and middle fingers and weakness of the thumb, can occur in up to 50% of patients in the cellular and inflammatory phases due to synovitis.

Table 15.2   Periarticular features in rheumatoid arthritis

Feature	Clinical manifestation
Nodules	Nodules, occurring in up to 30% of cases, are associated with seropositivity and severe disease. They commonly occur subcutaneously over points of pressure such as the olecranon (Fig. 15.9), finger joints, sacrum and occiput, as well as along tendons, especially the Achilles and flexors of the hand. May also occur in internal organs, for example the heart and lungs. Necrosing nodules can be a site for infection. Methotrexate therapy may exacerbate nodule formation and growth
Tenosynovitis	This is inflammation of the synovial tendon sheath, commonly affecting the extensor and flexor tendons of the hand and wrist, causing local pain, tenderness, swelling, deformity and functional impairment. Rupture is common at the extensor tendons around the ulnar styloids. Trigger finger (Fig. 15.10) is common, caused by tendon sheath thickening due to a nodule rather than inflammation
Bursitis	Bursae protect areas susceptible to friction. They have synovial membranes which become inflamed in active disease, causing swelling, tenderness and pain aggravated by movement. Sites commonly affected include the olecranon, subacromial, trochanteric, iliopsoas, gastrocnemius, sub-Achilles and calcaneus. Chronically active bursitis may be affected by nodules, particularly at the elbows
Synovial cysts	Cysts are associated with the knee. The Baker's popliteal cyst (Fig. 15.11) presents with posterior knee pain and 'tightness' due to swelling caused by overflow accumulation of synovial fluid from the joint. The cyst extends from the gastrocnemius bursa down into the calf. Rupture causes fluid to leak into the calf muscles, producing symptoms closely resembling deep vein thrombosis: severe pain, swelling, tenderness and positive Homan's sign

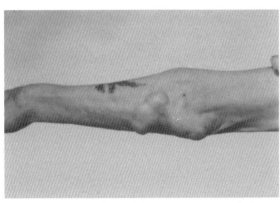

Figure 15.9   Rheumatoid nodules at the elbow joint. (From Dr R Jubb with permission.)

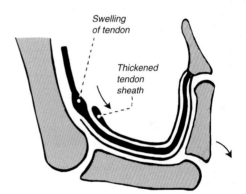

Figure 15.10   Trigger finger deformity. (From Adams & Hamblen 1990.)

EXTRAARTICULAR FEATURES

Rheumatoid arthritis does not limit itself to synovial joint involvement. Periarticular features are common (Table 15.2) and often spontaneously improve in parallel to improvements in disease activity. Local soft tissue infiltration of a steroid can be required if the pain and functional impairment persist from, for example, tenosynovitis and bursitis.

Systemic features (Table 15.3) are associated with seropositive patients, their presence indicating a more aggressive disease and less favourable prognosis. Ensuring patients are well informed about possible periarticular problems leads to the prompt reporting of these symptoms, enabling earlier investigation and intervention. The information needs to be given in context and with continued appropriate support to ensure it has a positive impact on patients' ability to cope and manage their disease.

Muscle atrophy and weakness are very common, noticeably affecting the fingers, but can be generalised. The cause is reflex inhibition of the muscles controlling the inflamed joint, disuse and occasionally

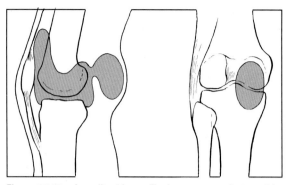

Figure 15.11   A popliteal bursa. The burse communicates with the synovial cavity of the knee. (From Dandy & Edwards 2003.)

steroid therapy. Whilst myalgia is fairly common, myositis is rare.

Oedema of the ankles and feet is usually predominant in the early disease phases.

Anaemia is common and often parallels disease activity. The haemoglobin is usually around 10 g/dl, the normal range being 13.5–18 g/dl for men and 11.5–16.5 g/dl for women. The anaemia is usually normocytic and normochromic with evidence of good iron stores. An iron deficiency anaemia is more common in later disease due to gastrointestinal bleeding.

Weight loss and anorexia occur during the active phases of the disease as a response to the

Table 15.3   Systemic features of rheumatoid arthritis

System	Clinical manifestation
Non-organ specific	Palmar erythema is common; do not confuse with that seen in liver disease. Lymphadenopathy occurs in about 30% of patients and is associated with active disease, the glands being mobile and non-tender. Felty's syndrome occurs in about 1% of patients, associated with marked neutropenia and leukopenia, increasing the risk of serious infection
Cardiac	Pericarditis is common but rarely of clinical importance. Constrictive pericarditis is rare. Valvular incompetence may result from myocardial or endocardial nodules. Coronary arteritis is rare
Hepatic	Elevated liver enzymes may parallel disease activity or be iatrogenic from NSAID or DMARD therapy. Liver abnormalities are common with Felty's or Sjögren's syndrome
Muscular	Muscle atrophy from chronic inflammation causing weakness is common. Inflammatory myopathy (muscle wasting from protein catabolism) is rare
Neurological	Peripheral entrapment neuropathies occur due to compression of local synovitis. The median nerve (wrist), radial and ulnar nerve (elbow) and posterior tibial nerve (ankle) are the most common sites involved. Atlantoaxial subluxation may lead to cervical myopathy
Ocular	Keratoconjunctivitis sicca occurs in up to 35% of patients, severity of symptoms often paralleling the severity of the RA disease. Tear production is quickly and easily measured with minimal discomfort by the Schirmer tear test. Episcleritis, characterised by painful, red eyes, is more common than scleritis. Scleritis is associated with long-standing RA and vasculitis; if left untreated leads to permanent blindness. Rarely uveitis and nodule formation occur. Steroid therapy may cause cataracts and glaucoma
Pulmonary	Pleurisy and pleural effusion occur in about 10% of patients, more commonly in men. Pulmonary nodules, located peripherally, are usually found in seropositive patients with nodules elsewhere. Caplan's syndrome is characterised by multiple pulmonary nodules. Fibrosing alveolitis and obliterative bronchiolitis are less common complications. However, pulmonary infiltration can occur with methotrexate and gold therapy
Renal	Renal involvement is rare but nephropathy and vasculitis have been reported. Renal abnormalities are more common as iatrogenic effects
Vasculitis	Raynaud's phenomenon occurs in about 10% of patients. Small vessel vasculitis usually affects the skin, causing splinter haemorrhage, nailfold infarcts, digital gangrene, leg ulceration and distal sensory neuropathy. The coronary, mesenteric and cerebral arteries may be involved. Systemic vasculitis is rare, associated with long-standing, severe disease. Vasculitis is associated with a poorer prognosis

inflammatory process. The cytokines interleukin 1 and tumour necrosis factor have direct catabolic effects.

A pyrexia is unusual. If present, it is associated with an active disease phase but the presence of an infection or neoplasm must be ruled out.

CONSTITUTIONAL FEATURES

Malaise and fatigue tend to be associated with active disease phases. The cause of fatigue is poorly understood but includes psychological and physical factors, for example poor motivation, lack of central drive, dysfunction in muscle physiology and anaemia. Fatigue can be acute in nature, especially at the start of the disease, but can become a chronic feature not relieved by sleep or rest (White 1998).

Psychological effects are very common in RA (Ryan 1998). They may manifest as irritability, anger, frustration, depression or helplessness which have far-reaching effects on the patient, their lifestyle and relationships.

EMOTIONAL EFFECTS

The impact of the diagnosis of rheumatoid arthritis, although unique to each individual, encompasses common elements affecting patients' physical, emotional, and socio-economic well-being. The way in which the patient is cared for following diagnosis will have a direct effect upon the way in which they come to terms with and manage the disease process. The nurse's role in providing this essential support and guidance for the patient and their family cannot be overemphasised.

The newly diagnosed person with acute-onset RA will find themselves at the centre of a barrage of sudden changes influencing their lifestyle. Often there is a sense of panic that nothing will ever be the same again, with only deformity and a wheelchair to look forward too. Ignorance about RA is a national problem and fear of the unknown is one of the first challenges the newly diagnosed patient and their family will face together, in parallel to the grieving process for their loss of health. Provision of accurate information and education about RA, its effects and available treatments is an essential therapeutic ingredient provided by the nurse.

The changes and challenges faced by newly diagnosed patients are numerous and complex. Pain, severe tiredness and stiffness have a direct impact upon their physical functioning and have far-reaching, simultaneous effects on their emotional status, self-esteem, the family and social interactions. The physical limitations caused by painful, swollen and stiff joints may lead to an inability to continue working and sudden role changes within the family unit. The impact of these changes will depend upon the level of support and the involvement of the family from the onset (Ryan 1998).

A sense of control may be lost in the early days from a lack of knowledge, understanding and management strategies; this also ties in with the loss of choice and expression of self. Altered ability in manual dexterity results in not being able to wear the clothes of choice because of difficulty in dressing, not being able to apply make-up, shave and wear jewellery because of swollen joints or to enjoy a meal out with friends.

The loss of perceived femininity or masculinity and ability to express sexuality can lead to lower self-esteem, self-consciousness and a sense that the patient is now different to what is accepted as 'normal'. It is common for sexual relationships to become strained and poor communication may lead to misunderstanding, the most common fear for partners being that touch will cause pain for the person with RA. This in turn may discourage closeness, support, communication and understanding.

The nature of sexuality is very complex. It is important that patients are aware early in their care that they can discuss with the nurse, in a discreet, confidential and sensitive manner, issues surrounding sexuality and sexual functioning. It is also important that nurses recognise that this area of counselling is highly specialised, requiring recognition of the nurse's own limitations and the level of resources available to support patients successfully (Prady et al 1998).

Understandably, lowness in mood and depression are common in RA (Creed et al 1990). These are disabling as energy levels fall and motivation dwindles. In conjunction with the physical symptoms and limitations, low self-esteem and loss of confidence can lead to a perpetually downward spiralling effect.

The interventions and support of the multidisciplinary care team are essential for favourable physical, emotional and socio-economic patient outcomes.

THE RHEUMATOLOGY CARE TEAM

Mutual cooperation and shared responsibility across the rheumatology care team (Fig. 15.12) help the

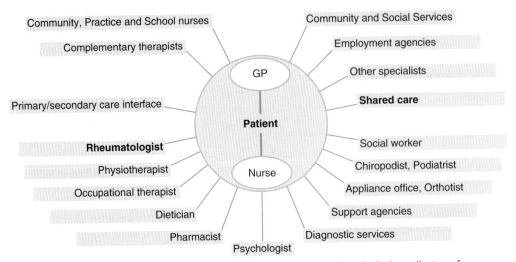

Figure 15.12   The rheumatology care team with the GP and rheumatology nurse as the principal coordinators of care.

patient to achieve their aims and positive health outcomes. Open and regular communication assists in providing continuity of care for the patient, as well as education for both the patient and across the professional groups involved in the care team.

The key aims of patient management and care are to:

- relieve symptoms where possible
- maintain or improve functional capability
- maintain psychosocial equilibrium
- minimise or correct deformity
- detect any side effects of treatment, systemic manifestations or complications of the disease early
- reduce the level of activity of the disease.

To achieve these aims and enable the patient to achieve their full potential, a collaborative care team approach is required.

GENERAL PRACTITIONER

The general practitioner (GP) is the first member of the team the patient goes to with their initial symptoms. As the disease progresses or becomes more complex, the GP will refer the patient on for a rheumatologist opinion. An early referral to the specialist rheumatology team is essential to ensure appropriate management strategies are used early in the patient's care, improving their initial care outcomes.

Shared care between the secondary and primary healthcare providers should be developed and

maintained; however, the service provision across this interface is variable nationally.

RHEUMATOLOGIST

The rheumatologist will see the patient on their first visit to the rheumatology unit, where a comprehensive medical history is taken and full examination performed with close attention to the musculoskeletal system. Investigations such as blood tests and radiographic imaging are also done at this stage. If an acute swelling or effusion is present, an intraarticular aspiration or injection may also be necessary at this initial visit.

Following the diagnosis of RA, the rheumatologist will discuss the therapeutic management options. Although the doctor initially provides information about the disease and drug therapy, the nurse should always support this with an in-depth discussion, to ensure the patient has fully understood their drug management and informed consent for therapy is gained.

The patient will continue to see the rheumatologist but the specialist nurse will in many cases provide the regular follow-up care and liaise closely with the rheumatologist regarding management issues.

RHEUMATOLOGY NURSE

In rheumatology healthcare, the nurse is often ideally placed within the rheumatology team to act as the point of contact and referral for the patient and their family, on an inpatient and outpatient basis, throughout the patient's lifespan (Fig. 15.12). The nursing role is an integral feature of the patient's care, beginning at their initial contact with the team.

All nurses working in rheumatology care must have a clear understanding of each team member's role and skills to act as an effective facilitator and coordinator of care. This requires a good understanding of the disease, its process and effects in order to provide appropriate patient information, education and support alongside the clinical care and comfort of the patient. As the nurse is pivotal within the team, good interpersonal and communication skills are essential for facilitating and maintaining high standards of care. Careful observation of the patient and their family allows progression or deterioration to be noted early and for constant reevaluation of the patient's care, enabling the nurse to instigate an early response to meet their needs.

The scope of professional practice (UKCC 1992) enabled the role of the specialist rheumatology nurse to evolve in response to the particular needs of the local population through role extension and expansion (Greenhalgh 1994). Although roles vary nationally depending on local needs, resources and the dynamics of the care team, the core elements remain the same (Arthur 1998).

The specialist nurse role is dynamic and complements that of the doctor, often including complex decision-making skills and care previously viewed as being within the domain of medicine (Flasher 1997). The role, key working areas (RCN 2000) and the positive impact of specialist nurse care provision have been well documented (Hill 1997, Hill et al 1994, Newbold 1996). These support a holistic approach to care where the nurse is the consistent point of referral for the patient and their family.

PHARMACIST

Pharmacists now have increasing responsibility in supplementing drug information provided by medical teams, advising the patient, nurse and medical staff on various aspects of medications, particularly their use, drug toxicity and interactions.

The pharmacy team assists in the production of drug information material for patients, accesses drug information resources and is a key member of 'self-medication' programmes, thus enabling the provision of a comprehensive pharmacology service.

OCCUPATIONAL THERAPIST

Occupational therapists (OT) are based in the hospital, Social Services and community teams. The OT will assess the problems faced by the patient during their normal activities of daily living. They can provide practical solutions, information, advice and support on how to approach problems in a positive manner, maintaining and promoting optimal patient independence, safety at home and work, for personal needs and leisure activities (Troman 1998).

The main emphasis of their care relates to upper limb assessment and function. The OT role can encompass aspects of:

- teaching and advising patients to carry out muscle-strengthening and range of movement exercises
- providing or making resting and joint protection splints
- giving advice and help on how to reduce stress on the patient's joints
- advising on energy conservation, relaxation and pain management strategies
- providing family and carer information, advice and support.

Most equipment the OT recommends will be supplied by the local Social Services department. However, they can offer advice on private purchasing of aids to daily living for making life more comfortable.

PHYSIOTHERAPIST

The chartered physiotherapist plays a vital role in educating the patient, reducing pain and swelling, strengthening muscles and mobilising joints to improve their function.

An initial history and functional assessment is carried out, usually in the outpatient setting. The patient's functional ability is regularly reassessed throughout their therapy, the most appropriate modality of treatment being discussed with the patient. Treatments can include: hydrotherapy, the why, how and when of exercise, rest, heat and cold therapies, transcutaneous electrical nerve stimulation (TENS), acupuncture, ultrasound, wax therapy, short-wave diathermy and assessment for, and provision of, walking aids.

Individualised programmes for maintenance of self-care at home are tailored to the patient's requirements. Close liaison with the GP and nurse will be maintained throughout the physiotherapist and patient partnership (Smruti-Riley 1998).

APPLIANCE OFFICER AND ORTHOTIST

The appliance officer and orthotist are skilled in assessing deformity and stresses across joints. A number of appliances and prostheses are available to correct, control and accommodate a deformity, stabilise joints and assist in mobilisation and the reduction of pain.

In RA the weight-bearing joints, particularly those of the ankle and feet, often warrant close attention. Metatarsalgia is a common problem, relieved with the use of metatarsal head supports, while an enthisitis, inflammation of a tendon or ligaments such as plantar fasciitis, may settle with the use of heel cups.

As the width and depth of footwear are a common difficulty for those with rheumatoid-related foot problems, shoes can be made to measure or shop-bought shoes adapted. Painful corns may develop over the fixed joints of a hallux valgus or hammer toe (Fig. 15.13a, c, d) deformities; these result from the pressure of ill-fitting shoes. Latex digital shields, silicone props and slings may help minimise the risk of ulcer formation.

Pain, often radiating up the shin due to a valgus deformity of the ankle (Fig. 15.13b), may respond to longitudinal arch supports.

Rigid braces, with or without movable joints, are also available to support and protect an inflamed or unstable joint. All patients should possess both resting and working wrist and hand splints (Fig. 15.14) to support the joints in an optimal position. Some appliances will be premanufactured but more often they are individually tailored to the person's requirement, which necessitates accurate assessment and several fitting visits for the patient.

A range of cervical collars is used, from soft for mild symptoms to rigid for more severe symptoms or when atlantoaxial instability is evident (Fig. 15.15).

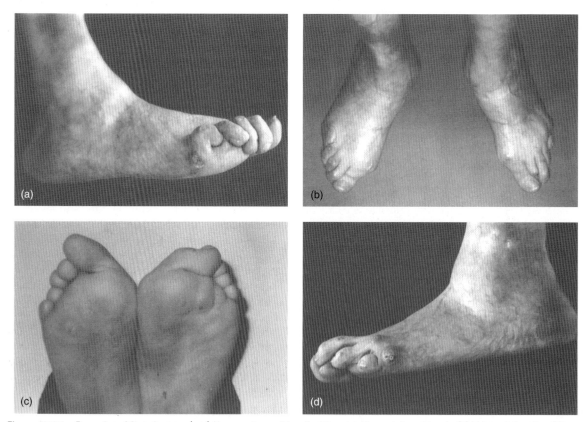

Figure 15.13 Examples of foot changes. (a, d) Hammer toes with callosities over the metatarsal heads. (b) Valgus deformity of the ankle. (b, c) Hallux valgus. (From Mr JL Plewes with permission.)

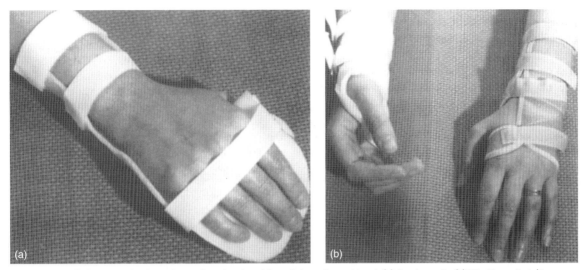

Figure 15.14   Splints to maintain optimum functional position of the wrist and hand. (a) Resting split. (b) Working splint. (From Turner et al 1992.)

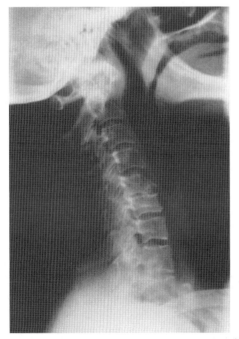

Figure 15.15   Rheumatoid changes of the cervical spine. (From Mr JL Plewes with permission.)

CHIROPODIST, PODIATRIST

Foot and toe problems are common in RA, frequently being the cause of reduced mobility.

The role of the chiropodist is to maintain the patient's foot health and to increase foot function, thereby improving mobility. The service provided includes the management of nail and skin conditions and redistribution of pressure by using padding and orthoses to correct or stabilise a deformity, thereby promoting a walking gait that is as near to normal as possible.

Podiatrists specialise in lower limb assessments and treatment; following postgraduate training, they can also offer surgical treatments.

An important role of both the chiropodist and podiatrist is to provide advice and information on footwear, foot and nail care (Hughes 1983). The need for regular visits to a chiropodist should be emphasised.

PSYCHOLOGIST

The chronicity and variability of RA often debilitate the sufferer emotionally. Many patients are able to work through the anxieties and problems they face with a member of the rheumatology team or with support groups. Occasionally, though, patients require support from a psychologist to skilfully enable their adjustment and acceptance of their disease and its far-reaching effects.

Psychologists also have a valuable educative role in identifying coping strategies, especially for pain management, personal and working relationships, and to support the family and carers' needs. In the absence of a psychologist, the nurse specialists may fulfil aspects of this role.

DIETICIAN

People with RA have to confront problems related not just to their diet but also to anorexia or obesity. Low body weight can be related to a number of factors including systemic illness, physical limitations and demotivation. On the other hand, inactivity, immobility and reduced energy levels can lead to an increase in body weight, thereby increasing the force placed through already weak joints, leading to increased pain and the risk of further damage. The dietician will provide expert advice on programmes for weight gain or loss.

As the nutritional status of people with this chronic and variable disease is an important aspect of their ongoing healthcare (Ryan 1995), an early referral to the dietician for assessment and support is an important management issue.

SOCIAL WORKER

The social worker not only coordinates social care for people with RA but also provides support, advice and counselling for the family and carers in the short term and in relation to long-term plans. It is ideal, although perhaps unrealistic in many healthcare settings, for there to be a dedicated rheumatology social worker providing continuity of care for the patient and their family via a therapeutic relationship.

Patients, particularly those in the later stages of RA, may have complex social needs, requiring lengthy social history reviews, assessments and planning.

Planning for safe discharge back into the community following inpatient care commences on admission with support from all members of the care team. Liaison with community Social Services will facilitate discharge and allow for the effective use of secondary care resources.

THE ROLE OF THE PATIENT

Holman (1996) describes the dramatic evolution in the patient role from a passive recipient of care, when the focus is on diagnosis, treatment and cure, to that of active participant in healthcare delivery when the chronic disease predominates (Pawlson 1994). Many people with RA will identify with the active patient role and this is where the patient needs support from the rheumatology care team.

The need for independence and the preservation of an acceptable lifestyle requires the patient to actively seek help and information. Sharing the decision-making process, responsibility for their disease and its management in a partnership (Charles et al 1997) increases patient satisfaction and improves care outcomes. It is important the care team encourage and support patients to participate actively in their care. This is now more commonplace with patients being involved in the development and review of services (DoH 2002).

PATIENT CARE AND MANAGEMENT

ACCESS TO CARE

Care delivery in the NHS is usually influenced by factors other than the needs of the client group it exists to serve; for instance, targets requiring a certain number of newly referred patients to be seen in a particular ratio to those attending follow-up care. In a specialty like rheumatology, the knock-on effects of this can be great, as a relatively small proportion of the patients seen are referred back to the care of their GP, as many will require regular ongoing care via the rheumatology team. This can mean that actual follow-up appointments with the medical team could become fewer and too widely spaced. Nurse-led clinics can provide some of the necessary continuity of care by monitoring DMARD therapy, continuing assessments, education, counselling, information giving and the administration of soft tissue and intraarticular injections.

SYMPTOMS EXPERIENCED

The course and effects of each person's rheumatoid arthritis are individual. Common features contribute to many of the problems experienced by sufferers but the effect of these varies with each person's background and individual life circumstances.

Joint and soft tissue pain, stiffness, reduced range of movement, paraesthesia, altered sensation, fatigue, varying degrees of deformity and relapses and remissions all add to the catalogue of potential problems. Figures 15.16–15.22 show some of the difficulties patients are confronted with related to specific joints and their surrounding tissues. The combined effects of one or more of these can lead to

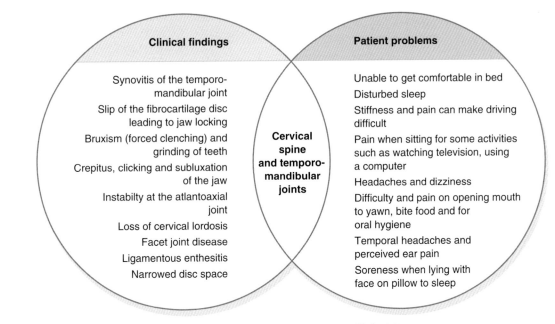

Figure 15.16   Presentation of symptoms at the cervical spine and temporomandibular joints.

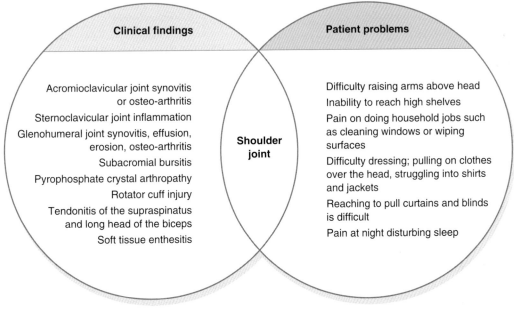

Figure 15.17   Presentation of symptoms at the shoulder.

being unable to run a household, continue in a chosen career, problems in caring for children, maintaining relationships or fulfilling previously perceived role functions such as being a parent, spouse, carer, lover or breadwinner, to name a few. In turn, loss of self-esteem, confidence, self-image, independence and the onset of depression may follow.

Added to these are the effects of feeling generally unwell, possible complications of osteoporosis, the systemic involvement and the potential for adverse effects of medications. These clearly illustrate the essential need for a team approach to care to be incorporated into the philosophy of rheumatology departments.

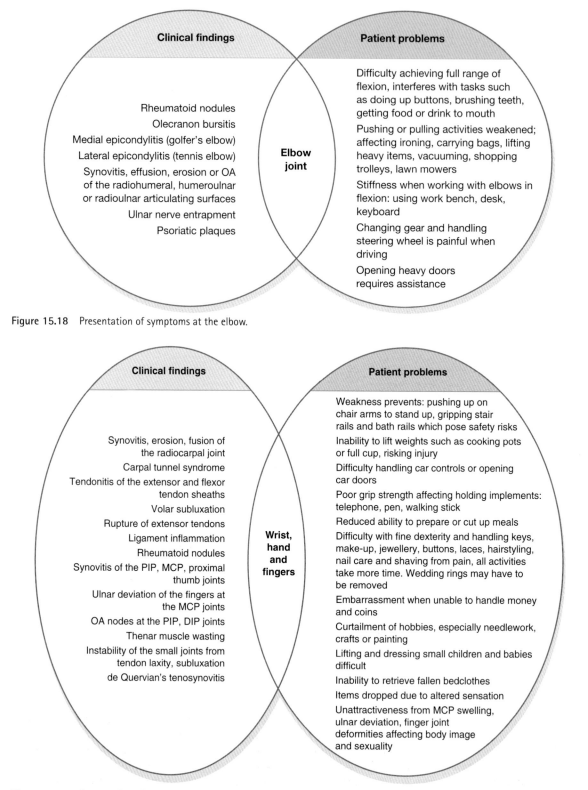

Figure 15.18   Presentation of symptoms at the elbow.

Figure 15.19   Presentation of symptoms at the wrist, hand and fingers.

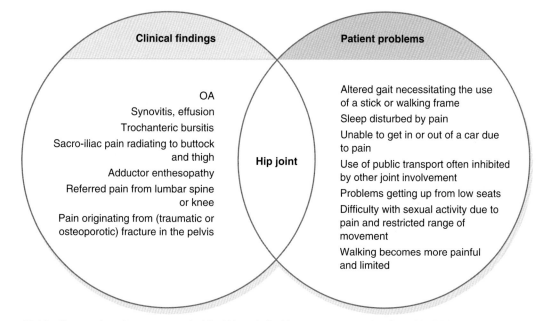

Figure 15.20 Presentation of symptoms at the hip. Although the hips are not commonly affected by RA itself, concomitant osteoarthritis is common. Soft tissue lesions may also be present; for example, trochanteric bursitis and adductor enthesopathy.

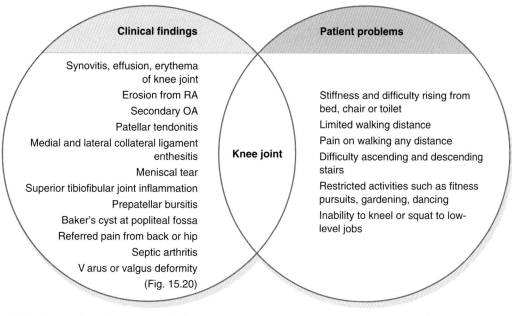

Figure 15.21   Presentation of symptoms at the knee.

ASSESSMENT TOOLS

A plethora of care models is evident in practice but one specifically designed for planning the management of rheumatology patients is that developed by White in 1998 (cited by RCN 2001), whose model is used to describe the standards for effective practice and audit in rheumatology nursing.

There are a significant number of tools (Table 15.4) used to assess various aspects of RA and other rheumatic disease progression, often being used alongside blood and radiological investigations to

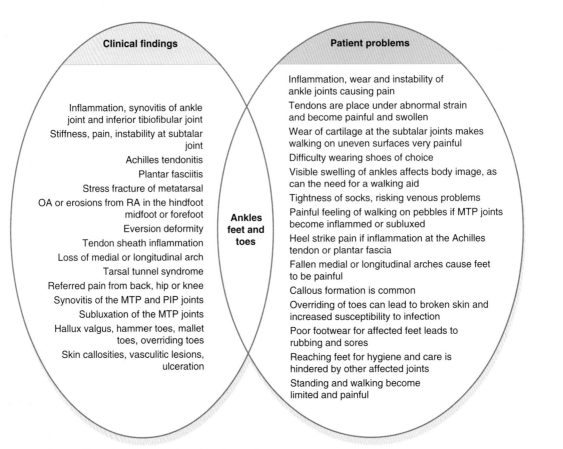

Clinical findings

Inflammation, synovitis of ankle joint and inferior tibiofibular joint

Stiffness, pain, instability at subtalar joint

Achilles tendonitis

Plantar fasciitis

Stress fracture of metatarsal

OA or erosions from RA in the hindfoot midfoot or forefoot

Eversion deformity

Tendon sheath inflammation

Loss of medial or longitudinal arch

Tarsal tunnel syndrome

Referred pain from back, hip or knee

Synovitis of the MTP and PIP joints

Subluxation of the MTP joints

Hallux valgus, hammer toes, mallet toes, overriding toes

Skin callosities, vasculitic lesions, ulceration

Ankles feet and toes

Patient problems

Inflammation, wear and instability of ankle joints causing pain

Tendons are place under abnormal strain and become painful and swollen

Wear of cartilage at the subtalar joints makes walking on uneven surfaces very painful

Difficulty wearing shoes of choice

Visible swelling of ankles affects body image, as can the need for a walking aid

Tightness of socks, risking venous problems

Painful feeling of walking on pebbles if MTP joints become inflamed or subluxed

Heel strike pain if inflammation at the Achilles tendon or plantar fascia

Fallen medial or longitudinal arches cause feet to be painful

Callous formation is common

Overriding of toes can lead to broken skin and increased susceptibility to infection

Poor footwear for affected feet leads to rubbing and sores

Reaching feet for hygiene and care is hindered by other affected joints

Standing and walking become limited and painful

Figure 15.22 Presentation of symptoms at the ankles, feet and toes.

Table 15.4 Commonly used assessment tools. Symmonds (1994) describes these in more detail along with other metrology tools used in quantifying outcomes of rheumatology treatment and care

Assessment tool	What the tool sets out to measure	How it is used
Health Assessment Questionnaire (HAQ)	Functional ability in relation to usual daily activities in the home	Questionnaire completed by the patient ticking appropriate answers to describe the degree of difficulty they have with specific daily activities
European League Against Rheumatism (EULAR) 28 joint count	Total number of painful joints and total number of swollen joints	Two diagrams of body maps, anterior and posterior, each showing 28 joints affected in inflammatory arthritis. These are marked when a joint is positive to swelling or pain following examination by applying pressure and moving the joint
Disease Activity Score (DAS)	Pooled indices: a combined score derived from the results of ESR results, VAS, tender and swollen joints	DAS calculators are available to complete the formula which provides the disease activity score
Visual Analogue Scale (VAS)	A subjective patient measurement, generally used for pain, well-being and disease activity measures	A horizontal 10 cm line going from 'best' to 'worst' score. The patient marks the point that represents the severity of their symptoms at that point in time. The distance of the mark along the line is measured and recorded in mm
Early Morning Stiffness (EMS)	For how long after rising in the morning the joints remain stiff	Simply ask the question and record in hours and/or minutes

measure clinical signs, responses to treatment and any improvement or deterioration between different points in time.

RHEUMATOLOGICAL INVESTIGATIONS

Various investigations are important in confirming the diagnosis of RA and in determining disease severity and activity.

Haematological investigations

Haematological investigations are important not only in diagnosing RA but also in monitoring its progression and the effects of treatment. The commonly used tests are listed in Box 15.1.

Biochemical investigations

Rheumatoid arthritis may cause renal and hepatic insufficiency but these are more commonly a

---

Box 15.1   Haematological investigations in rheumatoid arthritis

Rheumatoid factor (Rf)	Rf refers to some immunoglobulins (IgG) that act as antibodies to altered human gammaglobulins and produce autoantibodies. The Rose-Waaler or Latex tests detect the presence or absence of immunoglobulin M (IgM) antiglobulins (Rf). Although not conclusive, higher titres are typically found in patients with severe disease and indicate a less favourable prognosis. Seropositive RA and seronegative RA relate to the detection of IgM Rf in the serum. The number of false-positive tests increases with age
Acute-phase reactants: • Erythrocyte sedimentation rate (ESR) • Plasma viscosity (P. Visc) • C-reactive protein (CRP)	These are generally raised and broadly correlate to disease activity. P. Visc relates to the viscous quality of the serum and reflects the number of white cells in circulation. CRP is a small protein produced by the liver in the presence of inflammation. A sustained increase indicates a poorer prognosis. Acute-phase reactants are routinely used to assess the efficacy of treatment but are not specific to inflammation caused by RA alone, hence results will not always correlate to rheumatoid disease activity
Haemoglobin (Hb)	Hb results will indicate anaemia, common in chronic inflammatory disease. Anaemia is due to the nature of the disease or iron deficiency from treatment such as NSAID-induced gastrointestinal bleeding. Although red cell folate is often low, it may be unresponsive to replacement therapy because bone marrow stores are often normal or high: RA reduces the ability to mobilise stored iron for physiological use. Note that when investigating anaemia, serum ferritin may act as an acute-phase response in active disease, making levels normal to high
White blood cell count (WBC)	A raised WBC is from the inflammatory process and activation of the immune response. If a sudden rise occurs, exclude an infection or neoplasm. A low WBC may indicate drug-related immunosuppression, increasing the risk of infection. A low WBC and platelet count is commonly seen in Felty's syndrome
Platelets (PLT)	PLT levels are usually raised in response to inflammation. A low PLT can indicate drug-related immunosuppression. A low PLT, falling Hb and falling mean corpuscular volume (MCV) can indicate chronic occult blood loss
Antinuclear antibodies (ANA)	ANA are present in 20–40% of RA patients. They have no specific diagnostic or prognostic significance. ANA are more useful in monitoring disease activity in Sjögren's syndrome and systemic lupus erythematosus
Cryoglobulins	Useful to assess the vasculitic component of rheumatoid disease
Complement	The inflammatory process raises the complement serum levels. Circulating levels can be useful in predicting disease progression

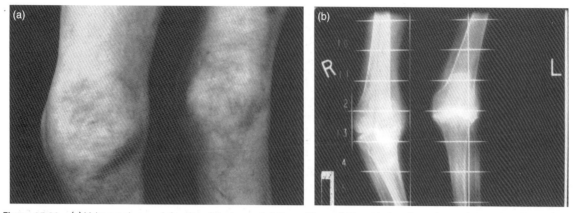

Figure 15.23 (a) Valgus and varus deformity of the knees; 'windswept' knees with evidence of muscle wasting on the left. (b) X-ray appearance of this deformity. (From Mr JL Plewes with permission.)

complication of NSAID and DMARD therapies. Renal and liver function tests should be performed according to local guidelines to monitor for toxicity.

Synovial fluid

The synovial fluid in the affected joints is typically turbid due to the presence of a high number of white cells and has a reduced viscosity. Analysis of the synovial fluid can prove useful in excluding conditions other than RA and determining the presence or absence of infection. A synovium biopsy is not useful as a disease-specific diagnostic tool but is used in immunological research.

Radiological investigations

Radiological techniques for imaging all have particular strengths and weaknesses related to the information they provide. Plain X-ray films remain the mainstay of musculoskeletal imaging, providing a valuable diagnostic and disease progression measurement tool (Figs 15.23, 15.24). However, MRI, bone density and ultrasound scanning are increasingly useful.

X-ray films. In the early stages, X-ray findings show periarticular osteoporosis and soft tissue swelling due to the inflammatory process and synovitis. These are noticeable at the PIP, MCP and MTP joints.

Marginal erosions of the bone, appearing as bony defects, are seen at the junction of the synovium and articular cartilage. These typically first appear in MCP joints of the index and middle fingers and MTP joints of the toes. Joint space narrowing may

well be evident. These changes can usually be observed within the first 6 months and if present, indicate a poorer outcome in terms of disability.

In established RA, large 'punched out' erosions become evident with complete loss of joint space. Severe damage to the periarticular structures, the tendons and ligaments causes joint instability leading to subluxation and dislocation. Marked joint destruction can lead to ankylosis, as seen in the carpus, osteolysis, such as protrusio acetabulae in the hip, or deformities at the MCP joints of the hand (Figs 15.24, 15.25).

Ultrasonography. This is particularly useful for assessing soft tissue changes in and around the joints, as it can highlight effusions, bursitis, synovitis, synovial cysts, calcification and erosions. Ultrasound is the tool most commonly used to identify a Baker's cyst of the knee (see Fig. 15.11) and more recently is proving a useful tool in assessing the shoulder joint.

Computed tomography (CT). Complicated bony anatomy is demonstrated well by CT scans, making it particularly useful for cervical spine assessment, where the effects of RA may cause spinal stenosis.

Isotope scanning. Evidence of malignancy, infection and inflammation is seen on isotope scans but the results are not specific enough to differentiate between these causes. It can be useful both pre and post diagnosis of RA, when the cause and extent of symptoms are unclear.

Magnetic resonance imaging (MRI). This is currently the best form of imaging and has superseded CT scanning. It identifies soft tissue changes and

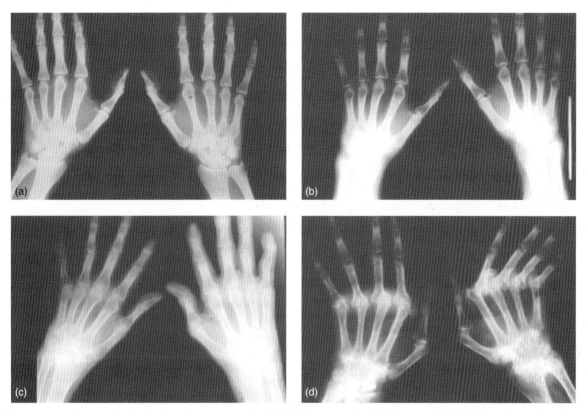

Figure 15.24 X-rays of hands showing disease progression. (a) Initial presentation. (b) Five years later. (c) Ten years later. (d) Advanced RA. (From Dr R Jubb with permission.)

erosions early, so is the best method for identifying cervical involvement.

THE CERVICAL SPINE

Radiological evidence of atlantoaxial subluxation (AAS) is seen in about 15% of patients after 3 years' duration of the disease. The normal space between C1 and C2 measures 3 mm or less, so any measurement greater than this defines AAS; flexion and extension plain X-ray views can delineate this.

If neck pain is present, it is usually high in the cervical spine and is associated with the more frequent symptom of occipital pain, which is worse in the morning. In most cases, symptom relief is gained from a soft cervical collar worn at night. As AAS can be a potentially disastrous defect, it requires regular radiological assessment.

Severe AAS of 7 mm and over with sudden weakness or clumsiness of the lower limbs, with or without sensory deficits, necessitates an MRI scan and often requires neurosurgical intervention. All patients

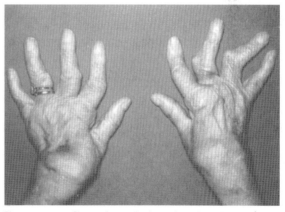

Figure 15.25 Shortening and telescoping of the fingers. (From Dr R Jubb with permission.)

with RA requiring general anaesthesia or hyperextension of the cervical spine must be assessed for AAS as a perioperative precaution. If found to be present, all members of the care team, especially those involved in surgical and postoperative care, must be alerted to minimise the risk of cervical cord damage.

INFORMATION AND SUPPORT

Knowledge, information and skills which health professionals possess are of little use to patients if they have no means to access them. A major factor in terms of timely access is the development of nurse-led telephone helpline services. By having a direct contact number, patients are immediately empowered to decide for themselves whether or not to seek help. For many, simply having the number and choice is enough as it provides the reassurance that help is there should they need it. For others the helpline is an important way of averting more serious problems, such as getting advice quickly when a medication causes side effects or to arrange to be seen within a few days of the onset of a severe flare of symptoms. When attendance at a hospital for appointments causes difficulty for the patient, telephone clinics can provide all the necessary information and a follow-up appointment can then be arranged if required. This can save resources for both the hospital and patient.

Whilst information and education form a large part of the nursing role, patients cannot retain everything they are told during a consultation. Sometimes information needs to be available for the individual to access when they feel ready. To this end a selection of educational leaflets covering many issues is now available for patients and their carers from the Arthritis Research Campaign. Additionally, specialist support groups are run for particular patient groups or are related to specific conditions. Self-help or peer support groups have a valuable role, as do charitable organisations, giving educational talks to the community. Patients also access support and information from the World Wide Web and other media.

The role of the nurse is to ensure that patients understand the information and take it in the correct context.

DRUG THERAPY

Drug therapy, although only one aspect of the care package required to treat patients with RA, plays a vital role in the control of the symptoms and ultimately the suppression of the disease process.

Aspirin, the archetypal antiinflammatory drug, has been replaced by an increasing number of safer antiinflammatory preparations. Increased understanding of the complex immunology of RA and the appreciation that joint destruction occurs early in the disease process have led to the much earlier use of more powerful immunosuppressive and cytotoxic drugs. The recent development of biological agents exemplifies the reversal of the previous pyramidal approach to drug treatment in inflammatory arthritis.

Analgesia

Pain relief is obviously high on the agenda for patients. A range of analgesia is available, including non-opioid, compound or opioid drugs. These are commonly used in conjunction with antiinflammatory drugs as they generally have limited value when used in isolation.

Education regarding the most effective use of analgesia enables the patient to gain the greatest realistic efficacy. Patients, particularly the elderly, must be well informed about the possible side effects, the most common being constipation from opioid preparations, dizziness and nausea. It is also worth considering other pain-modulating medicines such as antidepressants and topical preparations, for example the substance P-depleting agent capsaicin.

Non-steroidal antiinflammatory drugs (NSAIDs)

These do not have any impact on the rheumatoid disease process but they are widely used to reduce, in a relatively short time, the signs and symptoms of the inflammatory process. There should be a noticeable effect on the patient's pain and stiffness after a few days, with the maximum benefit seen within 2 weeks. As individual responses will vary, it is not unusual for patients to try NSAIDs from alternative classes or with a differing release mechanism until the most effective is found.

The mode of action of NSAIDs is by inactivation of cyclooxygenase (COX), leading to the reduction of prostaglandin synthesis, thereby suppressing inflammation. However, prostaglandins also play a vital role in maintaining normal physiological function; interference with this action may lead to a number of unwanted reactions (Box 15.2), some of which may be dose related.

Two enzymes have been identified as being involved in prostaglandin production.

- COX-1 enzyme produces prostaglandins used to maintain normal body function and tissue protection.

- COX-2 enzyme produces prostaglandins which are only activated in inflamed tissues.

This has led to the development of NSAIDs which are selective towards COX-2 inhibition. By ensuring the COX-1 enzyme is able to function relatively uninhibited, the incidence of adverse events, particularly in the gastrointestinal tract, is reduced.

The nurse's role of informing and educating is essential as patients armed with sound information and advice about their NSAID therapy are more likely to be compliant and seek advice and help appropriately, resulting in increased safety and efficacy of drug use.

Disease–modifying antirheumatic drugs (DMARDs)

DMARDs are the primary treatment for rheumatoid disease. They have the ability to suppress disease activity and progression, so are being used earlier in the disease process and in combinations (Van Der Heide et al 1996). Even though both short-term and long-term outcomes are more favourable with DMARD use (Egmose et al 1995), most patients will go on to develop bony erosions.

The choice of which DMARD to use (Table 15.5) is influenced by many factors such as the risk–benefit ratio of each drug, the severity of the disease, the medical team's knowledge and experience with each drug along with patient factors such as expectations, preference and commitment to the therapy, including any monitoring requirements.

In general, the greater the impact of the drug on the immune system, the higher the incidence of unwanted side effects. The clinical dilemma lies in balancing the risk of side effects with the potential therapeutic benefit. These drugs have a slow onset of action, making it difficult to predict which patient will respond well to which drug, when an effective dose has been reached and how long the effects will last.

The most common first-choice drugs are sulfasalazine and methotrexate (Drugs and Therapeutics Bulletin 1995); if these DMARD therapies are tolerated, the patient is likely to benefit. Mild side effects are relatively frequent, often being dose related, but as these drugs have the potential to cause serious toxicity, careful monitoring and management are essential. The British Society for Rheumatology (BSR 2000) has produced national guidelines for the monitoring of DMARDs. These provide the core requirements from which local protocols can be developed.

The majority of drug management is provided through outpatient clinics with the nurse being the key contact for information, advice and support on drug therapies, along with monitoring of the drug effects. The active involvement of the patient in their therapeutic options and decisions on drug regimes must be encouraged. This needs to be supported by current, clear, verbal and written information to ensure patients' consent to drug therapy is informed and to ensure they seek help and advice appropriately.

Antitumour necrosis factor α antibody therapy

The most recent additions to the biological therapies are treatments aimed at tumour necrosis factor α (TNF-α), a cytokine that plays a key role in perpetuating the inflammatory process in RA. Genetically engineered inhibitors block the action of TNF-α; this breaks the inflammatory cycle which if left intact would lead to joint damage.

Anti-TNF-α therapy rapidly reduces the signs and symptoms of RA (Maini et al 1998) and has

Table 15.5 Disease-modifying antirheumatic drugs

Agent	Dose range	Delay in therapeutic benefit	Possible side effects	Monitoring requirements	Patient and family education and advice
Hydroxychloroquine	400 mg daily Reduce to maintenance dose of 200 mg daily	4–6 months	Nausea, diarrhoea, abdominal cramps, tinnitus, hypotension, headache, fatigue, irritability, rash, myopathy, reversible visual disturbance	Pretreatment: full blood count (FBC), inflammatory marker, eye examination Follow-up: FBC, inflammatory marker, Amsler grid test every 3 months Clinical assessment	• Take medication as directed • Missed doses to be taken within 1 hour or omitted • On commencing medicine, avoid driving or other activities requiring alertness until the possible side effect of 'light headedness' is ruled out • Alcohol should be avoided • Perform once monthly Amsler grid test and report any changes in vision • Report and seek immediate advice in the event of: ringing in the ears or hearing difficulty, unusual bruising or bleeding, gastric upsets or marked muscle weakness • Keep out of reach of children • Be patient; potential therapeutic benefit may take up to 6 months
D-Penicillamine	125 mg daily, orally, before food Increasing to maintenance dose of 500 mg daily	4–6 months	Temporarily altered taste, rash, mouth ulcers, stomatitis, dyspepsia, nausea, muscle weakness, arthralgia, proteinuria, haematological effects, renal impairment Rarely shortness of breath, cough, wheeze	Pretreatment: FBC, inflammatory marker, urea and electrolytes (U&Es) and creatinine urinalysis Repeat urinalysis, inflammatory marker and FBC every 2 weeks until on a stable dose, then monthly thereafter U&Es repeated every 2 months Clinical assessment	• Take medicine as directed • If once-daily dose is missed take when remembered, but not the next day. If twice-daily dose is missed, take when remembered but do not double the next dose • Sense of taste may temporarily be disturbed • Report and seek immediate advice in the event of: rash, sore throat, mouth ulcers, unusual bruising or bleeding, fever, shortness of breath or new symptoms • Emphasise importance of attending appointments to check on progress in therapy and disease management • Dosage adjustment may be required • Inform dentist prior to treatment • Discuss over-the-counter medicines with pharmacists

Drug	Dose	Duration	Side effects	Monitoring	Patient advice
Gold injection: sodium aurothiomalate	IM injection: 10 mg test dose then 50 mg weekly up to a cumulative dose of 1 g. When remission is evident, treatment intervals are gradually increased to 50 mg monthly	4–6 months	Severe reactions are rare, most are reversible or dose related: rash, mouth ulcers, stomatitis, nausea, temporary altered sense of taste, diarrhoea, abdominal discomfort, arthralgia, photosensitivity, proteinuria, haematological effects. Rarely alopecia, renal effects	Pretreatment: FBC, inflammatory marker, U&Es and creatinine, BP, urinalysis. Repeat: FBC, inflammatory marker and urinalysis at the time of each injection or 1 week before. It is permissible to work with blood results 1 week in arrears. Clinical assessment	• Keep out of the reach of children • Be patient; potential therapeutic benefit may take up to 6 months • Good oral hygiene needed • Protection against the effects of the sun • Report and seek immediate advice in the event of: rash, mouth ulcers, sore throat, prolonged diarrhoea, fever, unusual bruising or bleeding, prolonged arthralgia following injection, suspected pregnancy or any new symptoms • Emphasise importance of attending appointments to check on progress and disease management • Discuss contraception and family planning • Be patient; potential therapeutic benefit may take up to 6 months • Dosage adjustments may be required
Oral gold (auranofin)	3 mg bd increasing to 3 mg tds if necessary	4–6 months	As for IM gold	Pretreatment: FBC, inflammatory marker, U&Es, liver function tests (LFTs), BP, urinalysis. Repeat: FBC and urinalysis monthly, BP and U&Es 3 monthly, LFTs every 6 months. Clinical assessment	• As for IM gold • Discuss the lower effectiveness: toxicity ratio in comparison to IM gold • Keep out of reach of children
Sulfasalazine	500 mg daily gradually increasing to a maintenance dose of 1.5–3 g daily	4–6 months	Nausea, diarrhoea, rash/ exfoliative dermatitis, headaches, dizziness, folate deficiency, oligospermia, photosensitivity, hepatic effects, haematological effects, rarely fibrosing alveolitis/ pneumonitis, may discolour urine and contact lenses orange	Pretreatment: FBC, inflammatory marker, U&Es and creatinine, LFTs. Repeat: FBC every 2 weeks, inflammatory marker and LFTs every 4 weeks for the first 12 weeks, then 12 weekly. If blood results are stable at 1 year, then repeat every 6 months. Clinical assessment	• Take medicine as directed • Do not crush or chew tablets • If a dose is missed, take it when remembered but if it is the next day omit the dose • On commencing medicine, avoid driving or other activities requiring alertness until the possible side effect of dizziness is ruled out • Discuss protection against the effects of the sun

(continued)

Table 15.5 (Continued)

Agent	Dose range	Delay in therapeutic benefit	Possible side effects	Monitoring requirements	Patient and family education and advice
					• Report and seek immediate advice in the event of: rash, fever, sore throat, mouth ulcers or soreness, any unusual bruising or bleeding, prolonged upset stomach, suspected pregnancy or any new symptoms • Discuss possible effect on urine and contact lenses • Discuss contraception and family planning • Emphasise importance of attending appointments to check on progress in therapy and disease management • Dosage adjustments may be required • Be patient; potential therapeutic benefit may take up to 6 months • Keep out of the reach of children
Methotrexate	5–20 mg once weekly, dose adjusted according to response	2–4 months	Nausea, dyspepsia, abdominal discomfort, diarrhoea, stomatitis, rash, photosensitivity, headaches, dizziness, malaise, reversible visual disturbance, reduction in male and female fertility, alopecia, immunosuppression, hepatotoxicity, pulmonary toxicity	Pretreatment: FBC, inflammatory marker, U&Es and creatinine, liver function tests. Chest X-ray and pulmonary function test if history of lung disease Repeat: FBC every 2 weeks until 6 weeks after last dose increase, then monthly. LFTs and inflammatory marker with each FBC. U&Es 6 monthly Clinical assessment	• Take medicine as directed • If a dose is missed, take within 2 hours or omit • Alcohol should be avoided, particularly on the day of medication • Unless advised otherwise, avoid medicines containing aspirin • Good oral hygiene needed • Maintain a fluid intake of at least 1.5 litres daily • Report and seek advice immediately in the event of: severe or ongoing episodes of nausea post methotrexate dose, unusual mouth ulcers or soreness, unusual bruising or bleeding, shortness of breath, cough or wheeze, fever, sore throat,

- suspected pregnancy, any new symptoms
- Avoid people with known infection
- Discuss potential of hair loss; unusual but normally dose related
- Dosage adjustments may be required
- Avoid live vaccines; discuss requirements with GP
- Discuss protection against the effects of the sun
- Discuss over-the-counter medicines with pharmacists
- Discuss contraception and family planning
- Emphasise importance of attending appointments to check on progress in therapy and disease management
- Be patient potential therapeutic benefit may take up to 6 months
- Keep out of the reach of children

Ciclosporin A	50–200 mg orally in divided dose. Dose dependent on body weight Maintenance dose adjusted according to response	2–5 months	Minor side effects are common in the first few weeks of treatment: fatigue, tremor, burning sensation in hands and feet, headaches, flushing, nausea, diarrhoea Other side effects include: rash, oedema, hypertension, cramps, hirsutism, muscle weakness, gum overgrowth, weight gain, dysmenorrhoea or amenorrhoea, haematological effects, nephrotoxicity	Pretreatment: FBC, U&Es, inflammatory marker, serum lipids, BP, urinalysis and weight should be normal on two separate occasions prior to treatment Repeat: U&Es, BP and inflammatory marker every 2 weeks for 3 months, then monthly FBC and LFTs monthly for 3 months, then 3 monthly Serum lipids 6 monthly Clinical assessment	- Take medicine as directed - If a dose is missed take within 12 hours, otherwise omit - Avoid grapefruit juice - Good oral hygiene needed - Initial minor side effects may occur but likely to settle spontaneously within a few weeks - Report and seek advice immediately in the event of severe, prolonged headaches, rash, fever, sore throat, unusual bruising or bleeding, suspected pregnancy, any new symptoms - Avoid people known to have an infection - Discuss the possibility of facial hair growth in women

(continued)

Table 15.5 (Continued)

Agent	Dose range	Delay in therapeutic benefit	Possible side effects	Monitoring requirements	Patient and family education and advice
					• Dosage adjustments may be required • Avoid live vaccines: discuss requirements with GP • Discuss over-the-counter medicines with pharmacists • Emphasise importance of attending appointments to check on progress and disease management • Be patient; potential therapeutic benefit may take up to 5 months to be evident • Keep out of the reach of children
Azathioprine	1–3 mg/kg daily, in a single or divided dose, adjusted to response	2–4 months	Rash, nausea, mouth ulcers, stomatitis, diarrhoea, malaise, dizziness, arthralgia, alopecia, bone marrow suppression, fever, chills, retinopathy, haematological effects, hepatotoxicity Rarely: pulmonary oedema, pancreatitis, nephritis	Pretreatment: FBC, inflammatory marker, UtEs and creatinine, liver function tests Repeat: FBC and inflammatory marker weekly for 6 weeks, then 2 and 4 weeks after a dose increase and monthly thereafter Monthly LFTs Clinical assessment	• Take medicine as directed • If a dose is missed, omit and take the next dose as normal • Report and seek immediate advice in the event of: severe or prolonged nausea or diarrhoea post dose, rash, unusual bruising or bleeding, sore throat, fever, suspected pregnancy or new symptoms • Avoid people known to have an infection • Avoid live vaccines; discuss requirements with GP • Discuss over-the-counter medicines with the pharmacist • Discuss contraception and family planning • Emphasise importance of attending appointments to check on progress and disease management • Be patient; potential therapeutic benefit may take up to 6 months • Keep out of the reach of children

| Cyclophosphamide | 50–200 mg orally daily. Dose is weight dependent and adjusted according to response | 2–4 months | Nausea, mouth ulcers, stomatitis, haematuria, haemorrhagic cystitis, alopecia, irregular menstrual cycles, reversible reduction in fertility, haematological effects, bone marrow suppression Rarely: secondary neoplasms, hypotension, pulmonary fibrosis | Pretreatment: FBC, inflammatory marker, U&Es, liver function tests, BP, urinalysis, weight Repeat every 2 weeks for 2 months, then monthly Clinical assessment | • Take medicine as directed
• If a dose is missed, omit
• Emphasise the need for increased fluid intake to 1.5 litres daily
• Good oral hygiene needed
• Report any severe or prolonged nausea, vomiting, unusual bruising or bleeding, especially blood in the urine, sore throat, fever, shortness of breath, sore mouth, rash, suspected pregnancy
• Discuss contraception and family planning
• Discuss potential of hair loss; unusual but normally dose related
• Avoid people with known infections
• Avoid live vaccines: discuss requirements with GP
• Alcohol should be avoided
• May cause darkening of the skin and nails
• Discuss over-the-counter medicines with pharmacists
• Dosage adjustments may be required
• Emphasise importance of attending appointments to check on progress and disease management
• Be patient; potential therapeutic benefit may take up to 4 months
• Keep out of the reach of children |
| Leflunomide | 10–20 mg daily, with or without a loading dose of 100 mg daily for 3 days | 4–6 weeks May improve further up to 4–6 months | Nausea, diarrhoea, weight loss, mouth ulcers, abdominal cramps, headache, dizziness, weakness, rash, dry skin, reversible hair loss, raised BP, haematological effects, hepatotoxicity | Pretreatment: chest X-ray, Heaf test (see local protocols), FBC, LFTs, BP Repeat: FBC every 2 weeks for 6 months, then 8 weekly LFTs and BP monthly for 6 months, then 8 weekly Clinical assessment | • Take medication as directed
• Missed doses should be taken within 2 hours or omitted
• Alcohol should be avoided
• Good oral hygiene needed
• Report and seek advice in the event of diarrhoea, nausea, vomiting, weight loss, fever, sore throat, cough, shortness |

(continued)

Table 15.5   (*Continued*)

Agent	Dose range	Delay in therapeutic benefit	Possible side effects	Monitoring requirements	Patient and family education and advice
					of breath, mouth ulcers, abdominal pain, headaches, dizziness, rash, unusual bruising or bleeding, suspected pregnancy or any new symptoms • Avoid people with known infections • Avoid live vaccines: discuss requirements with GP • Discuss potential of hair loss; unusual but normally dose related and reversible • Emphasise importance of attending appointments to check on progress and disease management • Dosage adjustment may be required • Discuss over-the-counter medicines with pharmacists • Keep out of the reach of children • In the event of serious side effect or pre-conception, a washout procedure of cholestyramine or activated charcoal may be required

disease-modifying properties (Bathon et al 2000). Although the choice is likely to increase as more drugs are developed and approved, there are currently two compounds licensed for use in the treatment of active RA in the UK:

1 etanercept, which is administered subcutaneously twice weekly
2 infliximab, which is administered by slow intravenous infusion every 8 weeks and is used in conjunction with methotrexate.

Integral to the NICE (2002) guidance on the use of anti-TNF-α therapy for RA are the recommendations by the BSR (2003) allowing treatment to be introduced in a systematic and planned way, to ensure the greatest possible benefit to patients. To assist nurses in the assessment, management and monitoring of biological therapies in arthritis, the RCN (2003) has produced guidelines for good practice.

Corticosteroids

Corticosteroids have been used to treat and control the symptoms of RA since 1950. Unfortunately, the initial hope that these drugs were the nearest thing to a cure was dashed when gradual increases in the doses required to maintain the powerful antiinflammatory effect led to the recognition of the long-term serious side effects (Table 15.6).

Corticosteroids have several routes of administration: oral, intramuscular (IM), intravenous (IV) and intraarticular injection. Oral steroids are used in various circumstances:

- as a short-term measure in the event of an acute flare, usually for a period no longer than 3 months
- when the effectiveness of DMARD therapy is awaited
- more commonly they are prescribed for elderly patients when quality of life outweighs the risks associated with long-term steroid use.

All patients taking oral corticosteroids must carry a steroid treatment card, which contains the prescription details and important information and instructions about the steroid therapy. Patients must be fully informed about the possible side effects and to never abruptly discontinue their therapy. They also need to know that supplementary doses of their steroid may be required in the event of an infection, trauma, surgery and serious illness.

Long-term use of oral prednisolone, usually 7.5 mg or less given daily during the first 2 years following

Table 15.6 Potential side effects of corticosteroids

System affected	Side effects
Cardiovascular	Oedema, hypertension, congestive cardiac failure
Central nervous system	Mood swings, psychosis, paranoia, euphoria, depression, benign intracranial hypertension
Endocrine/metabolic	Cushingoid features: moon face, truncal obesity, 'buffalo hump', hirsutism Hyperglycaemia and insulin resistance Electrolyte imbalance: sodium and fluid retention, hypokalaemia Also hepatic enzyme induction, adrenal suppression, impotence, altered menstrual cycle
Gastrointestinal	Peptic ulceration, pancreatitis
Growth retardation	
Immunological	Decreased resistance to infection, immunosuppression
Musculoskeletal	Osteoporosis, myopathy, avascular necrosis, tendon rupture, corticosteroid withdrawal syndrome
Ophthalmic	Cataracts, glaucoma
Skin	Acne, straie, bruising, impaired wound healing, skin atrophy

diagnosis, has been associated with fewer adverse events and a reduction in erosive changes (Kirwan 1995).

Intramuscular and intravenous 'pulse' steroid therapy has the ability to induce rapid remission in the event of an acute RA flare. Pulses of methylprednisolone 120 mg IM or 500 mg–1 g IV are administered as a single dose or as a course. Serious side effects are rare and minor side effects are self-limiting (Smith et al 1990).

Intraarticular injections (IAI) of steroids are the most effective method of reducing synovial inflammation and recurrent effusions whilst minimising the systemic effects. Adverse events are rare and response to treatment and improvement in function usually occurs within 1 week. Conclusive evidence on the effects and frequency between IAIs is awaited but generally, injections into the same joint are not repeated within a 2-month period. Traditionally, administration of IAIs was solely the remit of the doctor but role developments for nurse specialists and other practitioners have led to patients commonly receiving this treatment from a specialist nurse, physiotherapist or occupational therapist.

COMPLEMENTARY THERAPY

Patients with rheumatic conditions commonly use complementary therapies. It is important that patients are aware of the philosophy and evidence of the effectiveness of the therapy they wish to try, the financial costs involved, time commitments, who will carry out the therapy and how.

Commonly used therapies include acupuncture, homeopathy, herbal remedies, massage, reflexology, aromatherapy, spiritual therapies such as faith and Reiki healing, meditation, yoga and tai-chi. As osteopathy usually involves high-velocity manipulation, it has no place in the treatment of actively inflamed joints but it can produce very good results when used to treat mechanical problems, usually of the spine.

The use of complementary therapies is increasing. By having the opportunity to discuss and receive accurate information on the different therapies available, the patient can be protected against unqualified and unregistered practitioners. Patients should be advised against stopping their conventional treatments, as this can cause a disease flare, and to be very wary of anything declaring itself as a 'cure' (Cawthorn & Billington 1998).

SURGERY

Surgical interventions have a role within the management of RA, especially with the advances in surgical techniques. The aims of surgery are to:

- reduce pain
- maintain or improve function
- prevent or correct deformity
- maintain independence
- offer a cosmetic improvement.

The goal of surgical intervention is to enhance the quality of life experience. Some events require urgent surgical intervention, for example fusion or decompression of subluxed vertebrae that are causing neurological symptoms, and the repair of ruptured tendons of the hand.

Most surgery is elective (Box 15.3) with the decision to operate arising from the patient and team

Box 15.3	Common elective surgical procedures
Soft tissue surgery	Synovectomy, tenosynovectomy, contracture release, tendon repair, nerve decompression
Bone and joint surgery	Arthroscopy, osteotomy, excision arthroplasty, joint replacement, arthrodesis

collaboration, with close attention being paid to the advantages and disadvantages of each individual case. It is important to note that despite surgical intervention, disease progression will continue and it is therefore important that the patient and their family are well informed, have realistic expectations and ongoing support.

RHEUMATOID ARTHRITIS AND PREGNANCY

The ameliorating effect of pregnancy on the course of RA has been well documented since Hench (1938) first reported it. The mechanism, although possibly linked to immune response modulation by sex hormones, remains unknown.

Approximately 75% of women will experience remission of their symptoms during pregnancy, with the majority benefiting in the first trimester. Unfortunately, postpartum exacerbation is likely to occur within the first 3 months and often within the first 4 weeks of delivery.

There is no significant evidence to show that the mother's RA adversely affects the fetus. However, there are potential risks to the unborn child if the mother is taking drugs to control an active disease stage. Therefore, it is essential that careful planning along with counselling, education and support are provided before conception, during pregnancy and in the postpartum period (Le Gallez 1998).

A significant number of drugs used in the treatment of RA, particularly DMARDs, are known to be teratogenic; their use should be avoided due to the risk of damage to the fetus. This has equal importance for men as women. The recommendation that all DMARDs be stopped prior to conception, and in some cases for up to 6 months, can be devastating information for the patient who wants a child but knows significant deterioration in the control of their disease will be imminent.

Where disease activity is marked and pregnancy desired, low-dose prednisolone of 5–10 mg daily is often safely and effectively utilised.

Paracetamol is the recommended painkiller for use during pregnancy, as aspirin and many combined analgesics are known to cause side effects when taken during the course of pregnancy. NSAIDs are best avoided in early pregnancy, during fetal development and towards the end of the pregnancy as they are associated with delivery and postpartum complications.

All drugs taken by the mother will pass in small amounts into the breast milk, so generally they are avoided. However, some drugs may be taken with caution under medical advice and supervision (Needs & Brooks 1995). X-rays should be avoided throughout the course of pregnancy.

The nurse has an important role to help prepare the parents, psychologically and in practical terms, for the arrival of the baby and the return of the active disease. Early referral to the physiotherapist and occupational therapist will ensure expert assessments are done and appropriate needs met during the pregnancy and delivery and for managing life with RA and a baby.

COMPLICATIONS OF RHEUMATOID ARTHRITIS

Complications of RA are divided into those arising from the disease process and iatrogenic conditions that have arisen as a result of treatment. Three specific and common complications are addressed here: osteoporosis, septic arthritis and amyloidosis.

OSTEOPOROSIS

Rheumatoid arthritis is associated with both localised and generalised osteoporosis.

Local osteoporosis occurs in the juxtaarticular regions, around inflamed joints. It is an early X-ray feature presenting particularly around the small joints of the hand. It results from factors activated by the immune and inflammatory response that stimulate bone resorption.

In the early stage of RA, peripheral bone density loss correlates with disease activity. Bone density scanning has confirmed that generalised osteoporosis is a feature of established disease and can be seen at sites distant from the inflamed joints. It is unclear whether this is the consequence of the effects of RA, such as the level of disease activity and reduced mobility, or is a result of treatment therapies.

Corticosteroid therapy is known to cause generalised osteoporosis in up to 40% of patients, leading to a 25% increase in fractures, particularly in the spine.

SEPTIC ARTHRITIS

People with RA are more susceptible to bacterial joint infections, which require urgent medical care. The most common infecting organism is *Staphylococcus aureus*. The typical signs of joint sepsis are usually monoarticular (rarely polyarticular), redness, heat, swelling, severe tenderness and extreme pain on movement. In active arthritis these typical signs may not be so obvious.

If there is any suspicion of septic arthritis, the joint must be aspirated and the synovial fluid sent for microscopy and culture. It is worth remembering that if the infection has not extended to the joint space, the synovial fluid culture may be negative.

On confirmation of septic arthritis, treatment must begin immediately. Although there is no consensus on the duration of treatment, combined, parenteral antibiotics are recommended for a minimum of 2 weeks, possibly being required for up to 6 weeks, and followed by a further 6 weeks of oral antibiotic therapy.

The joint should be aspirated, and reaspirated as tolerated by the patient, until there is a positive response to treatment and synovial fluid cultures show no bacterial or other organism growth.

The joint is immobilised immediately following confirmation of sepsis and gently remobilised when the symptoms settle. X-rays are often required as a baseline. If the response to treatment is poor, an orthopaedic opinion should be sought. If left untreated, septic arthritis will cause significant joint destruction and can in extreme cases lead to septicaemia and death.

AMYLOIDOSIS

Amyloidosis is a rare complication of long-standing RA, resulting from chronic active inflammation. Almost all organs of the body are potentially involved but the most critical effect is on the kidney. Diagnosis is confirmed by biopsy of rectal or kidney tissue. The presence of amyloidosis indicates a poor prognosis but treatment with cyclophosphamide and chlorambucil can retard disease progression.

PROGNOSIS AND MORBIDITY

Following a diagnosis of RA, there is no accurate means by which its course can be predicted as the outcomes can vary immensely between individual cases. There are certain clinical and diagnostic features associated with a poorer outcome (Box 15.4).

Typically, in 100 people with RA, 25% will have little disability and will go into remission within a few years, 50% will continue to have exacerbations of their disease leading to moderate to severe disability and 25% will have progressive severe disease leading to marked disability. Studies by Silman et al (1983) have suggested that RA patients are less severely affected by the disease now than patients were 50 years ago. Whether this relates to early diagnosis and intervention or changes in the nature of the disease is under investigation.

Multiple studies assessing survival and death rates in RA have confirmed a shortened life expectancy for patients dying of the same causes as the general population, with a reduction of 3 years for women and 7 years for men (Vandenbroucke et al 1984). Higher mortality rates occur among those with more severe disease symptoms and rheumatoid-associated vasculitis. Although uncommon, death is most frequently associated with an infection and complications of drug therapies.

CONCLUSION

Rheumatology nursing in the 21st century is an exciting place to be. Patients are faced with huge personal challenges, which practitioners can only begin to understand. Nurses have much to offer patients in enabling them to regain some feeling of 'self' and in helping them fulfil their potential in terms of everyday life, their aspirations and goals for the future.

As nurses, we have the support of the multidisciplinary team to make important contributions to those under our care. The support and guidance from a variety of national and international professional and patient networks, such as rheumatology nursing forums, the Arthritis and Musculo-skeletal Alliance and specialist expert nurses in the field (Hill 1998, Le Gallez 1998, Ryan 1999), provide nurses with a unique network to learn from and really understand the patients who need their help.

Further reading

Arthritis Research Campaign. Reports on rheumatic diseases
    available at www.arc.org.uk
Doherty M, Hazelman BL, Hutton CW et al 1992
    Rheumatology examination and injection techniques.
    WB Saunders, London
Hart FD, Clarke AK 1993 Clinical problems in rheumatology.
    Dunitz, London

Hill J 1991 Assessing rheumatic disease. Nursing Times
    87(4): 33–35
Hunder GG (ed) 2001 Atlas of rheumatology, 2nd edn.
    Current Medicine, Philadelphia
Klippel JH, Dieppe PA 1998 Rheumatology, 2nd edn. Mosby,
    London

References

Adams JC, Hamblen DL 1990 Outline of orthopaedics,
    11th edn. Churchill Livingstone, Edinburgh

Arnett FC, Edworthy SM, Bloch DA et al 1988 The
    American Rheumatism Association 1987 revised

criteria for the classification of rheumatoid arthritis. Arthritis and Rheumatism 31: 315–324

Arthritis Research Campaign (ARC) 1998 Diet and arthritis. Arthritis Research Campaign, Chesterfield

Arthur V 1998 The role of the nurse specialist in rheumatology. In: Le Gallez P (ed) Rheumatology for nurses: patient care. Whurr, London

Bathon JM, Martin RW, Fleischmann RM et al 2000 A comparison of etanercept and methotrexate in patients with early rheumatoid arthritis. New England Journal of Medicine 343: 1586–1593

British Society for Rheumatology (BSR) 2000 Guidelines for second line drug monitoring. British Society for Rheumatology, London

British Society for Rheumatology (BSR) 2003 Working party guidelines 2003. Revised guidelines for prescribing TNF-alpha blockers in adult rheumatoid arthritis. British Society for Rheumatology, London

Carette S, Marcoux S, Gingras S et al 1989 Postmenopausal hormones and the incidence of rheumatoid arthritis. Journal of Rheumatology 16: 911–913

Cawthorn A, Billington J 1998 Complementary therapeutic interventions. In: Hill J (ed) Rheumatology nursing: a creative approach. Churchill Livingstone, Edinburgh

Charles C, Gafni A, Whelan T 1997 Shared decision making in the medical encounter: what does it mean? Social Science and Medicine 44: 681–692

Creed F, Jayson MV, Murphy S 1990 Measurement of psychiatric disorders in rheumatoid arthritis. Journal of Psychosomatic Research 34(1): 79–87

Dandy DJ, Edwards DJ 2003 Essential orthopaedics and trauma. Churchill Livingstone, Edinburgh

Darlington G, Jump A, Ramsey N 1990 Dietary treatment of rheumatoid arthritis. Practitioner 234(1488): 456–460

Denman AM 1995 Viral aetiology of arthritis. In: Collected reports on rheumatic diseases. Arthritis and Rheumatism Council for Research, Chesterfield

Department of Health (DoH) 2002 Patient and public involvement in the NHS. Department of Health, London

Dieppe PA, Doherty M, MacFarlane D 1985 Rheumatological medicine. Churchill Livingstone, Edinburgh

Drugs and Therapeutics Bulletin 1995 Methotrexate for rheumatoid arthritis. Drugs and Therapeutics Bulletin 33: 17–19

Edmonds J, Hughes G 1985 Lecture notes on rheumatology. Blackwell, Oxford

Egmose C, Lund B, Borg G et al 1995 Patients with rheumatoid arthritis benefit from early 2nd line therapy: 5 year follow up of a prospective double blind placebo controlled study. Journal of Rheumatology 22: 2208–2213

Flasher N 1997 Developing the scope of practice for rheumatology nurse practitioners. Journal of Orthopaedic Nursing 1: 123–126

Greenhalgh T 1994 The interface between junior doctors and nurses: a research study for the Department of Health. Greenhalgh and Co, Macclesfield

Gunn C 1992 Bones and joints, 2nd edn. Churchill Livingstone, Edinburgh

Hench PS 1938 The ameliorating effect of pregnancy on chronic atrophic arthritis, fibrositis and intermittent hydroarthrosis. Proceedings of the Mayo Clinic 13: 136–167

Hickling P, Golding J 1984 An outline of rheumatology. Wright, Bristol

Hill J 1997 Patient satisfaction in a nurse led rheumatology clinic. Journal of Advanced Nursing 25: 347–354

Hill J (ed) 1998 Rheumatology nursing: a creative approach. Churchill Livingstone, Edinburgh

Hill J, Bird HA, Harmer R et al 1994 An evaluation of the effectiveness, safety and acceptability of a nurse practitioner in a rheumatology out-patient clinic. British Journal of Rheumatology 33: 283–288

Holman H 1996 What would ideal care looks like? Invited address. In: Manning FJ, Barondess JA (eds) Changing health care systems and rheumatic diseases. National Academy Press, Washington DC

Hughes J 1983 Footwear and footcare for adults. Disabled Living Foundation, London

Isenberg D, Morrow J 1995 Friendly fire: explaining auto-immune disease. Oxford University Press, Oxford

Jacoby RK, Jayson MIV, Cosh JA 1973 Onset, early stages and prognosis of rheumatoid arthritis: a clinical study of 100 patients with 11 year follow up. British Medical Journal 2: 96–100

Kane WJ 1981 Current orthopaedic management. Churchill Livingstone, Edinburgh

Kirwan JR 1995 The effect of glucocorticoids on joint destruction in rheumatoid arthritis. The Arthritis and Rheumatism Council low-dose glucocorticoid study group. New England Journal of Medicine 338: 142–146

Kragg GR 1989 Clinical aspects in rheumatoid arthritis. Triangle 28(12): 15–24

Lawrence JS 1965 Surveys of rheumatic complaints in the population. In: Dixon A St J (ed) Progress in clinical rheumatology. Churchill Livingstone, London

Le Gallez P 1998 Patient education and self management. In: Le Gallez P (ed) Rheumatology for nurses: patient care. Whurr, London

Maini RN, Breedveld FC, Kalden JR et al 1998 Therapeutic efficacy of multiple intravenous infusions of anti-tumour necrosis factor alpha monoclonal antibody combined with low-dose weekly methotrexate in rheumatoid arthritis. Arthitis and Rheumatism 41: 1552–1563

National Institute for Clinical Excellence (NICE) 2002 Guidance on the use of etanercept and infliximab for the treatment of rheumatoid arthritis. National Institute for Clinical Excellence, London

Needs C, Brooks P 1995 Drugs, pregnancy and rheumatoid arthritis. In: Klippel JH, Dieppe PA (eds) Practical rheumatology. Mosby, London

Newbold D 1996 Coping with rheumatoid arthritis: how may specialist nurses influence it and promote better outcomes? Journal of Clinical Nursing 5: 373–380

Nicholas NS, Panayi GS 1988 Rheumatoid arthritis and pregnancy. Clinical and Experimental Rheumatology 6: 179–182

Patberg WR, Nienhuis RLF, Veringa F 1985 Relation between meteorological factors and pain in rheumatoid arthritis in a marine climate. Journal of Rheumatology 12: 711–715

Pawlson G 1994 Chronic illness: implications of a new paradigm for health care. Journal on Quality Improvement 20: 33–39

Prady J, Vale A, Hill J 1998 Body image and sexuality. In: Hill J (ed) Rheumatology nursing: a creative approach. Churchill Livingstone, Edinburgh

Rasker JJ, Peters HJG, Boon KL 1986 Influence of weather on stiffness and force in patients with rheumatoid arthritis. Scandinavian Journal of Rheumatology 15: 27–36

Royal College of Nursing (RCN) 2000 A charter for rheumatology nursing. Royal College of Nursing, London

Royal College of Nursing (RCN) 2001 Standards for effective practice and audit in rheumatology nursing: guidance for nurses. Royal College of Nursing, London

Royal College of Nursing (RCN) 2003 Assessing, managing and monitoring biologic therapeutics for arthritis. Royal College of Nursing, London

Ryan S 1995 Nutrition and the rheumatology patient. British Journal of Nursing 4(3): 132–136

Ryan S 1998 Psychological aspects. In: Hill J (ed) Rheumatology nursing: a creative approach. Churchill Livingstone, Edinburgh

Ryan S (ed) 1999 Drug therapy in rheumatology nursing. Whurr, London

Silman AJ, Davies P, Currey HLF et al 1983 Is rheumatoid arthritis becoming less severe? Journal of Chronic Diseases 36: 891–897

Smith MD, Ahern MJ, Roberts-Tompson PJ 1990 Pulse methylprednisolone therapy in rheumatoid arthritis, unjustified therapy or effective adjunctive treatment? Annals of Rheumatic Diseases 49: 265–267

Smruti-Riley H 1998 The role of physiotherapy in rheumatology. In: Le Gallez P (ed) Rheumatology for nurses: patient care. Whurr, London

Spector D, Brennan P, Harris P et al 1991 Does oestrogen replacement therapy protect against rheumatoid arthritis? Journal of Rheumatology 18: 1473–1476

Symmonds D 1994 Quantifying progression in arthritis. Topical Reviews: Reports on Rheumatic Diseases, series 3, no 1. Arthritis and Rheumatism Council, Chesterfield

Symmons DPM, Barrett EM, Bankhead C et al 1994 The incidence of rheumatoid arthritis in the United Kingdom: results from the Norfolk arthritis register. British Journal of Rheumatology 33: 735–739

Troman S 1998 The role of the occupational therapist in rheumatology. In: Le Gallez P (ed) Rheumatology for nurses: patient care. Whurr, London

Turner A, Foster M, Johnson SE 1992 Occupational therapy and physical dysfunction, 3rd edn. Churchill Livingstone, Edinburgh

United Kingdom Central Council (UKCC) 1992 Scope of professional practice. United Kingdom Central Council for Nursing, Midwifery and Health Visiting, London

Vandenbroucke JP, Havevoet HM, Cats A 1984 Survival and death in rheumatoid arthritis: a 25 year prospective follow-up. Journal of Rheumatology 11: 158–161

Van Der Heide A, Jacobs JWG, Bijlsma JWJ et al 1996 The effectiveness of early treatment with second line drugs: a randomised, controlled trial. Annals of Internal Medicine 124: 699–707

White CE 1998 Fatigue and sleep. In: Hill J (ed) Rheumatology nursing: a creative approach. Churchill Livingstone, Edinburgh

William DG 1998 Autoantibodies in rheumatoid arthritis. In: Klippel JH, Dieppe PA (eds) Rheumatology, 2nd edn. Mosby, London

Williams GH 1986 Lay beliefs about cases of rheumatoid arthritis; their implications for rehabilitation. Information Rehabilitation Medicine 8: 65–68

Chapter 16

Care of patients with rheumatic diseases

Sharon Church, Michelle Cage

CHAPTER CONTENTS

INTRODUCTION

Rheumatic diseases encompass some 200 different conditions and affect up to 8 million people in the United Kingdom alone (Arthritis and Musculoskeletal Alliance 2002).

People present at outpatient clinics with a spectrum of problems ranging from a transient, localised and self-limiting episode of tendonitis resulting from injury to the many inflammatory arthritides which can lead to chronic pain and reduced function, affecting mobility, increasing dependence on others and often accompanied by extraarticular features, systemic illness and altered body image.

Historically, many who suffered from the pain and disability of rheumatic conditions sought and received help only after the damage was done. Lasting impressions from the days when people 'had to learn to live with' their conditions do still exist today and many misconceptions about the lack of medical treatment and care available sadly still influence some people's ideas.

Long periods of inpatient care in spa-like surroundings have been replaced with care based largely in the community and outpatient settings. Similarly drug treatment for rheumatic conditions has almost turned on its head, with more potent medications now being used early in an attempt to arrest the disease process, rather than being reserved until simpler drugs had failed in a futile chase after the progressing symptoms and destruction. The recognition that early arthritis clinics play a major role in preventing morbidity (Emery & Salmon 1995) and the role of technology in providing more specific tests to enable an accurate diagnosis have led to the appearance of a higher incidence of rheumatic disease. In fact, problems are being identified that were previously unrecognised so early in the disease picture.

The conditions presented here are some of those encountered by specialist nurses in the outpatients department. Following initial consultations and diagnosis by a rheumatologist, the specialist nurses manage many of these patients, with medical support when required.

Nursing has pioneered in its move away from the medical-physiological model to one more aligned to addressing patients' needs. The specialist nurse faces challenges and situations that require knowledge and skills from nursing, medicine and other allied professions. For example, it may not be sufficient for the nurse to observe that a patient has a rash and to advise on skin care. Knowledge is needed about possible causes of rashes, which may include an adverse reaction to a medication, the pathology of the condition or a presenting feature of a hitherto undiagnosed condition. The ability to recognise the need for appropriate investigations, changes in medication or referral to other members of the multidisciplinary team is a necessary requisite.

The approach of this chapter is not therefore intended to be a departure from patient-centred care, but rather seeks to equip the nurse with the basics of each condition, in order that the patient's needs can be anticipated and dealt with knowledgeably and sensitively. We are not advocating that the nurse assumes the role of the physician, merely that nurse and patient together assess features and amass evidence for a proposed plan of care. Of paramount importance in this approach to care is that nurses have a sound awareness of their own limitations and recognise personal accountability (NMC 2002).

THE SERONEGATIVE SPONDYLARTHROPATHIES

The classification of the seronegative spondylarthropathies depends on the presenting clinical features. Initially the person may present with back pain but to avoid diagnosing a simple back strain, careful elimination of the relevance of any accompanying features is essential (Box 16.1).

Concomitant features to which the sufferer may not attach any relevance can include things such as oral or genital ulceration or inflammation of the eyes. These symptoms, along with sacroiliitis, may indicate Behçet's syndrome (Guillevin 2001). Similarly, a triad

---

Box 16.1   Classification criteria for seronegative spondylarthropathy (European Spondylarthropathy Study Group cited by Olivieri et al 2002)

Either   inflammatory spinal pain
Or   synovitis (asymmetric or predominantly in the lower limbs)

Plus one or more of the following
- Positive family history
- Psoriasis
- Inflammatory bowel disease
- Urethritis, cervicitis or acute diarrhoea occurring within the month before the onset of arthritis
- Alternate buttock pain
- Enthesopathy
- Sacroiliitis

---

of symptoms of polyarthritis, conjunctivitis and non-specific urethritis could constitute Reiter's syndrome (Olivieri et al 2002).

Examination of the patient must include a careful look at the degree of spinal involvement, areas of stiffness, pain and observing the ranges of movement; flexion, extension, side flexion, rotation and chest expansion. In addition, examination for tender or swollen peripheral joints is necessary.

Useful diagnostic markers include radiographic investigations using plain X-ray films and radio-isotope bone scans and where involvement of the gastrointestinal tract is suspected, barium studies are valuable.

Of the blood tests available, baseline measures of full blood count, haemoglobin, liver function, urea and electrolytes and a measure of inflammation such as erythrocyte sedimentation rate (ESR) or C-reactive protein (CRP) are required. Tissue typing is also useful; for example, there is a strong association between HLA B27 and ankylosing spondylitis. The serology referred to when stating that a person's status is seronegative is the absence of rheumatoid factor.

Management of the spondylarthropathies is mainly based on the use of non-steroidal anti-inflammatory drugs (NSAIDs), to help relieve symptoms of pain and stiffness. Where signs of disease are more severe, then disease-modifying antirheumatic drugs (DMARDs) can be an additional choice of treatment. Antibiotics may also feature if infection is an element, as in Reiter's syndrome.

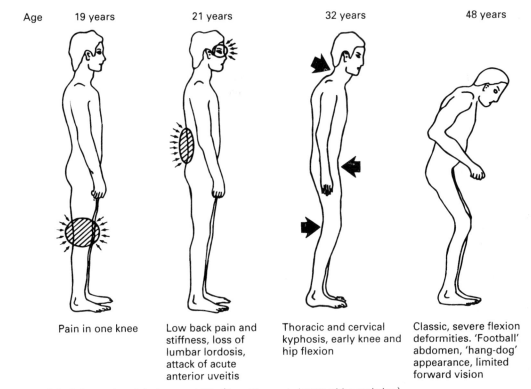

| Age | 19 years | 21 years | 32 years | 48 years |

Pain in one knee

Low back pain and stiffness, loss of lumbar lordosis, attack of acute anterior uveitis

Thoracic and cervical kyphosis, early knee and hip flexion

Classic, severe flexion deformities. 'Football' abdomen, 'hang-dog' appearance, limited forward vision

Figure 16.1   Spinal changes in ankylosing spondylitis. (From Dieppe et al 1985 with permission.)

Education, information, monitoring of the condition itself, how it affects the individual and the effects of medication are fundamental to the nursing support required in the care of people with these inflammatory conditions. Referral to a physiotherapist to assist in maintaining a good range of movement throughout the spine and affected joints is paramount in keeping patients as active and independent as possible. Patients often seek reassurance from the nurse that exercise is essential and not harmful.

ANKYLOSING SPONDYLITIS

Probably the one seronegative arthropathy that most nurses could name is ankylosing spondylitis (AS). Photographs of sufferers of end-stage disease with hunched and rigid back deformities (Fig. 16.1) and pictures of X-rays showing 'bamboo spine' will be familiar to many readers.

Given that patients today have access to information via the Internet, clear explanation of their diagnosis is essential to avoid them becoming misinformed about what may lie ahead.

Ankylosing spondylitis occurs in all areas of the world but race-related differences exist. Men are affected more commonly than women; 1 in 200 men and 1 in 500 women (National Ankylosing Spondylitis Society 2000). The age of presentation is young adults, at an average of 24 years. There are strong familial and genetic features.

Presentation

This is a chronic inflammatory arthritis affecting primarily the axial skeleton, with enthesitis (inflammation at the point of insertion of tendon into bone), sacroiliitis and synovitis of peripheral joints (Fig. 16.2).

Erosions occur at the sites of enthesitis and this is evident as 'squaring' of the vertebrae on X-ray. As the bones begin to heal, osteophytes form at the corners of the vertebrae, which can then bridge together to form syndesmophytes (Fig. 16.3). At the same time, inflammation can occur in the apophyseal joints of the spine, whilst interspinous ligaments are liable to calcification. All of these features lead to rigidity and fusion of the sections of the vertebral column

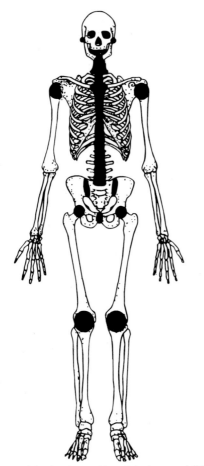

Figure 16.2   Joint involvement in ankylosing spondylitis. (From Dieppe et al 1985 with permission.)

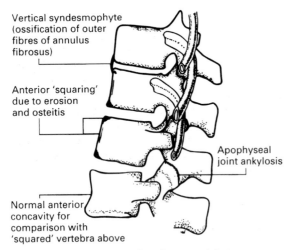

Vertical syndesmophyte (ossification of outer fibres of annulus fibrosus)

Anterior 'squaring' due to erosion and osteitis

Apophyseal joint ankylosis

Normal anterior concavity for comparison with 'squared' vertebra above

Figure 16.3   Classic progression of severe ankylosing spondylitis. (From Dieppe et al 1985 with permission.)

affected. Loss of lumbar lordosis and extension at the hip are also seen. Chest expansion can be impaired in advanced disease.

Ninety percent of white people affected will have a positive blood test for HLA-B27 (human leukocyte antigen). This differs between races but in most cases, a diagnosis of ankylosing spondylitis can be confirmed without this investigation. Other diagnostic tests include ESR, FBC, weight-bearing X-rays of the spine, pelvis and hips, a CT or MRI scan for clearer visualisation or differentiation of tissues involved.

Insidious onset of pain and stiffness in the back, sacroiliac region and hip are the first presentations. Symptoms do not improve with rest but are relieved by exercise. Inactivity then brings about a return of symptoms, particularly early morning stiffness. Fatigue and disturbed sleep are common.

Synovitis of peripheral joints such as the shoulder, knee or ankle can occur, leading to pain, stiffness, loss of range of movement and subsequently functional impairment. The need for total hip replacement within 20 years of disease onset is greater in those who experience juvenile onset. Temporomandibular joints may also be involved.

Eye involvement in the form of uveitis occurs in up to 30% of cases at some point in their disease; it is more common in HLA-B27 positive cases.

Treatment and care

Whilst there is no cure for ankylosing spondylitis, most patients' symptoms can be well controlled with the use of NSAIDs. If finding an NSAID that is efficacious enough proves difficult, there is still a role for the use of phenylbutazone, a drug previously removed from the formulary in view of adverse reactions seen in some patients. In the UK, this can be prescribed on a named-patient basis by the consultant rheumatologist.

Disease-modifying antirheumatic drugs (DMARDs), such as salazopyrin, are used when peripheral arthritis is involved. Injection of individual inflammatory lesions with steroid preparations may be helpful in some cases.

Physiotherapy plays an important role in teaching an exercise regime to preserve posture, strength and movement. Deep breathing exercises are taught. Swimming is a favourable form of exercise in this condition and where available, hydrotherapy may prove invaluable. In order to ensure adherence to vital exercise regimes, education and information are needed for the patient to understand their importance.

Occupational therapy referral can help to address postural influences such as seating, sleeping and working environments as well as assisting with individuals' daily living difficulties and joint protection measures.

Collaboration with orthopaedic teams may be needed.

PSORIASIS-ASSOCIATED ARTHRITIS

The word 'psoriasis' is derived from the Greek *psora*, meaning to itch. It was once believed that psoriasis-associated arthritis (PsA) was the chance occurrence of two relatively common disorders: psoriasis and a specific form of arthritis. However, over the last 50 years, concepts of the disease have evolved as a result of epidemiological and clinical investigations to suggest that PsA is a unique arthropathy, rather than the coincident occurrence of two common diseases (O'Neil & Silman 1994).

Epidemiology

The population prevalence of PsA is in the region of 2–10 per 10 000 although this is probably an underestimate as those with sacroiliac involvement only are not included. PsA is slightly more common in women than men, possibly due to hormonal factors, with a peak onset in the fourth decade of life. Between the ages of 36 and 45 more men are affected (O'Neil & Silman 1994).

PsA has been shown to be associated with the human leukocyte antigen (HLA) which explains the familial pattern of the disease. Environmental factors are also likely to play a role as predisposing factors, along with infection (Eastmond 1994).

In the majority of cases (75%), psoriasis precedes the joint disease. The arthritis then has an acute onset. More commonly affected are the distal interphalangeal joints, showing erosive changes, with nail involvement (Helliwell & Wright 1995).

In PsA the arthritis is due to the synovial membrane becoming thickened and inflamed, with an increase in synovial fluid. As the inflammation spreads to the joint cartilage, the outcome is erosion of the joint surfaces. The tendons are also lined with, and lubricated by, a synovial membrane which can become inflamed, causing painful soft tissue lesions.

The skin psoriasis is characterised by hyperproliferation of the epidermis, associated with increased tortuosity of the dermal blood vessels and an inflammatory cell infiltrate. The psoriasis can present as chronic plaques, gluttae or pustular lesions (Troughton & Morgan 1994).

Clinical features

Apart from the psoriasis and arthritis, fatigue is a common and recognised symptom associated with increased levels of inflammation. Patients need to be advised that their diet should include five servings of fresh fruit and vegetables per day, along with oily fish and foods rich in vitamin B, which all may help them to feel less exhausted. Tadman (2003) summarises some of the facts and fallacies surrounding diet and arthritis and may be a useful text for patients making initial enquiries into the subject. Minimising stress and regular gentle exercise also help reduce fatigue.

Ocular involvement can be seen in PsA in the form of conjunctivitis, requiring eyedrops which the nurse can teach patients to use effectively.

Dactylitis or 'sausage digits' is another feature of PsA, where swelling and pitting oedema are found in the distal extremities (Helliwell & Wright 1995). A rare form of PsA affecting the hands is arthritis mutilans, which can be very deforming. Patients can find this unsightly and distressing. The nurse will need to advise about treatment options and counsel on changes in body image to assist the patient to cope (Le Gallez 1998).

Enthesitis is inflammation at the attachments of tendons and ligaments to bone. Particularly common sites in PsA include the insertion of the Achilles tendon into the calcaneum and plantar fasciitis beneath the heel. Spondylitis affecting the spinal column itself may also be regarded as an example of multiple enthesitic sites (Helliwell & Wright 1995). When enthesitis occurs, patients are advised to rest the inflamed areas and take regular analgesia. Topical applications of NSAIDs may provide some relief. Depending on the site, the soft tissues are injected locally with corticosteroid to help reduce the swelling and pain, for example in plantar fasciitis. Reducing inflammation is important to minimise the risk of rupture of any tendons involved in the proximity of inflammation.

Several investigations used in the diagnosis of PsA are shown in Box 16.2.

Treatment and nursing care

Management of PsA depends largely on the presenting symptoms in each individual. As with

> **Box 16.2   Investigations used in the diagnosis of psoriatic arthritis (PsA)**
>
> - Rheumatoid factor: this is almost always negative but a positive factor does not rule out PsA
> - ESR and CRP: the acute-phase response increases with disease activity
> - Plain film X-rays: possible features observed include erosions, ankylosis of one or more joints, 'pencil-in-cup' deformity
> - Isotope imaging: abnormal uptake can be seen at affected sites

rheumatoid arthritis, early initiation of appropriate interventions may prevent development of joint deformity and its sequelae. Please refer to Chapter 15 for specific nursing management of joint inflammation.

Initial therapeutic management involves the use of NSAIDs. If the disease is progressing and musculoskeletal changes are occurring with a lack of response to NSAIDs, disease-modifying agents are required rapidly. Again the nurse provides education and information for the patient about the drugs of choice along with monitoring of efficacy and any adverse effects through the nurse-led clinics.

Emotional support for those facing changes in the integrity of their scalp and skin is an important aspect of care. Referral to the dermatology department may be pertinent.

In the presence of active synovitis, a balance between rest and activity is needed and opportunities for this need to be explored by the patient and nurse. Le Gallez (1998) explains how tasks which the individual needs to carry out at home, at work and in leisure pursuits need to be planned, paced and prioritised. Referral to the occupational therapy department can assist with difficulties the individual experiences now, as well as helping to anticipate and offer preventive advice against future problems.

Exercises taught by physiotherapists, with their importance reinforced by the nurse, include stretching movements to maintain the joint range, followed by strengthening exercises as synovitis resolves. The use of splints will help to preserve function and alignment of joints. Surgery may be indicated in the form of a synovectomy or total joint arthroplasty. Special attention to preoperative skin condition and preparation is paramount, as patients with PsA are more likely to develop an infection (Espinoza & Cuellar 1995).

Whilst disability is generally less severe than in rheumatoid arthritis, significant limitations occur for around 11% of sufferers. The nurse should be involved with the multidisciplinary team in the initiation of an early, comprehensive programme of care.

THE VASCULITIDES

There are many inflammatory vascular diseases, all characterised by inflammation within or through the vessel wall, resulting in damage to blood flow and sometimes to vessel integrity (Lightfoot 1995).

During 1988–1994 the Norwich Health Authority estimated an annual incidence of all the systemic vasculitides to be 8.5 per million population, the ratio of 2:1 men to women, commonly occurring after the age of 40 (Carruthers et al 1996).

The vasculitides present difficulties for many different specialties. Their impact on healthcare resources is out of proportion to their incidence, as patients are usually severely ill and often require intensive inpatient and follow-up care (Chakravarty & Scott 1993).

First described in the early 19th century, the vasculitides are described as occurring rarely. However, recent studies indicate that they are on the increase due to:

- the development of comprehensive classification of the vasculitides
- availability of investigations, especially the antinuclear cytoplasmic antigen (ANCA) test
- increased understanding and recognition of the various vasculitides (Chakravarty & Scott 1993).

WEGENER'S GRANULOMATOSIS

Wegener's granulomatosis (WG) presents as a triad of necrotising vasculitis of the upper and lower respiratory tract, associated with granuloma formation and glomerulonephritis. The aetiology is not as yet entirely understood but in the last 30 years much has been learned about a disease once deemed fatal. From a prognosis of 80% of sufferers dying within 1 year, this has now dramatically improved with the use of immunosuppressive drugs to a survival rate of 80% at 5 years, of which 93% will have complete remission 4 years after diagnosis (Hoffman & Fauci 1995).

Due to the increased use of immunosuppressive agents and the subsequent monitoring and follow-up care required, nurses are becoming increasingly involved in the care of those with WG.

The therapeutic goal of drug management is to reduce mortality. The initiation of early treatment is vital due to the potential for tissue destruction. Initially the nurse will monitor the patient's progress as they commence doses of immunosuppressive drugs high enough to induce a remission. The drug of choice to induce early remission is cyclophosphamide (Chakravarty & Scott 1993). The doses are reduced once the patient reaches a remission phase. Immunosuppressive agents may then be changed for a less potentially toxic DMARD, such as azathioprine, to aid the patient with maintenance of health.

Relapse in WG is common and the nurse must continue vigilance so that if this occurs immunosuppressive medications can be recommended. Patients need support from the nurse as they have to make choices between long-term drug therapy and the risk of relapse if they withdraw from treatment.

The nature of WG means that it can impose on family life, particularly if the affected person is the main wage earner for the family. Nursing care therefore includes addressing considerable psychological as well as physical needs. Counselling skills form part of the nurse's role but awareness of one's limitations and knowing when to call on more expert help are essential. The nurse can impart knowledge of practicalities such as financial help for which the patient may be entitled to apply, as well as assistance in completing application forms.

Pathology

Wegener's granulomatosis is characterised by:

- aseptic granulomatous necrosis of the upper or lower respiratory tract, or both
- small vessel vasculitis usually selectively in organs such as lungs and kidney
- focal segmental glomerulonephritis.

Clinical features

The main features focus on the respiratory tract, the lungs and the kidneys (Box 16.3). It is important that the patient is aware of the symptoms caused by their disease, as often they may not realise they are connected to WG. For example, mouth ulcers are a common problem but are also aggravated by the treatment. Patients are advised to use a regular mouthwash to reduce the discomfort and often the

---

Box 16.3   Patient's symptoms in Wegener's granulomatosis

Respiratory tract	Nasal crusting/blocking
	Epistaxis
	Weakened nose bridge (saddle deformity)
	Sinusitis
	Rhinorrhoea
	Nasal ulceration
Lungs	Shortness of breath
	Cough
	Chest pain
	Haemoptysis
Kidneys	Asymptomatic

---

doses of treatments are lowered if the ulceration is severe.

Education for patients and provision of information is again an essential nursing role, as an effective way of changing patients' knowledge, behaviour, psychological and health status. It is well illustrated by research that patients are able to cope more effectively with the outcomes of disease when they know and understand what is happening (Hill et al 1994).

The patient needs to be aware of the importance of their symptoms in relation to disease activity. For example, fatigue is a common and difficult problem for patients and the nurse can explain the importance of rest and provide reassurance that the fatigue will diminish as the disease activity reduces (Le Gallez 1998).

The investigations for Wegener's granulomatosis are shown in Table 16.1.

Specific nursing care

It is essential to realise that in the early stages of WG, patients are unable to cope with excessive amounts of information as they come to terms with the diagnosis (Le Gallez 1998). With the use of a carefully planned care package, the patient will gradually receive all the information needed regarding their condition and the need for continued monitoring in case of relapse.

The use of validated assessment tools provides objective information regarding each individual's progress and allows for planning of future care and treatment. The recorded values can provide a useful visual representation of changes over time.

Table 16.1   Investigations for Wegener's granulomatosis

Investigation	Potential findings
Full blood count	Low haemoglobin, raised white cell count, platelets raised
C-reactive protein	Positive and raised
ESR	Raised
Rheumatoid factor	Occasionally positive
ANCA	Positive
Plain film X-rays of chest and sinuses	Presence of nodules, fixed infiltrates or cavities
Urinalysis by routine dipstick testing	Haematuria and proteinuria If these are present urgent investigation should be carried out to determine the extent of renal involvement
Biochemistry of renal function	Raised levels of urea and electrolytes
24-hour urine collection	Raised creatinine and raised protein
Biopsy of tissues: nasal, lung, muscle, renal	Evidence of granulomatous inflammation, tissue necrosis, necrotising vasculitis or necrotising lesions

When diagnosed, patients face the prospect of potentially lifelong disease, the beginning of many hospital visits, tests and the start of potentially toxic treatments. These changes can have a huge impact on a person's ability to cope and the nurse is ideally placed as a point of contact to provide support where needed. Accessibility via telephone helplines and nurse-led clinics are important facets of care.

Treatment with immunosuppressive agents is used to manage disease outcome but individual patient's problems need to be addressed as they arise. Consideration of the asymptomatic features of WG should always be remembered, with routine urinalysis imperative at every hospital visit (Chakravarty & Scott 1993).

GIANT CELL ARTERITIS

Giant cell arteritis and polymyalgia rheumatica are closely related conditions, with the two forming a spectrum of disease affecting the same patient population and frequently occurring together. The nurse's clinical knowledge leads to vigilance in looking for new or changing symptoms which, if detected, enable speedy intervention should giant cell arteritis be suspected.

Patients should be encouraged to always report any alteration in symptoms, particularly those with rheumatoid arthritis or polymyalgia rheumatica who experience any of the symptoms described below.

Headaches are common, with 65% of giant cell arteritis patients experiencing them. They may be severe temporal or less well-defined occipital headaches. Scalp tenderness can be precipitated by brushing hair and may be enough to disturb sleep. Examination reveals tenderness over the temporal or occipital arteries, which can become thickened and nodular, with pulses often reduced or absent.

Visual disturbances occur, with eye problems in this group of patients being an ophthalmic emergency because blindness may follow but is preventable. Visual loss is sudden, painless and permanent, with the second eye becoming involved if treatment is not rapid. Whilst 25–50% of sufferers will experience visual disturbances, blindness is rare and occurs in less than 10% of patients due to early detection and treatment. Blindness does not usually occur as a presenting feature of giant cell arteritis as it is preceded by other symptoms by several weeks.

Pain on chewing food affects two-thirds of patients with giant cell arteritis. It is due to claudication of the muscles of mastication, resulting from vascular insufficiency. Tingling of the tongue, loss of taste and pain around the throat or mouth also occur.

Clinical diagnosis is based on temporal pain, tender thickening of the temporal artery with the loss of the pulse, scalp tenderness and the presence of a very high ESR. Where the diagnosis is in doubt, a temporal artery biopsy is carried out. Physicians vary greatly in their reliance on biopsy results but delaying steroid therapy to wait for histological reporting is unnecessary, as treatment is unlikely to change if the symptoms persist.

The treatment of giant cell arteritis is by administration of steroids. High doses are initiated during the presence of clinical signs and patients' symptoms. DMARDs such as methotrexate may enable later reduction in doses to succeed without relapse.

POLYMYALGIA RHEUMATICA

Polymyalgia rheumatica is a common condition. It occurs in women twice as often as men, affecting people aged between 50 and 90 years but occurring most commonly in those over 70 years (Hazelman 1995). The incidence is reported as 28–53 per 10 000 of the population over 50 years.

Polymyalgia rheumatica can occur on its own or as part of a broader picture of rheumatic disease. For example, it may be the presenting feature of rheumatoid arthritis. It can also occur in patients who have had rheumatoid arthritis for some years or it may be a precursor of giant cell arteritis.

The onset may be insidious, creeping up on the sufferer, or a person may describe having gone to bed feeling well but being unable to rise from the bed on waking in the morning. In both cases, constitutional symptoms of anorexia, weight loss, fatigue and depression may be concomitant features.

SYMPTOMS OF POLYMYALGIA RHEUMATICA

Eliciting descriptions from the patient about their symptoms is an important part of the nurse's assessment in the clinic setting. If the questions asked by the nurse are not detailed enough or if patients are not very forthcoming about how they are feeling, then changes in the nature of a person's pain may be missed and significant new features overlooked.

The use of a pain measurement tool such as the McGill Pain Questionnaire (Melzack 1975), which uses descriptive terms for pain, may elicit changes over a period of time, while more simple measures such as visual analogue scores (Arthur 1998a) change more rapidly. Assessments of functional ability, for example health assessment questionnaires (Fries et al 1980), can illustrate the changes resulting from polymyalgia rheumatica.

Pain and stiffness at night is an ongoing problem, with stiffness at any time of day being more severe following rest. Polymyalgia rheumatica typically affects the shoulder and pelvic girdle, with a symmetrical presentation. Predominantly there are muscular aches and pain, which can reach quite disabling degrees.

Whilst movement of the limbs is difficult due to accentuated pain, muscle strength is not usually impaired. Raising the arms can be so difficult as to render the patient dependent on others for tasks such as washing, dressing, tending to oral hygiene, hair brushing and even eating. Involvement of the pelvic girdle makes climbing stairs, rising from chairs, walking and driving difficult.

If there is a delay in making a diagnosis, physiological restriction of joint movement can occur due to secondary capsulitis. Whilst both axial and peripheral joint synovitis occur, these are usually transient, non-erosive and non-deforming but cause problems for the patient nonetheless.

DIAGNOSIS

A provisional diagnosis can often be made accurately on the history given by the patient and by the clinical findings on examination.

A major diagnostic feature of polymyalgia rheumatica is that the ESR is usually grossly elevated, often 100 mm/h or higher. In some cases, however, a normal ESR is present. Liver and thyroid function tests sometimes detect abnormalities and anaemia can occur.

Confounding the evidence is the muscle pain and stiffness along with the constitutional symptoms and raised ESR. This calls for the exclusion of several differential diagnoses including rheumatoid arthritis, osteoarthritis, connective tissue disease, multiple myeloma, hypothyroidism and malignancy (Dasgupta & Kalk 2000).

PATIENT MANAGEMENT

The treatment for polymyalgia rheumatica is corticosteroids. Response is rapid and remarkable. In fact, a poor response should prompt a second look at the diagnosis. Steroid dosage is titrated to symptomatic control and reduced as the ESR begins to fall. Hazelman (1995) states that studies of practice indicate that most physicians prescribe 10–20 mg prednisolone daily to treat polymyalgia rheumatica. Dasgupta & Kalk (2000) advocate intramuscular methylprednisolone administered at 3-weekly intervals in doses of 120 mg, this being as efficacious as oral regimes and may also procure more benefit in terms of reducing the incidence of adverse effects of steroid usage. Other advantages include increased compliance in administration and avoidance of self-adjustment of doses.

Continued management of patients taking steroids for polymyalgia rheumatica is by the patient's general practitioner or the specialist nurse.

Advice on optimising calcium and vitamin D intake, by both dietary and supplementary methods, is an important preventive measure in caring for any group of people requiring significant amounts of steroid therapy because of the potential risk of osteoporosis. The British National Formulary (BNF 2002) describes 7.5 mg or more of prednisolone over a 3-month period or more as amounting to a significant risk for bone density loss. Bone mineral density scans are done to provide both baseline and follow-up measurements. Options for prevention or treatment of loss of bone density should be discussed and include stopping smoking, taking weight-bearing exercise and treatments such as hormone replacement and bisphosphonates. For further information on bone loss and osteoporosis, see Chapter 19.

Regular patient assessment and observation for adverse effects related to the medication (BNF 2002), function and reports by the patient of any remission or relapse of their symptoms are essential along with monthly monitoring of ESR levels. The results of these will determine any adjustment to the drug dosage.

Hazelman (1995) states that the consensus from available studies into the duration of treatment required suggests that cessation of treatment is feasible from 2 years onwards. The primary consideration is to balance the risk of relapse with the risk of unwanted side effects from therapy.

Where dose reduction is difficult to achieve because of relapsing disease, then DMARDs such as methotrexate or azathioprine may have a steroid-sparing effect. In some cases long-term daily maintenance doses of 2.5–5 mg of steroid orally per day are required.

FIBROMYALGIA SYNDROME

Fibromyalgia syndrome is a term for a collection of symptoms, predominantly affecting women between the ages of 25 and 45 years. A study by Wolfe et al (1995) indicated that 3.4% of women are affected compared to only 0.5% of men.

Patients present with pain and tenderness over various sites, known as hyperalgesic sites. The pain is usually widespread and symmetrical, commonly affecting both upper and lower limbs and the base of the skull (Fig. 16.4). Pain and tenderness may affect any region and can indeed be felt all over.

Fatigue is a common symptom, associated with poor sleep patterns and tiredness on waking. The degree of fatigue is described as extreme, even after minimal exertion. Other presenting features include poor concentration, forgetfulness and feeling in a low mood and irritable. These symptoms increase the levels of stress experienced by sufferers and impair the ability to cope with daily living activities.

Fibromyalgia and chronic widespread pain syndromes are thought to be examples of somatisation (Bergman 2003). Somatisation is the expression of an emotional event as a bodily disorder.

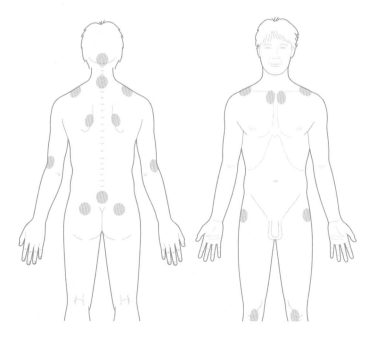

Figure 16.4 Sites of tender points in fibromyalgia.

All tests carried out, including radiological investigations, are performed purely to exclude differential diagnoses. As test results are almost always within normal range, a diagnosis is made on clinical findings; that is, the presence of excessive pain at the hyperalgesic points when firm pressure is applied. There is an absence of such sensitivity at the forehead, distal forearm and lateral fibula head.

The outlook of fibromyalgia is poor. The symptoms can persist for many years with little or no relief, making education for the sufferer and their family of utmost importance (Arthur 1998b). Reassurance that there is no serious underlying pathology will be called for and may be difficult for patients to believe.

Education and information are of more benefit than analgesics or antiinflammatory drugs, which often provide little if any relief. Encouraging the patient to undertake a physical exercise programme is beneficial for loosening tight paravertebral areas and increasing fitness levels. A warning that new exercise regimes may initially exacerbate symptoms should be given along with reassurance that this will settle and that exercise should be persevered with. Increased levels of activity should also aid sleep.

Achieving good-quality sleep can be a major problem requiring the use of tricyclic antidepressants. The aim is to improve the quality of sleep and influence the mechanisms of pain.

Supporting and empowering the patient to adopt a self-help approach will permit the patient to take control of their symptoms and to take positive action to improve things for themselves.

SYSTEMIC LUPUS ERYTHEMATOSUS

Lupus is a broad term covering several conditions.

- **Systemic lupus erythematosus (SLE)** is the most common and will be looked at in more detail here.
- **Discoid lupus** affects primarily the skin, causing a red, raised rash, predominantly but not exclusively found on the face.
- **Drug-induced lupus** is caused by medications. The symptoms are similar to those in SLE but disappear following cessation of the causative agent.
- **Neonatal lupus** can affect newborn babies of women who have SLE. These babies can have serious heart defects, skin rash, liver abnormalities or blood dyscrasia. Neonatal

lupus is very rare but requires prompt treatment at birth.

Systemic lupus erythematosus is a complex autoimmune disease of unknown aetiology. It is likely that rather than a single cause, there are a combination of genetic, environmental and possibly hormonal factors working together to cause the disease.

It is most common in women, with a ratio of 9:1 women to men. There are three times more black women affected than white. The age of onset is the child-bearing years, which suggests a hormonal element to the pathogenesis.

This inflammatory multisystem disease has diverse clinical and laboratory manifestations, with a variable course and prognosis. Immunological abnormalities give rise to excessive autoantibody production, some of which cause cellular damage, whilst others participate in immune inflammation (Edberg et al 1995).

Various organ systems are affected, either singly or in any combination. Figure 16.5 illustrates the clinical features; this gives the basis of the range of patients' problems.

INVESTIGATIONS

Diagnosis can be difficult and many months may pass before all the symptoms can be pieced together to form an accurate diagnosis.

There are some useful tests to aid diagnosis, including the presence of certain autoantibodies in the blood. The antinuclear antibody (ANA) is the most common, with the majority of SLE patients testing positive to this. Some drugs, infections and other diseases also produce positive ANA results, therefore individual types of antibody specific to SLE need to be tested for. These include:

- anti-DNA antibody
- anti-SM antibody
- anti-RNP antibody
- anti-Ro antibody
- anti-La antibody.

Not everyone with SLE will have positive tests. Other useful tests are shown in Table 16.2.

PATIENT MANAGEMENT

The medical treatment of SLE depends on the symptoms of the individual person. There is no

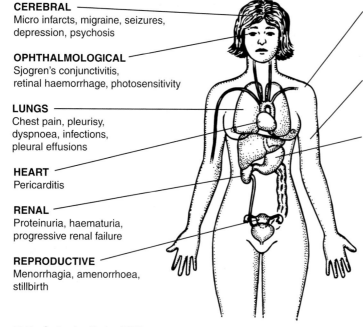

CEREBRAL
Micro infarcts, migraine, seizures, depression, psychosis

OPHTHALMOLOGICAL
Sjogren's conjunctivitis, retinal haemorrhage, photosensitivity

LUNGS
Chest pain, pleurisy, dyspnoea, infections, pleural effusions

HEART
Pericarditis

RENAL
Proteinuria, haematuria, progressive renal failure

REPRODUCTIVE
Menorrhagia, amenorrhoea, stillbirth

DERMATOLOGICAL
Butterfly rash, purpuric lesions, vasculitic skin lesion, alopecia

MUSCULOSKELETAL
Arthralgia/arthritis, myalgia, tenosynovitis

GASTROINTESTINAL
Anorexia, nausea and vomiting, diarrhoea, abdominal pain, hepatomegaly

HAEMATOLOGICAL
Anaemia, thrombocytopenia, abnormal auto-antibodies

NON-SPECIFIC FEATURES
Lymphadenopathy, splenomegaly, Raynaud's phenomenon, alopecia

Figure 16.5 Systemic effects of SLE.

Table 16.2 Investigations for systemic lupus erythematosus

Investigation	Result
ESR	Raised as part of acute-phase response and presence of inflammation
Complement levels	Reduced in active disease
FBC	Low haemoglobin and low platelet count
Urinalysis	Proteinuria and haematuria
Skin biopsy	Histological changes compatible with lupus
ANA	Positive in the majority of cases
Other autoantibodies: anti-DNA, anti-SM, anti-RNP, anti-Ro and anti-La	Variable results in individuals

cure so management concentrates on suppressing the activity of the disease. Analgesics and NSAIDS are useful in controlling symptoms. When a patient has a severe flare-up of the disease, steroids, DMARDs and cytotoxic drugs are used along with close monitoring of symptoms and response, which may or may not require inpatient care.

Nurses will encounter patients with SLE in a variety of clinical areas due to the homogenous nature of the disease. This includes rheumatology, general medicine, dermatology, orthopaedic and neurology nursing practice areas. Wherever the patient is cared for, there are three core components to their nursing care.

1 Monitoring the disease activity is achieved by using validated tools such as tender and swollen joint counts (Thompson & Kirwan 1995) and health assessment questionnaires (Fries et al 1980). These are useful indications of progress or relapse of symptoms.

2 Education is vital in any long-term illness. Awareness of the relationship between stress and flares in disease activity will assist patients to optimise their health chances. Advice on balancing activity with periods of rest, the importance of exercise, recognising the warning signs of a flare, such as increased fatigue, pain, rash, fever, headaches or dizziness, are all important in helping the patient to develop a coping strategy and to secure timely attention to problems.

3 Psychological support is a major requirement for SLE patients. Nurses can provide support and encouragement and, following training, are able to employ expert counselling skills. Empowerment of patients, family and carers enables better compliance

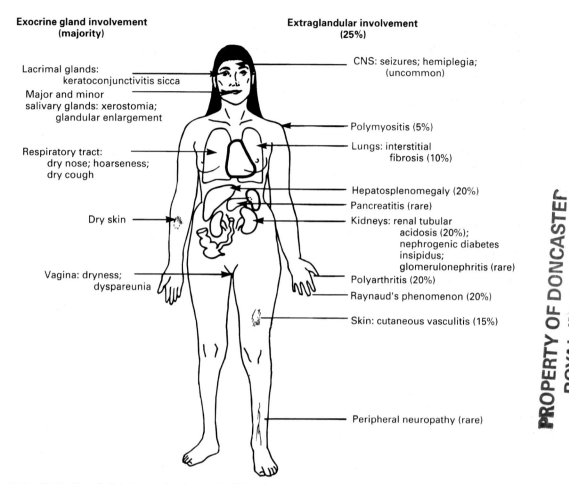

Exocrine gland involvement (majority)

Lacrimal glands: keratoconjunctivitis sicca

Major and minor salivary glands: xerostomia; glandular enlargement

Respiratory tract: dry nose; hoarseness; dry cough

Dry skin

Vagina: dryness; dyspareunia

Extraglandular involvement (25%)

CNS: seizures; hemiplegia; (uncommon)

Polymyositis (5%)

Lungs: interstitial fibrosis (10%)

Hepatosplenomegaly (20%)

Pancreatitis (rare)

Kidneys: renal tubular acidosis (20%); nephrogenic diabetes insipidus; glomerulonephritis (rare)

Polyarthritis (20%)

Raynaud's phenomenon (20%)

Skin: cutaneous vasculitis (15%)

Peripheral neuropathy (rare)

Figure 16.6 Distribution of clinical organ involvement in Sjögren's syndrome.

and personal control over their lifestyle and management regimes.

OTHER CONNECTIVE TISSUE DISEASES

SJÖGREN'S SYNDROME

Sjögren's is the second most common of the auto-immune rheumatic diseases. The disease features infiltration of exocrine glands by lymphocytes, causing atrophy and destruction, which results in the loss of secretory function (Fig. 16.6). The areas principally affected are the salivary and lacrimal glands, although the glands of the respiratory tract, vagina and sweat glands may also be affected.

Whilst this is rare in childhood, any age or race can be affected. It occurs most commonly in women in the fourth and fifth decades of life, with the ratio of women to men being approximately 9:1.

The exact prevalence in the general population is unknown. Symptoms may be a nuisance but are so slight they may not prompt sufferers to seek assistance. Hughes (1994) explains that even where symptoms are reported as causing considerable suffering, they are not dramatic. Recognition and appreciation of their clinical and immunological significance may pass undetected by the physician or may not be associated with the disease in question.

Approximately 25–30% of people with rheumatoid arthritis are thought to have Sjögren's disease.

The classification of Sjögren's disease centres on a triad of criteria.

- Dry eyes (keratoconjunctivitis)
- Dry mouth (xerostomia)
- Connective tissue disease.

Primary Sjögren's refers to the disease when it predominantly affects the exocrine glands, with any extraglandular features not numerous enough to

Table 16.3 The classification of Sjögren's syndrome

Classification	Symptoms
Primary	Dry eyes, dry mouth, parotid gland enlargement, arthralgia, Raynaud's phenomenon, fatigue
Secondary	As for primary but in association with rheumatoid arthritis, systemic lupus erythematosus, scleroderma, vasculitis, myositis, mixed connective tissue disease

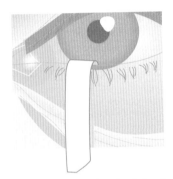

Figure 16.7 Schirmer tear test. A strip of absorbent paper is folded and inserted into the lower eyelid (as per individual product instructions). The level of moisture is measured after a given time. If the moisture, produced by tear secretion, does not reach an expected distance in millimetres, then a diagnosis of Sjogren's can be confirmed.

fulfil the criteria for other connective tissue disease. Where it is associated with other autoimmune diseases, for example rheumatoid arthritis, it is classified as secondary Sjögren's (Table 16.3).

If patients have dry eyes and mouth without the accompanying immunopathology, this is described as sicca syndrome. The incidence of this increases with age and it can be caused by other illnesses or the side effects of medicines.

Patient management

Problems for which the patient will usually seek advice are associated predominantly with the eyes or mouth. Improving comfort by the use of lubricant eyedrops and artificial saliva is the basis of symptomatic relief. Vigilance is required to enable early intervention for any infection occurring alongside the symptoms of grittiness, burning, difficulty opening the eyes in the morning, conjunctival stickiness and photophobia. Similarly, a dry, red, furrowed tongue and dental caries may encourage candida infection and require optimal oral hygiene and dental care. Frequent sipping of drinks may aid swallowing of food or relieve mouth dryness at night.

Sufferers of Sjögren's may be predisposed to drug hypersensitivity.

If Sjögren's syndrome is unsuspected, the diagnostic tests that should be considered include rheumatoid arthritis latex, anti-Ro and anti-La antibodies, antithyroid antibodies (present in 50% of sufferers) and the Schirmer tear test (Fig. 16.7).

Where systemic treatment is required, often the drug of choice is an antimalarial such as hydroxychloroquine. Steroids are prescribed either in low doses to reduce the troublesome effects of the disease or in larger doses to treat complications such as pulmonary fibrosis or peripheral neuropathy. Azathioprine is added as a steroid-sparing agent.

The role of the nurse includes monitoring of the efficacy and safety of such treatments along with ongoing education and information about disease and treatment.

Rare but serious complications of Sjögren's are renal tubular acidosis and lymphoma.

RAYNAUD'S PHENOMENON

This is characterised by episodic digital ischaemia provoked by cold and emotion. Raynaud's phenomenon is described by Belch (1987) as classically involving pallor of the affected digits, followed by cyanosis and rubor. The pallor relates to the decreased arterial flow, cyanosis is caused by deoxygenation of the static venous blood, while the rubor is a reactive hyperaemia following the return of the blood flow.

Raynaud's phenomenon affects women and men in a ratio of 9:1. If it occurs without an associated disease it is classified as primary Raynaud's; in this form the incidence in the general population is approximately 5%. Raynaud's phenomenon frequently occurs as a secondary feature in other diseases (see Box 16.4).

Careful questioning of the patient about what happens to their hands in the cold gives a good indication of whether Raynaud's is the cause of their problems. Investigations to be included when confirming a diagnosis of Raynaud 's phenomenon are shown in Box 16.5.

Within 2 years of onset of Raynaud's 60% of sufferers will develop a connective tissue disease. Scleroderma has the highest incidence of Raynaud's

Box 16.4   Conditions in which Raynaud's may feature as a secondary phenomenon

Connective tissue disease	Rheumatoid arthritis
	Systemic lupus erythematosus
	Systemic sclerosis
	CREST
	Polymyositis
	Dermatomyositis
	Mixed
Occupational	Vibration/percussion
	Work in a cold environment
Arterial disease	Thoracic outlet syndrome
	Cervical rib
	Thrombosis/embolism
Drugs and other substances	Beta-blockers
	Anti-migraine drugs
	Oral contraceptives
	Cytotoxics
	Smoking
Other disorders	Reflex sympathetic dystrophy
	Hypothyroidism
	Cryoglobulinaemia

Box 16.5   Investigations for Raynaud's syndrome

- Full blood count
- ESR
- Liver function test
- Serum protein electrophoresis
- Cryoglobulins
- Cholesterol
- Antinuclear antibody
- Anticentromere antibody
- Anti-Scl-70 antibody

with 95% of scleroderma patients being affected. The incidence in people with lupus is 20%. However, if primary Raynaud's has been present for many years only about 5% will go on to develop connective tissue disease. Mild scleroderma is the usual manifestation in this group (Maudsley 1994).

Vasospasm in response to emotional stress or the reduction in temperature is the initiating feature bringing on an attack. Toes and fingers are affected along with the nose, ear lobes and tip of the tongue. Symptoms are often mild, requiring little intervention, but can be severe, resulting in pain, ulceration of the digits, ischaemia and even loss of digits.

Patient management and care

The treatment varies according to severity, although in every case total abstinence from smoking is of greatest importance. Understanding that it is not the actual temperature itself but changes in the temperature leading to vasoconstriction will be of help. Patients with mild symptoms need advice on keeping warm generally, not just the extremities. Avoiding excessive cold, for example winter sports or air-conditioned environments, is beneficial. The use of ice packs for the relief of painful joints is avoided in those with Raynaud's.

Tips on clothing can be necessary, for instance, wearing several light layers for extra warmth or thermal garments. Insulated gloves and heat packs which fit into pockets or shoes are available. If a patient with Raynaud's is in hospital, it is important they are not moved from one area to another where the temperature may be different; for example, taking patients along outside corridors to departments where they may be required to undress without regard for their need to keep warm. Whilst they may require blankets for warmth at night, the weight of bedclothes on painful toes requires a bed cradle.

Where symptoms are more troublesome, requiring medication to help bring them under control, the treatment includes prazosin or nifedipine.

Digital ulcers are very painful. Where no infection is present then occlusive dressings help to avoid trauma and promote healing. Erythema, swelling, an increase in pain or the presence of pus indicates the ulcers are infected. Swabs are sent for microscopy enabling antibiotic sensitivities to be identified; *Staphylococcus aureus* is usually isolated. The ulcers are cleaned by soaking and the appropriate topical antibiotic is applied prior to the dressings.

Where digits have become acutely ischaemic, treatment with an intravenous infusion of prostacycline may help. As infusions are administered daily for up to 6 days and can cause significant adverse reactions, admission may be required depending on the adequacy of day-care facilities. Sympathetic blocks can be used to relieve pain. An arteriogram will indicate the need for microvascular hand surgery, surgical debridement or even amputation.

SYSTEMIC SCLEROSIS (SCLERODERMA)

Systemic sclerosis is a progressive generalised disorder of connective tissues of both the skin and internal organs. The aetiology is unknown.

The prevalence is approximately 10–20 individuals per 100 000, making this one of the less common rheumatic disorders. Women are affected four times more frequently than men are. The peak age of onset is between 30 and 40 years. Familial tendency is rare and genetic evidence is lacking.

Presentation

Systemic sclerosis is described by Seibold (1994) as being remarkably heterogeneous, with diverse initial presentations, a variable disease course and differing in each case in its pace, extent and severity of its clinical manifestations.

Black (1996) provides a classification into subsets describing the degree of tissue involvement.

- Pre-scleroderma
- Diffuse cutaneous scleroderma
- Limited cutaneous scleroderma
- Sine scleroderma.

The synonym CREST is sometimes used to describe the features of limited cutaneous scleroderma.

- **C**alcinosis
- **R**aynaud's phenomenon
- **E**sophageal (oesophageal) dismotility
- **S**clerodactyly
- **T**elangectasia.

Rather uncharacteristically for a rheumatic disease, flares and remissions of activity are not seen in systemic sclerosis. Identifying the person who presents with a pre-scleroderma picture is critical in helping to ensure the aims of therapy, which must be to halt the disease and prevent further spread (Black 1994). The presence of nailfold capillary abnormalities and disease-specific antinuclear antibodies should arouse suspicion. Zuffrey et al (1992) suggest that these will detect over 90% of those destined to develop systemic sclerosis.

Given the diverse and varied presentations that occur, the potential range of investigations required is extensive, including blood tests, urine tests, radiology (both external and barium studies), lung and cardiac function tests, electromyography (EMG), capillary microscopy and biopsy of skin, muscle or bowel tissue (Black 1994).

Some of the problems experienced by patients as a result of the physiological changes are outlined in Table 16.4.

Treatment

As there are so many combinations of symptoms, the treatment is variable and individual to each patient. Modification of the entire disease process is desirable, usually with DMARDs. Different drugs affect different aspects of the disease, so whilst prostacycline may be used for vascular changes, DMARDs such as methotrexate or ciclosporin may be needed to address immune abnormalities. Additional groups of drugs that are valuable for these patients include analgesics, NSAIDs and antibiotics.

POLYMYOSITIS AND DERMATOMYOSITIS

Polymyositis (inflammation of muscles) and dermatomyositis (where skin pathology is also present) are uncommon but serious inflammatory muscle diseases. There is a female predominance of 2:1. During the child-bearing years the ratio increases to 5:1. Whilst they are more common in the 50–70 age group, they affect people of any age, including children (Dorph & Lundberg 2002).

Drugs, toxins, excessive alcohol, infectious agents, trauma and genetic background can all be factors in the aetiology of inflammatory muscle disease (Butler & Nightingale 1998).

The onset can be either acute or chronic, with the predominance of presenting features occurring in the following pattern:

- 70% of patients present with primarily muscle involvement
- 25% with cutaneous involvement
- 5% with systemic features such as weight loss and fever.

The course of these diseases is one of exacerbations and remissions.

Presentation

Hughes (1994) describes the skin changes in dermatomyositis as collagenous thickening of the dermis, increased fibrosis that resembles scleroderma, calcium deposition and a thin atrophic epidermis. The muscle pathology includes degeneration of muscle fibre and the presence of chronic inflammatory cells

Table 16.4   Clinical features occurring in systemic sclerosis (adapted from Hughes 1994)

Tissues involved	Clinical feature	Examples of associated patient problems
Skin	Loss of tissue elasticity, thickening of tissue, reduced mobility of tissues, tightness around nose, pinched mouth, telangiectasia, hyperpigmentation, vitiligo, oedema, subcutaneous calcinosis	Poor grip, reduced hand function, increased dependence on others for daily activities Difficulty eating/yawning, changes in appearance/facial expression, body image issues Pain, discomfort, pruritus
Hair	Alopecia	Loss of confidence, self-esteem, body image issues
Vascular	Raynaud's syndrome, ulceration, infection	Pain, difficulty with changing environmental temperatures, poor hand function and mobility reduced if toes involved
Secretory glands	Sjögren's syndrome	Dry eyes, mouth, discomfort, infection, pain, difficulty eating, maintaining hygiene needs
Oesophagus and gut	Dysphagia, oesophageal reflux, shortening and stricture, hiatus hernia, fibrosis of stomach, malabsorption	Unable to manage preferred diet, indigestion, heart burn, pain and discomfort at mealtimes, anorexia, weight loss, poor nutrition
Liver	Primary biliary cirrhosis, portal hypertension	
Pulmonary	Fibrosis, crepitations, heart failure, pulmonary hypertension, cystic changes, pleural thickening, vasculitis, bronchiectasis, carcinoma (a rare complication)	Persistent cough, dyspnoea, recurrent infections, reduced exercise tolerance
Renal	Proteinuria, haematuria	Asymptomatic
Muscles and joints	Polyarthritis, inflammatory myositis, rigidity of tissues around joints	Pain, muscle weakness, reduced mobility and functional ability, affecting self-care, work, recreation, relationships
Haematological	Anaemia	Fatigue, dyspnoea
Cerebral	Vasculitis (rare)	

resulting in fibrosis and extensive muscle atrophy. The myocardium can be affected although this is usually asymptomatic.

Weakness and excessive fatigue are universal. The nurse can assist the patient to differentiate between muscle weaknesses, resulting in difficulty in carrying out tasks, from muscle fatigue following activities requiring endurance more than strength. Difficulty rising from a chair, inability to walk any distance or climb stairs and problems with brushing hair and dressing may ensue, making referral to occupational therapists an important part of care.

The muscles of the trunk and neck can also be involved, making it difficult to hold up the head. Respiratory muscles are affected in varying degrees with, in the most severe cases, patients needing temporary ventilation in intensive care.

The cause of pain in these conditions is calcium deposition around the muscle fibres and beneath the skin, for which there is no really effective therapy.

In dermatomyositis the degree of muscle involvement usually correlates to the severity of a rash, which typically occurs on the eyelids, over the knuckles and on the neck and chest (Fig. 16.8). Telangectasia may be present around the finger and toe nails.

Weight loss, fever, polyarthritis, arthralgia and Raynaud's can be present along with a low-grade anaemia. The question of whether polymyositis and dematomyositis are associated with malignancy remains unanswered.

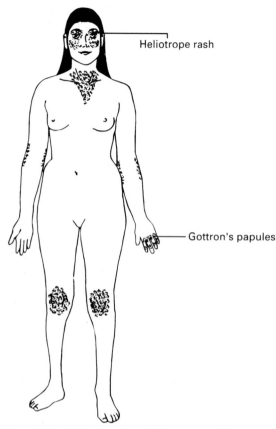

Figure 16.8 Distribution of rash in dermatomyositis.

Prompt diagnosis is believed to improve the prognosis. Appropriate clinical findings, laboratory testing and pathology findings are required to confirm the diagnosis (Table 16.5). Differential diagnoses include alcohol abuse, other connective tissue diseases, polymyalgia rheumatica, viral infections and muscular dystrophies or drug-induced myopathy. Malignancy should be excluded with baseline investigations.

Treatment and care

Treatment is based largely on the titration of medication to the severity of symptoms. For this reason, serial as well as baseline investigations are required to illustrate fluctuations in disease activity. Assessments include ability to cope with daily activities and muscle strength testing, respiratory peak flow rate, scores for pain and well-being, the extent and severity of any rash, serial haematology and biochemistry measures.

A return to normal serum enzyme levels is a favourable sign. Elevations later on may signify an exacerbation. However, they may remain normal

Table 16.5 Investigations for polymyositis and dermatomyositis

Investigation	Result
ESR and CRP	Raised due to muscle inflammation
Creatinine phosphokinase (CPK)	Raised in 95%, this enzyme leaks from damaged muscle
Liver function tests	Raised transaminases
Rheumatoid factor	May be present
Antinuclear antibodies Extractable nuclear antigens Myositis specific autoantibodies	Most commonly present is anti-Jo1 antibody
Muscle tests: • Electromyography (EMG) • Muscle biopsy	Abnormalities are found and vary in accordance with disease stage
Magnetic resonance imaging (MRI)	Can identify areas of muscle involvement, useful to indicate areas for biopsy

whilst new rashes or increased weakness indicate a flare. In some cases, enzymes may remain chronically elevated.

Corticosteroids are the mainstay of drug therapy. Whilst some physicians may designate daily oral doses ranging from 40 to 80 mg daily for 4–6 weeks, or until maximum benefit is achieved, others may favour intravenous bolus doses of 500 mg–1 g daily for 3 days. In addition, DMARDs such as azathioprine or methotrexate are used. Intravenous gamma globulins are used in acute disease stages.

Physiotherapy aims to maintain active movement of the muscles, with passive movements during a flare and strengthening exercises during periods of remission. Again individual needs must be taken into account.

Kagen (1995) explains that, whilst it has been shown clinically that treatment aimed at increasing strength and endurance can be successful, it should be borne in mind that where muscle fibres have become necrosed and replaced with connective tissue, the potential for recovery in that area is limited. Considering the muscles as having only limited fitness is advocated to enable achievable goals to be set.

GOUT

Gout is a syndrome caused by an inflammatory response to the monosodium urate crystals which develop secondary to hyperuricaemia. Both acute and chronic forms are recognised and both are treated differently (Cohen & Emerson 1995). Treatment is difficult to determine due to the remitting and relapsing nature of gout. The ratio of affected men to women is changing as a result of changes in lifestyle, available medication and increased longevity. It was formerly in the region of 20 men to each woman but is now between 2–7 men to each woman affected. Even so, gout is still recognised as the most common inflammatory arthropathy occurring in men over the age of 40.

Presentation

With sustained elevation of blood uric acid levels (hyperuricaemia), the result is the deposition of sodium waste in and around joints. In over half of the initial attacks of gout, the first metatarsophalangeal joint is affected, causing pain and erythema.

The uric acid can accumulate resulting in tophi that appear as firm nodular swellings at virtually any site, the most common being the digits of the hands and feet, the olecranon bursae and ear lobes. These may become infected as well as being sites of extreme pain.

Acute gout is characterised by the sudden onset and build-up of pain and swelling, with accompanying redness of the affected joint. It usually occurs in the early hours of the morning, disturbing sleep. The rapidly increasing pain reaches a peak within a few hours and remains at this level for between 1 and 3 days. There may be fever, chills and shivers, which increase with the levels of pain.

Symptoms often subside within 7–10 days but it can take up to several weeks for a severe attack to settle completely. Many patients have a single attack and therefore are not diagnosed but the majority will have more than one attack within 2 years.

Chronic gout occurs when the uricaemia is not controlled, with a lack of symptom-free periods. When this happens, gout becomes chronic from an early stage. The inflammatory process is mild, except when acute attacks supervene and it may then be associated with a destructive, deforming arthritis.

The diagnosis of gout depends largely on the history given by the patient. Examination and findings will include a large, red, swollen joint. Although any joint can be affected, the lower limb joints are involved more often. The swelling can be marked, potentially involving an entire body region.

Box 16.6 Gout: precipitating factors
• Acute illness
• Trauma
• Surgery
• Alcohol consumption
• Diuretic medications

As well as the history of how the acute attack affects the individual, it is important to identify other factors that are recognised precursors of an attack (Box 16.6).

Blood tests during the acute phase will reveal a raised ESR and raised levels of uric acid. Synovial fluid aspirated from the joints affected will show urate crystals along with low viscosity and a very high leukocyte count.

Plain film radiological findings include soft tissue calcification and possibly erosions.

Management and nursing care

Management of gout is different for acute attacks and chronic states.

Acute attacks can lead to inpatient treatment or are managed by the general practitioner. NSAIDs are administered to reduce inflammation and pain; the nurse must ensure advice is given on their correct use to avoid gastrointestinal side effects.

If NSAIDs are contraindicated, colchicine is the next drug of choice, being effective treatment for gout in up to 90% of patients experiencing acute attacks. Colchicine is administered orally, normally with an initial dose of 1 mg followed by 0.5 mg at 2-hourly intervals; it can be administered intravenously. Close observation is required to assess for toxicity, as the therapeutic dose and toxic dose of colchicine are very similar. Toxicity can present as abdominal pain, nausea and vomiting and more frequently diarrhoea. An effective dose rarely exceeds 8 mg before the attack subsides or before diarrhoea occurs. As colchicine can cause renal damage, observation of fluid balance is essential.

Colchicine is an effective prophylactic in smaller doses when used in the same way as for acute attacks. Prophylactic colchicine is normally continued for 9–12 months after hyperuricaemia is corrected and the patient is free from attacks.

Simple measures can offer significant relief, promote comfort and recovery, such as ensuring the person has a comfortable chair and footstool, pillows to elevate and rest the affected limb, a wheelchair to get to the bathroom or dining area to avoid weight bearing, paracetamol where necessary for relief of fever and a bed cradle to remove the weight of bed clothing.

Those with chronic gout may still suffer from intermittent acute attacks for which the treatment remains as above during acute flares. Chronic gout sufferers continue to have some pain in between the acute flares, which requires treatment. Continuous use of NSAIDs is indicated, along with an agent to lower the serum uric acid. Allopurinol is the drug of choice but should not be used during the acute phase, as it will cause a severe exacerbation. The dosage varies between 200 and 800 mg daily and the patient must be advised that a rash is a common side effect necessitating withdrawal of the drug. Once initiated, allopurinol should be given indefinitely, with monitoring of serum uric acid every 3–6 months. Renal and liver function tests should be monitored at the same time to note any signs of toxicity that might lead to organ failure, which is normally reversible on stopping the drug.

Nursing care in outpatient settings centres on drug information and monitoring for their efficacy and adverse effects, along with supporting the patient in necessary lifestyle changes to help avoid acute flares of gout.

Intraarticular aspiration and injection of steroid solution are used to relieve pressure and pain in acutely affected joints.

NURSING THE PATIENT WITH RHEUMATIC DISEASE

Nursing during the last decade has seen the development and expansion in the number of specialist nurse posts. Many of these were initially supported financially by non-governmental funds, particularly in rheumatology. This has led to a diverse group of practitioners, with an equally diverse range of skills and levels of qualifications.

All nurses are bound by the same professional code (NMC 2002), with personal accountability for professional practice remaining a cornerstone of all actions. This clearly sets out the principles on which any adjustment to the range of responsibilities for any individual nurse must be based. The emphasis is placed upon knowledge, skill, responsibility and accountability and when developing new roles, these need to be taken into account along with ensuring that each aspect of nursing practice is directed to meeting the needs and serving the interest of the patient or client. For specialist nurses in rheumatology this is inherent in their practice, as many have developed their role in response to the needs of the population they serve. They must, however, ensure they have the relevant knowledge and skills for carrying out each aspect of their role and never take on aspects they are ill prepared for or are not responsible or accountable for.

Flasher (1997) provides clear evidence of how evolving the scope of practice can effectively address the identification not only of problems experienced by sufferers of rheumatic disease but also the requirements of the nurse wishing to deliver and measure an effective care package.

Some of the vital components of care are addressed in the following services rheumatology specialist nurses provide.

- Nurse-led clinics
- Education and information giving
- Drug monitoring clinics
- Assessment and evaluation of treatment and care
- Providing timely access to care by, for example, telephone helplines
- Counselling
- Carrying out soft tissue and intraarticular injections, advising on aftercare of treated joints and reviewing outcomes
- Close working relationships with and referral to other members of the multidisciplinary team.

Patients are also changing. They no longer accept care without questioning it, are not always willing to conform to health professionals' advice or to hand over responsibility for their health to others. After all, as the largest stakeholders in healthcare provision, patients now expect to retain control over what happens to them. They require information, education and the opportunity to question, so that they become empowered to exercise choice in accepting treatment and therefore participate in decision making.

CONCLUSION

Having described only a few of the many rheumatic diseases, it becomes apparent that those working in the field of rheumatology are confronted by far more than a 'touch of rheumatism'. One sees that, despite the misconceptions of the uninformed, these conditions are not confined to the elderly alone, nor do they all end in severe disability.

One in four of the UK population will suffer, at some time, the consequences of a rheumatic condition. This makes it a significant problem for society in terms of lost employment days, financial cost and the provision of adequate resources for timely, appropriate treatment and care. Despite this, rheumatology is not one of the core services that authorities are bound to provide and to a degree, it has always been given low priority in comparison to other specialties.

Whilst the care of individuals requires a multidisciplinary approach, involving doctors, therapists and a gamut of other professionals, many of the facets of care and treatment called for in rheumatic disease management are increasingly being encompassed into the dynamic and exciting role of the specialist nurse in rheumatology.

Some patients will be facing a diagnosis of a potentially lifelong condition, the start of many tests, appointments and potentially toxic treatments. Whilst all involved strive to maintain a balance of health needs and the preferred lifestyle of the individual wherever possible, changes in life goals to varying degrees have to be faced by some. At times, the greatest and most effective skill the nurse can employ is to really listen, as this enables identification of the patients' problems for which we may be able to assist in finding solutions.

References

Arthritis and Musculoskeletal Alliance (ARMA) 2002 Information leaflet. ARMA, London

Arthur V 1998a The rheumatic conditions: an overview. In: Hill J (ed) Rheumatology nursing: a creative approach. Churchill Livingstone, Edinburgh

Arthur V 1998b The role of the specialist nurse in rheumatology. In: Le Gallez P (ed) Rheumatology for nurses: patient care. Whurr Publications, London

Belch J 1987 Collected reports on rheumatic diseases: topical reviews: Raynaud's phenomenon. Arthritis and Rheumatism Council for Research, Chesterfield

Bergman S 2003 Rheumatic disease in practice: a general practice approach to management of chronic widespread musculoskeletal pain and fibromyalgia. Arthritis Research Campaign, Chesterfield

Black CM 1994 Raynaud's phenomenon. Prescriber's Journal 34: 125–133

Black CM 1996 Reports on rheumatic diseases: topical reviews: systemic sclerosis series 3. Arthritis and Rheumatism Council for Research, Chesterfield

British National Formulary (BNF) 2002 Drugs affecting bone metabolism. British Medical Association and Royal Pharmaceutical Society, London (September)

Butler R, Nightingale S 1998 Reports of rheumatic diseases: practical problems. The assessment of muscle weakness and pain. No. 14. Arthritis Research Campaign, Chesterfield

Carruthers DM, Watt RA, Symmons DPM et al 1996 Wegener's granulomatosus – increased incidence or increased recognition? British Journal of Rheumatology 35: 142–145

Chakravarty K, Scott D 1993 Clinical aspects of systemic vasculitis in adults. Vascular Medicine Review 4: 195–220

Cohen MG, Emerson BT 1995 Crystal arthropathies: gout. In: Klippel JH (ed) Rheumatology. Mosby, St Louis

Dasgupta B, Kalk S 2000 Rheumatic disease: topical reviews: polymyalgia and giant cell arteritis. No. 2. Arthritis Research Campaign, Chesterfield

Dieppe PA, Doherty M, MacFarlane D et al 1985 Rheumatology medicine. Churchill Livingstone, Edinburgh

Dorph C, Lundberg MD 2002 Idiopathic inflammatory myopathies: myositis. In: Woolf AD (ed) Best practice and research. Clinical rheumatology, epidemiology of musculoskeletal conditions. Baillière Tindall, London

Eastmond CJ 1994 Genetics and HLA antigens. In: Wright V, Helliwell P (eds) Baillière's clinical rheumatology: psoriatic arthritis. Baillière Tindall, London

Edberg JC, Salmon JE, Kimberley RP 1995 Systemic lupus erythematosus. In: Klippel JH, Dieppe PA (eds) Rheumatology. Mosby, St Louis

Emery P, Salmon M 1995 Early rheumatoid arthritis: time to aim for remission? Annals of Rheumatic Disease 54: 944–947

Espinoza LR, Cuellar ML 1995 Psoriatic arthritis management. In: Klippel JH, Dieppe PA (eds) Rheumatology. Mosby, St Louis

Flasher N 1997 Developing the scope of practice for rheumatology nurse practitioners. Journal of Orthopaedic Nursing 1: 123–126

Fries JF, Spitz P, Kraines RG et al 1980 Measurement of patient outcome in arthritis. Arthritis and Rheumatism 23: 137–145

Guillevin L 2001 Vasculitides. In: Hunder G (ed) Atlas of rheumatology, 2nd edn. Current Medicine Inc, Philadelphia

Hazelman B 1995 Collected reports on the rheumatic diseases: polymyalgia rheumatica and giant cell arteritis. Arthritis and Rheumatism Council, Chesterfield

Helliwell P, Wright V 1995 Clinical features of psoriatic arthritis. In: Klippel JH, Dieppe PA (eds) Rheumatology. Mosby, St Louis

Hill J, Bird HA, Harmer R et al 1994 An evaluation of the effectiveness, safety and acceptability of a nurse practitioner in rheumatology outpatient clinics. British Journal of Rheumatology 33: 283–288

Hoffman GS, Fauci AS 1995 Wegener's granulomatosus. In: Klippel JH, Dieppe PA (eds) Rheumatology. Mosby, St Louis

Hughes GR 1994 Connective tissue diseases, 4th edn. Blackwell, Oxford

Kagen L 1995 Inflammatory muscle disease management. In: Klippel JH, Dieppe PA (eds) Rheumatology. Mosby, St Louis

Le Gallez P 1998 Patient education and self management. In: Rheumatology for nurses: patient care. Whurr Publications, London

Lightfoot R 1995 Overview of the inflammatory vascular diseases. In: Klippel JH, Dieppe PA (eds) Rheumatology. Mosby, St Louis

Maudsley AH 1994 Scleroderma: a handbook for patients. The Raynaud's and Scleroderma Association, Cheshire

Melzack R 1975 The McGill Pain Questionnaire: major properties and scoring methods. Pain 1: 277–299

National Ankylosing Spondylitis Society 2000 Guidebook for patients: a positive response to ankylosing spondylitis. Burleigh Press, Bristol

Nursing and Midwifery Council (NMC) 2002 The scope of professional practice. Nursing and Midwifery Council, London

Olivieri A, Van Tubergen A, Salvarani C, Van Der Linden S 2002 Sero-negative spondyloarthritides. In: Woolfe AD (ed) Best practice and research. Clinical rheumatology: epidemiology of musculoskeletal conditions. Baillière Tindall, London

O'Neil T, Silman AJ 1994 Historical background and epidemiology. In: Wright V, Helliwell P (eds) Baillière's clinical rheumatology. Psoriatic arthritis. Baillière Tindall, London

Seibold JR 1994 Systemic sclerosis: clinical features. In: Klippel JH, Dieppe PA (eds) Rheumatology. Mosby, St Louis

Tadman J (ed) 2003 Food for thought. Arthritis Today 119: 16–22

Thompson PW, Kirwan JR 1995 Joints count: a review of old and new articular indices of joint inflammation. British Journal of Rheumatology 34: 1003–1008

Troughton PR, Morgan AW 1994 Laboratory findings and pathology of psoriatic arthritis. In: Wright V, Helliwell P (eds) Baillière's clinical rheumatology. Psoriatic arthritis Baillière Tindall, London

Wolfe F, Ross K, Anderson T et al 1995 The prevalence and characteristics of fibromyalgia in the general population. Arthritis and Rheumatism 38: 19–28

Zuffrey P, Depairon M, Chamot AM et al 1992 Prognostic significance of nailfold capillary microscopy in patients with Raynaud's phenomenon and scleroderma – pattern abnormalities: a six year follow up study. Clinical Rheumatology 11(4): 536–541

Chapter 17

Osteoarthritis and total joint replacements

Rebecca Jester

INTRODUCTION

Over the last 20–30 years joint replacements have become well established in the field of orthopaedic surgery. Joint replacements, or arthroplasties as they are known, have revolutionised the treatment of patients with joint pain and dysfunction. Arthroplasties are available for almost every joint, with the hip and knee joints being the most frequently replaced. Indeed, total hip replacement (THR) is one of the most commonly performed orthopaedic operations with approximately 43 500 primary replacements being carried out each year in the UK (Frankel et al 1999) and 400 000 worldwide (Goldie 1992). Hip and knee replacements are predominantly performed on older people between the ages of 65 and 90 although occasionally, patients suffering with secondary arthritis following congenital hip dysplasia may undergo total hip replacement in their late 20s and 30s if the degree of pain and disability is severe.

Hip and knee replacements are performed primarily to relieve pain for patients suffering with a variety of degenerative, inflammatory and traumatic conditions such as primary and secondary osteoarthritis, rheumatoid arthritis, intracapsular femoral neck fractures and ankylosing spondylitis of the hip. The secondary reasons of joint replacement surgery are to restore function and reduce the degree of disability for the individual.

The condition that necessitates the largest number of joint replacements is osteoarthritis (O'Brien 1994). This chapter provides an overview of this degenerative and inflammatory disease that affects the joints. In addition, a review of the research-based literature pertaining to treatment interventions for joint disorders will be discussed, with a focus on total joint replacement. Rehabilitation options following total joint replacement will also be explored. This chapter reviews:

- osteoarthritis: the aetiology and epidemiology, assessment and examination, plus deferential diagnoses
- surgical and conservative treatment options
- risk management of complications following joint replacement
- ethical perspectives on selection of patients for total joint replacement
- rehabilitation following total joint replacement, focusing on home versus inpatient care.

OSTEOARTHRITIS

Osteoarthritis (OA) is the commonest cause of severe disability among the older population in the UK and North America (Martin et al 1988). It is the biggest cause of joint pain and provides a major challenge for healthcare providers (Jones & Doherty 1996). It has been estimated that 1 in 10 persons over the age of 65 years will consult their GP at least once a year because of osteoarthritis (P Croft, unpublished PhD thesis, 1993). The magnitude of the impact of this disease is illustrated by the fact that 11% of people diagnosed with OA are forced to work reduced hours and 14% will retire early (Hosie & Dickson 2000).

Osteoarthritis is frequently referred to as being a progressive process associated with getting older. Although it is estimated that 50% of those aged over 60 have radiographic evidence of osteoarthritis in at least one joint (Jones & Doherty 1996, Kumar & Clark 1990), there is little evidence to support either an 'ageing' or 'wear and tear' phenomenon (Ward & Tidswell 1994). Jones & Doherty (1996) affirm that OA is a complex, metabolically active process involving a varying balance between anabolic and catabolic processes that affects all the tissues of the joint, so is more than merely attrition of joint structures.

Despite a wealth of research into the aetiology of osteoarthritis, the exact cause remains uncertain. Mechanical causation of osteoarthritis is one school of thought: this advocates that abnormal load distribution on weight-bearing joints accelerates a wear and tear process within the joint itself. There are two broad ideas related to abnormal load bearing through the joint (Buckwalter 1996, Radin 1976). The first

possible cause is abnormalities of the joint at birth which, if left undiagnosed or incorrectly treated, alter the joint structure and initiate the osteoarthritic process. This theory is difficult to substantiate or dismiss in an adult presenting with osteoarthritic symptoms as the normal joint structures can be so altered that it would be almost impossible to diagnose a 'missed' congenital or developmental joint abnormality. This theory would also imply that all osteoarthritis was secondary to an earlier disease process.

The second theory, which suggests that osteoarthritis is caused by abnormal load bearing through the joints, proposes that normal joints become osteoarthritic due to abnormal external forces upon them. External forces are attributed to obesity and/or cumulative excessive exposure to overuse, resulting in abnormal repetitive strain being placed upon the joint. Obesity is the major risk factor for OA of the knee, particularly in middle-aged women in whom, for every 5 kg increase in weight, the risk increases by 30% (Jones & Doherty 1996). This second theory would therefore suggest that individuals 'at risk' of developing OA could be readily identifiable either through their occupational grouping or recreational activities or by their obesity status.

Aetiological studies of osteoarthritis using epidemiological methods are small in number. However, a study by Croft investigated a sample of 1367 men aged 60–75 years old and found that farmers within the sample had a higher prevalence of OA compared to other occupational groups which affirmed the theory that excessive cumulative overuse of joints leads to OA (P Croft, unpublished PhD thesis, 1993). The ramifications of this repetitive overuse theory are that 'at-risk' groups and individuals can be identified and preventive strategies instigated. It should be within the remit of a specialist orthopaedic nurse to identify at-risk individuals before the osteoarthritic disease process becomes too advanced. Liaison with nursing colleagues working within primary care and occupational settings is essential if the aim is to prevent and minimise the severity of this epidemic disease.

PHYSIOLOGICAL CHANGES

The physiological changes within the joint are explained as occurring in five stages (Dandy & Edwards 1998). Each joint may be showing two or more stages at any one time within different areas of the joint.

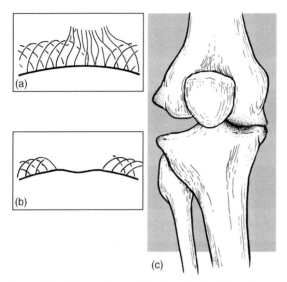

Figure 17.1   The development of osteoarthritis (a) Breakdown of articular surface with rupture of the collagen arcade. (b) Exposed bone with eburnation. (c) Deformity and collapse. (From Dandy & Edwards 1998.)

1 Breakdown of the articular cartilage occurs as the normally smooth joint surface is damaged by the breakdown of collagen fibres, giving a roughened surface (Fig. 17.1). Joint movement and friction cause some articular cartilage particles to break off into the joint. These are absorbed by the synovium and start an inflammatory response; this causes the patient to experience aching and stiffness in the joint after, rather than during, exercise.

2 Synovium irritation is probably due to the release of intracellular enzymes such as lysosomes. These cause hyperaemia and cellular responses in the synovial layers, leading to the synovium producing degradative enzymes such as interleukin-1.

3 Remodelling of the cartilage through repair is limited. The superficial lesions of the articular cartilage are unable to repair themselves but deeper lesions penetrating the cortical bone allow marrow cells to infiltrate and fibrocartilage formation to occur. In the subchondral bone there is an increase in the density of the bone tissue with an area of dense, hard, resilient bone developing below the cartilage. On the joint surface margins, new bone forms as osteophytes covered by fibrocartilage, probably in reaction to particles being swept to the joint edges by movements of the joint. These osteophytes will restrict joint movement. Together these changes affect the shape and congruity of the joint, termed 'remodelling'. The weight-bearing ability of the joints is affected and

results in the joint pressure now being taken by different areas of articular cartilage.

4 Eburnation of bone and cyst formation is the fourth stage. If the patient rests the joint, the wear particles will be gradually absorbed and fibrous tissue will develop on the joint surface but over time this will eventually fail, resulting in erosion of the articular surface to expose the subchondral bone which becomes polished and eburnated (Fig. 17.1). As a result of the loss of joint space, the patient experiences pain from bone rubbing on bone and as the eburnated bone is not as smooth as the original cartilage, there is friction and altered weight distribution across the joint. These changes cause excess loading on parts of the joint resulting in microfractures in the trabeculae of the underlying cancellous bone. As these microfractures heal with callus, the rigidity of the bone is increased, making it denser and less resilient, which in turn leads to more microfractures and the normal bone structure, or architecture, is lost. The synovial fluid is now able to enter the cancellous bone through the cracks in the articular surface and creates cavities seen on X-rays and cysts. These cysts are eventually lined by a thin layer of cortical bone and filled with fibrous tissue.

5 Disorganisation is the final stage where the disease progresses, the osteophytes enlarge and the bone surfaces are more worn, causing joint stiffness and deformity. The normal joint function is altered, leading to varus and valgus changes when one side of the knee joint, for example, is more affected as the joint tries to redistribute the load. In the upper limb the movement ranges will be affected along with the joint shape. This difference affects the strategies for treatment as lower limb surgery aims at restoration of ability to take weight without pain, while upper limb surgery aims to restore the range of movement. The ligaments and joint capsule become looser as the normal joint length is lost and on X-ray the disease progression is indicated by the narrower joint spaces, osteophytes, subchondral cysts and the altered shape of the bone (Fig. 17.2).

SIGNS AND SYMPTOMS

It is important to note that there is often disparity in the severity of symptoms experienced by patients compared to the radiographic evidence of the disease process (Nilsdotter 2001). Often patients with only slight evidence of osteoarthritic changes on X-ray will suffer with severe joint pain and disability.

Conversely, patients with almost total loss of the joint space and destruction of the articulating surfaces, apparent on X-ray, will complain of only a mild degree of discomfort and disability. It is therefore important that radiographic evidence alone is not used to determine the best treatment option.

An overview of the signs and symptoms relevant to osteoarthritis is presented in Box 17.1 and the radiographic changes are shown in Figures 17.3 and 17.4. These give an overview of the physical signs and symptoms that patients will experience in varying degrees and combinations. However, it is important to recognise the psychological and social effects of this disease process for the individual. How patients perceive chronic pain, stiffness, loss of mobility and function will depend upon their coping strategies and the degree of support and information they receive from their family and healthcare professionals.

ASSESSING AND EXAMINING THE PATIENT WITH OSTEOARTHRITIS

As orthopaedic nurses expand their scope of professional practice to respond to the complex needs of the patient, the opportunity to develop more specialist roles in the assessment and management of

patients diagnosed with OA will require nurses to develop advanced skills in clinical decision making.

An accurate and comprehensive history is essential to aid differential diagnostics and for making a

---

Box 17.1   Summary of the signs and symptoms of osteoarthritis

Signs
Crepitus
Restriction of range of movement
Shortening
Alterations in gait, for example Trendelenburg
Flexion and external rotation deformities of the hip joint
Radiographic changes: loss of joint space, osteophyte formation, varus deformity of the knee, subluxation, subchondral sclerosis, spurs at the joint margins, subchondral cysts

Symptoms
Pain on movement and at rest, disturbing sleep
Stiffness
Reduced mobility/walking distance due to pain, deformity and stiffness

---

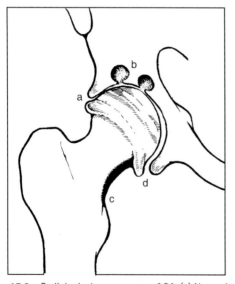

Figure 17.2   Radiological appearances of OA. (a) Narrowing of the joint space. (b) Cysts. (c) Sclerosis. (d) Osteophytes. (From Dandy & Edwards 1998.)

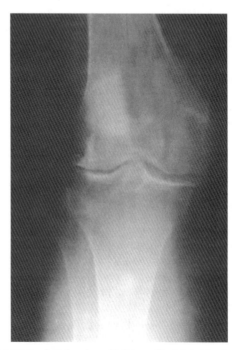

Figure 17.3   Anterior view of left knee. The joint space is reduced, particularly laterally.

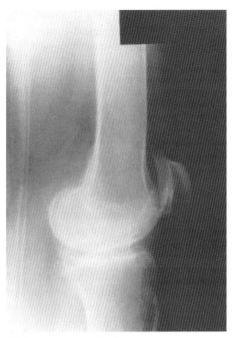

Figure 17.4 Lateral view of left knee.

clinical judgement on the most appropriate type of care or treatment for the patient presenting with joint pain and dysfunction. The assessment process must not be rushed as valuable information can be overlooked if the patient is not given sufficient time to answer questions. Box 17.2 provides an overview of the assessment of the patient presenting with osteoarthritic symptoms.

Following assessment and examination, the severity of the patient's symptoms is ascertained and the most appropriate treatment and care decided upon. The orthopaedic nurse has an important contribution in this process along with other members of the multidisciplinary team and the patient.

The patient should be empowered through support and the information they are given to make an informed choice about their treatment options.

TREATMENT OPTIONS

Patient care and management can be classified into two broad treatment categories: conservative and

---

Box 17.2   Overview of a comprehensive assessment of the patient presenting with suspected osteoarthritis

History of chief complaint	• Description of symptoms, in patient's own words • Onset of symptoms • Duration of symptoms • How are symptoms relieved, if at all? • Time of day or night when symptoms are worse or better
Past medical history, family history and social history	• Conditions such as rheumatoid arthritis have a strong familial trend, therefore family history is important • Use a genogram to document family history • A social history will help make a clinical decision on how the patient would cope with various treatment options • Include medications
Physical examination	• Always examine similar joints to make comparisons • Always examine joints above and below the joint of chief complaint, to differentiate for referred pain • Use a goniometer to assess range of movement • Ask patient to walk to assess for gait abnormalities
Use valid and reliable assessment tools such as the Nottingham Health Profile and Oxford Knee Score	• Quantify degree of pain, stiffness and difficulty with function
Allow patient time to express their anxieties and feelings	• Open-ended questions will help to ascertain how the patient is coping with their symptoms

surgical. As well as definitive treatments, options for interim relief of symptoms should be considered, for example pain relief and mobility support whilst the patient is on the waiting list for total joint replacement.

CONSERVATIVE MANAGEMENT

There are a range of non-surgical measures that can relieve joint pain and disability. Relatively simple measures may help the patient with joint disease, such as:

- the use of a walking stick in the opposite hand to the affected joint, to take some of the weight going through the joint
- monitoring of pain scores and effectiveness of analgesic and antiinflammatory drugs
- injection of local anaesthetic or steroid drugs to provide symptomatic relief
- adaptations to the home such as raised toilet seats or grabrails
- provision of aids such as long-handled shoehorns and stocking aids
- health education regarding weight and exercise.

Although these conservative measures may not prevent the patient from having a joint replacement in the long term they can provide relief in the short and medium term as either an alternative to joint replacement or whilst the patient is awaiting admission for surgery. The orthopaedic nurse has an essential role in providing such conservative measures in collaboration with other members of the multidisciplinary team.

SURGICAL INTERVENTIONS

There are a number of surgical procedures used in the treatment of OA, including joint resurfacing, osteotomy, arthrodesis and joint replacement.

Joint resurfacing is an alternative for younger patients with osteoarthritic joints. Nelson et al (1997, p736) states that 'Resurfacing of the femoral head is a time-buying first stage operation for younger patients'. It involves covering the femoral head with a cemented titanium shell, which protects the articulating surfaces and slows down the destructive processes associated with osteoarthritis and preserves bone stock within the joint. Many of the follow-up evaluative studies on the outcomes of

joint resurfacing are in the early stages, so at present there is little long-term empirical evidence to support the effectiveness of this procedure. One of the reported complications is femoral neck fracture (Brinker et al 1995).

An osteotomy is performed to reduce the load on the most severely affected areas of the joint. The procedure is typically performed to slow down the progression of joint destruction due to OA. Patients experience 30–90% pain relief up to 5 years following the procedure (Hosie & Dickson 2000).

Occasionally, when joint replacement surgery has failed or the joint is unsuitable for replacement surgery, an arthrodesis of the joint may be performed to alleviate pain. However, this procedure results in the patient having no or very little movement of the joint concerned.

The main surgical intervention for the treatment of osteoarthritic joints is total joint replacement. This involves the removal of the articulating surfaces of the affected joint and replacement with plastic or metal components. Joint replacements have been performed for several decades and over the years the design and reliability of prosthetic joints have been gradually improved. It is important to remember, however, that prosthetic joints will eventually wear out and the patient will require a revision of the joint replacement, which is a more complex procedure that needs to be carried out by a highly skilled orthopaedic surgeon. As Villar (1992, p3) states: 'All joints will fail eventually; and revision needs to be done by specialists'. Prosthetic joints will normally last 10–15 years depending on the subsequent load bearing through the joint and the amount of wear and tear it receives. The prosthesis may also loosen due to fracturing of the bone cement and loss of bone stock.

There are many types of prosthesis available on the market, which can be cemented or uncemented at the time of insertion. Examples of these are shown in Figures 17.5–17.8.

PREPARING PATIENTS FOR TOTAL JOINT REPLACEMENT

There is a great deal of empirical evidence to support the theory that comprehensive preoperative information increases patient cooperation and understanding postoperatively and reduces the incidence of postoperative complications. Many preoperative orthopaedic assessment clinics are nurse led and

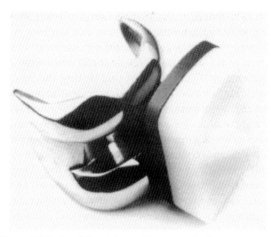

Figure 17.5   Insall Burstein total knee prosthesis.

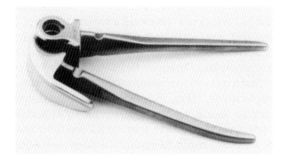

Figure 17.6   Stanmore total knee prosthesis.

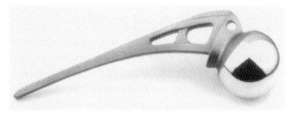

Figure 17.7   Austin Moore prosthesis, femoral component.

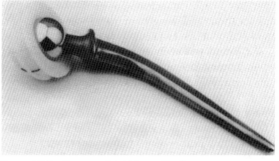

Figure 17.8   Stanmore total hip prosthesis.

give orthopaedic nurses an opportunity to enhance their skills and knowledge in patient assessment. The timing and method of preoperative information giving are vitally important if patients are to be as fully informed as possible about their surgery, care and postdischarge support needs. Information should be given in an appropriate format to meet the needs of the individual patient; for example, written information can be supported by a video the patient can view at home before their admission to hospital (Saroop-D'Souza 2001). Through the provision of support and education, the orthopaedic nurse has a vital role in preparing patients psychologically for total joint replacement.

Preassessment clinics, usually held 1–3 weeks before the date of the operation, provide the first opportunity to initiate good practice (Fellows 1998, 1999, Lucas 1998). Blood tests can be performed as required (full blood count, urea and electrolytes plus blood to cross-match for transfusion), urinalysis and blood pressure should be recorded. An electrocardiogram and chest X-ray are requested based on past medical history or clinical findings. A preoperative X-ray of the joint will also be taken. Those undergoing joint replacements tend to be older by the nature of the disease process. Consideration needs to be given to the likely systemic diseases that older patients suffer from that may affect their operative outcome or compromise the anaesthetic, such as atherosclerosis, hypertension, peripheral vascular disease, emphysema, bronchitis, asthma, intercurrent infection and chronic renal insufficiency. Following an explanation of the surgery and the potential risks, the operating surgeon will obtain written patient consent for the operation either at the preassessment clinic or on the day of operation.

The preassessment clinic is often the best forum in which to commence patient education as the patient will have time at home to digest the information, making this a better option compared to patient education on the day of admission for surgery. The factors to be considered in relation to patient education include the following (Hill & Davis 2000).

- Balancing patients' expectations with a realistic evaluation of the likely outcome of surgery. This is important in influencing a patient's overall satisfaction with the procedure, particularly in the long term.
- Information about the surgical procedure must be explained to the patient in terms they understand. Information should include whether the

operation will be under local or general anaesthetic, the location and length of the incision and the expected benefits, risks and complications.

- Patients will want to know how long they will be in hospital, how long they will be immobile and how long before they can return to work or resume normal activities. This will also include confirmation of whether they will be admitted the day before their surgery or on the same day to allow all the preoperative preparations to be completed.

- A subject often avoided is the issue of sexuality. Ageism can frequently result in healthcare professionals believing that elderly patients do not need or want to know about how undergoing total joint surgery will affect their sexual activity in the rehabilitation period. These misconceptions can often lead to avoidable anxiety and embarrassment on behalf of the patient and their partner. The nurse is in an ideal position through development of the therapeutic relationship to discuss issues pertaining to sexuality and sexual activity in a sensitive and safe environment.

- The extent of the patient's social support network can also be established; this is useful when negotiating discharge plans and care.

A significant number of patients who attend preassessment clinics are found to be unsuitable for surgery or anaesthesia due, for example, to uncontrolled hypertension, dental decay, local skin lesions such as leg ulcers or fungal infections of the feet. Although screening in the clinic prevents patients being admitted and cancelled on the day of surgery, the patient who is postponed or cancelled at this stage will, understandably, be distressed. In an attempt to minimise the number of patients cancelled or postponed at preassessment clinic, an initial screening process, through the outpatients clinic or by telephone, should be carried out as soon as the patient is put on the waiting list. The orthopaedic nurse in the preassessment clinic is in an ideal situation to prescreen patients and refer them to an appropriate member of the multidisciplinary team, including the primary healthcare team, to treat any conditions that would adversely affect their suitability for joint replacement surgery.

RISK FACTORS FOR PATIENTS UNDERGOING TOTAL JOINT SURGERY

Most patients who undergo total joint replacement exhibit excellent results regarding pain relief and restoration of function (Sarmiento et al 1990). However, joint replacement surgery is not without risk. Mortality within 1 year of total hip surgery is estimated at 2% (Goldie 1992). A study conducted by Seagroatt et al (1991) found that during the 90-day postoperative period there were 11 deaths per 1000 operations, for patients undergoing total hip replacement. Mortality is often difficult to attribute to a single cause when dealing with older people who often have multiple and complex pathologies. Seagroatt et al (1991, p1432) affirm this difficulty, stating 'Deaths in, say, the year after operation may be related to the operation or, particularly in elderly patients, may be independent of it'. So consequently the actual rate of postreplacement mortality is extremely difficult to quantify, especially if death occurs after the hospital discharge.

As well as mortality, morbidity following surgery must be considered. There are a variety of complications that can occur following total joint surgery. These can be grouped into: systemic, specific early and specific late. Orthopaedic nurses have an important part to play in managing the risk of postoperative complications. They have a major responsibility to ensure their practice is research based and related to preventive measures that avoid life-threatening and serious complications such as deep vein thrombosis, pulmonary embolism and infection of the prosthetic joint.

Systemic complications and prophylaxis

It is important to remember that patients who most frequently undergo joint replacement surgery are elderly and often have co-morbid states of health. It is therefore imperative that a comprehensive assessment is performed preoperatively to assess the patient's suitability for surgery and anaesthesia.

Orthopaedic patients tend to stay on the wards longer than other surgical patients do and get to know the staff better. Complications should be anticipated and any action taken immediately. The aim is to facilitate wound healing without a superficial or deep infection, to optimise mobility, particularly ambulation, and to reduce risks due to impaired physical mobility (Hill & Davis 2000).

Asking about chest pain, shortness of breath and calf pain and assessing the level of consciousness are as relevant as observations of temperature, pulse, respiratory rate and blood pressure. Peripheral pulses should be checked and the extremities examined for colour, temperature, sensation and movement. The wound is usually covered for 3–5 days and healing monitored.

Pulmonary embolus is still the most common cause of death following hip replacement surgery. After total joint replacement the incidence of venous thromboembolic disease (VTED) is reported to be 40–60% of all unprotected patients (Imperiale & Speroff 1994). Virchow's triad states the risk factors for VTED as being venous stasis, endothelial damage and an increase in clotting factors. Anticoagulant medication acts to reduce the clotting capacity of blood.

In 1994 a metaanalysis of the Medline database 1966–1993 demonstrated that low molecular weight heparin (clinically important bleeding occurs in less than 2% of patients) and pressure stockings reduced the risk of pulmonary embolism after THR; in addition the authors found that aspirin did not lower the risk of proximal deep venous thrombosis (DVT) (Imperiale & Speroff 1994). Treatment versus treatment comparisons indicated that low molecular weight heparin (LMWH) was the superior treatment to prevent all DVT. Metaanalysis of Medline 1986–1997, Embase and manufacturers showed that LMWH had considerable advantages over unfractioned heparin and warfarin to prevent DVT and proximal DVT after THR (Howard & Aaron 1998). LMWH is therefore indicated as providing effective protection against proximal DVT.

Warfarin takes 36 hours to have an effect, leaving the patient relatively unprotected in the early postoperative period. It requires daily dose adjustments and blood level monitoring.

Foot and calf compression systems are important in preventing the clinical consequences of venous stasis (Hartman et al 1982, Westrich & Sculco 1996). Combining foot compression and chemical prophylaxis is better than chemical prophylaxis alone. Graded pressure stockings may serve as a useful supplement to other thromboprophylactic measures in hip surgery but should not be used alone (Nilsen et al 1984).

Prophylaxis in any form should be continued until the patient is spending most of the day ambulatory. The highest incidence of DVT is on the fifth postoperative day, with the risk remaining high for about 30 days, indicating the need to continue prophylaxis following discharge home to cover this period.

While consensus groups such as that led by Scurr (1998) have attempted to produce guidelines to add consistency to prophylaxis for venous thromboembolism in hospital patients, there is still little agreement amongst those concerned. The orthopaedic nurse needs to understand the physiological changes and practice implications. They have an essential role in identifying patients at risk of thrombosis, in implementing preventive strategies and in supporting treatment measures (Davis 1998), all of which should be based on appropriate agreed practice protocols and guidelines derived from the current best evidence.

Specific early complications

Infection rates can be minimised to a rate of 1% for primary procedures by the prudent use of antibiotics and clean air operating theatres (Villar 1992), although Nade (1997) suggests figures of 0.23–8.8% are more realistic. Minimisation of infection requires an interdisciplinary approach to risk management during the perioperative and postoperative periods.

An initial pyrexic response occurs after total joint replacement surgery, as part of the normal inflammatory response (Shaw & Chung 1999). Usually this is maximal on the first postoperative day and gradually levels to normal by day 5. Knowledge of this may reduce unnecessary examinations and investigations for sepsis.

An early infection may occur in the first few days following surgery and is usually superficial, being limited to the dermal layers or within a haematoma. The early detection of a postoperative infection is essential to avoid a deep infection leading to the joint itself becoming infected. Prophylactic intra- and postoperative antibiotic regimes can significantly reduce the risk of an early infection. In addition, careful and regular observation of the surgical wound and monitoring of the patient's temperature should be undertaken for signs and symptoms indicative of a wound infection. Careful adoption of universal precautions and aseptic techniques for wound management is essential to minimise the risk of an early infection. Patient education is also needed to ensure that patients understand the importance of hygiene related to the surgical wound.

Deep infections are a dreaded complication of arthroplasty. They may arise from an incident during the operation, secondary to contamination from a discharging haematoma postoperatively or by the haematogenous route. Factors that increase the risk of infection are listed in Box 17.3. Appropriate initial investigations include a serum white cell count and erythrocyte sedimentation rate. The consequences of infected joint prostheses are a longer hospital

---

Box 17.3 Factors that increase the risk of infection (from Hill & Davis 2000)

- Poor-quality soft tissues or local infection
- Previous local surgery
- Joints close to skin surface with poor soft tissue coverage
- Previous sepsis
- Remote infection at the time of surgery
- Diabetes
- Sickle cell anaemia
- Rheumatoid arthritis
- Steroids
- Poor nutritional status
- Smoking
- Drains, IV lines, catheters

Table 17.1 Preoperative information for patients undergoing THR

Activity	Advice
Sitting	• Use a high chair with supportive arms
Getting out of bed	• Do get out on your operated side, remembering to keep your leg straight out in front of you
Dressing	• Use the dressing aids provided by the occupational therapist (OT) • Dress your operated leg first and undress it last
Picking things up from the floor	• Do use the long-handled tool provided by the OT • Ask someone to pick things up from the floor for you
Using the stairs	• Lead with your unoperated leg when ascending/going upstairs and lead with your operated leg when descending/going downstairs
Sexual intercourse	• In the absence of pain from your operation, sexual intercourse may be resumed 6–8 weeks after surgery unless your doctor informs you otherwise
Sleeping	• Sleep on your back for the first 6 weeks after the operation or until your doctor informs you otherwise
Using the toilet	• Use a raised toilet seat
Walking	• Use the correct walking aid • Lead with your feet when changing direction and avoid twisting your body

stay, wound dehiscence and the need for further surgery including excision arthroplasty, revision arthroplasty or arthrodesis.

Anaemia, poor nutrition (hypoalbuminaemia), obesity and diabetes adversely affect wound healing. Estimates as high as 50–80% are suggested for the rate of wound infections due to direct contamination at the time of surgery, usually from the patient's skin or by airborne bacteria (Nasser 1992).

Dislocation of the hip joint usually happens between the second and fifth postoperative day. Following a study by Li et al (1999), the incidence of dislocation is estimated to be 3.9%. The hip joint may dislocate posteriorly because of excessive flexion at the hip joint or because of poor surgical technique when performing the THR (Li et al 1999). If the hip prosthesis dislocates, the patient will complain of severe pain and the limb will appear internally rotated and shortened.

The nurse has an essential role in patient education to avoid postoperative dislocation. Information should be provided at the preoperative assessment and reinforced by nursing and therapy staff on a regular basis postoperatively. A list of advice is provided in Table 17.1. The patient should be advised to carry out these precautions until they are reassessed at their postoperative outpatient appointment, which is usually 6 weeks following surgery.

Specific late complications

Late sepsis around a prosthesis is a serious complication which may occur some 6–24 months after surgery (Nade 1997). The rate of late sepsis is estimated at 1–4% of prostheses (Duckworth 1995). Nade (1997) suggests that there are three surgical options for treating delayed deep infection.

1 If the causative organism is of low virulence and the bone stock is good, removal of the infected prosthesis may be followed by insertion of a new joint within the same operation.

2 If the organisms are of a high virulence then a two-stage replacement is needed with a period of at least 6 weeks between removal of the infected prosthesis and insertion of the new joint. During this period the patient is either non- or partially weight bearing through the hip or is immobile on bedrest, possibly on traction.

3 If the bone stock is poor, the patient may need to have the infected joint removed and an arthrodesis of the joint performed. This will leave the patient with

shortening of the limb and a stiff joint with very little range of movement.

Delayed deep infection of a joint replacement is costly to the health service and very distressing to the patient so it is essential that a multidisciplinary approach to infection control is maintained throughout the peri- and postoperative periods.

All primary total hip replacements will eventually fail. The length of time before a prosthesis begins to loosen will vary depending on a variety of factors including the age of the patient when the primary prosthesis is inserted, the weight of the patient, the surgical technique and type of prosthesis used. The average length of life for a prosthesis is generally estimated to be 10–15 years. Once a prosthesis becomes loose, causing pain and limited functioning of the joint, a revision arthroplasty will be needed.

Sonnabend (1996) suggests that the trialling of joint prostheses has not always been rigorous, resulting in disaster for some patients. In 1998 the 3M hip prosthesis was announced to be substandard and all patients who had received this type of prosthesis had to be contacted and faced possible removal of the joint and a further replacement. Joint replacements have become a highly profitable commodity not only for the care provider units but also for the commercial companies that manufacture them. Control of the production within strict guidelines and continued evaluation of the prostheses used is essential, this is being addressed by the use of national registers of prostheses.

MANAGING RISK AND PREVENTING COMPLICATIONS

Orthopaedic nurses have an important role in managing risk and preventing complications for patients undergoing total joint replacement. They must ensure that clinical protocols to minimise the risk of patients developing complications, such as wound infections and deep vein thrombosis, are research based and updated on a regular basis. It is no longer professionally or legally acceptable for practitioners to provide care that is based on custom and practice rather than evidence. However, clinical protocols should 'not be applied slavishly or automatically and are not a substitute for clinical judgement' (Tingle 1995, p28). Orthopaedic nurses who profess to be 'specialist' or 'expert' must be prepared to exercise higher levels of clinical decision making and to be able to justify such decisions as accountable practitioners.

ETHICAL AND PROFESSIONAL ISSUES

The issues related to eligibility for joint replacement surgery are complex and encompass ethical and economic considerations. With finite resources for healthcare provision, postoperative mortality and morbidity risk factors and an increasing elderly population, it is imperative that joint replacement surgery is only performed when and if it is warranted and determined by patient need. Goldie (1992) indicates that 90% of patients exhibit excellent results following THR in relation to pain relief and functional ability. Goldie also suggests that success has made it inevitable that the operation is on occasion used indiscriminately. Conversely, Fear et al (1997) concluded from their study that not all those warranting joint replacement surgery were put forward for operations. Their study demonstrated unequal access to joint replacement surgery related to age: 'With regard to the 75 year old and over this group, despite high levels of pain and disability and taking account of co-morbidity, seem to have relatively little chance of being put forward for surgery' (Fear et al 1997, p74). The National Service Framework for Older People (DoH 2001) stipulates that services must be provided on the basis of clinical need and that discrimination on the basis of age is not acceptable.

Currently, within the UK, patients are selected for joint replacement based on the clinical judgement of an orthopaedic consultant or one of their team following a brief examination and history, which is often limited due to the vast patient numbers to be seen during outpatient clinics. Objective assessment of the need for total joint replacement is crucial in order to avoid unfair access to surgery based on age or any other discriminatory factors and to avoid unwarranted joint replacements being performed. There are a number of valid and reliable disease-specific measures for assessing the severity of OA from the patient's perspective. These include the Western Ontario and McMaster Osteoarthritis Index (WOMAC), the Harris Hip Score and the Oxford Knee Score. Disease-specific measures such as these are a useful adjunct to comprehensive history taking, examination and clinical investigations.

REHABILITATION

To maximise the benefit of total joint replacement, it is essential the multidisciplinary team, including the patient, are all working towards agreed goals and outcomes during the rehabilitation period. Nurses historically have found it difficult to articulate their role within the rehabilitation process (Johnson 1995). This may be due to philosophical differences between the traditional definitions of nursing and the principles of rehabilitation. Henderson (1980, p242) defines nursing as 'care and support during illness, doing for others the things they would normally do for themselves'; in contrast, rehabilitation is defined as the planned withdrawal of support (Isaacs 1992), the aim being to maximise the patient's independence (Johnson 1995).

Specialist orthopaedic nurses have to tread a fine line between meeting the patient's needs in the early postoperative period and gradually withdrawing their support, encouraging independence during the restorative phase of care.

Research has shown that patients spend only a small percentage of their day engaged in useful rehabilitation activity. The estimates of time that patients spend in therapeutically useful activities ranges from 3.4% (Wade et al 1984) to 17% (Ellul et al 1993) of the total waking day. In order to maximise the patient's full potential and effectively utilise hospital beds it is essential that orthopaedic nurses incorporate therapy activities into the patient's activities of living 7 days a week, 52 weeks a year. Nurses are the only discipline to provide 24-hour cover and therefore are in an ideal position to close the gap in the rehabilitation cycle (Johnson 1995).

REHABILITATION OPTIONS

Rehabilitation following joint replacement should be a goal-directed, time-limited process that facilitates maximum patient recovery with effective use of finite resources. It is therefore essential that the rehabilitation process for this client group is patient focused and has an interdisciplinary collaborative approach. The term 'managed care' has been adopted to describe 'an organisational process which spells out the sequence of care and treatment that is to be delivered to a specific case type' (Hale 1995, p29). It is important that the tools of managed care, such as integrated care pathways, are developed by representatives from all disciplines involved in the patient's care and treatment and that the pathway is based on empirical evidence or, in the absence of valid research, a consensus of best practice. It should be remembered that the existence of integrated care

pathways for a client group is not a substitute for individualised care planning.

Traditionally patients have undergone their rehabilitation within the inpatient setting. This is gradually changing as the number of hospital at home and other early discharge schemes have increased within the UK in recent years, allowing the early discharge of patients back into their own homes following total joint replacement. Hospital at home schemes may be defined as 'schemes that provide intensive nursing, social and therapy care in the home to patients who would otherwise remain in hospital' (Elliot 1995). The genesis of the hospital at home scheme is due to several factors (Jester & Turner 1998).

- The reduction in the number of inpatient hospital beds available (Vaughan 1995).
- The recognition that hospitalisation can have negative psychological, social and physical effects on elderly patients.
- Patients can recuperate better in their own homes rather than hospital, given appropriate professional and social support.

Empirical evaluation related to outcomes of patients discharged early to hospital at home schemes following total joint replacement are still in the early stages (Black 1997, Palmer-Hill et al 2000). Current examples of this can be found in O'Brien & Beverland (1998), O'Brien et al (1999), Wong et al (1999), Wilde-Larsson et al (1999).

Other centres are developing supported early discharge with link nurses based either in the community or in the orthopaedic unit supporting patients in their home in the first few days post discharge. This latter approach does not always involve the multidisciplinary team in community-supported care.

Early discharge schemes may not be suitable for all patients after joint replacement surgery nor may it be suitable for their family. Careful assessment of the patient's suitability must be completed, ideally as part of their preassessment clinic visit, along with the availability and willingness of the family and carers to participate in the scheme. Patients who are not suitable may benefit from a period of intermediate care and rehabilitation.

It is imperative that comprehensive research is conducted to evaluate the effectiveness, cost and long-term outcomes of these types of rehabilitation before stakeholders make an informed choice about the best treatment option for patients.

Orthopaedic nurses must be prepared to transpose their specialist skills and knowledge to the community setting to meet the needs of patients discharged early and to support the centres providing intermediate care.

CONCLUSION

This chapter has provided an overview of issues pertaining to osteoarthritis and its treatment. The prevalence of osteoarthritis will continue to increase as the demographic proportion and number of elderly people within society continue to rise. The role of the orthopaedic nurse working in collaboration with other members of the multidisciplinary team is pivotal to ensure that patients with osteoarthritis

receive high-quality, evidence-based care and treatment.

Meeting the needs of patients with osteoarthritis requires a dynamic and flexible approach. This has led to orthopaedic nurses developing specialist roles and leading innovations such as nurse-led assessment clinics, the development of hospital at home and other early supported discharge schemes and liaison with primary care services to develop early screening and prevention strategies.

The future challenges of meeting intermediate care needs and those arising from developments in joint surgery will require further dynamic approaches to practice and create more opportunities for developing orthopaedic nursing roles.

References

Black C 1997 An evaluation of setting up an early discharge scheme. Journal of Orthopaedic Nursing 1(3): 119–122

Brinker M, Cook S, Skinner H 1995 Adjunct fibula strut bone graft in resurfacing hip arthroplasty. Journal of LA State Medical Society USA 147: 547–549

Buckwalter J 1996 Evidence for overuse/overloading of joints in the genesis and progression of osteoarthritis. Current Orthopaedics 10: 220–224

Dandy DJ, Edwards DJ 1998 Essential orthopaedics and trauma, 3rd edn. Churchill Livingstone, Edinburgh

Davis P 1998 The hidden threat: deep vein thrombosis. Journal of Orthopaedic Nursing 2(1): 45–51

Department of Health (DoH) 2001 National Service Framework for Older People. Department of Health, London

Duckworth T 1995 Lecture notes on orthopaedics and fractures, 3rd edn. Blackwell, Oxford

Elliot M 1995 There's no place like home. Nursing Times 91(34): 36–37

Ellul J, Watkins C, Ferguson N et al 1993 Increasing patient engagement in rehabilitation activities. Clinical Rehabilitation 7: 297–302

Fear J, Hillman M, Chamberlain A et al 1997 Prevalence of hip problems in the population aged 55 years and over: access to specialist care and future demand for hip arthroplasty. British Journal of Rheumatology 36: 74–76

Fellows H 1998 Orthopaedic pre-admission assessment clinics: part 1. Journal of Orthopaedic Nursing 2(4): 209–218

Fellows H 1999 Orthopaedic pre-admission assessment clinics: part 2. Journal of Orthopaedic Nursing 3(2): 60–66

Frankel S, Eachus J, Pearson N et al 1999 Population requirement for primary hip replacement surgery: a cross-sectional study. Lancet 353(9161): 1304–1309

Goldie I 1992 Arthritis surgery in the elderly. In: Newman R (ed) Orthogeriatrics: comprehensive orthopaedic care for the elderly patient. Butterworth-Heinemann, Oxford

Hale C 1995 Key terms in managed care. Nursing Times 91(29): 29–31

Hartman JT, Pugh JL, Smith RD et al 1982 Cyclic sequential compression of the lower limb in prevention of deep vein thrombosis. Journal of Bone and Joint Surgery 64A(7): 1059–1062

Henderson V 1980 Preserving the essence of nursing in a technological age. Journal of Advanced Nursing 5: 245–260

Hill N, Davis P 2000 Nursing care of total joint replacement. Journal of Orthopaedic Nursing 4(1): 41–45

Hosie G, Dickson J 2000 Managing osteoarthritis in primary care. Blackwell, Oxford

Howard AW, Aaron SD 1998 Low molecular weight heparin decreases proximal and distal deep vein thrombosis following knee arthroplasty. Thrombosis and Haemostasis 79: 902–906

Imperiale TF, Speroff T 1994 A meta-analysis of methods to prevent DVT following total hip replacement. Journal of the American Medical Association 271(22): 1780–1785

Isaacs B 1992 The challenge of geriatric medicine. Oxford University Press, Oxford

Jester R, Turner D 1998 Hospital at home: the Bromsgrove experience. Nursing Standard 12(20): 40–42

Johnson J 1995 Achieving effective rehabilitation outcomes: does the nurse have a role? British Journal of Therapy and Rehabilitation 2: 113–118

Jones A, Doherty M 1996 Osteoarthritis. In: Snaith M (ed) ABC of rheumatology. BMJ Books, London

Kumar P, Clark M 1990 Clinical medicine. Baillière Tindall, London

Li E, Meding J, Ritter M et al 1999 The natural history of a posteriorly dislocated total hip replacement. Journal of Arthroplasty 14(8): 964–968

Lucas B 1998 Orthopaedic patients' experiences and perceptions of pre-admission assessment clinics. Journal of Orthopaedic Nursing 2(4): 202–208

Martin J, Meltzer H, Elliot D 1988 The prevalence of disability among adults. OPCS surveys of disability in Great Britain, Report 1. HMSO, London

Nade S 1997 Infection after joint replacement. Current Orthopaedics 11: 129–133

Nasser S 1992 Prevention and treatment of sepsis in total hip replacement. Orthopedic Clinics of North America 23(2): 265–275

Nelson C, Walz B, Gruenwald J 1997 Resurfacing of the femoral head. Long-term follow-up study. Journal of Arthroplasty USA 12: 736–740

Nilsdotter D 2001 Radiographic stage of OA or sex of the patient does not predict one year outcome after THA. Annals of the Rheumatic Diseases 60: 228–232

Nilsen DWT, Naess-Andersen KF, Kierulf P et al 1984 Graded pressure stockings in prevention of deep vein thrombosis following total hip replacement. Acta Chirurgica Scandinavica 150: 531–534

O'Brien S 1994 The hip factory. Nursing Times 90(37): 34–35

O'Brien S, Beverland DE 1998 Setting up a hip and knee replacement outcomes team. Journal of Orthopaedic Nursing 2(4): 196–201

O'Brien S, Dennison J, Breslin E et al 1999 A review of an orthopaedic outcome assessment telephone follow-up helpline and nursing advice service. Journal of Orthopaedic Nursing 3(1): 18–23

Palmer-Hill S, Flynn J, Crawford EJP 2000 Early discharge following total knee replacement, a trial of patient satisfaction and outcomes using an orthopaedic outreach team. Journal of Orthopaedic Nursing 4(3): 121–126

Radin E 1976 Mechanical aspects of osteoarthritis. Bulletin of Rheumatology 26

Sarmiento A, Ebramzadeh E, Gogan WJ et al 1990 Total hip arthroplasty with cement. A long term radiographic analysis in patients who are older than fifty and younger than fifty years. Journal of Bone and Joint Surgery 72A(10): 1470–1476

Saroop-D'Souza 2001 Patients' views on screening of a videotape on osteoarthritis in an orthopaedic outpatient department. Journal of Orthopaedic Nursing 5(4): 192–197

Scurr T 1998 Risk of and prophylaxis for venous thromboembolism in hospital patients. Phlebology 13: 87–97

Seagroatt V, Tan H, Goldacre M et al 1991 Elective total hip replacement; incidence, emergency readmission rate and postoperative mortality. British Medical Journal 303: 1431–1435

Shaw JA, Chung R 1999 Febrile response after knee and hip arthroplasty. Clinical Orthopaedics 367: 181–189

Sonnabend D 1996 New joints for old: a surgical perspective for osteoarthritis. Current Orthopaedics 10: 225–229

Tingle J 1995 Clinical protocols and the law. Nursing Times 91(29): 27–28

Vaughan B 1995 Who cares? Hospital, home or somewhere in between: the case for intermediate services. Journal of Clinical Nursing 4: 341–342

Villar R 1992 Failed hip replacements. British Medical Journal 304: 3–4

Wade D, Skilbeck CE, Langton H 1984 Therapy after stroke: amounts; determinants and effects. International Rehabilitation Medicine 6: 105–110

Ward D, Tidswell M 1994 Osteoarthritis. In: Cash J (ed) Cash's textbook of orthopaedics and rheumatology for physiotherapists. Faber and Faber, London

Westrich GH, Sculco TP 1996 Prophylaxis against deep vein thrombosis after total knee arthroplasty. Journal of Bone and Joint Surgery 78A(6): 827–834

Wilde-Larsson B, Baath C, Larsson G et al 1999 Patients' perceptions of quality care, self-rated functional ability and health one year after total knee arthroplasty. Journal of Orthopaedic Nursing 3(1): 11–17

Wong J, Wong S, Brooks E et al 1999 Home readiness and recovery pattern after total hip replacement. Journal of Orthopaedic Nursing 3(4): 210–219

Chapter 18

Care of patients with spinal conditions and injuries

Mike Smith

CHAPTER CONTENTS

INTRODUCTION

The bones, ligaments, muscles and nerves that enable movement of the spinal column are at the basis of most functional and consequently social activities. Therefore, musculoskeletal injuries and conditions affecting the spine are amongst the most debilitating of all healthcare events.

Knowledge of spinal anatomy is essential for understanding the underlying pathophysiology and appropriate management strategies that will produce optimum patient outcomes for those with spinal conditions. This chapter aims to furnish the nurse with an overview of spinal anatomy, the more commonly related conditions and skeletal fractures, along with their nursing and collaborative management.

THE VERTEBRAL COLUMN

The vertebral column forms part of the axial skeleton and is composed of seven cervical, 12 thoracic, five lumbar, five fused sacral and four fused coccygeal vertebrae. The column is shaped in two convex and two concave curves that develop in the fetus and early childhood. It comprises the vertebrae, spinal ligaments and intervertebral discs, with movements facilitated by the musculature of the upper body.

The major functions of the vertebral column are to permit movement, protect the spinal cord and provide attachments for muscles, tendons and ligaments, and an exit for the spinal nerves from the spinal cord. Stability of the vertebral column is provided through three elements:

- articulation of the vertebrae between one another
- fusion of the sacral and coccygeal vertebrae
- longitudinal ligaments which support the spinal column throughout its length.

Any damage to the vertebrae or ligaments through injury or disease can threaten this stability, potentially resulting in damage to the spinal nerves or delicate spinal cord beneath. The most common back problems are degenerative, particularly in the ageing adult, involving disc problems with associated spinal nerve irritation, reduction in ligament elasticity and thickening of the facet joints. Such gradual changes may result in the loss of space for the neurological structures, as seen in spinal stenosis. Patients with spinal conditions will therefore present with a variety of symptoms such as leg pain, numbness, tingling, weakness, back pain, unsteadiness and fatigue. In severe cases, neurological impingement can lead to severe disabling pain or may affect functional movement and sensation, occasionally with a permanent paralysis.

THE VERTEBRAE

With the exception of C1, all vertebrae have a number of common features (Fig. 18.1). An individual vertebra is made up of several parts. The primary areas of weight bearing are the vertebral bodies, each separated by a fibrous intervertebral disc. The vertebral foramina of all the vertebrae form the vertebral canal. The spinous processes are felt when running a hand down someone's back. The paired transverse processes are oriented 90° to the spinous process and provide attachment for the back muscles.

There are four facet joints associated with each vertebra, one pair facing upward and another pair facing downward. These interlock with the adjacent vertebrae.

The first cervical vertebra, the atlas, supports the head. Unlike the remaining vertebrae, the atlas does not have a body or true spinous process and its superior articular facets are 'kidney shaped' to support the occipital bone.

SPINAL LIGAMENTS

The two major ligaments in the vertebral column are the anterior and posterior longitudinal ligaments.

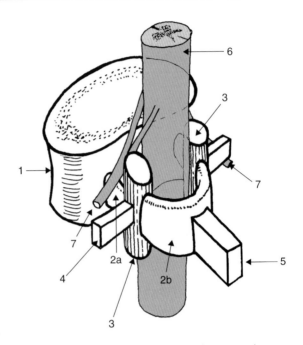

The components of a typical vertebrae comprise:

1 Vertebral body
2 Horseshoe-shaped neural arch comprised of 2a the pedicles and 2b the laminae
3 Facet (interarticular) joints
4 Transverse processes
5 Spinous process
6 Spinal cord
7 Nerve roots

Figure 18.1 Typical features of a vertebra. (Adapted from McRae & Esser 2002.)

The anterior longitudinal ligament runs from the anterior tubercle of the atlas to the anterior surface of the sacrum; it is attached to the anterior surface of the intervertebral discs and the bodies of the vertebrae. The posterior longitudinal ligament runs inside the vertebral canal from the axis to the sacral canal, attached to the posterior surface of the intervertebral discs and vertebral bodies.

Other ligaments that to a lesser degree facilitate stability of the column are the:

- ligamentum flava joining the laminae of adjacent vertebra
- supraspinatus ligament joining adjacent spinous processes from C7 to the sacrum
- interspinous ligaments which are weaker fibrous tissues joining spinous processes

- intertransverse ligaments that join the transverse processes of adjacent vertebrae
- in the neck, the ligamentum nuchae, which replaces the supraspinatus and interspinous ligaments.

INTERVERTEBRAL DISCS

Two components comprise the intervertebral discs: the annulus, a fibrous outer layer allowing excess movement to be resisted, and the inner nucleus pulposus, the inner framework of type II collagen fibres that has a more fluid consistency. The discs have four main functions to act:

- as shock absorbers
- as spacers between vertebral bodies
- to facilitate movement
- to prevent excessive movement.

PATIENT ASSESSMENT

PHYSICAL ASSESSMENTS

A physical assessment (Box 18.1) is needed in combination with a full history of the patient's back problem(s). The important questions to ask patients or their parents in the case of children and adolescents may include the following.

- If a progressive condition is suspected, at what age was the spinal condition first noted?
- Did they meet normal developmental milestones?
- Has the patient had other illnessess in the past or present? This may indicate the potential of other underlying illnesses or syndromes.
- Is there a family history of any spinal or related conditions?
- Whether the changes are caused by trauma or are developmental, ascertain the current level of spinal development and the presentations of symptoms.

The above are by no means exhaustive and other condition-specific questions and assessments are also needed. A complete head-to-toe health assessment, assessment of functional implications regarding the ability to independently perform self-care activities and assessment of the patient's social environment and desired roles are essential to guide intervention.

> **Box 18.1   Physical assessment areas**
>
> - Symmetry of spine
> - Range of movement: rotation, flexion and extension
> - Presence of another deformity, for instance asymmetry of the scapula or rib prominence in scoliosis
> - Limb length equality when standing
> - Gait pattern and ability to walk on heels and toes
> - Motor, sensory and reflex function of the lower extremities
> - Skin and back for signs suggestive of other underlying disorders such as skin tags and hairy patches
> - Scoliosis from either a neuromuscular cause or with a curve greater than 60%
> - Pulmonary function testing performed for cervical spinal cord injury

IMAGING STUDIES

As with the majority of orthopaedic conditions, X-ray is the standard imaging study for spinal conditions. Antero-posterior (AP) and lateral views of the lumbar and thoracic spines usually are the minimum studies needed. Often evaluation of the entire spine is important. Additionally, lateral flexion and extension studies, standing if possible, may give essential information regarding actual or potential problems with stability.

A computed tomography (CT) scan is an invaluable tool to evaluate the complexity of spinal conditions and spot subtle changes not easily identifiable on X-ray. CT scans accurately visualise the amount of spinal canal compromise and middle canal involvement. This is the best test to visualise fractures of the posterior elements and laminae of the neural arch, often making this invaluable for making decisions about surgery.

Magnetic resonance imaging (MRI) scans produce the best visualisation of the neural and ligamentous structures of the spine. Additionally, the MRI, when performed with contrast enhancement, can visualise haemorrhage, tumour and infection with the greatest sensitivity.

A myelogram involving injection of iodine into the spinal theca, though less commonly used due to the widespread use of MRI, can be employed to outline the spinal canal and nerve roots in those patients with a prolapsed intervertebral disc.

ADDITIONAL INVESTIGATIONS

In some patients, neurophysiological testing may be helpful for diagnosing the cause of back pain. These tests include electromyography (EMG) and nerve conduction velocity (NCV) evaluation, which help determine whether a particular nerve root and the muscle that it supplies are abnormal.

Assessment of the patient's functional ability in performing daily living tasks indicates the degree to which a person has been affected by a particular condition. This may form a more useful patient-orientated evaluation to ascertain the success or otherwise of interventions. It is vital these are tested in a number of environments, rather than just in a physiotherapy gym, as it is likely that an unrealistic picture will be presented, which bears little reality to how an individual may perform in their own environment. There are established outcome measures used by spinal rehabilitation teams such as the Barthel Index or Functional Independence Measure (FIM). These provide a 'score' that is used to ascertain progress by repeating the measurements over time.

SOCIAL ASSESSMENT

In the author's opinion, of equal or more importance is a social assessment of the patient. If asked what it is that makes life worth living, most patients are unlikely to mention a health issue or ability to move a particular joint but would mention that family, work, social contact, sports and leisure activities, travel or other 'social roles' are the major life pleasures. It is therefore essential that the patient's social desires are at the forefront of the healthcare intervention. If these are ascertained then functional rehabilitation and therapy can be geared towards these goals. Nursing and collaborative interventions related to health will optimise the patient's ability to participate in such rehabilitation.

The social implications of spinal conditions, particularly those resulting in chronic pain, have profound effects on the individual's ability to function within their social world. As the pain becomes the focus of the patient's life, all forms of relationships with family and friends may suffer. It is likely that employment and hence financial independence will also be affected. These merit different approaches from other healthcare situations where the patient is in acute pain.

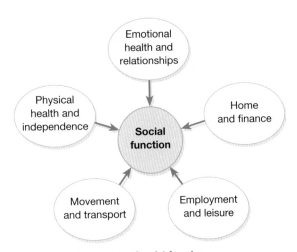

Figure 18.2   Dimensions of social function.

There are few formal tools which offer user-friendly frameworks for a social assessment; however, asking questions related to the dimensions outlined in Figure 18.2 (Smith 1999) may prove beneficial. By utilising these dimensions, meaningful patient goals can be set, forming the basis for rehabilitation programmes.

BACK PAIN: AN OVERVIEW

With few exceptions, the symptom leading the patient to seek medical assistance is back pain, although the cause can be complex to diagnose (Fig. 18.3).

The most common type of back pain is mechanical in origin, resulting from a problem with the back muscles, bones, joints or ligaments. In essence, back problems are most commonly a result of abuse, overuse or underuse of the back. People working in industries requiring excessive lifting, bending and heavy work on a routine basis are more prone to develop this condition. Nurses were prime candidates in previous years due to poor handling techniques, underinvestment and underutilisation of manual handling equipment, and of course the unique nature of the load being lifted (Scott 1994).

When rheumatoid arthritis affects the back, it usually involves the cervical and lumbar spine. This causes severe neck and back pain as well as the inability to move these normally very mobile parts of the back. If bony spurs (osteophytes) grow from the vertebrae, then spinal stenosis may result, exerting pressure on the spinal cord and nerves.

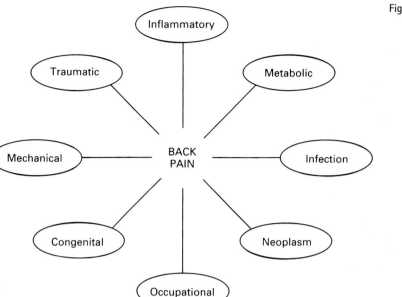

Figure 18.3   Causes of low back pain.

Primary tumours can develop in the bone marrow, the vertebra itself, the nerve roots, spinal cord or meninges. Metastatic tumours commonly originate from tumours in the lung, breast, prostate or kidney but can be from anywhere else in the body. Both primary and metastatic tumours can compress the spine or nerve roots and cause significant pain. The spinal cord has only a limited amount of space inside the spinal column, so even a very small tumour can cause enough pressure to become problematic.

An infection can arise in the vertebrae, discs, meninges or spinal fluid. In addition to back pain, patients usually have a fever and serum abnormalities indicative of an infection. Some infections can compress the spinal cord and result in serious neurological deterioration if not diagnosed and treated immediately.

Osteoporosis is the most common cause of vertebral fractures in the elderly, especially older women. Patients may develop chronic back pain, as well as multiple bony fractures.

Back pain can also result from various non-musculoskeletal disorders in other parts of the body and may be mistaken for spinal musculoskeletal syndromes. These include bleeding from the aorta (aortic dissection), pancreatic disease, pneumonia, bladder disorders, uterine abnormalities and kidney diseases, including acute renal stones. However, these only account for about 1 in 200 people who seek medical consultation for low back pain.

CONSERVATIVE MANAGEMENT OF ACUTE BACK PAIN

The main treatment for back pain caused by muscle or ligament strain or stiffness is a restricted duration of bedrest combined with appropriate back-strengthening exercises and pain control. It is worth stressing that too much bedrest can make the situation worse. Gentle exercise is important for increasing circulation to the area and for strengthening the muscles to minimise likelihood of recurrence.

A variety of medications are used to relieve acute back pain, from mild pain relievers such as aspirin and ibuprofen to stronger prescription drugs for more severe pain. Medication is also prescribed to treat muscular spasm or related neurological problems.

- Non-steroidal antiinflammatory drugs (NSAIDs), including ibuprofen, help relieve pain and decrease inflammation in the soft tissues and other structures. They can be used to treat rheumatoid arthritis flare-ups, disc diseases, muscular pain and traumatic injuries. Usually they are taken orally, though some can be given by injection. The major side effect of NSAIDs is that they can cause significant gastrointestinal problems, particularly ulcers. Patients with previous gastrointestinal problems may be advised to use alternative methods of pain relief as a general rule, although the latest breed of NSAIDs, the COX-2 inhibitors such as celebrex, may be less of a problem and are tolerated well in such a case.

• Tramadol is used to treat both musculoskeletal and neuropathic pain such as the pain from a tumour exerting pressure on the spinal nerves. The side effects of dizziness and light-headedness can be distressing for some patients.

• Narcotics are used for short-term pain relief, especially for patients experiencing severe pain from disc herniation or trauma.

• Muscle relaxants, for example orphenadrine and diazepam, are often used to treat muscular spasm and in combination with NSAIDs for pain relief. A major side effect of muscle relaxants is extreme sleepiness, making them helpful for patients having difficulties sleeping due to the discomfort in their back.

CONSERVATIVE MANAGEMENT OF CHRONIC BACK PAIN

A range of drugs are used in treating chronic back pain.

• Tricyclic antidepressants, for instance amitriptyline, are often used in low doses. Their use is indicated for patients who experience numbness, burning, aching, throbbing or stabbing pains that shoot down the limbs. The side effects include drowsiness, dry mouth and constipation.

• Gabapentin has proven extremely helpful in the management of many forms of chronic pain. It is taken orally, three times a day in slowly increasing doses, until the pain is relieved. Like the tricyclic antidepressants, it is especially helpful if there are any signs of irritated nerve roots. It is often taken in combination with a tricyclic antidepressant. It has minimal side effects, including mild drowsiness.

• Tramadol is usually reserved for short-term back pain but can be used to treat chronic pain if other drugs are having no effect.

• Tizanadine is a relatively new drug prescribed to treat muscular spasticity, as well as chronic back pain, especially musculoskeletal back pain. The side effects include drowsiness and light-headedness.

• If no other drugs work, narcotics are sometimes necessary to relieve chronic back pain, either orally or via a skin patch. The potential complications from narcotic usage include drug addiction, withdrawal reactions, an altered mental status and constipation.

Pain clinics

Even with all of the above, it may not be possible to completely remove the patient's pain. In such circumstances, the patient enters a chronic pain cycle where the focus of their attention in life becomes almost exclusively the pain itself, resulting in not only physical symptoms but also major changes to the social aspect of the patient's life (Tripp 1999). Employment and relationships both at home and outside may suffer.

Dedicated chronic pain clinics attempt to enable the person to live with their pain, by applying the principles of rehabilitation goal-setting techniques. They encourage patients to change their focus away from the pain by empowering the patient to get on with their life. The pain experience, although often still an issue, gradually becomes less disabling, enabling the patient to be a more participative and constructive member of society (Hansson et al 2001).

Such clinics are interdisciplinary in nature, involving the input of many professionals. Psychologists have a valuable role in supporting patients to break the cycle of chronic pain and offer advice on relaxation techniques. Occupational therapists will usually lead occupational retraining programmes and may help individuals slowly get back to the kind of work they were previously doing.

The nurse's role is dependent on the particular treatment modality employed, generally acting as a case manager within the rehabilitation process. The patient education role relates to techniques that enable the patient to perform daily living activities despite the pain. Other aspects of the role include the administration of analgesia or other pain management techniques and dealing with the psychosocial aspects associated with the chronic back pain (Davis & White 2001). Patients are referred to nurse counsellors within some specialist rehabilitation units. In recent years postgraduate courses in rehabilitation counselling have become available to offer formal academic support to professional staff in such roles.

The goals of physiotherapy, both for conservative management and pre- and postsurgical care, are to minimise discomfort, restore normal movements and help return patients to their previous level of functioning or their highest possible level of functioning. The particular techniques used depend on personal choice, the severity of the pain and extent of patient immobility. For some of these techniques there is little clear evidence for their benefit but they appear to be helpful for some patients, for example spinal manipulation. They include the following.

- Exercises involving bending and stretching the muscles and spine, as well as endurance strengthening.
- Massage to increase circulation to the area; this includes traditional techniques, neuromuscular massage therapy and the use of hand-held devices.
- Ultrasound will increase blood flow by heating and vasodilating vessels within the skeletal muscles.
- Applying an ice pack helps to relieve pain within the first 48 hours. After a couple of days, using a hot water bag or heating pad on the painful area, or soaking in a hot bath, can provide some relief.
- Spinal manipulation to move and adjust the vertebrae in relation to each other.

Further research is required to determine the potential benefits of these approaches, as there are authors who cast doubt on their usefulness in achieving outcomes.

For those who progress to surgery, preoperative care ensuring fitness for surgery and postoperative assistance with activities until the patient is able to resume these are key areas of nursing intervention. Additionally the patient will often be prescribed a brace to wear for a specified period of time.

NURSING THE PATIENT WITH AN ORTHOTIC DEVICE

In general terms, an orthosis is an external device utilised to correct, control or counteract the effect of an actual or developing deformity. When used following spinal surgery, the aim is to provide postoperative restriction of movement to facilitate healing and reduce potential complications. Other orthoses such as splints and callipers are used if there are multiple musculoskeletal conditions.

Ideally, a qualified orthotist should be involved in the design and fitting of the appropriate device to meet the specific needs of the individual patient. Formal follow-up by an orthotist to solve both actual or potential problems should be organised and contact details should be available if the nurse or client suspects the device is not functioning properly.

General nursing care of the client wearing an orthosis comprises a few key points. These demonstrate the need for education for patients, their carers and those nurses involved directly in their care.

- The patient should be educated regarding the donning, removal and care of the orthosis as appropriate. Although this is provided initially by the orthotist, constant reinforcement is essential.
- Relevant exercises both in and out of the orthosis should be taught.
- Practical advice is needed relating to the effects and potential restrictions on the client's life and activities from wearing the orthosis, including issues relating to the maintenance of personal hygiene, elimination and dressing.
- After initial prescription and wearing of a new orthosis, the skin condition should be checked regularly. Most orthotic devices are made to fit tightly if they are to achieve their purpose but if too tight, this may cause undue pressure and ultimately may result in the development of a pressure ulcer. In the long term, any weight gain may result in the same outcome. This is a particularly vital observation if the patient has a degree of sensory impairment of the affected limb or body part.
- Patients may need constant psychological support, particularly in the early stages of wearing the orthotic device. Although significant improvements have been made in achieving a more acceptable cosmetic effect, many clients may find the altered body image resulting from wearing a new orthosis requires some time to adjust to. In the author's experience, a tactic that has been successfully utilised in such situations is constant reference to the benefits of wearing the device, particularly if the orthosis is designed to enable increased function. Additionally, preparation of the patient for wearing the device through the provision of pictures or contact with similar patients may aid in reducing anxiety.
- The client must be instructed to report immediately any numbness or pins and needles, as these may indicate the onset of neurological impairment.

SPINAL SURGERY

Many spinal conditions ultimately progress at some stage to surgical intervention. The following section outlines the common approaches to clarify the techniques and offer guidance on the related nursing care.

SPINAL DECOMPRESSION

There are many different techniques used by surgeons to perform a decompression, yet the common goal is to ensure a careful freeing of the affected nerves by removal of bone, disc and facet capsule. The common procedures include:

- discectomy for a herniated disc
- laminotomy to open up more space posteriorly in the spinal canal
- laminectomy to unroof the spinal canal posteriorly
- foramenotomy to open up the neuroforamen.

In many cases a combination of techniques is used to ensure a proper decompression of the nerve elements.

SPINAL FUSION

Spinal fusion procedures aim at restoring stability and proper spinal alignment. In the simplest terms, a spinal fusion is the growing together of bone structures to create a solid bone bridge between the vertebrae involved.

There are many different methods employed to create a fusion of the spine. The ideal technique for a particular patient will depend upon a number of factors, including the levels to be fused, degree of instability or deformity, age of the patient, risk factors for non-union and experience of the surgeon.

Anterior spinal fusion

An anterior spinal fusion involves removal of the intervertebral disc between two or more levels and replacing this with pieces of bone. Over time, the bone develops a firm bone bridge between the desired levels of the spine. This approach is used universally for cervical disc herniations, with great success. In the lumbar spine, anterior fusions without the support of either additional instrumentation or a posterior fusion are less successful.

Posterior fusion without spinal instrumentation

Posterior spinal fusion with an autologous graft was the 'gold standard' of spinal surgery for many years. Recent developments in instrumentation systems now facilitate earlier, successful stabilisation of the spine, improving the success rate for spinal fusions further. Patients generally need to wear a brace or cast after surgery to provide an exterior support and protection from inappropriate movements until the graft or fixation has had time to heal. This method does carry a rare risk of incomplete or unsuccessful fusion (pseudarthrosis).

Posterior spinal fusion with instrumentation

Posterior bilateral fusion with instrumentation, using pedicular screws and rods or plates, generally offers a high rate of successful spinal fusion. However, these procedures require a large area to be exposed and involve muscle stripping that may cause weakness, stiffness and prolonged recovery.

Circumferential fusion

Circumferential or an anterior and posterior fusion is a combination of interbody and posterolateral fusion. This technique is usually performed with instrumentation, the disc space being packed with a cage filled with an allograft or autologous bone graft. To stabilise the spine one of several systems is used: pedicle screws and rods, screws and plates, hooks and screws, facet screws, or cables and wires with screws. The ideal instrumentation technique depends on the degree of instability, the amount of bone structure present and the experience of the surgeon.

In general, circumferential fusion leads to a very high fusion rate. The disadvantage, compared to anterior or posterior procedures alone, is the invasiveness of the surgery with anterior and posterior incisions to access the spine. This invariably requires a period of postoperative high-dependency nursing.

Posterior circumferential fusion

An alternative to the circumferential front and back surgery involves a circumferential fusion and interbody fusion through one incision in the back. There are two common versions: posterior lumbar interbody fusion (PLIF) and transforaminal lumbar interbody fusion (TLIF).

In both techniques, the disc is removed from the back by manoeuvring around the delicate nerve structures. A bone graft or mesh cage is used in the disc space, supported by posterior instrumentation and a posterior bone graft. The success rate in terms of fusion and pain relief is excellent, in carefully selected patients. The advantages of these techniques over the anterior and posterior circumferential fusion include avoidance of the potential complications from an anterior approach, decreased operating time, decreased blood loss and reduced recovery time.

REVISION SURGERY

The need to operate on the spine a second time is unfortunately fairly common. This stems from the spine being a tremendously complex structure, subject to the ravages of time and further degeneration.

Even if a surgical procedure appears to have effectively treated a problem, over time there can be a failure of other segments along the spine, with progression of symptoms being experienced by the patient. These later problems can develop months or years after the initial surgery.

DISC REPLACEMENT SURGERY

Disc replacement surgery remains unproven in the treatment of discogenic pain, mainly because of the considerable difficulty in identifying the painful level or levels, although it may improve in time as techniques and technology continue to develop. The standard discectomy, normally a fenestration with discectomy, appears to give consistently better success rates than a microdiscectomy, which in turn has better success rates than chemonucleolysis. A review by Zigler et al (2001) of current thinking and the latest surgery is recommended for further reading on this area of practice.

OTHER SPINAL SURGERY

Some surgical procedures involve implanting specialised systems that deliver a constant rate of medication or stimulation to the spinal area. These implantable 'pumps' can deliver narcotics or other substances directly to the spinal area to relieve pain. The advantage of this direct drug delivery, as compared to taking the drug orally, is that it creates fewer side effects. Surgically implanted spinal cord stimulators modulate the pain response, so that a person feels less pain than they would otherwise.

Surgery is often necessary for people with spinal infections, spinal tumours and trauma patients when the spine is clearly unstable. Infections, tumours, trauma and spinal instability are normally all treated with spinal fusion surgery.

PRINCIPLES OF POSTOPERATIVE MANAGEMENT

Spinal surgery is a major surgical event, in many cases requiring a period of close monitoring often in a high-dependency environment. Clearly there is a period of immobilisation following surgery. Pain control is a major nursing care issue prior to any movement. The complications associated with enforced mobility, such as the increased risk of pressure ulcer

---

Box 18.2   General principles of body mechanics following spine surgery

- Sleep on the side with knees bent and a pillow between the legs
- Avoid sleeping prone
- Place a pillow under the knees for support when sleeping supine
- Unless otherwise indicated, use a flat pillow under the head and neck when lying down following cervical surgery
- When getting up from the bed, the patient should turn to the side, using their arms to push up while the legs should swing over the side of the bed
- Avoid movements that will twist the neck or lower back

Box 18.3   Causes of poor outcomes from spinal surgery

- Recurrent disc herniation
- Recurrent spinal stenosis
- Chronic nerve injury
- Infection
- Incomplete decompression
- Pain from the bone harvest site following fusion
- Failure of fusion to develop
- Loosening of instrumentation
- Nerve irritation from instrumentation and subsequent pain
- Incomplete diagnosis of problem
- Poor postoperative alignment of the spine
- Junctional failure of the spine where there is collapse or instability of a segment of the spine adjacent to a previously operated area

---

formation and thrombosis, are key elements of the nursing role.

Once mobilisation has commenced, there are general principles that will assist in the healing of and comfort of the majority of patients (Box 18.2). It is worth strongly pointing out that these are general principles and should not be utilised without prescription from relevant members of the patient's healthcare team. Clearly these will change over time and be dependent on the individual patient.

Unfortunately, despite high success rates for spinal surgery, poor patient outcomes occur for a variety of reasons (Box 18.3).

ANKYLOSING SPONDYLITIS

Ankylosing spondylitis is an inflammatory progressive disease of unknown origin, more common in men than women. It primarily involves the spine but may involve other joints.

Onset is usually gradual but leads to a marked difference in the patient's physical appearance, resulting in an altered body image. Typically, the thoracic spine becomes stiff and 'rounded' and the cervical spine grows rigid. A variety of potential problems occurs from patients having reduced mobility, being unable to perform daily living activities and debilitating pain. Breathing is affected if there is significant thoracic spine involvement, impinging on chest expansion and vital capacity.

An acute phase is managed by the use of NSAIDs and analgesia, with respiratory problems being treated by intravenous antibiotics. The provision of a firm mattress is essential and the patient may be advised to wear a spinal orthosis to maintain the best possible alignment of the affected areas.

Key to the nursing management is to limit bedrest, as this may encourage further fusion of the vertebrae; this must be borne in mind if the patient is admitted for another medical problem as long-term immobility can result from prolonged periods of enforced immobilisation. Good posture and an exercise programme designed to increase muscle strength are of benefit, the nurse's role being to reinforce these and to provide assistance for patients to meet hygiene, nutrition and elimination needs. Prior to discharge, the patient is taught the correct use of any spinal orthosis, their medication and strategies to maintain mobility and optimum respiratory function.

SPONDYLOLYSIS AND SPONDYLOLISTHESIS

Spondylolysis results from a defect in the pars interarticularis, usually presenting in adolescents as a fatigue fracture from repetitive hyperextension stresses in some sports, for example gymnastics, weight lifting and javelin throwing (Moeller & Rifat 2001). In rare cases, acute spondylolysis is seen in adulthood. For those with a lesion developing late into adolescence at the L4–5 level, further progression of the condition may occur as an adult.

Non-union of this type of fatigue fracture is a relatively common cause of spondylolisthesis. Literally, 'spondy' refers to the vertebrae and 'listhesis' means to slip. This slipping of the vertebrae usually occurs at L4–5 and L5–S1 levels. There are many potential causes of spondylolisthesis, including: congenital causes, especially spina bifida occulta, spondylosis, degeneration of the facet joints, trauma or a tumour (Fig. 18.4). This condition is twice as common in women as men and often occurs during the first and second decades of life. Younger patients have a higher risk of developing progressive spondylolisthesis than older patients (Box 18.4).

Degenerative spondylolisthesis around the L4–5 level occurs commonly after the age of 40 years and is five times more common in women. The pain, located in the low back and posterior thighs, begins insidiously, often presenting as an ache. Neurogenic claudication may be present, with the lower extremity symptoms increasing with activity and improving with rest. In most cases, symptoms are chronic and progressive, although patients may experience periods of remission.

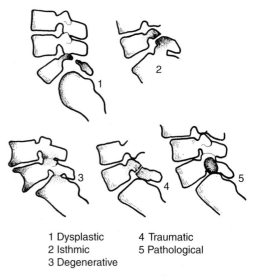

1 Dysplastic	4 Traumatic
2 Isthmic	5 Pathological
3 Degenerative	

Figure 18.4 Types of spondylolisthesis. (Adapted from Dandy & Edwards 1998.)

Box 18.4   Classification of spondylolisthesis

Grade 1: 1–25% slippage
Grade 2: 26–50% slippage
Grade 3: 51–75% slippage
Grade 4: 76–100% slippage
Grade 5: greater than 100% slippage

Although trauma is a relatively uncommon causative factor, it must be ruled out in any trauma patient presenting with acute pain and, in severe cases, neurological symptoms.

AP and lateral X-rays, along with flexion and extension views, give some idea of the degree of instability present. A classic spondylolysis is seen as a 'Scotty dog whose neck is broken' on the oblique films. A bone scan is useful; if positive, the lesion is metabolically active and healing is still in progress, in which case the physician may consider bracing. CT scan and MRI may help visualise any defect and ascertain its severity.

MANAGING SPONDYLOLYSIS AND SPONDYLOLISTHESIS

Most patients with low-grade isthmic spondylolisthesis and degenerative spondylolisthesis can be treated conservatively. Treatment choices should focus on three main outcomes:

1 elimination of pain
2 preparation for return to full activities
3 prevention of recurrence.

With an acute lesion, the patient is advised to stop potential aggravating activities or sports until they are free from symptoms. An exercise programme to improve abdominal strength and increase flexibility is ideal, along with appropriate hamstring stretches as patients often present with 'tight' hamstrings. Pelvic tilt exercises may help reduce any postural component caused by an increased lumbar lordosis.

Patients with degenerative spondylolisthesis are often older and have co-existing medical issues that need consideration when deciding appropriate treatment. Their management is dependent primarily on the percentage of slip (Box 18.4). A slip of less than 30%, which is not progressing, is generally helped by reducing the predisposing sporting activity, pain management and 6-monthly radiological follow-up.

Surgical treatment is indicated when any type of spondylolisthesis is accompanied by a neurological deficit involving a motor or sensory loss. Persistent unresponsive disabling back pain after conservative management is often considered an indication for surgical intervention. High-grade slips of greater than 50% and progressive slips invariably require surgical intervention. Traumatic spondylolisthesis almost always requires surgical stabilisation. The surgical intervention is usually decompression with or without fusion, depending on the degree of slip.

INTERVERTEBRAL DISC DISEASE

There are age-related changes in the intervertebral disc, resulting in degeneration and increased likelihood of a clinical problem. Proteoglycan synthesis decreases with age, causing a loss of water content which, along with the concurrent increase in collagen content, results in stiffening of the discs. As the nucleus dries out and becomes more fibrous, the annulus has to play a greater role in load transmission, subjecting the annulus to greater stresses. The cumulative stresses on the discs contribute to degeneration, increasing the likelihood of herniation or prolapse.

DISC HERNIATION

A 'slipped disc' or, more correctly termed, a herniated or prolapsed intervertebral disc commonly occurs in the lumbar and cervical areas (Figs 18.5,

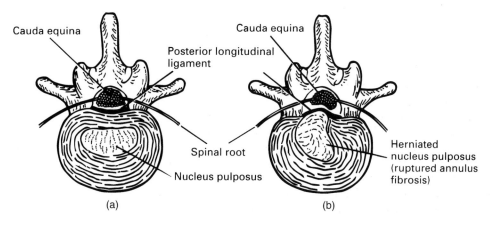

Cauda equina

Cauda equina

Posterior longitudinal ligament

Spinal root

Nucleus pulposus

Herniated nucleus pulposus (ruptured annulus fibrosis)

(a)   (b)

Figure 18.5   Normal (a) and herniated (b) intervertebral disc.

Example of possible
disc prolapse and root
compression at the
L4–5 junction

(a)

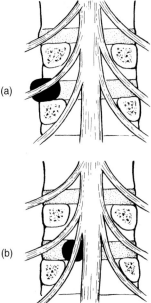

(a) Lateral prolapse may
compress the L4 root

(b)

(b) Central prolapse will
compress either L5

(c)

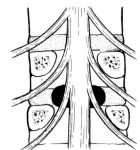

(c) or the cauda equina

(d)

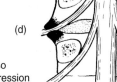

(d) Osteophytes in the
lateral canal will also
produce root compression

Figure 18.6 Types of disc prolapse. (Adapted from Dandy & Edwards 1998.)

18.6). These areas of the spine have the most mobility, putting the discs at high risk of damage.

The primary symptom of pain is intermittent in both severity and frequency. Sciatica is experienced if the damage is in the L4 region where a herniation irritates the sciatic nerve. The pain here may differ in both intensity and type, being described by patients as numbness, tingling, burning, aching or a shooting pain down a limb as the sciatic nerve extends down the leg to the foot. Such descriptions offer a baseline for determining the success of interventions and offer clues to more specific aetiology. Depending on the site of the disc prolapse and the nerve involvement, the patient will typically have intense radicular (nerve root) pain: 25% from the sciatic nerve and 75% from the femoral nerve. The pressure that the disc puts on the nerve roots often causes neurological symptoms in addition to the pain, with some patients developing motor weakness.

MANAGEMENT OF DISC DISEASE

Conservative methods of back pain management are used initially. Localised epidural steroid injection has been shown to benefit many patients; in the study by Weiner & Fraser (1997) a sustained relief of symptoms occurred for 27 out of 30 patients.

In contrast, although rare with an incidence of 0.5%, patients with a disc prolapse in the thoracic spine require a posterior fusion.

Central disc prolapse

Central disc prolapse represents a medical emergency, requiring an immediate MRI scan. Decompression within 24 hours of the onset of symptoms is needed as the disc presses on the cauda equina, causing the following motor and sensory problems:

- loss of perianal sensation known as saddle anaesthesia
- bilateral motor weakness in the legs
- sphincter disturbance to bowel and bladder, causing a reduced ability to sense the bladder filling, painless retention and overflow with consequent urinary incontinence and loss of anal tone with resultant faecal incontinence.

The conservative management of a central disc prolapse includes the use of NSAIDs, exercise programmes and epidural injections of local anaesthetics or steroids.

The decision to operate depends on the presence of three key indicators:

- unrelenting leg pain despite adequate conservative measures
- neural damage
- cauda equina syndrome.

A combination of spinal fusion and discectomy adds considerable risk of secondary postoperative complications and the benefit of this over a simple discectomy is not proven.

SPINAL STENOSIS

By definition, a stenosis is the narrowing of a hollow tubular structure. In this context, a spinal stenosis is a narrowing of the spinal canal, nerve root canals or intervertebral foramina. Lumbar and cervical stenoses are far more common than those in the thoracic vertebrae (Esses 1995). Three types of stenosis occur:

1 local, affecting only one nerve root on one side of the body (Fig. 18.6d)
2 segmental, involving one specific area in the lumbar spine
3 generalised, involving a large part of the lumbar spine from excess bone, soft tissues or a combination of the two.

As spinal stenosis is often part of the general spinal arthritic degeneration that occurs with ageing, it commonly affects those over 60 years. Other causes are (Fritz et al 1998, Garfin et al 2001, Hilibrand & Rand 1999):

- congenital in patients born with a tight spinal canal, as seen in certain syndromes like achondroplasia (dwarfism)
- developmental, forming during growth and development
- trauma from a fracture pushing bone or soft tissue into the spinal canal or neural foramen
- tumours.

Many authors have described the events involved in the pathophysiology of the ageing spine in degenerative conditions (Best 2002).

1 The intervertebral disc in the spine desiccates (dries up) and loses height.
2 The disc loses its mechanical integrity, making it unable to perform functions such as resisting motion. The annulus bulges into the vertebral canal, causing pressure on the spinal cord, cauda equina or nerve roots.
3 The ligamentum flavum, the soft tissue covering the back of the spinal canal, thickens in reaction to the additional movement caused by the loss

of integrity and tends to buckle towards the canal space.
4 Formation of osteophytes and hypertrophy of the facet joints may occur, resulting in a stenosis primarily pinching the nerve roots (Jenis & An 2000).

A battery of tests using diagnostic imaging will aid the confirmation of a spinal stenosis. Plain X-rays can show facet joint arthritis, degenerative disc spaces and spondylolisthesis. Further studies, routinely ordered for preoperative and perioperative planning, will assist in the determination of the levels of compression, exact aetiology and hence potential management strategies. CT scans show the bony anatomy and stenosis, with the presence of spurs and facet joint arthritis. An MRI scan is taken to demonstrate the impact on soft tissue such as the ligamentum flavum and the nerve roots.

In general, patients have a progressive yet slow development of symptoms. The most common complaint is back pain, with any or all of the three distinct symptom patterns associated with spinal stenosis:

- neurogenic claudication
- radicular pain in the distribution area of a nerve root such as the leg pain from sciatica
- chronic cauda equina syndrome, although this is rare.

The most common pain pattern is neurogenic claudication, presenting as leg pain after walking, which is relieved by sitting or squatting. The severity of pain varies between patients but as a rule, it is worse in the morning, is exacerbated by exercise and will disappear when the patient sits down or bends forward at the waist. Patients can have leg pain with or without a nerve root deficit.

TREATMENT OF SPINAL STENOSIS

The majority of patients will be treated conservatively by medication and exercise programmes. Patients need reassurance that a mild degree of back pain is not dangerous and can be a normal aspect of the ageing process of the spine. Clearly patient education forms a key part of the nursing role in enabling patients to maximise their independence in daily living tasks.

The range of drugs used generally includes:

- NSAIDs and regular analgesics
- muscle relaxants such as diazepam

- antidepressants for chronic radicular pain
- epidural and nerve root block steroid injections, which are successful in reducing the swelling of the soft tissues and thecal sac for some patients.

Non-medication pain-relieving techniques may be of some use, for example nerve stimulators, acupuncture and hot or cold packs.

An exercise programme focusing on flexion and building strength in the paravertebral muscles is good practice; this may be formally in groups or on an individual basis, in a back pain clinic.

A spinal brace may offer support and be particularly beneficial for those with multilevel pathology or degeneration as seen in the elderly.

Surgical intervention is indicated if conservative methods do not produce a satisfactory patient outcome, especially if the pain is increasingly affecting daily living and social activities or progressive neurological deficits exist (Krismer 2002). Operative interventions include decompression with or without fusion and instrumentation, depending on the specific aetiology and radiological picture. Contraindications to surgery are regular recurrent infections and patients with a nutritional deficit. A nutritional assessment should be part of any elective preoperative assessment. Anecdotal evidence suggests this is currently ad hoc and informal rather than a standard assessment for these patients.

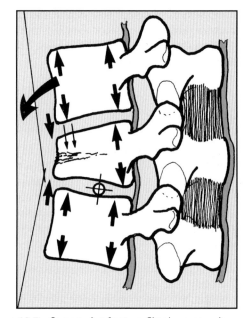

Figure 18.7 Compression fracture. Simple compression fractures are common stable injuries involving the anterior column only. Hyperflexion of the spine around an axis passing through the disc space leads to mechanical failure with either an anterior (shown here) or lateral wedge fracture. The height of the posterior vertebral body is maintained. Severe wedging often indicates damage to other columns, and a burst fracture or fracture dislocation. (Adapted from McRae & Esser 2002.)

LUMBAR COMPRESSION FRACTURES

In young and middle-aged adults, the most common cause of lumbar compression fractures (Fig. 18.7) is trauma, with high-velocity falls from a height and motor vehicle accidents being the most common modes of injury. Such fractures require substantial force; they are invariably very painful in nature and are often associated with other traumatic injuries such as head injuries, rib fractures and abdominal trauma.

There is an obvious risk of damage to the spinal cord and cauda equina resulting in a spinal cord injury (see Chapter 20 for spinal cord injuries). All compression fractures require a thorough patient examination to make certain that the fracture is not a secondary manifestation of a systemic illness such as malignancies, infections or renal disease.

OSTEOPOROSIS

This is a silently progressive disease, with a progressive reduction in the bone mass, the decrease in bone density predisposing patients to a pathological fracture.

Osteoporosis occurs mainly in postmenopausal women of 51–65 years as a result of oestrogen deficiency: this is often termed type I. The rate of bone density reduction dramatically increases in women after the menopause. In those over 75 years of age, senile or type II osteoporosis occurs. Taking hormone replacement or other medications can substantially reduce the risk or degree of bone density loss and the risk of fractures occurring. For men the same risk factors apply, as low testosterone levels are associated with an increased risk of the typical osteoporotic vertebral compression fractures. As the bone is thin and weak, very little force may be needed to cause the fracture. The predisposing factors, prevention and management of osteoporosis are discussed in depth in Chapter 19.

Other medical conditions are associated with osteoporotic changes of the vertebrae, including bone metastases, renal failure and liver failure, which can lead to painful compression fractures. Nutritional deficiencies can decrease the rate of bone remodelling and increase osteopenia, leading to similar fractures.

COMPRESSION FRACTURES

A compression or wedge fracture will result in the loss of height of that vertebral body. Patients present with back pain in the area of the broken vertebra, although it may be painless and the patient may not remember any injury. Occasionally patients describe a history of bending over or lifting a moderately heavy object and feeling a 'pop' or a sudden pain in the back. The most common regions for these types of fractures are the thoracic and lumbar spine: they are rare in the cervical region.

About 75% of women over 65 years, who have a spinal curve, have at least one osteopenic wedge fracture. A patient may therefore present with back pain or other spinal conditions and on X-rays, previous small osteoporotic fractures may be seen. After multiple wedge fractures, the patient may develop a hunched appearance from the accumulative effect of the decrease in the anterior vertebral body height, causing a kyphosis or rounding of the back (Fig. 18.8).

Although mortality from this cause is rare in elderly patients, any prolonged period of reduced mobility may result in secondary complications, for example pneumonia, deep vein thrombosis and pulmonary embolism, problems with skin integrity and gastric ulceration.

Conservative management of compression fractures comprises pain control, possibly the use of a brace and a rehabilitation programme to optimise the patient's functional capability whilst minimising the risk of secondary complications. Mobility and strengthening rehabilitation programmes are individualised to each patient's capabilities and focus on their desired social activities. Additionally, it is essential that the patient receive education on minimising their risk of a future fracture. A programme involving advice on posture and lifting is essential as poor techniques will undoubtedly increase a patient's risk (Myers & Wilson 1997).

In some areas, rehabilitation begins with the patient in a thoracic-lumbar-sacral orthosis (TLSO).

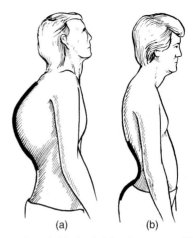

Figure 18.8   Rounded kyphosis (a) and exaggerated lordosis (b). (From Dandy & Edwards 1998.)

To facilitate progress, patients are treated in a less restrictive corset if their pain is well controlled but this is dependent on the fracture severity. It may be necessary to restrict mobility to a degree whereby no daily living activities can be performed independently. The reasons for this should be explained to the patient and support provided to accommodate their needs. Patient compliance is essential if an orthosis is to be used, especially following discharge from hospital. Although there is no significant evidence, it seems logical that patient education relating to their condition will increase compliance with wearing the prescribed brace.

Early mobilisation and weight-bearing exercises prevent the secondary complications of immobility and minimise progression of any osteoporosis present. Extension exercises are also considered beneficial. Continuing physiotherapy through outpatient clinics and radiographic monitoring of fracture healing are essential to optimise long-term function and because some fractures can worsen over the ensuing months, potentially requiring surgical intervention.

Treatment of osteoporotic compression fractures is based on individual symptoms. Restricting activities such as lifting and bending helps alleviate some of the immediate pain and concomitant spasms; antiinflammatory and antispasmodic medications are used if indicated.

Whether managed surgically or conservatively, if a patient is neurologically compromised following a traumatic injury, they will require a comprehensive assessment, an early transfer to a specialist unit and a complex rehabilitation programme to enable them to reintegrate into the community. This care is addressed in Chapter 20.

The surgical options for correcting a lumbar fracture depend on the:

- degree of bony canal compromise
- angulation
- level of the fracture
- neurological status
- patient's preinjury health.

Most fractures of the lumbar spine requiring surgery occur at the thoracolumbar junction.

As well as the standard surgical techniques described earlier for spinal surgery, the relatively recently developed vertebroplasty technique is being used for osteoporotic compression fractures. This technique involves the injection of methylmethacralate (bone cement) into the vertebral body via an X-ray guided needle or a small incision. Although becoming more widely employed, vertebroplasty is still relatively limited compared to other surgical techniques. Although it is viewed with cautious optimism, its use is still debated within the orthopaedic world (Spivak 2002, Zigler et al 2001).

Once a patient has undergone surgery, a brace is often prescribed in the postoperative period depending on the cause of the fracture and surgical technique employed.

A progressive kyphosis can occur when the pattern of fractures progresses. Serial X-rays for 1 year after the initial injury can help monitor any progression of this condition.

Generally, the prognosis after a simple compression fracture is excellent, with most patients having little or no residual back pain and no functional impairments. Once a lumbar fracture has occurred there is a high risk of a subsequent injury occurring. Weight-bearing exercises become extremely important to prevent any further progression of osteoporosis and to prevent future fractures. The use of outpatient therapy must also focus on fall prevention and functional activities.

SPINAL DEFORMITIES

When viewed from behind, a normal spine appears straight and the trunk is symmetrical but when viewed from the side, curves are seen in the neck, upper trunk and lower trunk. The gentle, rounded, convex thoracic contour and convex sacral curve are normal kyphoses, while the lower lumbar concave

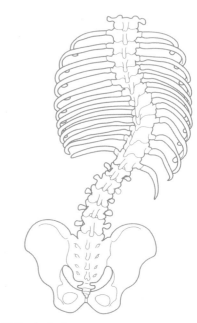

Figure 18.9 Scoliosis.

curve is a normal lordosis; these curves are needed to maintain appropriate trunk balance over the pelvis. A smaller cervical concave curve is also present to enable head control and movement.

Deviations from this normal alignment include an abnormal kyphosis, lordosis (see Fig. 18.8) and, more commonly, a scoliosis (Fig. 18.9).

SCOLIOSIS

Scoliosis is traditionally defined as a side-to-side deviation from the normal frontal axis view of the body. However, this definition is limited as the deformity may occur to varying degrees in all three planes: back to front, side to side or top to bottom.

In the majority of patients with a scoliosis, no specific cause is found; these cases are termed idiopathic. Conditions known to cause spinal deformity are congenital spinal column abnormalities, neurological disorders and genetic conditions. Spinal deformities are common and often severe in patients with a neuromuscular disease, especially those unable to walk because of their underlying neurological disease, for instance muscular dystrophy and spina bifida. Contrary to some beliefs, a scoliosis does not result from carrying heavy loads, participation in sports, posture or minor lower limb length inequality.

A clinical evaluation of the patient focuses on their medical history and physical examination. Family histories of spinal deformity can occur. In children, the circumstances surrounding the child's birth, delivery and development histories are investigated. Abnormalities in these areas may lead to consideration of the potential for a neuromuscular or congenital cause. If one congenital abnormality is found, the patient must be examined further to eliminate others; for example, kidney abnormalities are often associated with congenital scoliosis.

There have been many attempts to classify scoliosis and readers are encouraged to consult Lenke et al (2001) and King et al (1983) for further information on this.

Physical assessment

The physical examination focuses on assessment of trunk symmetry.

The Adams forward bend test is where the patient bends forward with their arms extended and knees straight. The trunk when viewed from the front or the back will show the presence of any asymmetry while any increase or decrease in the normal lordosis and kyphosis is viewed from the side. This test is used during school screening for scoliosis. Although indicative, any positive result showing the probable presence of an abnormality merits further investigation for scoliosis.

Further physical findings depend on where the changes to the spinal structures are and the magnitude of the curve involved. The heights of the shoulder may be uneven, along with an increased space between the elbow and trunk due to the thoracic or lumbar deviation. Prominence of one hip or breast or a pelvic tilt are also seen.

In addition to the amount of spinal deformity, the patient's physiological age is assessed to determine whether growth is completed or if there is more potential spinal growth. In the latter case, the potential curve progression is related to the time remaining until skeletal maturity. In the adult, progression of a curve is often associated with degenerative intervertebral disc disease, joint disease of the spine in middle-aged or older patients or a previously untreated scoliosis.

Examination of the skin overlying the spine may show the presence of dimples, sinuses, hairy patches and skin pigmentation changes. The effect of any limb length inequality is also tested. Neurological examinations will include evaluation of the muscles and nerve function of the upper and lower limbs.

Pulmonary and cardiac changes are never affected in patients with lumbar curves, unless there is another underlying condition. However, pulmonary and cardiac function tests are required to assess lung and heart function if there is a severe thoracic scoliosis, especially preoperatively. Changes of pulmonary function are not seen until the thoracic curve is severe, reaching a level greater than 70°. This amount of curve and subsequent cardiac and pulmonary changes are often seen later in life in untreated idiopathic infantile and juvenile scoliosis patients and present a threat to life.

With the older patient, during adolescence and early adulthood, intermittent backache may occur from idiopathic scoliosis but complaints of pain radiating into the legs, night pain or systemic complaints, for example changes in bowel or bladder habits, are not usual and may be more indicative of other spinal conditions.

Imaging studies

Anteroposterior (AP) and lateral X-rays of the entire spine are taken, if possible with the patient in a standing position. The curves are measured using the Cobb system as this method allows a physician to track the curve progression over time.

An MRI or CT scan is carried out if the patient has a neurological abnormality, unusual curve patterns, rapidly progressive curvatures or congenital scoliosis.

Neuromuscular scoliosis

Various neurological disorders affect the development of the spine, the spinal curves and the function of the spinal nerves.

- Patients with muscular dystrophy often find the curve increases as their walking ability diminishes.
- Myelodysplasia (spina bifida) often produces major progressive deformities from both paralytic and congenital factors, particularly in patients with high levels of paralysis.
- Progressive spinal deformity is seen in patients with cerebral palsy, leading to difficulty with seating and care, especially for patients who do not walk.

Unfortunately modification of seating and a bracing regime appear to have no long-term effect on the natural course in the majority of cases. Such techniques may improve sitting ability but do not alter the curve progression. Surgical correction and stabilisation are therefore used to prevent further curve progression. This is carried out early for patients with muscular dystrophy while their pulmonary function is still adequate. Best surgical outcomes may be obtained with earlier intervention if there is curve progression. Developments in spinal surgery now mean that many patients will not require postoperative immobilisation in braces or casts.

Idiopathic scoliosis

Idiopathic scoliosis is considered in three age groups, with treatment generally being dependent on the patient's age:

- infantile, from birth to 3 years of age
- juvenile, from 3 to 9 years of age
- adolescent, from 10 to 18 years of age. The adolescent type is the most common, representing about 80% of idiopathic scoliosis patients.

Infantile. In patients with infantile scoliosis, left-sided curves are more common, particularly in boys; these may resolve spontaneously with growth. The potential for progression is observed using repeat X-ray evaluation every 4–6 months. The use of braces and surgery is uncommon.

Juvenile. Juvenile idiopathic scoliosis may progress rapidly, especially in children over the age of 5. This group may require orthotic management using a brace, with surgical intervention should curve progression be poorly controlled by bracing. Although surgery on a significantly skeletally immature spine will produce some decrease in ultimate spine height, it is better to have a shorter spine with a more normal alignment than a progressive curve where height is lost because of the deformity.

Adolescent. The most common of all types is adolescent idiopathic scoliosis, occurring in 2–4% of adolescents (Reamy & Slakey 2001). In low curve magnitudes, it is seen with equal frequency in boys and girls. Girls, for unknown reasons, have a significantly higher risk of developing a progressive curve than boys, the time of highest risk for curve progression occurring around puberty when the growth rate is fastest. It appears that thoracic curves carry a higher progression risk than curves in the thoracolumbar and lumbar regions of the spinal column. Patients whose curves are of greater magnitude prior to the onset of their adolescent growth spurt also have a higher curve progression risk.

The treatment choice in adolescent idiopathic scoliosis is determined by a complex equation that includes the patient's physiological (rather than chronological) maturity, the curve magnitude, the curve location and the potential for progression. Treatment options include observation, bracing or surgery.

General guidelines include a reevaluation of the condition every 4–6 months, including X-rays for patients who are skeletally immature and have curves of less than 25°. In patients who are more skeletally mature and have a curve of less than 45°, similar observations are carried out to assess for any change at 6 months.

Brace management for adolescents is restricted to those with a spinal deformity, curve magnitudes of 25–40°, who are skeletally immature and have a period of significant growth remaining. The primary goal of brace management is to stop curve progression; any curve correction seen at the end of brace treatment must be considered a bonus.

Surgery for adolescents is suggested when the curve magnitude is 50° or more, for patients previously untreated or where brace treatment fails and the curve is progressing. Surgery is undertaken with two goals in mind:

- the primary goal is to prevent spine deformity progression
- the secondary goal is to diminish spinal deformity.

The natural history of idiopathic scoliosis during adulthood is one of continued progression. If the curve is more than 50° at the end of growth, surgery using a posterior spinal fusion with instrumentation and bone grafting is the most frequent option for preventing this scenario. With current surgical techniques, postoperative casting and bracing are not required in many cases. Patients are rapidly mobilised and usually discharged from hospital within 7 days, with progressive resumption of their routine daily activities, including returning to school.

Bracing in idiopathic scoliosis. There are a range of orthoses used, usually underarm or the higher-reaching Milwaukee-type braces. These may be off the shelf but are commonly custom made by an orthotic or plaster room team. The type of brace and amount of time the braces are worn each day vary according to the prescription of the specific orthopaedic surgeon. Modern bracing techniques provide cosmetic braces, allowing patients to continue their routine daily activities and minimise the impact of body image changes associated with wearing a brace. Removing the brace so the patient can participate in sports and exercise is often strongly encouraged.

A common alternative to full-time brace wear is the use of a nighttime 'bending' brace for the management of a single curve. This may increase tolerance and compliance with a bracing regime. Success and ending the use of a brace are determined by the achievement of skeletal maturation, usually indicated by the patient having no further changes in height, no curve progression and evidence of maturity on spinal X-ray. It is worth pointing out at this stage that there appear to be an increasing number of studies which question the success of bracing (Karol 2001, Wright 1997), although many would put this down to poor compliance by patients (often quoted as being less than 40%). This raises questions regarding the value of putting patients through this form of management.

Nursing role in the patient with scoliosis

As the majority of patients with a scoliosis are of school age, the general challenges of working with children and their parents over a long period time, usually for several years or most of their life until skeletal maturity, require a specialist unit approach to optimise the outcomes for all patients.

The nursing role within the rehabilitation team includes education of the patient and family where appropriate, in relation to the treatment, means of undertaking daily living activities when wearing a brace and pre- and postoperative management to minimise complications for those progressing to surgery.

There appears to be little strong evidence supporting the effectiveness of manipulation or electrical stimulation in the management of scoliosis, although these approaches are used to some degree in many centres. Additionally, a review by Negrini et al (2001) suggested, theoretically and from reviewing studies performed to date, that exercise has a positive influence on disability associated with scoliosis. As well as this, the fitness associated with exercise can only benefit the patient generally and will certainly influence postoperative recovery should the patient progress to surgery.

ABNORMAL KYPHOSIS

Congenital kyphosis is much less common than congenital scoliosis but potentially more serious due to the potential for rapid progression of the curves. If untreated, this can lead to spinal cord compression and paraplegia. Any change in the normal thoracic kyphosis warrants investigation.

Examination of the patient will include a thorough history and physical assessment. The examination includes the same forward bend test as for scoliosis, with the spine being viewed from the side to see if the normal spine contours are present. Any prominence of the patient's thoracic kyphosis or failure to reverse their lumbar lordosis with bending requires further investigation.

Similar imaging guidelines are used as described above for scoliosis. With the patient erect, X-rays are taken to show the side-to-side alignment. Spinal X-rays, taken with the patient in both erect and supine positions, are helpful to document the flexibility of a rigid deformity. CT, MRI and bone scans are used as required. Surgical management is best performed before the age of 5 years in those who have a congenital deformity. Arthrodesis with potential instrumentation is a common surgical approach used in such cases (McMaster & Singh 2001).

Postural round back

This condition is defined as an increase in the thoracic kyphosis while standing. A flexible curve is seen when the patient stands erect but resolves when the patient is prone or supine. It is a nonprogressive condition commonly observed in mid adolescence, more common in girls, and almost always resolves by itself with no specific treatment. Once diagnosed, it is essential that patients are educated regarding the condition as there may be a tendency to nag a child with a perceived 'poor posture'.

Scheuermann's disease

Scheuermann's disease is a condition of unknown cause, which produces a usually painless increased thoracic kyphosis of greater than 40°. There are true structural changes within the thoracic vertebra, with 5° of wedging in each of three adjacent vertebrae as measured on lateral X-rays.

Treatment is dependent on the degree of deformity, the existence of pain and the maturity of the patient. Regular monitoring is required if the deformity is less than 60°. A brace is usually prescribed for curves between 60° and 80° if the patient is skeletally immature. Surgery is rarely required but is indicated if the brace management is unsuccessful.

Congenital kyphosis and lordosis

Deformities arising from congenital failure of vertebral formation are progressive and require early surgical treatment. Renal ultrasound is recommended because of the potential for associated renal abnormalities to occur. MRI of the spinal canal may also be needed to rule out associated spinal cord abnormalities.

CONCLUSION

Spinal conditions create health, functional and social implications for the patients who present with these debilitating problems. Physical, functional and social assessments are vital to ensure an accurate diagnosis, to plan patient management and to guide meaningful rehabilitation goals.

Nursing these patients creates challenges requiring a range of skills from the management of an acute injury, preoperative care, immediate postoperative management and participation in the interdisciplinary rehabilitation process.

The range of skills required and the variety of spinal conditions that occur have implications for patient care to be coordinated by a nurse specialist. Although there is little evidence of the effectiveness of such a post, it seems logical that the nursing role is ideally placed to provide the skills and knowledge required to develop the seamless service that maximises patient outcomes.

Further reading

Levine AM, Eismont FJ, Garfin SR et al (eds) 1998 Spine trauma. WB Saunders, Philadelphia

Vaccaro AR, Betz RR, Zeidman SM et al (eds) 2003 Principles and practice of spine surgery. Mosby, St Louis

Wetzel FT, Hanley EN 2002 Spine surgery: a practical atlas. McGraw-Hill Professional, New York

References

Best JT 2002 Understanding spinal stenosis. Orthopaedic Nursing 21(3): 48–56

Dandy DJ, Edwards DJ 1998 Essential orthopaedic and trauma, 3rd edn. Churchill Livingstone, Edinburgh

Davis GC, White TL 2001 Nursing's role in chronic pain management with older adults. Topics in Geriatric Rehabilitation 16(3): 45–55

Esses SI 1995 Spinal stenosis. In: Esses SI (ed) Textbook of spinal disorders. Lippincott, Philadelphia

Fritz JM, Delitto A, Welch WC, Erhard RE 1998 Lumbar spinal stenosis: a review of current concepts in evaluation, management and outcome measurements. Archives of Physical Medicine and Rehabilitation 79(6): 700–708

Garfin SR, Yuan HA, Reiley MA 2001 New technologies in spine: kyphoplasty and vertebroplasty for the treatment of painful osteoporotic compression fractures. Spine 26(14): 151–155

Hansson M, Bostrom C, Harms-Ringdahl K 2001 Living with spine-related pain in a changing society: a qualitative study. Disability and Rehabilitation 23(7): 286–295

Hilibrand AS, Rand N 1999 Degenerative lumbar stenosis: diagnosis and management. Journal of the American Academy of Orthopaedics 7(4): 239–249

Jenis LG, An HS 2000 Spine update: lumbar foraminal stenosis. Spine 25(3): 389–394

Karol LA 2001 Effectiveness of bracing in male patients with idiopathic scoliosis. Spine 26(18): 2001–2005

King HA, Moe JH, Bradford DS, Winter RB 1983 The selection of fusion levels in thoracic idiopathic scoliosis. Journal of Bone and Joint Surgery 65A(9): 1302–1313

Krismer M 2002 Fusion of the lumbar spine: a consideration of the indications. Journal of Bone and Joint Surgery 84B(6): 783–794

Lenke LG, Betz RR, Haher TR et al 2001 Multisurgeon assessment of surgical decision-making in adolescent idiopathic scoliosis: curve classification, operative approach, and fusion levels. Spine 26(21): 2347–2353

McMaster MJ, Singh H 2001 The surgical management of congenital kyphosis and kyphoscoliosis. Spine 26(19): 2146–2155

McRae R, Esser R 2002 Practical fracture treatment, 4th edn. Churchill Livingstone, Edinburgh

Moeller JL, Rifat SF 2001 Spondylolysis in active adolescents. Physician and Sportsmedicine 29(12): 27–33

Myers ER, Wilson SE 1997 Biomechanics of osteoporosis and vertebral fracture. Spine 22(24S): 25S–31S

Negrini A, Verzini N, Parzini S, Negrini S 2001 Role of physical exercise in the treatment of mild idiopathic adolescent scoliosis: review of the literature. Europa Medicophysica 37(3): 181–190

Reamy BV, Slakey JB 2001 Adolescent idiopathic scoliosis: review and current concepts. American Family Physician 64(1): 29–31, 111–116

Scott J 1994 Spinal problems. In: Nursing the orthopaedic patient. Churchill Livingstone, Edinburgh

Smith MJ 1999 The nature of rehabilitation. In: Smith MJ (ed) Rehabilitation in adult nursing practice. Churchill Livingstone, Edinburgh

Spivak JM 2002 Vertebroplasty: weighing the benefits and the risks. American Family Physician 66(4): 565

Tripp S 1999 Providing psychological support. In: Smith MJ (ed) Rehabilitation in adult nursing practice. Churchill Livingstone, Edinburgh

Weiner BK, Fraser RD 1997 Foraminal injection for lateral lumbar disc herniation. Journal of Bone and Joint Surgery 79B(5): 804–807

Wright A 1997 The conservative management of adolescent idiopathic scoliosis. Physical Therapy Reviews 2(3): 153–163

Zigler JE, Anderson PA, Bridwell K, Vaccaro A 2001 What's new in spine surgery. Journal of Bone and Joint Surgery 83A(8): 1285–1292

Chapter 19

Osteoporosis nursing implications

Ann Allsworth

INTRODUCTION

Osteoporosis is the most common form of bone disease, affecting 1 in 3 women and 1 in 12 men over the age of 50 in Britain, costing the NHS and government £1.7 billion each year (NOS 2003a). It is therefore a significant health issue for both the primary and secondary healthcare services.

The World Health Organisation (WHO) defines osteoporosis as a bone disease characterised by a low bone mass with microarchitectural deterioration of the bone tissue, leading to increased bone fragility and a consequent increase in the risk of a fracture (WHO 1994). Although it usually affects the whole skeleton, the most common sites are those with a high trabecular content, typically the vertebrae, distal forearm and femoral neck.

As the development of osteoporosis is age related, the extended life expectancy of women and men has led to an increase in the number of people diagnosed each year. Kessenich (2000) describes osteoporosis as a long-term, debilitating metabolic bone disease historically considered a disease of ageing women.

Osteoporosis fractures now account for more days in hospital for women over 45 years than any other disease (Healy 2000). Yet many women admitted with a hip fracture are not, automatically screened for osteoporosis, assessed for their risk of falling, being made aware of the underlying skeletal changes or how to prevent the further progression of their osteoporosis or how to prevent future fractures.

Men have larger, denser bones than women so are often mistakenly thought not to suffer osteopenia and osteoporosis. They do not undergo the rapid bone loss associated with the female menopause but can be at equal risk of developing the condition as they age (Kessenich 2000). Unfortunately, the disorder remains underdiagnosed, undertreated and less well researched in middle-aged and elderly men. It is predicted that by the year 2025, 1.2 million men worldwide are likely to sustain an osteoporotic hip fracture (Rosen & Kessenich 1997). Regrettably men experience greater morbidity and mortality following an osteoporotic hip fracture (Orwoll 1998) from a combination of co-morbidity, age and mental confusion whilst hospitalised.

The best strategy for dealing with osteoporosis is prevention rather than treatment, the aim being to restore and maintain the patient's bone strength and reduce the risk of a fracture occurring. Osteoporosis specialist nurses are involved in a variety of roles and strategies related to the continuing care and support of patients with this condition. Many are involved in hospital and community-based care, addressing the needs of the individual, family and society, the promotion of good bone health in adults and children, prevention and monitoring of the patient's condition, reducing the risks of accelerated osteopenia and assessment of fracture risk. This area of practice is continually developing, requiring practitioners to keep abreast of the advances in patient management, current research and recommendations for best practice. This chapter focuses on the effects of the condition, the medical management options and nursing implications.

OSTEOPOROSIS AND OSTEOPENIA

Both osteoporosis and osteopenia (low bone mass) occur when the rate of bone resorption is faster than the rate of bone formation. The rate of renewal of bone tissue decreases with age, leading to this imbalance but osteoporosis is not only seen in the elderly. Additional factors affect the rate of bone formation and resorption throughout life, leading to primary and secondary osteoporosis.

The term 'primary osteoporosis' refers to there being no other known disease contributing to the development of the condition. This definition mainly refers to postmenopausal oestrogen deficiency and consequent loss of bone density seen in the majority of women with the condition.

Secondary osteoporosis describes the situation when a preexisting disease or drugs prescribed for another condition, particularly corticosteroids, contribute to the development of the condition

Box 19.1 Causes of secondary osteoporosis	
Endocrine abnormalities	Hyperthyroidism, hyperparathyroidism, Cushing's disease, diabetes mellitus, hypogonadism in men
Drugs	Corticosteroid therapy, heparin therapy (over a long term), anticonvulsants
Neoplastic conditions	Multiple myeloma, bone metastases
Others	Alcoholism, anorexia nervosa, post transplantation, malabsorption syndromes, e.g. coeliac disease

(Box 19.1). The majority of male patients will develop osteoporosis following a predisposing illness, a significant number may have a history of hypogonadism.

A geographical difference in the incidence of osteoporosis is evident with a higher prevalence in Caucasian and Asian populations. It is rarely found in African and black American populations. One explanation for this is the racial differences in the density of bone structure. Due to this difference, the majority of research in osteoporosis, its prevention and treatment, has involved Caucasian women. Similar studies on wider population groups, especially in relation to drug therapies, are needed in the future.

Osteoporosis is frequently referred to as a silent disease because the first evidence of its presence is when the patient has a fracture. Due to the gender discrepancy, there is a higher incidence of fractures in women than men.

CORTICOSTEROID THERAPY RISK

When first introduced, corticosteroids were widely believed to be a revolutionary new treatment for a variety of conditions including rheumatoid arthritis, respiratory and skin problems. Although a short course of corticosteroid treatment can be life saving during acute events, long-term therapy is associated with various complications including osteoporosis.

The reason why bone loss occurs in relation to these drugs is not fully understood but reduced calcium absorption, secondary hyperparathyroidism, hypogonadism and inhibition of bone remodelling are known to occur. If long-term corticosteroids are necessary the patient should be maintained on the minimum possible dose and regularly monitored for side effects, including bone loss.

Before commencing corticosteroids, the issue of bone loss and preventive therapy must be discussed with the patient and a bone density scan carried out. As with any form of osteoporosis, a low bone mass prior to treatment will carry a higher risk of a fracture occurring. As women routinely have lower bone density than men, they are likely to be more at risk, especially if the woman is also postmenopausal. The risk of a hip fracture occurring is 50% higher for patients on long-term corticosteroid therapy (Meunier 1993), resulting in as many as 40% of patients on high-dose or long-term corticosteroids suffering fractures.

Although long-term oral therapy is known to cause bone loss, less is known about the effects of inhaled and topical steroid use.

LOW BONE MASS IN CHILDHOOD

Low bone mass is rarely found in children but may result from a range of conditions (Box 19.2). Although clinicians are increasingly aware of this condition, patients will require specific investigation, information and education on how to decrease their risk of a reduced bone mass and the implications this may have for adult skeletal health.

DISUSE OSTEOPOROSIS

Those unable to take regular weight-bearing exercise are at greater risk of osteoporosis and sustaining a fracture. Weight-bearing exercises require the skeleton to support the body weight against gravity (Bonnick 1994) and the forces involved put stress through the bones, encouraging their development and strength.

Prolonged bedrest following surgery, illness or a spinal cord injury are likely to result in extensive bone loss. This loss is greater in trabecular than in cortical bone and can be reversed if the period of immobility is just a matter of a few weeks. Nurses need to be aware of this potential complication and ensure patients are immobilised for the minimum time required. This applies if the whole body is immobilised or just one part, for example a limb in a cast or on traction.

GRAVITY

The zero gravity experienced during space travel results in significant bone loss. The research data provided by the National Aeronautical Space Agency will potentially provide valuable information on the effects of osteoporosis on otherwise healthy adults. This will be beneficial for future patients.

PATIENT ASSESSMENT

Orthopaedic and trauma nurses need to understand how patients are assessed for the presence of osteopenia and the risk of developing osteoporosis. This primarily involves a thorough patient assessment with bone densitometry and the identification of risk factors.

Obtaining a detailed patient history and examination are essential. A thorough history may provide clinical evidence of the secondary causes of osteoporosis and a physical examination may show indicators such as loss of height, a dorsal kyphosis and back pain that indicate vertebral osteoporosis.

Bone densitometry

There have been major advances in the diagnosis of osteoporosis, particularly with the ability to detect

Box 19.2	Causes of childhood osteoporosis
Inherited disorders	Osteogenesis imperfecta
	Ehlers–Danlos syndrome
	Marfan's disease
	Gaucher's disease
	Glycogen storage disease
	Severe congenital neutropenia
	Galactosaemia
	Musculodystrophy
	Idiopathic juvenile osteoporosis
Acquired disorders	Steroid-induced osteoporosis
	Cerebral palsy
	Anorexia nervosa
	Inflammatory bowel disease
	Acute lymphoblastic leukaemia
	Post transplantation

and measure bone mass before a fracture has occurred at the main fracture sites: vertebrae, hip and wrist.

Peak bone mass is reached during early adulthood, around the age of 30. Achieving an optimal bone mass is influenced by genetic factors, adequate calcium intake, weight-bearing exercise and the absence of risk factors. The changes in bone mass are categorised as a statistical value of bone density:

- osteopenia: -1.00 to -2.5 standard deviations below the young adult mean
- osteoporosis: more than -2.5 standard deviations below the young adult mean.

Bone densitometry is the key to diagnosis but it has limitations. Some of the earliest attempts to quantify bone mineral density (BMD) used plain skeletal X-rays; these have limited value as demineralisation is only notable after 30% or more bone density has been lost. The most widely used methods in Britain are dual energy X-ray absorptiometry (DXA), quantitative computed tomography (QCT) and quantitative ultrasound (QUS) (Table 19.1). These screening tools provide an indicator of future fracture risk (Raisz 1999).

DXA scanning is currently considered the gold standard for assessing BMD, predicting future risk of fracture and assessing the response to treatment. It is precise, increasingly available, is a relatively quick procedure with superior precision, high resolution and a low exposure to radiation.

QCT is unique in providing a three-dimensional image, allowing the direct measurement of bone density and the spatial separation of trabecular from cortical bone. The drawbacks are the expense of the procedure and patient exposure to higher levels of radiation.

QUS has a role in the assessment of bone micro-architecture, independent of the BMD (Keen 2000). The calcaneum is the preferred site of measurement as it is easily accessible, has a high percentage of measurable trabecular bone loss and is a weight-bearing bone. The benefits of QUS are that it does not use ionising radiation, is less expensive and more portable than conventional bone densitometers that scan the spine or femur. When used by a skilled operator, this is an effective substitute and may prove a more appropriate technology for assessing fracture risk in larger populations.

At present screening everyone is not considered cost effective. Elderly patients presenting with a typical femoral, vertebral or radius fracture and those with multiple risk factors do not need screening, they can be started on treatment (Stephen & Wallace 2001). The guidelines for referring patients for bone densitometry are:

- a history of oestrogen deficiency; this is only an indicator for screening after an early natural or surgical menopause, prolonged amenorrhoea or if the results will influence a decision to commence drug treatment
- to confirm a diagnosis following a low-impact fracture, especially a Colles' fracture or vertebral deformity
- to confirm a diagnosis of osteopenia
- following a history of long-term corticosteroid use, for example 5 mg daily for more than 6 months
- secondary osteoporosis risk factors are present
- to monitor response to treatment
- some practitioners recommend screening for any dosage of corticosteroids over a prolonged period.

Risk factors

A variety of factors are known to increase the risk of osteoporosis. Apart from the conditions and drugs identified in Box 19.1, the most frequently occurring risk factors for women are amenorrhoea for 6 months or more and an early natural or surgical menopause before the age of 45 years. For both men and women, additional risk indicators are:

- long-term immobility and inactivity
- history of excess exercise causing amenorrhoea
- low body mass index, especially with a low body weight of 70 kg or below (Cadarette et al 2001)
- history or risk of falling and low-impact fractures

Table 19.1   Bone density assessments

Assessment	Site measured
Dual energy X-ray absorptiometry (DXA)	Axial and appendicular skeleton, particularly the spine, femur or radius
Single energy X-ray absorptiometry	Forearm, calcaneum
Single photon absorptiometry (SPA)	Radius
Quantitative computed tomography (QCT)	Femur, spine, radius
Broadband ultrasound attenuation (BUA), also known as quantitative ultrasound (QUS)	Calcaneum and patella

- maternal history of hip fracture or kyphosis
- premature menopause or oophorectomy before the age of 45 years
- poor dietary calcium intake
- high alcohol intake, as alcohol reduces the absorption of calcium
- smoking, as this reduces osteoblast activity and changes the oestrogen metabolism in women.

PREVENTION AND TREATMENT

The strategies for preventing osteoporosis are also used for reducing the risk of a fracture occurring when a patient has osteoporosis. The benefits of treating patients at high risk are greater than for treating those at lower risk as they have fewer osteoporosis and fracture risk indicators.

LIFESTYLE CHANGES

A variety of changes in lifestyle can prevent the progression of osteoporosis and reduce the risk of a fracture occurring. The possible changes need to be discussed with the patient. As these changes are not easily achieved the level of internal motivation to accept and act on these changes must be established. Continued support from the healthcare team and the patient's family is essential. Lifestyle changes include:

- reducing and stopping smoking
- reducing or stopping alcohol intake
- increasing weight-bearing exercises
- increasing dietary intake of calcium and vitamin D
- adjusting the home environment to reduce the risk of falling.

EXERCISE

The purpose of any non-pharmacological intervention for osteoporosis is to prevent, treat or alleviate the consequences of osteoporosis (Lips & Ooms 2000). Exercise plays a vital role in preventing and treating osteoporosis as well as fracture prevention (Hertel & Trahiotis 2001). In addition to exercise having an impact on the disease process, it improves general health, well-being and quality of life, and preserves independence (Sharkey et al 2000).

A more active lifestyle can be adopted at any age as an appropriate exercise programme can increase

bone mass in adolescents and adults. Studies have shown that while moderate exercise protects against osteoporosis, both too little and excessive exercise may accelerate the rate of bone mass loss (O'Brien 2001).

It is important when starting or increasing exercises to ensure they are carried out at an appropriate pace for the person's ability and age (NOS 2003b). For the elderly, the main emphasis needs to be on improving muscle strength and balance in order to decrease the risk of falls (Lips & Ooms 2000). The NOS (2003b) recommends the following ground rules for appropriate exercises (Box 19.3), which are applicable to all ages.

- Patients must not rush into unaccustomed exercise too fast.
- Some muscle stiffness is likely to occur at first but persistent pain may indicate an overuse injury. If this occurs the person should stop exercising until the injury heals.
- Exercise needs to be taken regularly to be beneficial.
- Regular exercise needs to become a way of life. If stopped, any benefit gained will be lost.
- It is possible to take too much exercise, with very intensive training potentially causing damage to the musculoskeletal system. If the level of training results in a very low body weight and low body fat levels, women will be at risk of amenorrhoea, which increases the risk of osteoporosis.
- Although exercises such as swimming and cycling are excellent, especially for the cardiovascular system, they are not weight bearing and have no effect on bones.

Box 19.3   Recommended exercises (NOS 2003b)

- Jumping or skipping: 50 jumps a day for young people
- Stair-climbing: 10 flights a day for older people
- Jogging: 3 times a week for young people or intermittent jogging 3 times a week for older people
- Exercise to music classes
- Weight training using high loads and few repetitions
- Field sports
- Racket sports
- Dancing

Where possible patients are referred for a physiotherapy exercise programme. This will incorporate the principles of pain management, graduated exercises, resistance and stamina. Many exercises are demonstrated and practice while sitting or lying. Particular attention is paid to exercises that can be continued at home. Circuit training exercises to increase cardiovascular fitness and exercises requiring balance will help as they generally involve weight-bearing exercises and reduce the risk of falling if continued long term (Lewis 2002). The use of hydrotherapy encourages muscle and joint movements by using gentle exercises but unless resistance activities are involved, there is little benefit for bone structure.

DIET

A varied and balanced diet is essential for musculoskeletal health. The average human body contains more than 1 kg of calcium, of which 99% is stored in the bones. To maintain this level and optimum bone health, men and women need an adequate dietary intake of calcium and vitamin D throughout their life (Box 19.4).

Supplements are beneficial if the dietary intake is inadequate, especially for older people to reduce the risk of sustaining a hip fracture. Calcium supplementation has been regarded as a vital part of the prevention and treatment of postmenopausal osteoporosis and the impact it has on

---

Box 19.4   Calcium and vitamin D intake (recommended daily intake)

Calcium:

women under 45 years	1000 mg
women over 45 years	1500 mg
women over 45 years taking HRT	1000 mg
men over 60 years	1500 mg
Vitamin D	800 international units

Calcium-rich foods:
milk (full fat, semi-skimmed and skimmed), cheese, yoghurt, spinach, parsley, nuts (almonds, brazil, hazel), figs, sesame seeds, tofu, fish (sardines, whitebait, salmon, pilchards)

Vitamin D-rich foods:
fish oils, liver, egg yolks, fortified cereals

---

bone mass has now been shown through research (Reid 1996).

Vitamin D is needed for the absorption of calcium. Deficiency in vitamin D is widespread in the frail elderly, because of their low exposure to sunlight or malabsorption problems due to gastrointestinal disease (Reid 1998). Calcitriol, an active form of vitamin D that improves the absorption of calcium from the gastrointestinal tract, may be recommended as a supplement for postmenopausal and frail elderly women with a history of vertebral osteoporosis.

The metaanalysis by Homik et al (2003) on calcium and vitamin D for corticosteroid-induced osteoporosis found they had a significant preventive effect on bone loss at the lumbar spine and forearm. As both these have a relatively low cost and toxicity, the authors recommend all patients started on corticosteroids should receive both supplements.

DRUG TREATMENT

The majority of drugs prescribed to relieve patients' symptoms and reduce the risk of further fragility fractures work by reducing osteoclastic bone resorption. Generally treating patients at high risk of a hip fracture has proven cost effective (Royal College of Physicians 1999). New treatments are constantly being developed, tested and introduced worldwide; for example, parathyroid hormone is licensed for use in the USA and in the UK. The National Institute for Clinical Excellence (NICE 2003) is anticipating publishing guidance in 2005 on the effectiveness and cost effectiveness of drug therapies, including bisphosphonates and parathyroid hormone, for the prevention and treatment of osteoporosis and prevention of fractures in postmenopausal women.

Bisphosphonates

This group of drugs is widely prescribed and generally well tolerated. They are designed to bind to the calcium in bones. It is important they are taken on an empty stomach with a full glass of tap water. Mineral water is not suitable as it contains added calcium. The patient must be upright, that is standing or sitting upright, after taking the medication otherwise oesophageal irritation may occur. They are not appropriate for patients with a history of gastric problems or poor kidney function. Three drugs are licensed for the prevention and treatment of osteoporosis in Britain.

1 Cyclical etidronate (Didronel PMO). The recommendation is 400 mg taken for 14 days, followed by effervescent calcium carbonate 500 mg for the following 76 days. It must be taken in the middle of a 4-hour fast. This is recommended for postmenopausal women to prevent the development of osteoporosis in patients with osteopenia and for the prevention and treatment of corticosteroid-induced osteoporosis. The Cranney et al (2003a) review suggests that etidronate increases bone density at the lumbar spine and femoral head, reducing the risk of a vertebral fracture but with no apparent effect on non-vertebral fractures.

2 Alendronate (Fosamax) is available as a 10 mg tablet taken once daily or 70 mg once weekly. Alendronate is generally well tolerated and effective for both the spine and hip bone.

3 Risedronate (Actonel) is available as a 5 mg tablet taken once daily or as a once-weekly 35 mg preparation. It is taken either first thing in the morning on an empty stomach in the same way as alendronate or in the middle of a 4-hour fast but not within 30 minutes of going to bed. This is recommended for patients with established postmenopausal osteoporosis, for preventing osteoporosis in postmenopausal women who have a high fracture risk and for postmenopausal women on long-term corticosteroid therapy.

Calcitonin

Calcitonin is effective during the acute phase of a vertebral fracture. The drawbacks are the expense of this drug and the side effects of nausea, vomiting, headaches, dizziness and diarrhoea.

Cranney et al (2003b) suggest there is an average of 14% bone loss at the hip following 1 year on corticosteroids. Their review of the efficacy of calcitonin in preventing and treating corticosteroid-induced osteoporosis suggests that this is not yet established although they did find it had a role in preserving bone mass in the lumbar spine but not at the femoral neck.

Hormone replacement therapy (HRT)

HRT is now a well-established therapy given to women during or immediately after the menopause. It was widely prescribed for the treatment and prevention of osteoporosis, particularly for women experiencing menopause symptoms with a high risk of developing osteoporosis, as it provides a low dose of natural oestrogen. However, it is no longer recommended for the prevention or treatment of osteoporosis and is only used to manage menopause symptoms.

Women who have undergone a hysterectomy are able to take oestrogen-only medication. Women who have not had a hysterectomy are prescribed an oestrogen and progestogen medication as the progesterone has a protective effect on the endometrium lining of the womb, reducing the risk of endometrial carcinoma. The recommended period of treatment is for a minimum of 5 years. Longer use for 10 years or more will give added protection but it is up to each woman to decide the period of their treatment.

HRT preparations are divided into three groups:

1 oestrogen only
2 cyclical or sequential HRT which contains both oestrogen and progestogen
3 continuous combined or period-free HRT recommended for postmenopausal women who have not had a period for at least a year.

These are available in a variety of formats as a skin patch, implant, cream, pessary or tablet, making this a flexible medication. Some patients find the side effects of breast tenderness, nausea and leg cramps reduce or disappear if they change their prescription to a different mode of drug delivery.

The short-term benefits include the reduction of symptoms such as hot flushes, night sweats and vaginal dryness. Additional long-term benefits are protection against the effects of oestrogen deficiency causing osteoporosis and cardiovascular disease. The contraindications to the use of HRT are pregnancy, recent thrombosis, abnormal genital bleeds, liver damage, renal disease and if the patient has a known carcinoma risk, especially oestrogen-dependent carcinomas.

Selective oestrogen receptor modulators (SERMs)

These drugs are designed to mimic the effect of oestrogen on bone to maintain bone density and reduce the risk of fracture (NOS 2003a) by binding to oestrogen receptors found in the tissues of the breast, reproductive system, liver, brain and bone. Raloxifene (Evista) inhibits bone resorption and is known to be effective in preventing postmenopausal bone loss and to significantly reduce the incidence of vertebral fracture but it has little effect on incidences of wrist and hip fracture (Keen 2000).

Testosterone therapy

This is prescribed to men known to have low testosterone levels to help maintain their bone density levels (NOS 2003a). The underlying cause needs to be identified and treated where possible. Testosterone therapy is ideally given by injection every 2 weeks to ensure more accurate serum level control, although patches are generally more convenient for patients. The potential side effects must be discussed with patients prior to starting treatment as these include priapism, weight gain, reduced fertility and an increased risk of prostate problems and heart disease.

FALLS

The majority of osteoporosis-related fractures are the result of a fall. There are numerous reasons why individuals fall (Box 19.5); fortunately most will not result in major injuries but for the elderly the risk of sustaining a fracture is extremely high. Those aged 75 years and above suffer at least one fall a year with many requiring hospital treatment for their injuries.

Elderly people living in nursing homes are particularly vulnerable and many become 'repeat fallers'. Hip protectors are now available and have been shown to reduce the risk of hip fracture occurring as a result of a fall by forcing the energy away from the trochanter (Lips & Ooms 2000). Parker et al (2003) recommend their use for those living in institutional care, especially if there is a high incidence of falls. Compliance in wearing hip protectors is essential. There is no evidence for the effectiveness of hip protectors for those living in their own home, principally because they are likely to be more active and have fewer risks and incidences of falling.

The National Service Framework for Older People outlines standards of care along with examples of service and performance models from a range of health service providers (DoH 2001). The framework includes a standard on falls related to osteoporosis and fractures. This advises that patients with osteoporosis, especially those who have experienced a fall or fracture, be referred to a falls clinic. Here a full assessment can identify the risks and reasons a patient has fallen or had a fracture and recommend any relevant preventive steps. Advice on simple prevention measures such as footwear, removal of rugs, sight tests, encouragement to use walking aids and ensuring correct prescriptions for glasses can significantly reduce the risk of falling.

The proactive involvement of the osteoporosis nurse in the assessment of older people will reduce the number of osteoporotic fractures in the future. The National Osteoporosis Nurse Initiative falls and fracture risk assessment programme (NOS 2003c) is one such UK strategy. This aims to encourage the assessment of nursing and care home residents through training the care home staff to carry out risk assessment and alert the general practitioner to the residents' risk status.

Box 19.5 **Factors affecting the risk of falling**
• Age
• Female
• Physical impairment: poor gait, balance and muscle strength
• Sensory impairment, e.g. visual impairment
• Cognitive impairment, e.g. confusion
• Other medical conditions, e.g. Parkinson's disease, stroke
• Medications used, e.g. night sedation, multiple medications
• A history of falling and low-impact fractures
• Social and physical environment, e.g. stairs, uneven surfaces, cluttered walking space
• Excess alcohol intake

OSTEOPOROSIS SPECIALIST NURSE

The role of nurses working within the field of osteoporosis varies depending on the focus and area in which they work in the primary or secondary healthcare setting. The majority of roles are within secondary care and require a range of management, research, education and clinical practice skills. Many specialist nurses have a Master's degree, are expected to work autonomously and be innovative in their approach to care and practice in this field.

They work within a multidisciplinary team that includes physiotherapists, occupational therapists, community teams and researchers. It is essential for all members of the team to have good communication skills and an open collaborative approach to practice and the team needs to forge links with other disciplines, departments and agencies involved in the medical, nursing and social care of these patients. The nature of the nursing role often means the senior nurse is responsible for the coordination and management of the team and may control a substantial budget to support the work of the team.

Medical research into the causes, prevention and treatment of osteoporosis is substantial. It is essential nurses recognise the contribution they can make by getting involved in research-based activities and not dismissing or underestimating the value of reviewing and implementing research practices or being actively involved in research studies. By taking part in these activities, practice is reviewed to ensure it is based on relevant research or other evidence, enhancing their own understanding of the condition and a patient-focused approach to care.

The nurses provide information and education in a variety of different ways, each requiring different approaches.

- For health professionals in the academic arena and clinical practice, especially to practitioners in related specialties, for example in accident and emergency departments, elderly care, school nursing forums, rheumatology and gynaecology.
- For patients and carers who have or are at risk of osteoporosis in both hospital and community settings.
- For the public through interest groups, women's groups and the media.
- For children in schools and youth clubs.

Many patients are proactive in the management of their condition and welcome the opportunity to receive support from the nurse and other patients, especially through specialist support networks and healthcare user groups. This often provides a forum for discussion and allows patients to share concerns and anxieties in a safe supportive environment. The support required will vary but generally allows the nurse to influence skeletal health and ensure people understand the condition, treatment options, lifestyle changes and practical advice. The educational opportunities are relevant across all age groups, for example:

- **children**: diet and exercise advice, particularly to raise awareness of calcium-rich foods

- **adolescents**: advice relating to diet, exercise, smoking, alcohol and specific risk factors such as anorexia
- **adults**: advice on how to maintain peak bone mass, preconception advice, diet advice during pregnancy, recognition of risk factors, pre- and postmenopausal advice
- **older people**: advice on diet, exercise and recognition of risk factors, especially falls and fracture risks.

As with any chronic or long-term condition, the nurse–patient relationship is of paramount importance. This is enabled in part through nurse-led clinics and direct contact facilities for patients and carers. The nurse-led clinics offer a service that supports and complements the medical clinics by allowing additional time for discussion of relevant personal issues and patient education. Patients are also encouraged to contact the nurse directly between clinic visits using telephone or email facilities if they have any concerns. Knowing they can directly contact the nurse offers patients reassurance and may avoid additional clinic visits.

CONCLUSION

Osteopenia and osteoporosis are natural progressive changes in bone quality that can have major effects on the lifestyle, health and mobility of those affected. The consequences are often fractures that affect their level of independence in the short and long term and have huge cost implications for the health service. The rates and effects of osteoporosis will increase as the number of older people in the population continues to rise and life expectancy is extended, resulting in it having an even larger impact on future healthcare provision.

The osteoporosis nurse has a vital role in enabling patients to understand the need for lifestyle changes, the effects of which are not seen for many years. This is one of many facets of a role constantly expanding and evolving in response to developments in healthcare. Through involvement in the primary and secondary care sectors, osteoporosis nurses can influence all age groups to prevent the rapid progression of the condition and reduce their risk of fractures occurring. Recommendations for best practice in the prevention and treatment of the condition vary but patients most at risk must be offered support to decide on the best options for them.

References

Bonnick SL 1994 The osteoporosis handbook. Taylor Publishing, Dallas

Cadarette SM, Jaglal SB, Murray T et al 2001 Evaluation of decision rules for referring women for bone densitometry by dual-energy x-ray absorptiometry. JAMA 286(1): 57–63

Cranney A, Welch V, Adachi JD et al 2003a Etidronate for treating and preventing postmenopausal osteoporosis (Cochrane review). Cochrane Library Issue 3. Update Software, Oxford

Cranney A, Welch V, Adachi JD et al 2003b Calcitonin for preventing and treating corticosteroid induced osteoporosis (Cochrane Review). Cochrane Library Issue 3. Update Software, Oxford

Department of Health (DoH) 2001 National Service Framework for Older People. Department of Health, London

Healy P 2000 Bone of contention. Nursing Standard 14(48): 11

Hertel KL, Trahiotis MG 2001 Exercise in the prevention and treatment of osteoporosis: the role of physical therapy and nursing. Nursing Clinics of North America 36(3): 441–453

Homik J, Suarez-Almazor ME, Shea B et al 2003 Calcium and vitamin D for corticosteroid-induced osteoporosis (Cochrane Review). Cochrane Library Issue 3. Update Software, Oxford

Keen R 2000 Rheumatic disease topical reviews no 1. Osteoporosis and metabolic bone disease. Arthritis Research Campaign, Chesterfield

Kessenich C 2000 Update on osteoporosis in elderly men. Geriatric Nursing 21(5): 242–244

Lewis R 2002 A physiotherapy programme for osteoporosis management. Osteoporosis Review 10(2): 11–14

Lips P, Ooms ME 2000 Non-pharmacology interventions. Best practice and research. Clinical Endocrinology and Metabolism 14(2): 265–277

Meunier P 1993 Is steroid induced osteoporosis preventable? New England Journal of Medicine 328(24): 1781–1782

National Institute for Clinical Excellence (NICE) 2003 Scope: prevention and treatment of osteoporosis. Available online at: www.nice.org.uk/article.asp?a=35472

National Osteoporosis Society (NOS) 2003a Osteoporosis. Available online at: www.nos.org.uk/osteo.asp

National Osteoporosis Society (NOS) 2003b Exercise and osteoporosis. Available online at: www.nos.org.uk/ecom/prodlistpub.asp

National Osteoporosis Society (NOS) 2003c Scope Osteoporosis Nurse Initiative. Available online at: www.nos.org.uk/health info_ni.asp

O'Brien M 2001 Exercise and osteoporosis. Irish Journal of Medical Science 170(1): 58–62

Orwoll ES 1998 Osteoporosis in men. Endocrinology and Metabolism Clinics of North America 27(2): 349–367

Parker MJ, Gillespie LD, Gillespie WJ 2003 Hip protectors for preventing hip fractures in the elderly (Cochrane Review). Cochrane Library Issue 3. Update Software, Oxford

Raisz LG 1999 Osteoporosis: current approaches and future prospects in diagnosis, pathogenesis and management. Journal of Bone and Mineral Metabolism 17(2): 78–79

Reid I 1996 Therapy of osteoporosis: calcium, vitamin D and exercise. American Journal of Medical Sciences 312(6): 278–286

Reid I 1998 The roles of calcium and vitamin D in prevention of osteoporosis. Endocrinology and Metabolism Clinics of North America 27(2): 389–398

Rosen C, Kessenich C 1997 Risk factor for osteoporosis in men. Clinical Geriatrician 5(4): 87–95

Royal College of Physicians 1999 Osteoporosis: clinical guidelines for prevention and treatment. Royal College of Physicians, London

Sharkey NA, Williams NI, Guerin JB 2000 The role of exercise in the prevention and treatment of osteoporosis and osteoarthritis. Nursing Clinics of North America 35(1): 209–221

Stephen AB, Wallace WA 2001 The management of osteoporosis. Journal of Bone and Joint Surgery 83B(3): 316–323

World Health Organisation 1994 Assessment of fracture risk and its application to screening for post-menopausal osteoporosis. WHO, Geneva

Chapter 20

Care of patients with acute spinal cord injuries

Mike Smith

INTRODUCTION

Despite the lack of accurate published UK statistics, using an estimate based on available figures, there appear to be 650–750 people per year in the UK who sustain traumatic damage to the spinal cord. A more accurate picture may be obtained from Australia where full adult national spinal cord injury figures are kept. The 1998–9 figures suggested an incidence of 14.5 per million of population (O'Connor 2002).

These injuries invariably follow direct injuries to the bones and ligaments forming the vertebral column, which protect the delicate spinal cord beneath. Clinical areas at the sharp end of trauma services, the trauma, neurosurgical, intensive care and accident and emergency units, are responsible for the initial management of those with a spinal cord injury from the time of hospitalisation. This period of responsibility will often exceed 48 hours post injury while the patient awaits transfer to a specialist spinal injury unit (SIU). The implications of inappropriate management are substantial, potentially resulting in the exacerbation of an already undesirable situation.

The key points relating to the management of spinal cord injury patients in the acute stage are that:

- a spinal cord injury is a multisystem, life-changing event for an individual
- the long-term outcome is directly affected by the quality of the interventions in the first 48 hours following injury, often the care taking place in a general hospital setting
- nurses have a vital role in the provision of quality acute care for patients with a spinal cord injury

- nurses require practical advice in all aspects of acute spinal injury care underpinned by knowledge of normal and altered neurophysiology
- early referral to a specialist centre is essential, to meet the short-term and long-term needs of the individual patient and to act as a resource for advice and support prior to transfer.

This chapter gives the reader the background knowledge and practical advice in relation to these key issues. The nature and types of spinal cord injury (SCI) are discussed along with the effects of post-injury physiology changes. The assessments and nursing interventions related to the whole-body effects of this injury are described. The organisation of SCI services is discussed with specific reference to the situation in the UK, along with practical advice relating to the referral and transfer of a patient to a specialist spinal injury unit.

THE NATURE OF SPINAL CORD INJURY

SCI of traumatic origin occurs as a result of an insult to the vertebral column via various mechanisms (Box 20.1), causing damage to the spinal cord or the cauda equina that runs within the vertebral canal (Fig. 20.1). Spinal cord lesions also occur from non-traumatic sources, including tumours, infection and disturbances of the cord circulation.

MECHANISM OF INJURY AND TRENDS IN SCI INCIDENCE

Road traffic accidents remain the major cause of spinal cord injury in most developed countries. Published records are not available for the UK but figures provided by the Royal National Orthopaedic Hospital Trust (RNOHT), Stanmore, and the Duke of Cornwall spinal treatment centre in Salisbury,

Box 20.1 Mechanisms of vertebral injury resulting in SCI
- Compression
- Flexion
- Extension
- Rotation
- Direct trauma

(Grundy et al 1995) suggest this is still the case. Again anecdotally from the experience of the Stanmore unit, SCI attributable to motorcycle injury has declined, accounting for only 3% of the overall incidence. It is conceivable that restriction on the engine capacity for learner riders has contributed to this decrease.

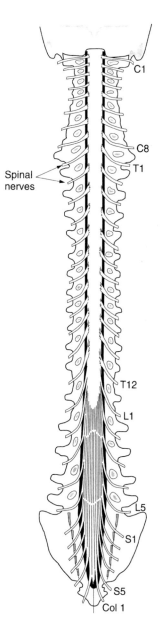

Figure 20.1 The spinal cord and spinal nerves viewed from the back. The laminae of the vertebrae have been removed to reveal the spinal cord in the vertebral canal and the spinal nerves in the intervertebral foramina. (Adapted from Palastanga et al 1998.)

Falls, often taking place in the home such as down stairs, are a common mechanism of injury, particularly among older patients.

Building sites seem to be a frequent location for SCI from industrial accidents, with falls from roofs and scaffolding being common causes.

SCI resulting from sports injuries appear to be seasonal in nature. In the winter months rugby and skiing injuries both provide a significant number of injured clients, whereas the summer brings diving injuries necessitating, in some cases, repatriation following injury on holiday and initial treatment to ensure stability of the spine before travelling.

There appears to be an anecdotal increase in the number of patients sustaining SCI following failed suicide attempts in recent years. The combination of mental illness and a major physical disability causes extreme difficulties in the rehabilitation stage and reintegration back into the community. The reason for this increase is not known but it does raise questions relating to the amount of support provided for those with mental health problems in the community. Supporting patients with the combination of SCI and existing mental illness is challenging as the psychiatric problems are a barrier to standard models of physical rehabilitation. However, once their symptoms are under control there is no reason why these patients should not benefit from rehabilitation (Liang et al 1996).

A relatively small percentage of injuries occur as a result of an assault, primarily from stabbing and shooting incidents. Such assault injuries are significantly higher in some areas of the USA, often as high as 30% (Go et al 1995). They appear to be increasing often as a result of drug-related criminal activity. The presence of police in the clinical area for fear of retribution or repeat attacks by the parties responsible, plus the reported increase in verbal and physical abuse towards nurses, are clearly unsettling and, in severe cases, disturbing and potentially dangerous for the nurse.

A summary of the mechanisms of SCI relating to patients admitted to the RNOHT Stanmore spinal injuries unit can be seen in Figure 20.2. These appear congruent with other figures available from the Duke of Cornwall spinal treatment centre, Salisbury (Grundy et al 1995).

Traditionally a 4:1 male to female ratio has been quoted for incidences of spinal cord injury. One must, however, bear in mind that such figures originate from the USA where there is a high incidence of assault as a cause of SCI in young men, which has

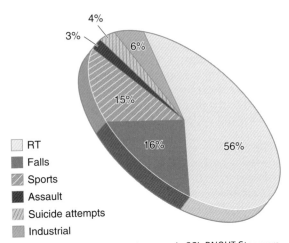

Figure 20.2   Mechanisms of traumatic SCI, RNOHT Stanmore 1994–6.

the potential to skew the figures somewhat. It appears that figures in the UK and Australia (unpublished data from Sir George Bedbrook spinal unit in Perth) may be in the region of a 3:1 male to female ratio, though again this figure cannot be corroborated with complete data.

The age distribution of the main group sustaining traumatic SCI has traditionally been in the 20–40 year range. Recently there has been an increase in those who are 60 years and over; in this age group the main implications for care can relate to their previous medical history, which invariably creates further complications in the acute stage. SCI in children is comparatively rare, probably in the region of 2–3% of those injured annually. Not only are children more flexible than adults but also they rarely take part in high-risk activities such as driving cars or high-risk sports. Figure 20.3 illustrates age ranges of clients admitted to the SIU, RNOHT, in 1994–5.

CLASSIFICATION OF SPINAL CORD INJURY

Spinal cord injuries are classified in different ways. There are three generally recognised classifications: by level of injury, by severity of injury and by level of motor neuron injury.

Level of injury

The most common broad classification of SCI is related to the extent to which limbs have been affected by the injury (Zedjlik 1992).

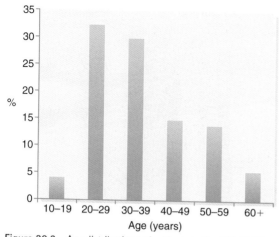

Figure 20.3   Age distributions of patients in the SIU, RNOHT 1994–5.

The term 'paraplegia' is defined as the loss of, or reduced function in, the lower limbs caused by damage to the thoracic, lumbar and sacral vertebral areas resulting in injury to the spinal cord or the cauda equina. The synonymous terms 'quadriplegia' or 'tetraplegia' are defined as loss of or reduced function in all four limbs and results from injury to the cervical portion of the spinal cord. Unpublished data from 1995–6 from the SIU at the RNOHT, Stanmore, indicated an approximate 1:1 ratio of quadriplegia (51%) to paraplegia (49%).

Severity of injury

The severity of the injury relates to the amount of nerve fibres affected and the level of injury sustained. A complete injury refers to a total absence of motor or sensory function below the injury level; an incomplete injury refers to some function remaining intact. There is an increasing trend towards a greater number of injuries being classed as incomplete. Unpublished data from the SIU at RNOHT, Stanmore, suggest a reversal of the traditional 3:1 ratio of complete to incomplete injuries (1984–5) compared to 1994–5 figures showing a 1:3 ratio. The reasons for this very positive change are not clear but there appear to be two contributory factors.

1 Improved prehospital care at the accident scene and during transportation to hospital with the increased number and training of paramedics within the ambulance service.

2 From the author's personal experience, medical and nursing personnel have increased knowledge and understanding related to the identification of SCI and use of correct handling techniques within the accident and emergency departments and intensive care units responsible for the care of SCI patients in the critical hours following injury.

Spinal cord injuries are classified by neurological level, according to the segment of the spinal cord that is damaged or the spinal nerves affected in the case of the cauda equina. Neurological examination to determine the level and severity of injury incorporates testing sensory, motor and reflex function. Examination of sensory function involves testing of the dermatomes, the areas of cutaneous tissue supplying information to a specific spinal nerve (Fig. 20.4). Testing sensation using touch and pinprick tests is particularly relevant in those who have incomplete injuries, as the fibres that carry these sensations travel differently within the cord. From this it may be possible to determine which part of the cord is damaged (Table 20.1). Motor function is tested through examination of myotomes, the muscle groups supplied by a specific spinal nerve. Such information is recorded using the ASIA system (ASIA 2001), the international standard allowing injuries and the effects of interventions to be compared across many centres. Abdominal, anal and somatic reflexes are also tested and recorded although these will often be absent due to spinal shock (Box 20.2).

Although nurses will perform neurological tests in some centres, this is not the case within all units. It is essential, though, for nurses to be aware of the patient's neurological status along with the level and severity of the injury, as changes must be acted on swiftly. This is particularly important if the patient has deteriorating function. Due to the working patterns of nursing compared to other disciplines, it is often the nurse who will be in a position to detect such changes early.

The severity of the injury will determine the motor, sensory and reflex functions that remain intact and give an indication of the expected degree of disability the SCI patient has sustained.

Upper motor neuron versus lower motor neuron

The final method used, although less commonly these days, is to classify an injury as an upper or a lower motor neuron injury. An upper motor neuron runs entirely within the central nervous system: the brain and spinal cord. Injuries above the first lumbar

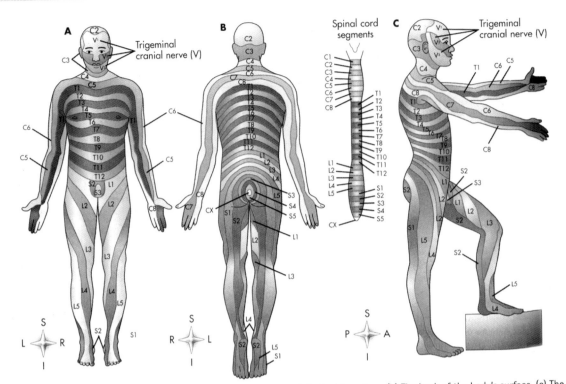

Figure 20.4   Dermatome distribution of spinal nerves. (a) The front of the body's surface. (b) The back of the body's surface. (c) The lateral view of the body. Inset segments of the spinal cord associated with each spinal nerve and the sensory dermatomes shown. (From Thibodeau & Paton 1999.)

Table 20.1   Incomplete syndromes

Syndrome	Description and clinical picture
Central cord	A lesion that exclusively occurs in the cervical region, often due to hyperextension injuries in older patients. Results in sacral sensory sparing and a greater weakness in the upper limbs than lower limbs
Brown Sequard	Damage to one half of the spinal cord resulting in motor loss on the same side as the lesion and sensory loss on the opposite side
Anterior artery	The anterior artery supplies the front two-thirds of the cord. This syndrome results in a variable loss of motor function and pinprick and temperature sensations. Proprioception is usually preserved

vertebra will damage the cord itself and are classified as upper motor neuron (UMN) injuries. The implication for this type of injury is that after the period of spinal shock, the patient will regain spinal reflex activity, as the reflex arc will remain intact. Conversely, a patient with an injury damaging the lower motor neurons, that run from the spinal cord to the periphery via the spinal nerves which form the cauda equina, will have a flaccid paralysis with no reflexes, as the sensory and motor neurons that form the reflex arc will be damaged.

Due to spinal shock the main issues for management occur in the postacute phase. Additionally, for patients with UMN injuries, when the reflexes return they will be exaggerated due to the lack of moderation from the higher centres. The patient is said to be in a hyperreflexic state; spasticity (exaggerated tonal reflexes) will occur and the bladder reflex will be initiated at a lower residual volume.

THE PATHOPHYSIOLOGY OF SCI

Through an understanding of the exact pathophysiology of spinal cord injury, it may be possible to provide early interventions to influence the degree of damage to the cord.

The damage to the spinal cord occurs as a two-stage process.

Box 20.2   Spinal shock

Spinal shock can be defined as a transient loss of all reflex activity below the injury level. Onset is immediate or within minutes following cord damage and will last from 6 days to 6 weeks. To date there is no hard evidence that the presence of spinal shock affects sensory and motor function or the patient's long-term prognosis (Ko et al 1999). To claim that a prognosis cannot be suggested until spinal shock has subsided is incorrect. Spinal shock will affect both somatic and autonomic reflexes; in all patients who have complete injuries there will be an absence of:

- somatic reflexes below the injury level
- bladder and bowel reflexes
- vasomotor tone below the injury level.

In patients with injuries above T6 level there will be major disruption of autonomic reflexes resulting in: bradycardia, hypotension, hypothermia.

The return of reflexes in patients with damage above L1 level (those with upper motor neuron injuries) signifies the end of spinal shock. There is an apparent major diuresis in most patients as spinal shock subsides, the reason for which is not entirely understood.

1 The primary injury occurs at the time of the accident. The major emphasis on preventing primary injury is through health promotion related to accident prevention. There are continuous attempts to enact this, in some cases backed by legislation and television advertisements relating, for example, to the wearing of seatbelts and poster campaigns emphasising the need to drive with care.

2 The second stage of injury occurs in the hours following the initial injury and this has been the focus of much research over the last few years. This secondary damage occurs as a result of a complex biochemical cascade of events, leading to a process called lipid peroxidisation, which ultimately culminates in further neurological deterioration. The emphasis of research has therefore been to attempt to influence various points within this cascade, to positively affect outcomes for the patient by reducing the potential degree of long-term disability.

Following the NASCIS II multicentre trial in the USA (Bracken et al 1990), it was suggested that this biochemical cascade can be influenced positively through pharmacological means, by administration of massive doses of the corticosteroid methylprednisolone. This only appeared to be the case if treatment was commenced within the first 8 hours following injury (Bracken et al 1990). This early intervention is increasingly being adopted, although cannot yet be described as widespread internationally. More recently, a third NASCIS trial has utilised tirilazad mesylate as well as methylprednisolone with some effect and reinforced the positive results from the earlier trial (Bracken et al 1997). Additionally this study suggested a longer infusion period was needed if there was a delay of more than 3 hours post injury. The protocol for all SCI patients within 8 hours of injury is:

- methylprednisolone 30 mg/kg as a bolus over 15 minutes, followed by a 45-minute break then,
- commence an infusion of 5.4 mg/kg per hour as an IV infusion:
  — either for 23 hours if less than 3 hours since injury
  — or extend this infusion period for a further 24 hours (47 hours in total) if 3–8 hours since injury.

Associated injury

As the mechanism of spinal cord injury often involves significant force, major trauma resulting in multiple injuries is common. The injuries commonly associated with SCI relate to the levels of the vertebral injury:

- a cervical injury is associated with head and facial injuries
- thoracic injuries are linked to chest injuries to the ribs or sternum with an associated risk of pneumothorax
- lumbar injuries are linked to abdominal injury
- sacral injuries are associated with pelvic fractures and damage to the lower gastrointestinal and urinary tracts.

All the above have additional medical and nursing implications in the acute stage of patient care.

The autonomic nervous system and SCI

Before discussing the patient implications and nursing care interventions it is worth reviewing the autonomic nervous system as it has a major influence on patients with a high SCI.

The autonomic nervous system (ANS), so called because it was thought to be autonomous in relation

Table 20.2 Autonomic nervous system effects

Effector	Sympathetic response	Parasympathetic response
Heart rate	Increase	Decrease
Bronchioles	Dilate	Constrict
Peripheral blood vessels	Constrict	No parasympathetic innervation
Skeletal muscle vessels	Dilate	Constrict
Gastric and bronchiole secretions	Inhibit	Increase
Detrusor (bladder) muscle	Relax	Contract
Internal anal and bladder sphincters	Contract	Relax

to the rest of the nervous system, controls the involuntary functions of the body, including smooth and cardiac muscle contraction and the activity of glands. Controlled by the hypothalamus and responding to internal and external stimuli, the ANS can be divided into two branches: the sympathetic and parasympathetic nervous systems.

With a couple of exceptions, the effectors, organs and glands have dual innervation from both branches, each having opposite results. The sympathetic nervous system effects can be related to what happens to the body in an emergency situation: the fight-fright-flight response. The parasympathetic nervous system initiates effects that are more calming. Knowing this, the practitioner can work out the effect each branch has on each effector. To illustrate this, imagine being faced with a charging rhinoceros. The heart rate would rise, the bronchioles dilate to assist oxygen intake, the iris would open to facilitate seeing an escape route and skeletal muscle blood vessels would dilate to facilitate oxygen reaching the muscles. These are sympathetic nervous system responses. There would be little need for peripheral blood vessel dilation, the production of gastric or bronchial secretions, bowel and bladder activity or sexual arousal, all of which are initiated by parasympathetic activity. Table 20.2 provides an overview of the autonomic nervous system responses.

The implications for physiological changes relate to the outflow of the respective branches. The parasympathetic outflow is via the cranial nerves; of particular importance is the vagus nerve, and the second to fourth sacral nerves as part of the bladder

and bowel reflexes. The sympathetic outflow is via the T1–L2 spinal nerves, the implication being that in high SCI above T6 level, there will be major sympathetic nervous system disruption resulting in unopposed parasympathetic outflow in the acute stage following SCI. Referring back to Table 20.2, the patient with an injury at C6 level, for example, will have a low heart rate, increase in secretions and loss of peripheral vasomotor control resulting in a state of passive vasodilation.

In summary, the implications of an acute SCI will be dependent on:

- level of injury
- severity of injury
- associated trauma
- the patient's previous medical history.

MANAGEMENT OF SKELETAL SPINAL INJURY

OBJECTIVES OF ACUTE MANAGEMENT

The principal objectives relating to management of the patient are as follows.

1 **Preserving existing neurological function.** This is primarily concerned with the management of the vertebral column injury, including correct manual handling of the fracture site and minimising the likelihood of damage to the cord. There may be some scope for reducing the damage to the cord through pharmacological intervention as described earlier.

2 **Physiological resuscitation.** Of primary concern in the initial management is awareness and management of the potential life-threatening effects related to respiratory and cardiovascular implications of spinal cord injury.

3 **Prevention of secondary complications.** As SCI is a multisystem event, secondary complications are commonplace. These may be physical or psychological and can either be prevented entirely or their effect minimised by appropriate monitoring and nursing intervention.

SKELETAL STABILITY

The simple classification of the mechanism of injury (Box 20.1) is inadequate from the clinical perspective. The first broad classification is whether the injury is stable or not. Stability relates to whether the vertebral

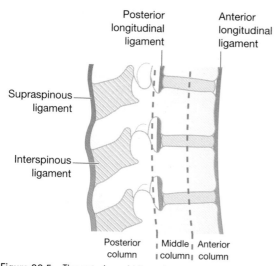

Figure 20.5   *The anterior, middle and posterior spinal columns.*

column structures are able to maintain the column in normal alignment and allow function without further damage to the spinal cord. This is determined using the three column rule: if only one column is disrupted the injury is stable, if two or three are disrupted the injury is classed as unstable (Fig. 20.5).

There have been attempts to provide more refined standards for classifying injury. Most examine the number of columns affected, the extent of displacement, degree of loss of vertebral height, the degree of angulation or amount of impingement on the canal space.

SKULL TRACTION

It remains common for a patient with a cervical vertebral column injury to have skull traction inserted, either presurgery or for a period of 8–12 weeks if being managed conservatively. The principles of traction and pin-site care discussed in Chapter 6 are transferable to the patient with skull traction.

There are various types of skull traction utilised; three are briefly described here.

Halo traction

Halo traction is becoming the most commonly used method. Many systems are now MRI compatible, contributing to their popularity. They can be used with a fixed jacket for patients with intact neurological function, facilitating early discharge. The screws holding the traction in place will need to be tightened on an outpatient basis.

Skull callipers

These are situated in the side of the skull. There are several types, the two common ones being Cones and Gardner Wells. They have been popular for patients who are being conservatively managed or on the rare occasions where skull traction is used to reduce the fracture by adding weights. In such cases every increase in the weight applied requires a repeat X-ray and neurological test. This method of management is less commonly used due to the increased popularity of halo traction.

Crutchfield tongs

In contrast, the Crutchfield tongs are placed in the top of the skull. These are only suitable for maintenance traction as increased weight may result in the traction becoming dislodged.

MOVING AND HANDLING THE PATIENT WITH AN UNSTABLE FRACTURE

This area of practice causes a great deal of concern for nurses caring for patients outside specialist spinal injury centres. The implications of mishandling a patient with acute SCI are clearly the prospect of worsening the neurological function, either through increasing severity at the existing injury level or even causing neurological damage at a higher level, especially in those with cervical cord damage.

As a guide to handling techniques the following are general principles for handling the patient with an unstable vertebral injury.

- Patients should be treated as having multilevel fractures until a full set of spinal X-rays has been undertaken and verified by an appropriate member of the medical staff. The results of this should be recorded in the patient's notes prior to any changes in turning regimes.
- The aim when handling the patient with vertebral injury is to maintain the fracture site in spinal alignment.
- All patients with possible or confirmed injuries above T5 vertebral level should be treated as cervical patients for the purposes of handling to protect the fracture site and should have their neck supported by a head hold.
- Any cervically injured patient should have the fracture site protected by pushing down on the shoulders when performing manoeuvres such as passive limb movements, washing, applying antiembolic

stockings to the lower limbs or providing an assisted cough. Any procedure which may result in movement of the upper part of the patient's body necessitates this precaution.

- Surface-to-surface transfers should be performed using a device with a solid base, as with the Mo-lift or a scoop stretcher, not sliding sheets such as the Easislide or Pat-slide type devices.
- Patients should not be sat up or put on a bedpan. Eliminatory functions are performed by placing the patient, still in alignment, on their side and using an incontinence pad for bowel care. Consider using a temporary indwelling catheter or intermittent catheterisation for urinary output.
- The team member at the patient's head must coordinate the manoeuvre. Other team members must listen and follow instructions and not attempt to lead as this may result in an uneven, uncoordinated turn with an increased risk of moving the fracture site. The patient should be given clear instructions to ensure cooperation for the same reason.
- Cervical collars need not be worn by the majority of patients when in bed as pointing out the potential risks to the patient will normally ensure compliance. For those patients who may be confused due to other injuries such as a traumatic brain injury or a preexisting confusion state, a collar is advisable; such situations may be an indication for early surgical stabilisation. If a collar is worn, it should be a properly measured hard collar, which is adjustable to ensure a good fit; for instance, the Stiff Neck collar. This should be removed at least daily to observe for potential skin problems around the collar.
- The general principles of manual handling should be followed to maintain the personal back safety of the team.

For specific turning regimes the reader is encouraged to consult either of the descriptions provided in *The ABC of spinal cord injury* (Grundy et al 1995) or an article written by McCarthy (1998). Additionally most spinal units will run study days for interested professionals if requested.

MANAGEMENT OF THE NEUROLOGICAL IMPLICATIONS

For each of the implications of acute SCI identified in Figure 20.6, the relevant nursing assessments and interventions will be explored. Additionally, brief reference will be made to the longer term management,

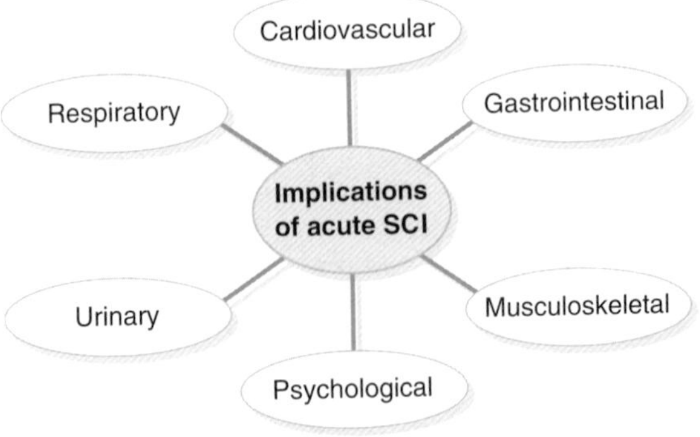

Figure 20.6   Implications of acute SCI.

Table 20.3   Respiratory muscle innervation

	Muscle	Spinal nerve
Inspiration	Diaphragm	C3–5
	External intercostal muscles	T1–7
	Accessory muscles	C1–8
Expiration (forced), e.g. coughing and exercise	Internal intercostal muscles	T1–7
	Abdominal muscles	T6–12

where appropriate, to equip the nurse to deal with queries from the patient or relative, as these are often voiced at a very early stage.

RESPIRATORY IMPLICATIONS

Respiratory implications are primarily dependent on the level and severity of injury and the related effect on respiratory muscle function (Table 20.3). Respiratory problems are the most common cause of death in early SCI (DeVivo et al 1999).

In simple terms, the higher the level of injury, the greater the degree of respiratory insufficiency (Jackson & Groomes 1994). All cervically injured patients will therefore have a need for respiratory intervention. For example, the patient with a complete C6 lesion will have an intact diaphragm and accessory muscle spinal innervation but will have a decreased vital capacity and an ineffective cough. With the loss of intercostal muscle function, such a patient will exhibit a greater reliance on accessory muscle use to maintain effective respiration. As with any muscle which is used more frequently, there will be a tendency for that muscle to tire until an increased tolerance is developed. Additionally, the loss of sympathetic nervous system inhibition of secretion production causes bronchial secretions to be increased. These factors and the enforced immobility of the patient are a recipe for a potential chest infection due to mucus stasis.

Associated chest injuries appear frequently. Fractures of the ribs are common, along with the potential for a pneumothorax, which further complicates the situation. If the mechanism of injury was diving, it is likely the patient will have aspirated some water, with possible respiratory implications.

Those who have lesions above the C3 level will need lifelong mechanical ventilation. There may be scope for insertion of diaphragmatic pacing later for such patients, dependent on the suitability of the individual (Oo et al 1999).

Potential nursing diagnoses related to respiratory function may include:

- ineffective airway clearance
- ineffective breathing pattern
- high risk of chest infection.

Respiratory assessment

Assessment of the high SCI patient related to the above covers the following points.

- Observation of chest movement for symmetry and expansion, particularly in those with an associated chest injury.
- Monitoring of respiratory rate to assist the nurse in detecting potential respiratory tiring, a rate of 30–35 per minute indicating potential problems.
- Vital capacity monitoring. It would not be unusual for the vital capacity in a newly injured patient to be as low as 1200 ml. This level is acceptable but a decreasing vital capacity later on should alert the nurse that the patient is becoming tired. A drop to 1000 ml will merit the use of positive pressure breathing via a BIRD respirator. A drop to below 800 ml may indicate the need for elective mechanical ventilation, although Tromans et al (1998) suggest that using a biphasic positive airway pressure (BIPAP) system might lower the numbers of those who require this outcome.
- Measuring oxygen saturation through the use of pulse oximetry and serial arterial blood gas analysis via an arterial line are standard interventions for patients with high SCI. These are useful indicators of how tired the patient is becoming and the need for early ventilatory intervention.

- Increased accessory muscle use, with the patient's shoulders rising visibly on inspiration, is another indication that a degree of respiratory distress is being experienced.
- Bilateral auscultation of air entry at the apex and bases should be performed on a 4-hourly basis and more frequently in those who are exhibiting some respiratory deficit, to assist in early detection of a developing chest infection.

Respiratory intervention

Regular positional change will not only minimise the likelihood of tissue viability problems but will assist in reducing mucus stasis. A rigorous programme of chest percussion and clearance on each turn, 2–3 hourly initially, will be instrumental in facilitating a clear chest.

Associated with this is the need for the nurse to perform an assisted cough technique. Patients with cervical injury, resulting in the loss of abdominal and intercostal nerve function, will not be able to expectorate effectively (Dicpinigaitis et al 1999). The technique involves placing the forearm underneath the ribs of the patient and, on an agreed signal, the patient attempts to cough while the nurse pushes the forearm inwards and upwards.

Incentive spirometry has been used to demonstrate that an improvement in respiratory function occurs if an inspiratory muscle-training programme is utilised (Liaw et al 2000, Uijl et al 1999).

Intermittent positive pressure breathing utilising a BIRD respirator is usually prescribed on a 1–2 hourly basis when the vital capacity drops below a litre.

Oxygen should be given in high concentrations in the immediate postinjury stage and continued if respiratory complications exist. Not only is this essential to prevent general systemic hypoxia but it is vital in minimising hypoxia to the injured part of the spinal cord which otherwise could potentially exacerbate ischaemic changes.

CARDIOVASCULAR IMPLICATIONS

In all patients there will be a loss of vasomotor control below the level of injury, resulting in a state of passive vasodilation in the affected vessels. Particular attention should be paid to those patients whose injury is above the T6 level as there will be major sympathetic nervous system disruption, affecting heart rate, and the effects of the vasodilation will be more pronounced.

Additional consideration will be required if the clinical picture is complicated by:

- previous cardiac and cardiovascular medical problems, especially in older patients
- an increased risk of arrhythmias
- anaemia which can develop in some individuals
- the multiply injured patient who has sustained significant blood loss or may do so.

Generally there are four main potential cardiovascular implications that present depending on the level and severity of injury (Glenn & Bergman 1997): hypotension, bradycardia, hypothermia and an increased risk of deep vein thrombosis (DVT) and pulmonary embolus (PE). Each will be briefly described in terms of their neurophysiology, the assessment techniques required and related nursing interventions.

Hypotension

Three factors are involved in the regulation of blood pressure. As well as circulating blood volume and cardiac output, the key issue in the patient with a SCI above T6 level of injury is peripheral resistance. This is normally controlled via the autonomic nervous system which regulates the size of the arterioles through contraction of the smooth muscle within the vessel walls. Unlike most effectors, there is no dual innervation to the peripheral vessels, vasomotor control being controlled solely by the sympathetic nervous system. Since the parasympathetic nervous system has no role to play, if no sympathetic innervation is present following SCI, there is a state of passive vasodilation. Consequently there is a decreased peripheral resistance and therefore a low blood pressure. It would therefore not be unusual for a young patient with cervical SCI to have a normal blood pressure of 90/60 mmHg. Clearly if they have suffered associated injuries involving major blood loss, this will be lower still. In such cases, central venous or preferably pulmonary artery pressure monitoring should occur.

There are two key issues in which nurses should be involved. First, for patients who present with a low blood pressure following trauma, it is common practice for an IV line to be inserted and fluids run through at a high rate, the assumption being that the patient is hypovolaemic. As hypotension in the patient with SCI without major blood loss is due to

changes in the nervous system rather than hypovolaemia, there is a risk of overinfusing the patient. One of the effects of this will be a pulmonary oedema. Bearing in mind the respiratory implications discussed previously, there is the potential to exacerbate any problems being experienced. Although it is often junior medical staff who will order such interventions, the nurse is in a position to question such practice with an appropriate rationale.

The second concern relates to the effects of hypotension on renal function. Some patients, especially when their systolic pressure has dropped below 80 mmHg, may develop problems with renal perfusion. If untreated, acute renal failure will eventually occur. Therefore a standard intervention for those with cervical SCI should be hourly urine volume monitoring, observing for an output of at least 30 ml per hour. Two consecutive recordings below this level will require intervention.

Bradycardia

Neurophysiological control of the heart rate is via the autonomic nervous system. To increase the heart rate and contraction force, sympathetic nervous system impulses travel from the cardio-accelerator centre in the medulla oblongata down the spinal cord and to the heart via the accelerator nerves which run within the T1–5 spinal nerves. To decrease the heart rate and contraction force, parasympathetic impulses travel from the cardio-inhibitory centre in the medulla oblongata via the vagus nerve.

In patients with a cervical SCI, the result will be a loss of sympathetic innervation, so the parasympathetic nervous system will be operating unopposed. As a consequence, such a patient will present with a lower than usual heart rate, 50–60 bpm not being unusual for younger patients. Although this rate is of little concern, two interventions have been reported to exacerbate the bradycardia to a point where it may become dangerous:

1. performing endotracheal suction (Mathias 1976)
2. turning patients onto their left side or prone, for example when patients are on a Stryker frame.

In both cases it appears from anecdotal evidence that this is a particular risk within the first 48 hours post injury, although the exact reason is not fully understood.

Nursing interventions should involve ECG monitoring in the first 48 hours in cervical injury patients or longer if the patient either has a previous history of cardiac problems or is displaying problems within that 48-hour period. Endotracheal suction as described in the respiratory section should be short and frequent rather than longer and occasional periods of suction. The short and frequent approach is therefore indicated from a chest management point of view and to limit the likelihood of exacerbating a bradycardia. It is recommended that intravenous atropine 0.5 µg be available at the patient's bedside for quick emergency administration if a bradycardia is noted during endotracheal suction.

Hypothermia

The state of passive vasodilation experienced through loss of peripheral sympathetic nervous system innervation will result in a reduced ability to control body temperature, as this is the key mechanism by which temperature control is achieved.

Although those with SCI may experience hypothermia, they more commonly experience a variation in body temperature control failure known as poikilothermia. By definition, this is when the patient will have a tendency to mimic the temperature of the environment. Therefore if a patient presents with a pyrexia, the first intervention is to ensure that the environment is not too warm. Other interventions are common-sense nursing care actions such as reducing exposure during care.

DVT and PE risk from loss of muscle activity

Deep vein thrombosis has been described earlier in this book with reference to general orthopaedic nursing. However, it is worth briefly discussing it further with reference to the increased risk following spinal cord injury. Three factors exist which require nursing consideration.

1 The loss of motor function in the lower limbs reduces the effect of muscle activity on venous return.
2 The loss of sensory function causing the loss of the key symptom of pain from both a monitoring and early intervention point of view.
3 The loss of vasomotor control in the lower limbs resulting in a decreased blood flow.

Additionally, there are two other points. First, there is a need to prevent dehydration and the consequent state of hypercoagulability. The second point relates to the need to avoid the insertion of IV cannulae into feet if possible. Although it may seem

kinder to cannulate the patient in an area without sensation, the increased risks of a DVT mean there is a greater likelihood of the venous puncture site becoming the focus for thrombosis formation. Clearly in an emergency situation one may more reasonably disregard this.

Nursing intervention is fivefold and relates to monitoring and prophylaxis.

1 Temperature recording is needed at least twice daily, as an unexplained pyrexia can indicate DVT development.
2 Leg measurements of the calf and thigh circumference. There is some debate in the literature regarding this as a monitoring technique, with particular concerns regarding reliability, but it remains common nursing practice across SCI units due to a loss of the symptom of pain. A unilateral difference of 2 cm appears to be the standard for further diagnostic investigation.
3 Anticoagulation measures.
4 Antiembolic stockings.
5 Lower limb passive movements every time the patient is turned. These consist of foot pumps and 'frog' exercises. Frog exercises are where the nurse supports the leg, bends the knee and brings the foot towards the opposite knee (Fig. 20.7). The leg is then straightened out again. Standard practice appears to be to do this 10–12 times on each leg, every 2–3 hours, usually being performed when the patient is turned. Patients with lumbar injuries should have their frog exercises restricted to a knee flexion of 30% as further flexion may impact on the fracture site.

GASTROINTESTINAL COMPLICATIONS

There are five main gastrointestinal implications which merit discussion (Halm 1990, Weingarden 1992): paralytic ileus, gastric ulceration, vomiting, abdominal injury and management of the neurogenic bowel. Each of these will be discussed with reference to the appropriate related physiology, assessment and nursing intervention.

Paralytic ileus

Available literature suggests that around 60% of patients with complete SCI will develop a paralytic ileus (Halm 1990). The onset is within 48 hours, depending on the injury level. In paraplegic patients the onset tends to be immediately or very soon after

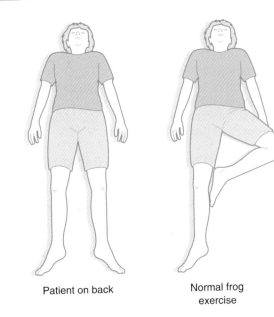
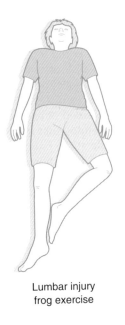

Figure 20.7   Frog exercises.

Patient on back   Normal frog   Lumbar injury
                         exercise   frog exercise

injury. With tetraplegic injuries, an ileus may take up to 48 hours to develop. The exact cause of a paralytic ileus is unknown but is likely to be connected to the sudden disruption of the autonomic nervous system. Apart from the nutritional concerns relating to the need to be nil by mouth, the concern relates to the potential for abdominal distension. If major distension occurs in the cervically injured patient, this may contribute to respiratory problems due to a possible splinting effect on the diaphragm.

Nursing assessment involves the monitoring of bowel sounds. This should be performed in all four quadrants and medical staff informed if concerns exist.

Until fairly recently measuring abdominal girth was common practice in spinal injury units with the aim of detecting any abdominal distension. This practice is no longer recommended due to problems of reliability but there may still be spinal injury units utilising this form of assessment and requesting a baseline measurement from a referring hospital.

The passage of a nasogastric tube should significantly reduce the likelihood of abdominal distension. It is worth reinforcing the need to aspirate the nasogastric tube with particular care, in view of the increased risk of gastric ulceration these patients are subjected to.

As with any patient with a paralytic ileus, concern regarding the nutritional status of the individual is paramount. Anecdotal evidence suggests that the standard in spinal units has been to commence an IV infusion for fluids and to start parenteral feeding if there is a prolonged ileus of greater than 3 days. However, this is not based on any clear clinical evidence. This author would encourage a more aggressive approach with formal assessment, earlier intervention and referral to a dietician and nutritional nurse specialist.

Gastric ulceration

The literature available suggests an incidence of gastric ulceration of 4–5.5% of patients with complete SCI (El Masri et al 1982, Kewalramani 1979). Two main factors contribute to the formation of a gastric ulcer. First, there are changes in circulation resulting from autonomic nervous system disruption. Second, and more significantly, unopposed parasympathetic activity results in increased gastric secretions. The increase in hydrochloric acid production may erode the mucosal lining. Detection can be difficult in those with a complete injury due to the absence of pain, although some authors have described reports of referred right shoulder tip pain in patients with an acute abdomen (Bar-on & Ohry 1995). If perforation is to occur as a direct result, 10–14 days post injury seems the most common timescale. Again detection requires vigilance on the part of the nurse due to the absence of pain. Intervention is through the administration of intravenous ranitidine for the first 48 hours and then orally for up to 12 weeks post injury.

Vomiting

There are still instances of patients with high-level SCI who, following aspiration of vomit, require a period of mechanically assisted ventilation. The scenario seems obvious but merits reinforcing: the patient is lying on their back, head immobilised in skull traction with a reduced ability to cough. Three nursing actions are suggested:

1 keep suction by the bedside of all SCI patients with a cervical injury
2 antiemetics must be prescribed PRN and administered at the slightest report of nausea and while the patient remains on enforced bedrest
3 utilise an emergency turn manoeuvre if the patient starts to vomit when lying on their back. The reader is encouraged to refer to the aforementioned texts (Grundy et al 1995, McCarthy 1998) in relation to moving and handling patients in the emergency situation.

Abdominal injury

Abdominal injury is not uncommon in patients with paraplegia, particularly with injuries to the lumbar vertebrae, and should be suspected in all patients with neurological loss (Berlly & Wilmot 1984). There is an obvious potential problem in early detection due to:

- the absence of pain in patients with sensory loss, although there may be referred right shoulder tip pain
- systemic haemodynamic changes due to a SCI.

For all patients who are suspected of having some abdominal injury, an abdominal X-ray and ultrasound are indicated and in some cases peritoneal lavage.

Bowel management

After manual handling issues, the second most common query from practitioners relates to bowel management. Although the focus of this section is on the acute stage following injury, there is brief reference to long-term management to supply the reader with information to pass on to patients within their care.

During the period of spinal shock, the patient will have no defaecation reflex, commonly termed a flaccid bowel. In this situation the regime is:

- a daily per rectum check until faeces is present in the rectum

- manual evacuation daily, initially on the bed which is
- reduced to alternate days if the results indicate this is satisfactory.

Even in the acute stage the emphasis is on regularity and aiming to establish a pattern of defaecation. This philosophy prevents the likelihood of accidents and continues throughout the rest of the patient's life. It is somewhat unfortunate that, from anecdotal evidence, some nurses and hospitals are reluctant to undertake what is a necessary and relatively simple procedure. Clearly in light of the UK *Code of professional conduct* (NMC 2002) there is no excuse for this not being undertaken.

Broadly speaking, despite slower gastrointestinal transit times following SCI (Krogh et al 2000), the key factor in long-term bowel management will be whether the patient has defaecation reflexes or not. Table 20.4 summarises bowel management for patients with a bowel that is either reflex or flaccid.

URINARY IMPLICATIONS

Here reference will be made to long-term issues as well as the focus on the acute stage of bladder management. The primary aim during the acute stage is protecting renal function and maintaining continence through the use of catheters. Long term, the method of management chosen will take into account the patient's desired lifestyle and ability.

Much has been written on the neurogenic bladder and formal reviews of the literature have been performed (Madersbacher 1999, Shekelle et al 1999).

During the period of spinal shock the bladder is flaccid, occasionally termed areflexic. If the patient is hypotensive the potential for a decreased output is a major concern. A 3 litres per day intake should be strictly adhered to and hourly urine volumes recorded. A urethral catheter, size 14 G with 5 cc balloon, should be used, as this is less likely to cause trauma to the bladder neck. Using larger catheter balloons should be avoided as these may result in long-term problems to the bladder neck.

At this stage it is important to only treat a urinary tract infection if systemic symptoms are present, such as the patient feeling unwell or pyrexic. The reason for this approach is that many patients will be catheter dependent for life, resulting in the risk of regular infections. If every bacteriuria is treated, the range of antibiotics available to treat a serious infection may quickly be reduced as resistance develops.

Table 20.4   Long-term bowel management in SCI

Reflex bowel (injury above L1)	Flaccid bowel (injury below L1)
Reflex arc intact: distension of the rectum will result in contraction of the rectal muscles and opening of the involuntary internal sphincter	No reflex present
No voluntary use of abdominal muscles: massage of the abdomen may initiate an abdominal reflex, which encourages faeces to move into the rectum	Innervation of the intact abdominal muscles (spinal nerves T6–12): this allows the patient to 'bear down' and may be sufficient in time for rectal emptying
Suppositories can be inserted to stimulate reflex: long-term use with glycerine suppositories only, as other varieties can cause damage in the long term	Can be reliant on manual evacuation initially: patient taught to perform this and to check if bowel is empty
Injuries above C6 level: will lack the dexterity and mobility to be independent	Independent in all aspects of bowel care
Gastrocolic reflex may assist in emptying: there is mass movement of faeces into the rectum 20–30 minutes after eating or drinking	Requires the use of aperients in most cases in the early months after injury, e.g. diotyl 100 mg bd, lactulose 10 ml tds

Table 20.5   Options for bladder management

Device	Management
Intermittent catheter	A catheter is passed to empty the bladder and is then removed. Usual regime is 4 catheters per day. A fluid restriction of 2 litres will limit the residual bladder volume to less than 500 ml. Advantages include a positive body image compared to other methods, allows sexual activity and a lower infection risk. A major disadvantage is the hassle factor: remembering to perform catheterisation and limit fluids. It is more difficult for women and patients with high injuries
Indwelling catheter	A permanent catheter. Initially it is urethral but a suprapubic catheter is commonly used long term to allow for urethral access (see autonomic dysreflexia) and improves sexual activity. The predominant advantage is the comparatively low hassle factor. Disadvantages include a higher infection risk, the need for an external collecting device and potential long-term risk of bladder cancer
Condom drainage	Usually involves an operative sphincterotomy, which involves cutting the internal sphincter to allow micturition. Advantages include lower bladder pressures and low hassle factor. The disadvantages are that it is only available to men, it requires an external collecting device, has a potential negative effect on fertility and many patients require repeated sphincterotomy
Tapping	The patient initiates the reflex by tapping over the suprapubic area. Commonly used 20–30 years ago but currently less popular due to the success of other methods and potential safety problems. There may be a risk of high bladder pressures in those patients with detrusor–sphincter dyssynergia, where the sphincter does not open as the bladder muscle contracts
Sacral anterior root nerve stimulator	An electronic implanted device that initiates voiding. It has given variable success to date but is improving with recent technology. There is a risk of infection with the implant

Long-term bladder management may be performed by a number of different methods (Table 20.5) and is determined by a number of factors (Table 20.6). The bladder can be described as reflex or flaccid. Those with a reflex present will be hyperreflexic. This means that a patient who before injury had a reflex initiated when the bladder contained 400–500 ml after injury will have a reflex initiated at reduced volume of 200–250 ml. This has implications relating to maintaining continence for those undertaking an intermittent catheter regime. Hyperreflexia is usually managed through the administration of anticholinergic drugs, for example oxybutynin 2.5–5 mg tds, which delays the volume at which the reflex is initiated. Side effects from such medication include blurred vision and a

Table 20.6   Considerations in the choice of bladder management

Factor	Effects
Gender	The anatomical differences between men and women make some forms of management either impossible, e.g. condom drainage, or difficult, e.g. intermittent catheterisation
Body image	Some patients find the idea of a 'tube' and leg bag abhorrent and prefer a management method that does not have a permanent reminder, e.g. intermittent catheter
Sex	Having a urethral catheter in situ makes intercourse more difficult. For patients who have sphincterotomy, fertility may be affected, as the patient is likely to have a retrograde ejaculation into the bladder, ejaculation being initiated through perineal vibratory stimuli or electro-ejaculation
Urodynamics	A radiological investigation required after spinal shock has subsided to test bladder and sphincter function. Potential medication options and the risk of long-term problems, e.g. from high bladder pressures, can be determined by urodynamics
The 'hassle factor'	With an intermittent regime the individual must restrict fluid to 2 litres per day if a 4-catheter regime is chosen or undertake the procedure more frequently
Level of injury	This will determine whether the individual has a reflex or flaccid bladder and affects the ability to be independent in bladder management

dry mouth; the former may prove problematic for some individuals.

Autonomic dysreflexia

Autonomic dysreflexia is defined as an abnormal sympathetic reflex response to a noxious stimulus and constitutes a medical emergency, as the eventual outcome could be death. It can occur in patients with a cord lesion above T6 level and, using the above definition, may occur after spinal shock has subsided, as it is a reflex response.

The most common noxious stimulus resulting in autonomic dysreflexia is bladder distension (approximately 80%) due to either a blocked indwelling catheter or excessive fluid intake. Bowel distension is the other main cause while other causes include anything that would cause pain or discomfort in someone without a SCI, for example burns, fractures, haemorrhoids, pressure ulcers or even an ingrowing toenail. Prior to describing management of this condition it is worth briefly outlining its pathophysiology, illustrated in Figure 20.8.

The treatment is as follows.

- Sit the patient up.
- Remove tight clothing and any abdominal binder, if the patient is wearing one.
- Check the bladder. If an indwelling catheter is in situ then ensure no kinking is present in the

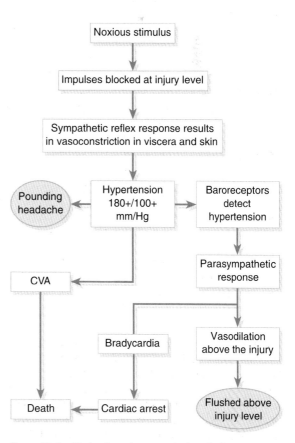

Figure 20.8   Mechanism of autonomic dysreflexia.

tube. If the catheter is blocked, remove it and recatheterise. If the patient is on an intermittent catheter regime then pass a catheter.

- If not resolved then next check bowels: insert a gloved finger into the rectum using lidocaine (lignocaine) as a lubricant. Any faeces must be manually evacuated.
- It will be clear if the problem has resolved, as the patient will immediately have relief from the symptoms outlined in Figure 20.8.
- If the patient remains autonomic, administer nifedipine or GTN sublingually and contact the local spinal injury unit for advice and transfer.

MUSCULOSKELETAL MANAGEMENT

PAIN IN ACUTE SCI

Pain management is discussed in a previous chapter but specific issues are outlined here that relate to the types of pain the patient with acute SCI may experience (Demirel et al 1998, Siddall et al 1997).

Fracture pain. The pain from the fracture site can occur both pre- and postoperatively. Clearly this is one of the key symptoms of someone who has sustained a vertebral injury and responds well to the use of PCA pumps.

Shoulder pain. Musculoskeletal pain in the shoulders of the quadriplegic patient is commonplace. Management is usually with NSAIDs and mechanical methods of pain relief such as TENS. However, this is not always successful. Prevention or minimising any pain experienced is best achieved through good handling techniques of the paralysed upper limb and assisting the patient in the correct performance of active or passive exercises.

Phantom pain. A few patients experience a phantom-like pain similar to the patient who has had an amputation. The aetiology is not clearly understood and although treatment is usually not particularly successful, the nurse may reassure the patient that this is normally fairly short-lived.

Hypersensitivity. Some patients, particularly those with incomplete injuries, can develop a quite distressing hypersensitivity around the injury site. Again the nurse may reassure the patient that this is usually of short duration and can also minimise the distress caused through ensuring that if the patient is touched, even by sheets and blankets, a firm rather than light touch is used.

HANDLING THE PARALYSED LIMB

Correct handling of the paralysed limb is essential for three main reasons:

1 maintaining joint mobility
2 minimising the risk of problematic spasticity through overextension of the joint
3 minimising the risk of musculoskeletal pain, particularly in the shoulder joint.

It is not within the remit of this chapter to discuss issues surrounding splinting and caring for the paralysed hand. It is sufficient to point out that the hand must also be taken through its normal range of movement as part of a passive exercise programme. The occupational therapist should prescribe any splints used. If splints are required, the nurse should check the area around the splint regularly and carefully to determine any potential or actual problems with skin integrity.

SKIN CARE

A full skin check, at least every 3 hours, of all the bony prominences is essential for those with neurological impairment. Their position should be changed utilising the left and right sides and the back. Any impairment of skin integrity should be recorded, monitored and the turning regime altered to avoid placing the patient on that surface until the problem is resolved.

There are specific implications for the patient in relation to skin care.

- Loss of sensation causes a decreased awareness of pressure and temperature changes that potentially cause damage.
- The loss of motor function and, in the acute stage of care, a period of enforced immobility result in a decreased ability to change position to relieve pressure.
- Changes in circulation will decrease the tolerance of the skin to pressure and there can be changes in the skin's collagen quality in the long term.
- Finally there are psychological effects of not being able to feel touch.

The nursing goals of skin care relate to the need to:

- perform skin checks on vulnerable areas on a regular basis
- assist the patient to alter position using the manual handling techniques described earlier.

Anyone touching a patient during nursing procedures, or relatives when they visit, should ensure the touch is on an area of intact sensation.

PSYCHOLOGICAL IMPLICATIONS

SENSORY DEPRIVATION

The effects of sensory deprivation are very individual in nature but the patient may exhibit one or more of the following signs:

● confusion
● restlessness
● decreased concentration
● hallucinations.

The mechanisms causing these are not fully understood but are thought to relate to the level of sensory input received in the reticular activating system above the midbrain. It appears that a certain level of stimulus is required for this complex part of the brain to operate. If there is an insufficient sensory stimulus, then distorted images are obtained from the cerebral cortex, resulting ultimately in the individual believing or behaving according to another stimulus.

Sensory deprivation is far from being a spinal injury-specific issue and may affect anyone within a critical care or acute environment. However, the effect of SCI on all the senses may contribute to this being a common situation (Crossman 1996). The following outlines, for each sense, the effect of a SCI and potential interventions that may limit the likelihood of contributing to a sensory deprivation.

SMELL

Secretions within the respiratory tract are increased due to autonomic disruption and the loss of sympathetic inhibition of secretion production. The nose is likely to become blocked: Guttman's nose. The remedy is quite simply administration of ephedrine nasal drops.

SIGHT

Sight is restricted for cervical injury patients when the head is immobilised in skull traction. The average hospital ward ceiling gives little in the way of visual entertainment. The primary way to improve visual stimulus is by nursing the patient on their side rather than supine. When they are supine, the judicious use of mirrors may enable the patient to see events going on around the bed and ward. The provision of reading frames and ensuring staff and visitors approach the patient from the side on which they are lying also facilitate visual stimuli.

HEARING

Hearing is affected by an alteration in the level of familiar stimuli to which new patients may be subjected, particularly those on skull traction. Explanations of unfamiliar sounds and the measures described above in reference to sight will improve the situation.

TOUCH

Many authors have written about the importance of touch in a health context. A patient with a high complete injury will have a greater touch stimuli deficit. Common sense indicates the need to touch a patient in an area they can feel. Relatives and partners may require gentle reminders that if a patient is unable to feel a hand being held, far more benefit for both parties will be gained from placing a hand on, for example, the shoulder.

TASTE

The alteration in the level of taste stimuli is usually related to appetite. The hospital food may be less palatable than the individual's normal diet, the patient may be feeling generally unwell or there can be restrictions imposed by trying to eat during the period of enforced bedrest. Simple measures can improve the situation such as altering the patient's turning times so they are on their side to eat rather than lying flat. Relatives may bring in food the patient enjoys, certainly in early dependent stages when the patient cannot order or prepare their own food.

EFFECTS ON SEXUALITY

It is common for the question after 'Am I going to walk again?' to be one related to sexual function. This is particularly the case with younger male patients, who form a significant proportion of those injured.

From a general sexuality perspective the patient may have concerns regarding their attractiveness to either their current or prospective partner. Perceptions of gender roles may be affected and concerns relating to social roles within peer or family groups, for example their role as a parent or provider.

Behaviourally, for both genders, a change in sexual activities may be required due to the loss of motor function, for instance a change of sexual positions. The loss of sensory function limits the ability to feel a caress, genital sensation will often be absent and orgasm may not be possible. However, previous erogenous zones may have exaggerated sensation and some people with SCI have described orgasm-like sensations from stimulation of these. Additionally bladder and bowel issues may need a degree of pre-planning. It is the lack of spontaneity which appears to be a major loss reported by patients of both genders.

For women, although fertility will not be affected, additional lubrication may be required.

In men both erection and ejaculation are often affected. For men with erectile disruption vacuum devices, intercavernosal injections (for example, Cavijet) or rings placed around a reflex erection for those with upper motor neuron lesions may be possibilities to overcome the disability. Ejaculation is a more difficult situation to deal with. Those who wish to father children following injury must rely on vibratory stimuli around the perineal area or, more commonly, an electro-ejaculation procedure in a hospital situation. In either case IVF will be required.

Despite the above, like most impairments resulting from SCI, it is worth stressing to the patient that although there will be changes, there are means by which to overcome these and a fulfilling sexual relationship remains an undoubted possibility.

BREAKING BAD NEWS

SCI is a life-changing event for the individual and their family with the prognosis for recovery generally being poor. Nurses are often placed in the position of being the bearers of such bad news or reinforcing a prognosis given by medical staff (Dewar 2000). Talking to patients can be stressful for practitioners as well as the patient and their family. The following are a few key pieces of advice for these situations.

- Be honest.
- Ensure all the facts are known and available before breaking the news to the patient.

Box 20.3 UK and Ireland spinal injury units	
Belfast	Salisbury
Cardiff	Sheffield
Dunlaoghaire	Southport
Glasgow	Stanmore
Hexham	Stoke Mandeville
Middlesbrough	Wakefield
Oswestry	

- Document what the patient is told to facilitate consistency, not only amongst all nursing staff but also amongst other members of the team. Failure to do this can result in the patient believing the scenario they view as 'best'.
- It is always worth stressing the worst scenario as the most likely final picture. Unless the patient is told that any changes are likely to be small and that full recovery will not occur, they appear often to cling to unrealistic hopes that they may walk or feel again. As rehabilitation of such individuals will only be possible if they begin to adjust to their new health status, such beliefs of significant recovery will prove a huge barrier to the patient taking on information relating to living with the consequences of SCI.

ORGANISATION OF SCI SERVICES

There are 13 specialist spinal injury units within the UK and Ireland (Box 20.3). With the exception of the three units in Cardiff, Dublin and Belfast, all provide an integrated service. Through this system it is possible to manage patients during the initial acute stage of injury, with hospital-based rehabilitation and it provides continuity through the support of community professionals when the patient returns to their home environment.

This system has proven popular internationally and is adopted by the majority of European units and in Australia. There are differences within the USA where patients are managed in acute units and then transferred to rehabilitation units in different hospitals. The three UK and Irish exceptions indicated above also follow this model.

The efficacy of these approaches has not been fully investigated, although the first integrated model seems to possess certain advantages.

- Management of SCI in this manner provides a continuum of care, allowing a client-centred approach to be adopted with rehabilitation and acute interventions occurring simultaneously. Additionally the interrelationship and effect of interventions on others is more easily measured.

• A specialist unit provides an aggregation of professional expertise and allows focused education and research. Outcomes are better in specialist spinal injury units from the health, functional and social perspectives (Smith 2002).

• The peer support provided by other patients in the same position is something healthcare professionals can never provide. From the anecdotal evidence of patients and a focus group project undertaken by this author (Smith 1996), it appears to be a vital part of the emotional rehabilitation of the patient. This seems particularly to be the case when patients further along the process of rehabilitation interact with the more acute patient.

REFERRAL OF PATIENTS

Early referral to spinal injury units is the optimum course of action from the perspective of the patient with neurological impairment. It is evident that the health, functional and social outcomes are better when the patient is nursed in a specialist spinal injury unit rather than on a general rehabilitation area (Smith 2002).

An early referral will ideally facilitate the early transfer of the patient to the spinal unit and consequently their access to specialist services. For patients unable to be transferred immediately, the specialist centre can be used as a resource by the referring hospital. Ideally, referral should be done as soon as a patient with a cord injury has been admitted to an accident and emergency department. When a referral is made, the respective unit will require a complete clinical picture. The infor-

> **Box 20.4 Referral information**
>
> • Demographic information regarding the patient
> • Date, time and mechanism of injury
> • Type of vertebral column injury
> • Neurological status
> • Respiratory function
> • Cardiovascular function
> • Gastrointestinal function including bowels
> • Bladder function
> • Skin condition
> • MRSA status
> • Medical interventions since injury, including medication
> • Previous medical history, including mental health if appropriate
> • Social situation

mation required mirrors the assessment issues covered in this chapter; these are listed in Box 20.4.

CONCLUSION

In summary, a spinal cord injury is a multisystem, life-changing event requiring a multitude of clinical skills to ensure that the objectives of acute management and care of these patients are met. Ideally this is achieved within an integrated specialist spinal injuries unit. In reality it is nurses within acute settings in general hospitals who are first to be involved in meeting some of the patient needs outlined in this chapter. For readers in this position at any stage within their nursing career, the best advice one could give is to utilise the local specialist centre to gain appropriate and maximum support until the patient is able to be transferred.

References

American Spinal Injury Association (ASIA) 2001 Standards for neurological and functional classification of spinal cord injury. Available online at: www.asia-spinalinjury.org/publications/2001_Classif_worksheet.pdf

Bar-on Z, Ohry A 1995 The acute abdomen in spinal cord injury individuals. Paraplegia 33(12): 704–706

Berlly MH, Wilmot CB 1984 Acute abdominal emergencies during the first four weeks after spinal cord injury. Archives of Physical Medicine and Rehabilitation 65(11): 687–690

Bracken MB, Shepard MJ, Collins WF et al 1990 A randomised controlled trial of methylprednisolone or naloxone in the treatment of acute spinal cord injury. New England Journal of Medicine 322: 1405–1411

Bracken MB, Shepard MJ, Holford TR 1997 Administration of methylprednisolone for 24 or 48 hours or tirilazad mesylate for 48 hours in the treatment of acute spinal cord injury. Results of the Third National Acute Spinal Cord Injury Trial. Journal of the American Medical Association 277: 1597–1604

Crossman MW 1996 Sensory deprivation in spinal cord injury: an essay. Spinal Cord 34(10): 573–577

Demirel G, Yllmaz H, Gencosmanoglu B et al 1998 Pain following spinal cord injury. Spinal Cord 36(1): 25–28

De Vivo MJ, Krause JS, Lammertse DP 1999 Recent mortality trends among persons with spinal cord injury. Journal of Spinal Cord Medicine 22(1): 35

Dewar A 2000 Nurses' experiences in giving bad news to patients with spinal cord injuries. Journal of Neuroscience Nursing 32(6): 324–330

Dicpinigaitis PV, Grimm DR, Lesser M 1999 Cough reflex sensitivity in subjects with cervical spinal cord injury. American Journal of Respiratory and Critical Care Medicine 159(5 Pt 1): 1660–1662

El Masri WE, Cochrane P, Silver JR 1982 Gastrointestinal bleeding in patients with acute spinal injuries. Injury 14(2): 162–167

Glenn MB, Bergman SB 1997 Cardiovascular changes following spinal cord injury. Topics in Spinal Cord Injury Rehabilitation 2(4): 47–53

Go BK, De Vivo MJ, Richards JS 1995 The epidemiology of spinal cord injury. In: Stover SL, DeLisa JA, Whiteneck GG (eds) Spinal cord injury: clinical outcomes from the model systems. Aspen Publishers, Gaithersburg, Maryland

Grundy D, Swain A, Russell J 1995 ABC of spinal cord injury. BMJ Publications, London

Halm MA 1990 Elimination concerns with acute spinal cord trauma. Assessment and nursing interventions. Critical Care Nursing Clinics of North America 2(3): 385–398

Jackson AB, Groomes TE 1994 Incidence of respiratory complications following spinal cord injury. Archives of Physical Medicine and Rehabilitation 74(11): 1199–1205

Kewalramani LS 1979 Neurogenic gastroduodenal ulceration and bleeding associated with spinal cord injuries. Journal of Trauma 19(4): 259–265

Ko HY, Ditunno JF Jr, Graziani V, Little JW 1999 The pattern of reflex recovery during spinal shock. Spinal Cord 37(6): 402–409

Krogh K, Mosdal C, Laurberg S 2000 Gastrointestinal and segmental colonic transit times in patients with acute and chronic spinal cord lesions. Spinal Cord 38(10): 615–621

Liang HW, Wang YH, Wang TG et al 1996 Clinical experience in rehabilitation of spinal cord injury associated with schizophrenia. Archives of Physical Medicine and Rehabilitation 77(3): 283–286

Liaw MY, Lin MC, Cheng PT et al 2000 Resistive inspiratory muscle training: its effectiveness in patients with acute complete cervical cord injury. Archives of Physical Medicine and Rehabilitation 81(6): 752–756

Madersbacher HG 1999 Neurogenic bladder dysfunction. Current Opinions in Urology 9(4): 303–307

Mathias CJ 1976 Bradycardia and cardiac arrest during tracheal suction mechanisms in tetraplegic patients. European Journal of Intensive Care Medicine 2(4): 147–156

McCarthy L 1998 Safe handling of patients on cervical traction. Nursing Times 94(14): 57–59

Nursing and Midwifery Council (NMC) 2002 Code of professional conduct. Nursing and Midwifery Council, London

O'Connor P 2002 Incidence and patterns of spinal cord injury in Australia. Accident Analysis and Prevention 34(4): 405–415

Oo T, Watt JW, Soni BM et al 1999 Delayed diaphragm recovery in 12 patients after high cervical spinal cord injury. A retrospective review of the diaphragm status of 107 patients ventilated after acute spinal cord injury. Spinal Cord 37(2): 117–122

Palastanga N, Field D, Soames R 1998 Anatomy and human movement: structure and function, 3rd edn. Butterworth Heinemann, London

Shekelle PG, Morton SC, Clark KA et al 1999 Systematic review of risk factors for urinary tract infection in adults with spinal cord dysfunction. Journal of Spinal Cord Medicine 22(4): 258–272

Siddall PJ, Taylor DA, Cousins MJ 1997 Classifications of pain in spinal cord injury. Spinal Cord 35(2): 69–75

Smith MJ 1996 Presentation. Conference of the American Association of SCI Nurses

Smith MJ 2002 Efficacy of specialist versus non-specialist management of spinal cord injury. Spinal Cord 40(1): 10–16

Thibodeau GA, Paton KT 1999 Anatomy and physiology, 4th edn. Mosby, St Louis

Tromans AM, Mecci M, Barrett FH et al 1998 The use of the BIPAP biphasic positive airway pressure system in acute spinal cord injury. Spinal Cord 36(7): 481–484

Uijl SG, Houtman S, Folgering HT et al 1999 Training of the respiratory muscles in individuals with tetraplegia. Spinal Cord 37(8): 575–579

Weingarden SI 1992 The gastrointestinal system and spinal cord injury. Physical Medicine and Rehabilitation Clinics of North America 3(4): 765–781

Zedjlik C 1992 Management of spinal cord injury. Jones and Bartlett, New York

Chapter 21

Care of patients with upper limb injuries and conditions

Brian Lucas

INTRODUCTION

Upper limb injuries and chronic conditions can have profound effects on patients' lives, potentially affecting many of their activities. It is essential that orthopaedic nurses have an understanding of all aspects of care for patients with injuries to, or conditions of, the upper limb.

This chapter discusses the principles of assessment, diagnosis and care of patients with upper limb problems, together with the common conditions and injuries seen in practice. Brachial plexus injuries and nerve conditions of the hand such as carpal tunnel syndrome and repetitive strain injuries are addressed in other chapters.

The focus of this chapter is the nursing care and interventions that aim for restoration of function and mobility. The care of a patient with an upper limb condition or injury requires an interprofessional approach. Apart from medical interventions, the roles of the physiotherapist and the occupational therapist are of particular importance in the initial assessment, treatment and rehabilitation stages of care. The orthopaedic nurse plays a vital role in the coordination of care for patients with upper limb problems; the importance of this coordination or 'mediator' role (Santy 2001) should not be underestimated.

Although many patients with chronic upper limb problems are not admitted to an acute orthopaedic ward, they still need to have access to skilled nursing and other therapy care (Lucas 2002). Similarly, many patients with upper limb injuries are cared for through a primary care, fracture clinic or outpatient setting. Orthopaedic nurses need to work with their nursing colleagues in these areas to share their expert orthopaedic nursing knowledge.

The impact on a patient's life of an upper limb condition or injury can be substantial; they may be able to walk but still have significant difficulties with many other activities of life. The patient's motivation and involvement in all aspects of their care are vital if treatment is to be successful.

PATIENT ASSESSMENT

Assessment of the patient with an upper limb injury or condition needs to encompass a holistic approach with a particular focus on mobility. The Balcombe model of orthopaedic care (1994) is used as the framework for discussing the assessment and planning of care, with the focus on aspects of particular relevance to patients with an upper limb condition or injury.

Assessment needs to begin as soon as possible; this means when a patient is first listed for elective surgery or, for those with traumatic injuries, as soon as the patient's condition allows.

ASSESSMENT OF MOVEMENT

The joints of the upper limb are more complex in their anatomy and physiology than comparable joints in the lower limb. Active and passive movements of the affected limb need to be assessed both as an indication of the severity of the problem and as a baseline on which to measure any improvement following treatment. The medical staff, a physiotherapist or a nurse practitioner will carry out an assessment of the range of movement. However, all orthopaedic nurses need to understand the normal range of joint movements so they can detect abnormalities.

The neurological status of the affected limb and any muscle weakness are assessed in comparison to the normal or unaffected limb. As Metter et al (1997) have shown, both women and men over 40 years experience strength and power decline in the upper extremities, whether or not they have underlying musculoskeletal problems. This is accentuated in those who have a chronic or acute upper limb disease or injury. Patients with chronic conditions such as osteoarthritis may have both upper and lower limbs affected, which may impact on, for example, their ability to use walking aids; this needs to be taken into consideration when assessing patients.

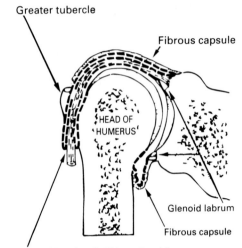

Figure 21.1   Anatomy of the shoulder. (From Smith et al 1983.)

The shoulder complex

The shoulder complex consists of four joints.

- The glenohumeral joint is a synovial ball and socket joint between the head of the humerus and the glenoid of the scapula (Fig. 21.1). The joint has a wide range of movement, with stability provided by a group of muscles that cross the joint: the rotator cuff.
- The sternoclavicular joint is a synovial modified saddle joint between the sternum and clavicle.
- The acromioclavicular joint is a small synovial plane joint between the acromion and the clavicle. This allows the acromion to glide over the lateral end of the clavicle, allowing the glenoid fossa to face the glenoid head continually.
- The scapulothoracic joint is not a true joint. The scapula has no bony or ligamentous attachments to the thorax; instead they are separated by the subscapularis and serratus anterior muscles with the scapula suspended by its muscular attachments.

The movements allowed at the above joints make the shoulder capable of many complex movements. Only the most common are shown in Box 21.1.

In injuries or conditions affecting the shoulder, it is important the muscles are assessed for strength; this allows a baseline to be established. The physiotherapist or nurse practitioner usually carries this out. The strength is measured on isometric contraction against manual resistance, being recorded as

Box 21.1   Movements of the shoulder joint

Starting with the arm straight at the side and keeping the arm straight:

- 180° of forward flexion (takes arm forward and up),
- 60° of backward extension (takes arm back and up),
- 180° of lateral abduction (takes arm out to the side),
- 50–75° of medial adduction (takes arm across the chest)

Starting with upper arm at the side of the body and elbow flexed to 90°:

- internal rotation 90° (to place arm across the chest),
- external rotation 60–90° (to position lower arm out to the side)

Starting with arm held straight out to the side at shoulder height:

- horizontal extension (adduction) through horizontal flexion (abduction), a range of 130° (takes arm from side to in front of the body)

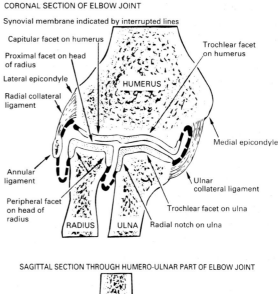

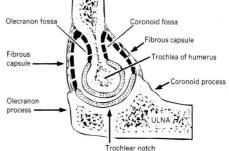

Figure 21.2   Anatomy of the elbow joint. (From Smith et al 1983.)

normal, weak or very weak. A Constant score (Constant & Murley 1987) may also be recorded; this assesses the patient's pain, range of movement, function and power and is repeated at intervals post treatment to monitor the patient's progress.

The elbow

The elbow is a synovial hinge joint. The radial head articulates with the lateral humerus at the capitulum while the olecranon process of the ulna articulates with the trochlea of the medial humerus (Fig. 21.2). The joint space includes the superior radioulnar joint, which allows pronation and supination of the forearm. Lateral and medial ligaments strengthen the joint capsule, allowing flexion and extension. Box 21.2 demonstrates the normal range of movements possible at the elbow joint.

The wrist

The wrist is a synovial ellipsoid joint between the proximal ends of the scaphoid, lunate and triquetral bones and the distal end of the radius (Fig. 21.3). The ulna is separated from the joint cavity by a disc of fibrocartilage, which articulates with the carpal

Box 21.2   Movements at the elbow joint

Movements taken from position of arm in extension (elbow straight):

- hyperextension of 10–15°
- flexion of 140–150°
- supination of the forearm 90°
- pronation of the forearm 90°

bones. It also separates the inferior radioulnar joint from the wrist joint. For the normal range of movements, see Box 21.3.

The hand and fingers

Synovial joints are present between the carpal bones, between the carpal and metacarpal bones, the metacarpal bones and the proximal phalanges

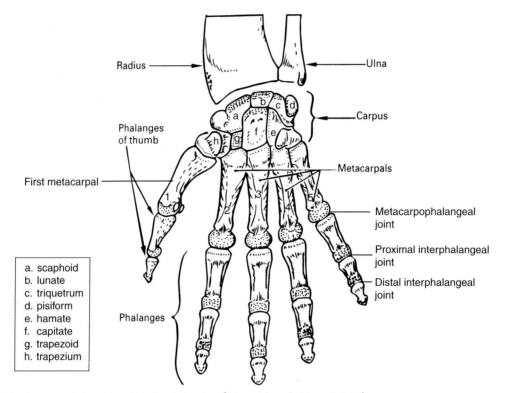

Figure 21.3   Anatomy of the wrist and hand, anterior view. (Adapted from Smith et al 1983.)

Box 21.3   Movements at the wrist joint

Ulnar flexion (adduction) 35°
Radial flexion (abduction) 20°
Flexion 75°
Hyperextension 75°

Box 21.4   Movements of the fingers

Adduction taken as 0° (fingers straight and closed together)
Abduction 20–30° (fingers straight but separated)
Extension (starting with fingers straight):

- metacarpophalangeal joint 30–45°
- proximal interphalangeal joint 0°
- distal interphalangeal joint 20°

Flexion (making a fist):

- metacarpophalangeal joint 85°
- proximal interphalangeal joint 100–115°
- distal interphalangeal joint 80–90°

---

and between the phalanges (Fig. 21.3). The muscles in the forearm provide the powerful movements of these joints. Like the shoulder, the fingers are capable of many complex movements; the most common are shown in Box 21.4.

ASPIRATIONS FOR HEALTH

Central to the model for orthopaedic nursing is the patient's desired state of health. With upper limb injuries or conditions it is important to ascertain what benefits the patient feels they will gain and to assess whether these are achievable from their orthopaedic treatment and care. A good knowledge of what is realistic is vital to provide effective care for patients with upper limb problems; for example,

a professional pianist may have very different aspirations for health following an elbow fracture from those of an office manager.

HOME ENVIRONMENT

Upper limb conditions and injuries may have a profound effect on the patient's ability to carry out physical activities important to their lifestyle. Those with a chronic condition, such as a rotator cuff tear, may have adapted their lifestyle to incorporate reduced mobility. Osteoarthritis most commonly affects the joints of the hand and impairs the ability to carry out everyday tasks (Stamm et al 2002).

The home environment encompasses important areas of life such as the patient's financial position, their social relations, work and hobbies. If the patient is the carer for a friend or relative, arrangements are needed to ensure the friend or relative is cared for; such care may need to be continued when the patient is discharged from hospital if they have limited upper limb mobility following surgery. Financial problems can be ongoing for patients with a chronic condition if they have been unable to work for many months or years, while a sudden financial crisis can arise for patients suffering traumatic injury.

Activities such as driving or using public transport may be difficult or impossible with a chronic shoulder condition or following trauma and this can affect a patient's ability to maintain their social network.

DIET

The ability to maintain an adequate diet may be impaired. Function deteriorates with age and even in the healthy older person, there is a decrease in manual dexterity, strength and the performance of functional tasks (Rahman et al 2002).

With a chronic disease such as osteoarthritis or an acute injury, this function will deteriorate further. Reduced or painful mobility of the shoulder, elbow, hand or fingers may affect a person's ability to obtain food (carry shopping), prepare food (cut vegetables, open cans), cook food (carry food to oven, turn gas or electricity on) or eat (carry food from oven to table or use cutlery). For patients with a traumatic injury requiring hospital admission or those who have had surgical treatment, the ability to eat food is often impaired in hospital.

Assessment of the ability to maintain adequate nutrition on discharge is needed.

HYGIENE

Patients may find it difficult to maintain their hygiene to a level acceptable to themselves. They may not be able to get in and out of the bath, turn taps on and off, wash all areas of the body or dry themselves adequately. Linked to this, they may find it difficult to dress and undress. Observing a patient performing these tasks is a good assessment method for identifying their independence status. The ability to wash clothes can be affected also.

MENTAL STATE, BEHAVIOUR AND SELF-CONCEPT

As well as ascertaining the patient's desired health state, the nurse needs to assess their mental state to establish if the injury or condition has affected them in terms of anxiety, depression or grief from reduced or lost function.

Body image is important to consider in many upper limb conditions, such as the hand joint deformities in rheumatoid arthritis or muscle wasting in rotator cuff disorders. These can affect a patient's self-concept, their sexuality and their interaction with others. Price (1990) suggests that body image has three components:

1 body ideal: a mental picture of how the body should look
2 body presentation: how the body is arranged, adjusted or presented to others
3 body reality: the body as it really is, affected by ageing, illness and environment.

The nurse needs to assess what the patient feels the limb should look like, how they present the limb, for example whether a patient hides their hands because of the rheumatoid changes, or how the injury, condition or treatment will affect how the arm appears. Within Price's (1990) model, assessment is also made of the patient's:

● coping style: their habitual or preferred ways of responding to change
● social support network: people who provide psychological and practical support.

Interaction with others is impaired if the dominant arm or hand is affected, thus restricting motor activities, such as the ability to write or use a computer easily. The effect is compounded if the patient has a sensory impairment from loss of sight or hearing, which leads them to rely on using their hands as an important source of communication.

PAIN

Patients with chronic and acute upper limb conditions or injuries may have pain that restricts their ability to carry out activities of living. Pain can also make it difficult for them to maintain adequate levels of sleep. Assessment of the type and location of pain is needed, using both a general pain score and a specific one, such as the pain element of the Constant score for shoulder problems (Constant & Murley 1987).

BREATHING

Trauma to the upper limb may accompany rib trauma, which causes difficulties in breathing. Patients with chronic or acute upper limb conditions who require medication for chronic respiratory disease may find they have difficulties in managing their disease because of loss of dexterity in opening medicine bottles or difficulties in using inhalers.

SLEEP

Typically, sleep is disturbed by pain or the loss of movement, making it difficult to attain and maintain a comfortable position in bed. The ability to maintain a comfortable body temperature whilst in bed might be lost if a patient cannot easily put on or remove bedding.

NURSING DIAGNOSES AND CARE

Although each patient is an individual and their treatment and nursing care will be unique, there are certain principles of care that apply to many. The general aspects of care and the specific considerations for particular upper limb injuries and conditions are discussed here. The nursing diagnoses are adapted from the North American Nursing Diagnosis Association classification (NANDA 2001).

IMPAIRED PHYSICAL MOBILITY: THERAPEUTIC RESTRICTION

A patient's physical mobility can be impaired by the injury or condition itself or by treatment, especially in the postoperative phase. Patients often need to have the limb immobilised or elevated to promote healing or rest. The focus here is on the methods of immobilising the arm; general issues surrounding restrictions of movement are discussed in Chapter 6.

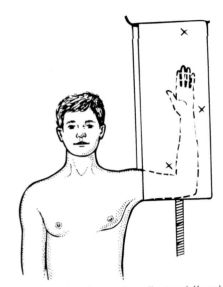

Figure 21.4 Elevation of arm using roller towel. X marks position of safety pins.

The goal of care is to ensure immobilisation is carried out safely and effectively.

Application of a roller towel

Arm elevation is achieved using a foam sling such as the Bradford sling, a roller towel or a pillowcase. Figure 21.4 demonstrates the use of a roller towel to elevate the arm, keeping the shoulder in abduction and achieving a high elevation of the hand. The patient should sit towards the appropriate side of the bed, with the upper arm supported horizontally. An adjustable dripstand supports the towel, with the bed height adjusted accordingly. A pillow placed under the upper arm gives added support, reducing pressure on the ulnar nerve at the elbow.

Broad arm sling

This sling is used to support an injured hand or arm, spreading the weight evenly across the neck and shoulders. The elbow is flexed at 90° and supported across the chest (Fig. 21.5). When applying the sling, the patient should be standing if possible and supporting their affected hand (Wheeler 1994). The sling is placed across the chest with the 90° angle of the triangle pointing towards the elbow and the long edge of the sling towards the unaffected arm. The affected arm is placed across the patient's chest, on top of the sling, with the elbow flexed at 90°. The sling is then folded up over the arm and tied in a reef knot, a strong weight-bearing knot, on the same side

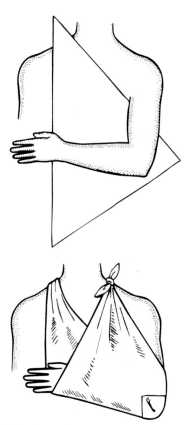

Figure 21.5 Broad arm sling.

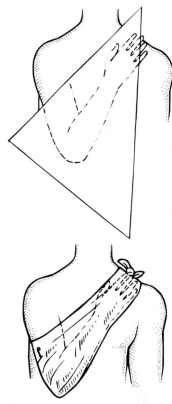

Figure 21.6 High arm sling.

of the neck as the affected arm; this avoids pressure on the spine. The elbow edges are then tucked in and held in place with a safety pin.

The hand must be supported in the sling to prevent oedema; this also reduces the risk of pressure and rubbing at the wrist (Wheeler 1994).

The patient must be educated about the importance of maintaining the range of movement of the upper arm joints, depending on the nature of the injury or condition.

High arm sling

A high arm sling (Fig. 21.6) is used to reduce oedema postoperatively or post injury. To apply the sling, the patient should be standing with the fingers of the affected arm touching the shoulder of the other arm. The sling is placed as before but on top of the arm. The sling is then folded below the arm, then upwards underneath the arm to encase it, then tied behind the patient's shoulder with a reef knot (Wheeler 1994). Finally the corner at the elbow is tucked in and secured with a safety pin.

Collar and cuff

This is often used to support an upper limb and can be applied in a variety of ways (Fig. 21.7). It must not constrict the limb and the patient needs to be taught how to remove and reapply it.

Abduction wedge

This method of immobilisation allows the patient to be ambulant whilst holding the arm in a fixed position. It is ideal for patients who require immobilisation of the upper limb for a length of time, for example following rotator cuff repair (Fig. 21.8).

INCREASING PHYSICAL MOBILITY

Whilst physical mobility can be restricted immediately postoperatively, for the majority of patients increased mobility of the upper limb is required as part of the treatment. The physiotherapist, occupational therapist and nursing staff are involved in

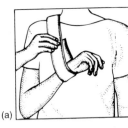
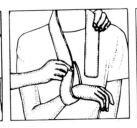
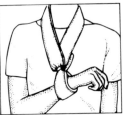

1. Take approx. 75 cm of Collar 'n' Cuff and place arm in required position.

2. Support the wrist with one end of the Collar 'n' Cuff, the other end being taken round the neck.

3. Bring the two ends together and fasten with tie provided, ensuring sufficient room for the hand to be withdrawn from the Collar 'n' Cuff.

  Excess tie can be cut off and cut edge tucked into the Collar 'n' Cuff to make a neat finish.

(a)

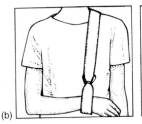
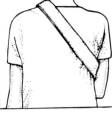
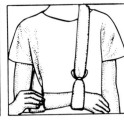
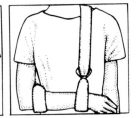

(b)

1. To support an arm in a balanced position, often in conjunction with forearm casts, take approx. 1.5 m of Collar 'n' Cuff and tie one end around the wrist.

2. Take the Collar 'n' Cuff around the neck and over the opposite shoulder, bringing it across the back of the patient.

3. Bring the loose end through, and over the arm at the elbow.

4. Secure and tie behind, again ensuring there is sufficient room for the arm to be removed from the Collar 'n' Cuff.

Figure 21.7 Collar and cuff. (a) To fit as a traditional sling. (b) To support the arm in a balanced position. (From Seton & Co. with permission.)

Nursing actions

Orthopaedic nurses play an important part in reinforcing the advice given by other health professionals with regard to increasing physical mobility, the 'guide' role in Santy's work (Santy 2001). In some centres, orthopaedic nurse practitioners have taken on the primary role of teaching patients how to increase physical mobility of the upper limb.

For chronic conditions such as osteoarthritis, attention to issues such as the type of exercise being undertaken is essential, as daily low-load resistance exercises will improve the muscle endurance and the contraction velocity.

Following surgery patients can require assistance to perform their exercises. Rehabilitation exercises are divided into three categories (Wheeler 1994).

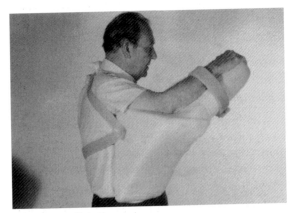

Figure 21.8 Abduction wedge.

treating muscle disuse arising from chronic upper limb conditions or trauma. The goals of care are decided in consultation with the medical and physiotherapy staff, often being expressed in terms of measurable ranges of movement.

1 Passive movements aim to help maintain the patient's range of joint movements and prevent the development of adhesions or soft tissue contractures,

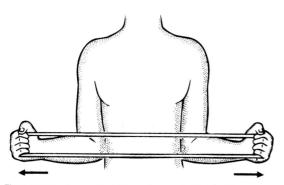

Figure 21.9   External rotation using graded latex strip.

whilst at the same time preventing excessive strain on repaired muscles postoperatively. This is particularly important after operations such as total shoulder replacement and rotator cuff repairs.

2 Active assisted movements are designed to maintain and increase movement, often with the assistance of the good hand, a pulley or a stick.

3 Strengthening exercises are active exercises designed to strengthen the muscles. They are usually commenced when any soft tissue damage has healed, 4–6 weeks following surgery or used by patients with a chronic upper limb disorder. They are resisted exercises, using equipment such as a latex strip (Fig. 21.9).

Evidence for the effectiveness of formal therapy in increasing function is variable. With reference to physical exercise after distal radial fractures, Handoll et al (2002a) found that there was only weak evidence of better short-term hand function in patients given physiotherapy than in those given instructions for home exercises to be performed unaided. For more complex surgery or injuries, however, patients need clear guidance and instructions about the correct exercises to undertake.

It is important to ensure the patient has had sufficient analgesia prior to exercising the upper limb, so that maximum benefit can be gained from the exercise session.

RISK OF PERIPHERAL NEUROVASCULAR DYSFUNCTION

Patients with traumatic injuries to their upper limb and those having upper limb surgery are at risk of disruption to the circulation, sensation or movement in part of the arm. It is vital orthopaedic nurses understand the importance and correct assessment of neurovascular status.

The aim of nursing care is to reduce the risk of neurovascular changes, detect any early disruption by neurovascular observations (see Chapter 6) and prevent any deterioration, especially by reducing the risk from arm elevation.

ACUTE AND CHRONIC PAIN

Pain may be chronic, as with osteoarthritis, or acute following a fracture or soft tissue injury. The aim of care is for the patient to indicate that their pain is controlled to a level acceptable to them.

Nursing actions

Assessment and interventions for pain relief generally are discussed in Chapter 7. Specific management of upper limb pain is complex and often there is insufficient evidence to justify the use of one intervention over another. Green et al (2002a), in their Cochrane Review of interventions for shoulder pain, concluded there was little evidence to support or refute the efficacy of common interventions such as NSAIDs, intraarticular or subacromial glucocorticosteroid injection, physiotherapy, manipulation under anaesthesia or surgery.

Evidence does exist for certain conditions. For example, Green et al (2002b) conclude that in the short term, topical NSAIDs relieve lateral elbow pain (tennis elbow) and that a steroid injection may also be more effective than oral NSAIDs in the short term.

Orthopaedic nurses need to be aware of such evidence so that they can help patients to make informed choices about their pain relief.

SELF-CARE DEFICIT

Patients may have self-care deficits with regard to toileting, bathing, dressing, preparing and eating food. The aim of care is to help patients overcome any deficit so they can carry out activities to their satisfaction, with or without assistance.

Nursing actions

Following surgery, patients may not be able to wash the unaffected arm and are often wary of washing the affected one. Patients with hand conditions or those who have had hand surgery may not be able to get the hand wet. The nurse needs to provide help in the initial postoperative stage, for example by washing under the arm of a patient with a shoulder replacement.

Education and support on dressing and the choice of clothes are needed. For patients with chronic conditions, this should be provided as early as possible; the support of the community occupational therapy services could be required for some patients. For elective surgery patients this is discussed in the preoperative clinic, allowing the patient to prepare for their postoperative needs in advance.

Patients are advised to wear clothes with wide or short sleeves, as it can be difficult to get any clothes over a splint or cast. They need to be taught to put their affected arm into the sleeve first and may require help initially. Relatives or friends need to be taught how to do this ready for the patient's discharge from hospital.

Patients will have restricted ability to prepare and cook food; this will obviously have implications if they have no help in the community. Simple questions such as how they will get food from the oven to the plate and then to where they will eat the food need to be asked as part of the overall assessment. For patients with rheumatoid arthritis, which commonly affects the hands, adapted cutlery can be provided.

The occupational therapist will be involved in assessing self-care issues, offering supervised dressing practice, providing mobility and other aids such as a trolley on wheels and large-handled cutlery as required.

INEFFECTIVE ROLE PERFORMANCE

An upper limb condition or injury can affect a patient's ability to perform successfully the roles expected of them. These include roles within the family or relationships such as providing physical care for young children, social roles such as the playing of amateur sports or work roles, including the ability to perform all or some aspects of a job. The aim of care is to allow the patient to feel that they can adequately fulfil their role expectations or adapt to their altered role performance.

Nursing actions

Identification of the patient's desired health status is important; for example, the level of sport they wish to play at the end of treatment or the tasks they need to carry out at work or in the home. These desires may be unrealistic and the nurse will therefore be involved in helping the patient to accept a redefined health status.

Discussion with the patient about how their life can be adapted in order to cope with an upper limb disorder or trauma in the short or long term may be necessary. This might involve a change of job or role within a particular job, the use of help from family and friends or referral to an outside agency such as Social Services for specific help. The nurse needs to have a thorough knowledge of what is, and is not, available in their local area. The multidisciplinary team must remember the patient has the right to decide that they do not wish to comply with restrictions, although they should be aware of the possible consequences of this.

ALTERED BODY IMAGE

The patient may have been living with an altered body image for many years due to a chronic condition such as rheumatoid arthritis but progressive changes or treatment can lead to a further change in body image, which the patient will need help to adjust to. Following a traumatic injury, both the injury and the treatment, such as an external fixator being applied, will suddenly alter the patient's own body image.

The aim of care is to help the patient achieve a body image they are comfortable with. This can be expressed, for example, in terms of the patient demonstrating they are willing and able to care for their arm in an abduction splint for 6 weeks following repair of a rotator cuff lesion and are willing to continue social activities whilst wearing the splint. These actions indicate the patient has accepted the altered body image caused by the changes imposed.

Nursing actions

In Chapter 6, issues relevant to altered body image and orthopaedic conditions or trauma are discussed. In addition to these are particular issues to consider with regard to the upper limb.

- Upper limb surgery may result in scars that are difficult to conceal, although shoulder surgery on women is performed through a bra-line incision, making it less visible. Where possible, the nurse must ensure the patient is aware of this preoperatively and given the opportunity to voice any anxieties postoperatively.
- Upper limb trauma or conditions can result in a patient feeling they have lost control over many of

their life activities, especially if their normal coping strategies have left them feeling inadequate. Patient education is vital to ensure independence is maximised and it can help to restore faith in a patient's normal coping strategies.

- Patients on a specialist upper limb unit are generally more comfortable with their body image as there are other patients in a similar situation. However, when this support is no longer available, for example following discharge from the acute unit, body image problems can be more apparent. By involving the patient's family in their care, the nurse can help develop a vital support system for the patient to use on discharge.

KNOWLEDGE DEFICIT

Practitioners should never assume that a person has a thorough knowledge or understanding of their chronic upper limb condition, even if they have been living with it for many years. Equally, a patient with a traumatic injury is unlikely to have an understanding of what their treatment will entail.

The goal of care is for the patient to explain the rationale for their care and the activities they must perform, in terms of exercises for example, and the activities they should avoid, such as driving immediately after shoulder replacement surgery.

Nursing actions

There is much research on the benefits of information giving and patient education, although questions such as the most appropriate timing of education have not been definitively answered. The education of adults is dependent on awareness of adult learning principles (Knowles 1990), including using the person's previous experiences.

Patient education needs to cover the three domains of learning: cognitive, affective and psychomotor. Cognitive learning is the understanding of facts and concepts necessary for intellectual learning; for example, a patient may need to understand why an arm needs to be immobilised post rotator cuff surgery. Such learning can take place through the provision of verbal information, written and audiovisual materials.

Affective learning relates to attitudes; for example, helping a patient to accept they may not return to their job following trauma. This learning occurs through discussion and allowing the patient to express their fears and feelings.

Psychomotor learning involves the development of physical skills, for example being able to carry out postoperative exercises prior to discharge. This occurs through the demonstration of skills and practising them until the skill is perfected. The physiotherapist or occupational therapist may demonstrate and teach the skill initially but the orthopaedic nurse is involved in enabling the patient to practise the skill and ensuring they will be able to manage at home.

SUMMARY OF NURSING CARE POINTS

These principles of nursing care are applicable to individual patients with particular upper limb problems. Specific aspects of care are discussed below in relation to chronic conditions and acute injuries of the upper limb. Before this, a brief discussion of the implications of arthroscopic surgery on the upper limb is given, as this is an expanding area of surgery with specific implications for orthopaedic nursing.

UPPER LIMB ARTHROSCOPY

There is a move towards minimally invasive surgery of the upper limb for both chronic and traumatic injuries. For the shoulder, arthroscopic surgery enables the surgeon to view both the rotator cuff and the glenohumeral joint, the main sources of shoulder problems. Other advantages of an arthroscopic approach are smaller skin incisions, no deltoid detachment, less soft tissue dissection, less pain and quicker rehabilitation (Gartsman 2001).

Elbow arthroscopy is useful as a diagnostic procedure, for the removal of loose bodies, excision of bony spurs and evaluation of the joint function. Wrist arthroscopy claims to have a positive place in the treatment of lesions of the triangular fibrocartilage complex and scaphoid fractures (Gupta et al 2001).

The implications of these procedures for orthopaedic nursing are great, not least because arthroscopic procedures are often carried out on a day case basis with the patients not being admitted to an orthopaedic ward. It is important that patients are prepared adequately for the surgery and postoperative rehabilitation; orthopaedic nurses have an obligation to liaise and communicate with staff working in day surgery units and in outpatient departments to ensure that patients receive optimal care.

PRE- AND POSTARTHROSCOPY CONSIDERATIONS

Knowledge deficit. Patients require information about the nature of arthroscopic surgery and their postoperative rehabilitation.

Therapeutic restriction and increasing physical mobility. Patients are generally encouraged to mobilise the arm following surgery so adequate analgesia is important. If required, a sling is used for the first few days, for comfort.

Impaired skin integrity. The patient will have 3–4 portal holes, with either a suture or Steristrip securing each. The patient can remove the Steristrips after 2–3 days, otherwise arrangements are made for sutures to be removed and the wound checked in a nurse-led orthopaedic clinic, fracture clinic or in the community.

Risk of peripheral neurovascular dysfunction. There is potential for neurovascular damage following surgery, particularly following an elbow arthroscopy as any radial nerve damage can lead to long-term wrist drop. This must be observed for after surgery and on discharge, the patient should be taught the warning signs to look for.

SHOULDER CONDITIONS

TOTAL SHOULDER ARTHROPLASTY

A shoulder arthroplasty is indicated for patients with a painful shoulder and destruction of the glenohumeral joint (Deuschle & Romeo 1998). This is commonly due to rheumatoid arthritis or other inflammatory arthropathy, osteoarthritis or fractures of the proximal humerus. Other indications may be avascular necrosis of the humeral head, mal- or non-union of a proximal humeral fracture and chronic deficiency of the rotator cuff causing destruction of the glenohumeral joint. The main aim of surgery is to provide pain relief and pain-free movement of the joint.

This is an evolving area of surgery and consequently there are a variety of prostheses available:

- cemented or uncemented
- unconstrained with two separate components
- semi-constrained with a hooded glenoid component or subacromial spacers that restrict superior migration of the humeral component, the latter usually being reserved for deficiencies of the rotator cuff as there is more danger of dislocation

- fully constrained prostheses for very unstable shoulders. Many of these have been withdrawn because of problems with aseptic loosening, glenoid fracture and component dissociation (Zadeh & Calvert 1998).

There are a variety of shoulder prostheses. The Neer Mark II, an unconstrained shoulder replacement, is one of the most commonly used (Redfern & Wallace 1998). There is a lack of long-term follow-up studies for shoulder prostheses compared with hip prostheses but it appears that one which closely approximates to normal anatomy and which can be securely fixed to an eroded glenoid is most likely to be successful (Redfern & Wallace 1998). In a study of 102 patients following shoulder arthroplasty for primary glenohumeral osteoarthritis, patients on average regained approximately two-thirds of the functions that had been absent preoperatively (Fehringer et al 2002).

Whilst the orthopaedic nurse will not be obtaining patients' consent for surgery, they have a professional responsibility to act in the patient's best interests. Therefore they must have an understanding of the particular prostheses being used in their practice area, so that any patient concerns can be adequately addressed or referred to the appropriate healthcare professional.

As with all surgery, there are potential problems which patients need to be aware of. Loosening of the components, in particular the glenoid component, is the most commonly reported problem in shoulder arthroplasty surgery. Wallace reports a revision rate of 18% on 300 arthroplasties carried out between 1983 and 1993 (Wallace 1998a); these were required because of loosening of the components, subluxation, dislocation, rotator cuff tears, infection and nerve injury. Of these, two anterior dislocations were associated with the abduction splint slipping posteriorly during the postoperative period; this is avoidable with good nursing care (Wallace 1998a).

Preoperative care

Much of the preoperative preparation will be similar to that of any orthopaedic surgery. The specific considerations are as follows.

Knowledge deficit. Even though a patient may have lived with pain and disability for many years, they may have no knowledge of what a shoulder replacement entails. The information provided should include the type of immobilisation necessary post surgery to enable the patient to fully prepare for the restrictions.

Ineffective role performance and self-care deficit. The patient will have some degree of reduced or lost function postoperatively. The long-term aim will be to improve their level of function but in the short term this may be restricted as the patient recovers from surgery. Patients should be aware of this before they consent to surgery and be helped to make provision for the immediate postdischarge period.

Postoperative care

Impaired skin integrity. Following surgery a drain is inserted at the wound site; this is removed after 24–48 hours depending on the amount of drainage. The drain needs to be closely monitored, as the amount lost in theatre and in the immediate postoperative period can be extensive, requiring transfusion of one or more units. The initial wound dressing is left in situ for 48 hours and then it is changed to provide more comfort for the patient as they mobilise with a sling on.

Acute pain. Patient-controlled analgesa (PCA) is ideal if the patient has no decreased physical mobility in the other arm. Alternatively, a subacromial catheter can be used to give bupivacaine (Damrel 1998a). Step-down analgesia needs to be carefully planned, as continuous effective pain relief is necessary to ensure patients are able to take part in their rehabilitation programme.

Self-care deficits. Patients require help to ensure they have an adequate nutritional intake in the immediate postoperative period. Consideration is needed of the patient's ability to reach, hold, cut up and take their food and fluids from their unoperated side. Assistance is needed in the first few days with hygiene and dressing.

Risk of peripheral neurovascular dysfunction. Regular neurovascular observations are needed to identify any problems early, particularly as there is risk of axillary nerve damage during surgery. The frequency of these observations should be dictated by the findings and any local policies.

Therapeutic restriction and increasing physical mobility. Both an initial restriction and a gradual increase in movement are necessary if the patient is to gain maximum benefit from surgery and to reduce the risk of complications. The shoulder is rested for the first 48 hours in a sling or abduction wedge, although the patient is encouraged to walk around and use the other arm as much as possible.

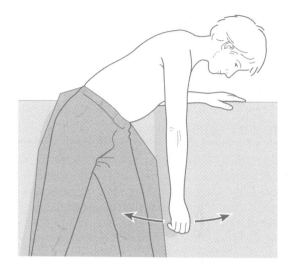

Figure 21.10   Pendulum exercise. (From Wallace 1998c.)

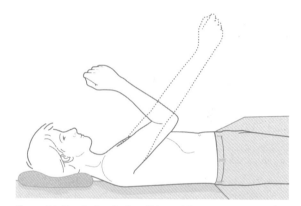

Figure 21.11   Active flexion. (Adapted from Wallace 1998c.)

Following this a range of passive motion exercises are commenced (Fig. 21.10), the aim being to achieve 140° of forward elevation and 40° of external rotation (Deuschle & Romeo 1998, Owens 1997).

Whilst physiotherapists will initially supervise these exercises, suitably trained orthopaedic nurses can take this over, particularly at weekends and evenings (Damrel 1998a). Assisted exercises to gain rotation and isometric exercises to strengthen the rotator cuff and deltoid muscles are started 10 days following surgery, with active abduction and flexion (Fig. 21.11) at 14 days to increase deltoid muscle strength (Damrel 1998a). After 3 weeks, resisted exercises and passive stretching are performed to increase muscle power and improve the range of both active and passive joint movement (see Fig. 21.9) (Damrel 1998a). These should continue for at least 6 months so that the patient gains full benefit from surgery.

Ineffective role performance. Patients are discouraged from returning to sedentary work and driving for the first 6 weeks. Patients with more strenuous jobs may not be able to return until 12–16 weeks post surgery. Housework must not be recommenced until at least 4 weeks post surgery.

IMPINGEMENT SYNDROME

Subacromial impingement syndrome is one of the most frequently seen causes of shoulder pain. It is caused by impingement of the supraspinatous tendon (part of the rotator cuff) under the acromio-clavicular joint when the arm is abducted (Fig. 21.12) or forward flexed. It can be caused by bony anatomy from a curved or hooked acromion, a trauma injury, shoulder instability or rotator cuff weakness, all of which decrease the available space for the rotator cuff (Lyons & Orwin 1998). Commonly patients complain of pain when the arm is abducted 60–120°, with no pain before or after this arc of movement. The pain is often localised to the anterolateral border of the acromion and is increased by overhead or repetitive work. Impingement can be classified as stages 1–3 (Table 21.1). Both conservative and surgical treatments may be tried.

Conservative treatment

In the absence of an acute injury, the initial treatment is conservative, generally carried out within an outpatient or primary care setting.

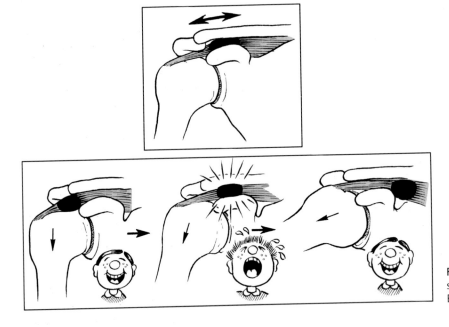

Figure 21.12   Impingement syndrome. (From Dandy & Edwards 2003.)

Table 21.1   Impingement classification (Neer 1983, cited by Lyons & Orwin 1998)

	Aetiology	Signs and symptoms	Typical patient profile
Stage 1	Reversible oedema and haemorrhage within the rotator cuff	Mild activity-related pain, no weakness or limitation in movement	Any age but typically less than 25 years old, following excessive overhead use of shoulder from sports or work
Stage 2	Fibrosis and thickening of the subacromial bursa and chronic supraspinatus tendinitis	Pain that may occur during activities of daily living or at night	Athletes aged 25–40
Stage 3	Partial or full-thickness tears of rotator cuff and biceps tendon lesions	Weakness of rotator cuff muscles	Patients over 40 with long-standing impingement

Knowledge deficit. The nurse is involved in helping patients understand about the benefits and necessity of rest, NSAIDs medication and avoidance of activities that cause pain.

Increasing physical mobility. To prevent long-term problems of joint stiffness, a programme of active exercises is begun; if movement is limited this may start with a passive stretching programme. Whilst the physiotherapist will probably initiate such exercises, nursing staff may provide support and reinforcement for patients.

Pain. Effective pain management is achievable using subacromial corticosteroid injections but these must only be administered by suitably trained and experienced medical, physiotherapy or nursing staff.

Conservative treatment can be successful for stage 1 and stage 2 patients, with approximately two-thirds of patients obtaining good or excellent results (Lyons & Orwin 1998). Even full-thickness rotator cuff tears can be improved with conservative treatment (Lyons & Orwin 1998).

If such treatment has not benefited a patient after 6–12 months, surgery is generally considered, in particular a subacromial decompression.

Surgical treatment: subacromial decompression

In order for tendons to move freely within the sub-acromial space, surgery is required to increase the available space. The exact nature of this surgery will depend on the cause of the impingement, for example removal of a bursa, opening the joint by cutting the coracoacromial ligament, partial resection of the anterior acromion or trimming the acromion from anterior to posterior. The surgery is performed arthroscopically or as an open procedure. An open reduction carries the risk of deltoid detachment if the deltoid muscle has not been adequately reattached at the end of surgery, leaving cosmetic and functional problems. The procedure requires only a short hospital stay of 48–72 hours.

The postsurgery care must address the following areas.

Impaired skin integrity. Arthroscopic repairs have small incisions that are Steristripped, the Steristrips being removed by the patient after 48 hours. An open decompression results in a suture line, dealt with as with any surgical incision.

Acute pain. Good pain management is often achieved using an indwelling catheter to deliver morphine and a local anaesthetic such as bupivacaine;

suitably trained nurses can top this up. Research has shown this is an effective way of providing pain relief following decompression (Park et al 2002) and other shoulder surgery (Yamaguchi et al 2002).

Risk of peripheral neurovascular dysfunction. Regular neurovascular observations are essential to detect any problems, in particular axillary nerve damage.

Self-care deficit. Patients require assistance with personal hygiene and maintaining their nutritional needs during the immediate postoperative phase.

Increasing physical activity. Although the patient will return from theatre in a PolySling, this is for comfort rather than immobilisation. When the patient's pain is controlled the emphasis becomes maintenance of shoulder mobility to prevent any complications from shoulder stiffness. Physical activity begins with a passive range of movement progressing to active assisted exercises when the patient has recovered from the anaesthetic. The patient needs to be able to reach full shoulder elevation prior to discharge. At 4–6 weeks, the physiotherapist or nurse practitioner will start the patient on resisted active exercises to build up the muscle strength.

Ineffective role performance. Patients are able to return to driving within 3 weeks and carry out light work within 6 weeks. Returning to manual work, overhead activities and contact sports is not advised until 12 weeks.

ROTATOR CUFF TEARS

Tears of the rotator cuff generally affect the tendon of the supraspinatus muscle (Box 21.5). Most lesions are secondary to impingement but are also found in patients with glenohumeral instability or following trauma.

The commonest cause of damage is from repetitive injury (see Chapter 26 for the causes of overuse injuries). It is most prevalent after the age of 40. Ageing or unaccustomed use may be a hidden factor along with shoulder dislocation and direct-impact injury to the tip of the shoulder. In younger adults, the tendinous part of the cuff–bone complex is stronger than the bone, causing avulsion fractures.

Most tears start at the point of insertion of the supraspinatus tendon. Tears result in limited abduction beyond 25°. Due to a common insertion point, the injury can affect the actions of the infraspinatus and teres minor, limiting backward extension and external rotation of the arm. This affects activities such as putting the arm into a jacket sleeve, causing pain and disablement.

Box 21.5   Muscles of the rotator cuff

The rotator cuff comprises four muscles: supraspinatus, infraspinatus, subscapularis and teres minor. They are part of the muscle complex that stabilises the shoulder joint. The tendons of the supraspinatus, infraspinatus and teres minor fuse at the point of insertion to the greater tuberosity of the humerus. They receive additional support from the coracohumeral ligament.

The anterior portion of the supraspinatus tendon has the greatest mechanical strength and performs the main functional role of the tendon, being responsible for locating the head of the humerus within the glenoid cavity. The infraspinatus and teres minor are responsible for external rotation and arm extension and the subscapularis is responsible for internal rotation and arm adduction.

Activities that put most strain on the supraspinatus are abduction positions when the arm is carrying out an additional activity such as throwing a ball. Assessment of movement reveals that the patient has problems raising their arm in abduction (Fig. 21.12); they tend to shoulder shrug in order to abduct the arm. If the arm is passively raised, the patient can then hold it in that position using the deltoid muscle but otherwise they are unable to perform overhead activities. A provisional diagnosis is confirmed by a magnetic resonance imaging (MRI) scan, arthrogram or shoulder arthroscopy.

Conservative management of rotator cuff tears

An injured tendon may never recover its normal structure and strength. The healing process can include the development of scar tissue that restricts rather than improves movement. To avoid this, where possible, the aim of treatment is to relieve pain and restore function using physiotherapy and analgesia.

Knowledge deficit. Patients must understand the importance of activity modification, their anti-inflammatory medication, cortisone injections and exercise programme that improves the muscle strength of the unaffected shoulder and scapular muscles (Gartsman 2001).

Therapeutic restriction and increasing physical mobility. These are managed along with good acute pain control. It is important to begin a programme of graduated exercises to retrain the intact muscles. If this is not successful and the patient cannot maintain an adequate quality of life, surgery is required

to repair the damaged cuff. The exercise regime requires a high level of commitment from the patient if it is to be fully effective and this must be explained at the start of any treatment.

Surgical repair of torn rotator cuffs

Rotator cuff surgery is not without risks, the main complications being a deep infection, deltoid detachment or failure of the repair, especially if the cuff is badly damaged. Some large tears may not be repairable and amenable only to decompression and debridement.

Preoperative preparation. This includes patient education to ensure they are aware of the need to wear an abduction splint postoperatively to rest the repaired muscles. Patients with no social support will have problems with this therapeutic restriction and self-care deficit, requiring referral to local agencies.

Postoperative care. An open or arthroscopic approach can be used, the latter having the advantage that the deltoid is left attached. For patients with partial-thickness tears, the rehabilitation is the same as following a subacromial decompression.

Therapeutic restriction and increasing physical mobility. Initially patients have a period of postoperative rest to promote tissue repair prior to rehabilitation and consequently the arm is immobilised in a splint. In some centres, an abduction wedge is used following repair of massive tears (see Fig. 21.8). Patients are started in passive elevation and external rotation exercises prior to discharge and continue these at home for 6 weeks. After this, active exercises can begin with the aim being to mobilise the shoulder and strengthen the muscle when the tendons have healed; this can be as an inpatient or outpatient. To promote comfort, a PolySling can be worn between exercise periods. For 3 months following surgery, the patient is encouraged to lift their arm with a bent elbow to create a short lever and less stress on the shoulder muscles; they must not lift the arm over shoulder level.

Self-care deficit. The abduction wedge will cause a major disruption for the patient, as one arm is totally immobilised in the splint and cannot be removed except for short periods by a carer for hygiene. When removed, the shoulder position must remain the same with the arm supported on a table and pillows. The patient and carers need to be taught about management of the splint and the limb prior to discharge.

The patient will require maximum support in hospital and at home for personal hygiene and dressing; advice such as wearing loose-fitting clothes makes dressing easier. The cosmetic position of the scar along the bra line in women makes wearing a bra uncomfortable until it is healed.

Ineffective role performance. The lengthy rehabilitation period means that patients are unable to drive or work for at least 6 weeks, affecting their ability to fulfil many of their responsibilities. The implications of this need to be considered before surgery is performed.

SHOULDER INSTABILITY

Instability of the glenohumeral joint occurs because of the anatomical position of the joint, namely the shallow glenoid cavity and the role of the rotator cuff in providing stability. Instability can take many forms.

- Anterior instability is most common, occurring when the arm is abducted and externally rotated. This risks damage to the axillary nerve or artery as they run near to the neck of the humerus.
- Posterior instability is generally due to a lax shoulder joint. It is associated with swimming and gymnastic activities that stretch the joint capsule. Epileptic fits and electrocution can also cause posterior dislocation.
- Inferior instability occurs when the humeral head subluxes or dislocates into the inferior area of the joint. Although rarely seen, it can occur in the first week after a fractured neck of humerus. It is also associated with neuromuscular conditions such as deltoid paralysis or palsy.
- Superior instability occurs when the humeral head dislocates superiorly when muscle control of the humeral head is lost, as with rotator cuff tears.
- Multidirectional instability occurs when the humeral head can dislocate in a number of directions. It is generally seen in patients with acquired or congenital joint laxities and in high-performance athletes.

The direction of the dislocation is confirmed by an X-ray. A scan may be required if damage to the glenoid labrum is suspected following repeated dislocations.

Achieving stability

Reduction of a dislocated joint may be achieved by manipulating the arm so that the humeral head returns to the glenoid cavity, for example by the hanging arm technique (Fig. 21.13). To reduce the risk of future dislocation, the arm is supported in either a sling or body bandage for 3–4 weeks. After

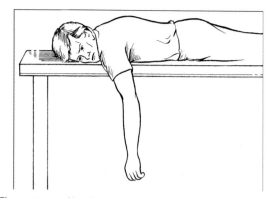

Figure 21.13   Hanging arm technique for reducing dislocation of the shoulder. (From Dandy & Edwards 2003.)

this physiotherapy exercise to strengthen the rotator cuff, deltoid and periscapular muscles may be sufficient to stabilise the joint.

For repeated dislocations, a surgical repair is likely, the choice depending on the classification of instability and the exact nature of the problem. For anterior instability with glenoid labral tear, the favoured repair is Bankart's, as others have a higher rate of complications; for example, the Putti-Platt procedure which limits external rotation and leads to degenerative changes within the glenohumeral joint (Gill et al 1997). A Bankart repair involves using anchors to secure the labrum or capsule to the glenoid and has a good success rate of up to 93% (Gill et al 1997). This can be performed as an open procedure or as an arthroscopic one if there is a discrete lesion without capsular laxity or injury (Fealy et al 2001). For recurrent posterior dislocations a posterior bone block or glenoid osteotomy is performed, although both are unreliable procedures (Dandy & Edwards 2003).

Patients need to be aware preoperatively that although they may only remain in hospital for 24–48 hours, the rehabilitation is lengthy and they need time to adequately prepare for this.

Impaired skin integrity. If a drain is used, it is removed at 24–28 hours.

Acute pain. A subacromial catheter used to instil analgesia directly into the area is generally effective.

Self-care deficit. The patient is likely to require assistance in dressing and personal hygiene because the arm is immobilised in a PolySling with a waistband attachment for 2–4 weeks. To wash under the affected arm, the patient is encouraged to hang their arm down by their side and lean forward slightly to allow access to the axilla without moving the shoulder. The patient needs to be taught to dress and undress one-handed and how to remove and replace the sling.

Restricting movement and increasing physical mobility. Elbow and hand exercises are commenced on the first day to prevent muscle wastage and joint stiffness. At 2 weeks, pendulum exercises are begun (see Fig. 21.10) and the waistband of the PolySling is discarded. At 3–4 weeks, the sling is removed and active movement initiated. By week 6, external rotation at 90° is initiated and progressed to a full range of movement (Fealy et al 2001).

Ineffective role performance. Restrictions from the surgery and rehabilitation affect the patient's ability to undertake such activities as driving and working for about 6 weeks. The patient can usually return to non-contact sports at 3 months and contact sports at 4 months.

THE ELBOW

As a less mobile joint than the shoulder, the elbow joint is less at risk of chronic disease. The commonest lesion is tennis elbow (Dandy & Edwards 2003).

TENNIS ELBOW

A tear occurs in or near the insertion of the common extensor tendon on the lateral condyle and humerus (Fig. 21.14). It is caused by sharp extension of the wrist whilst the extensors are contracted, such as an awkwardly hit backhand in tennis or in activities such as gardening or lifting (Dandy & Edwards 2003).

Treatment is by rest and NSAIDs if tolerated by the patient. A systematic review of the use of anti-inflammatories for tennis elbow found some support for the short-term use of topical NSAIDs, insufficient evidence to recommend or discourage oral NSAIDs and that an injection may be more effective than oral NSAIDs in the short term (Green et al 2002b).

ELBOW ARTHROPLASTY

Total elbow replacement is less common than lower limb or shoulder replacement and is usually performed for patients with a rheumatoid arthritis who have muscle wasting or, more recently, for post-traumatic arthritis in older patients (Gschwend 2002). Results of replacement for primary osteoarthritis

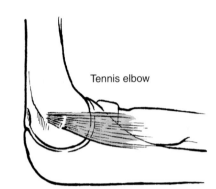

Figure 21.14   Tennis elbow. (From Dandy & Edwards 2003.)

are generally poor because of the heavier loading applied by patients following reconstruction (Radford & Carr 2003).

The aim of surgery is to provide a stable, painless range of motion during activities of living (Moro & King 2000). Prostheses are linked or unlinked; most are stabilised by the use of bone cement. Unlinked prostheses require the presence of good bone stock with little deformity and stable capsuloligamentous support, which is uncommon after trauma (Moro & King 2000).

Wallace (1998b) has reported that following surgery, transient ulnar nerve damage occurs in up to 65% of patients with a 10% risk of permanent damage, the risk of a deep infection is 10%, elbow dislocation is 4–10% and aseptic loosening at 10 years is 10%. Wound healing is an additional specific problem for these patients.

There are few long-term follow-up results but 10-year results in rheumatoid arthritis patients have shown 90% survival rates for the prosthesis (Gschwend 2002). However, the results are less good in younger patients who place greater demands on the prosthesis.

Preoperative preparation

The main issue for preoperative care is addressing the patient's knowledge deficit. They need to understand the risks and benefits of surgery in order to balance these and make an informed decision about whether to proceed or not. The orthopaedic nurse therefore has to have an understanding of the issues if caring for these patients on a regular basis.

Postoperative care

Therapeutic restriction and increasing physical mobility. Immediately post surgery, the new joint is protected in 90° of flexion, with a backslab or firm crepe bandage and padding (Wallace 1998b). On removal at 48 hours, a polyurethane splint is applied, which maintains the elbow at 90° flexion with the forearm in full pronation (Moro & King 2000). This splint is used for 6 weeks, except during exercises. Active assisted elbow flexion and passive gravity extension are performed to protect the triceps repair. It is important that elbow extension past 30° is avoided to prevent subluxation or dislocation (Moro & King 2000). The physiotherapist may use an elbow continuous passive movement (CPM) machine. At 6 weeks extension is encouraged, with a nighttime extension splint being used for a further 6 weeks (Moro & King 2000).

Risk of peripheral neurovascular dysfunction.   Regular neurovascular observations of the hand are required, particularly to detect ulnar nerve neuropraxia. If a partial ulnar nerve lesion has not improved within 10 days, it may be explored and decompressed (Wallace 1998b).

Impaired skin integrity.   The skin around the elbow is thin, with little subcutaneous fat, so the wound is prone to complications. The use of a CPM and the fragile skin of many rheumatoid patients further increase the risk of wound breakdown, as do multiple skin incisions that can result in poorly vascularised skin flaps. The risk of a haematoma is reduced through the use of vacuum drainage and a firm postoperative dressing. Careful observation is required for early detection of wound breakdown or infection.

Ineffective role performance.   It is not until at least 4 weeks post surgery that patients can begin to resume normal activities; light housework is allowed at 4–6 weeks, light gardening at 6 weeks and driving at 8 weeks. Strenuous activities, such as carrying heavy shopping, should be avoided after an elbow replacement (Damrel 1998b).

WRIST AND HAND CONDITIONS

There are a variety of conditions affecting the bones, cartilage and tendons of the hand, the more common ones being addressed here.

OSTEOARTHRITIS AND RHEUMATOID ARTHRITIS

As with other synovial joints, the wrist and hand joints are prone to both forms of arthritis.

The wrist in particular is prone to rheumatoid arthritis as it affects the synovium around the wrist and inferior radioulnar joints; see Chapter 15 for discussion of rheumatoid arthritis. There is damage to the adjacent tendons, leading eventually to a loss of carpal height and stability, development of ulnar-palmar translocation and supination of the carpus on the distal forearm (Shapiro 1996).

Osteoarthritis of the wrist may follow trauma, particularly a scaphoid fracture, and is common in the interphalangeal joints. The resultant nodules are known as Heberden's nodes if they involve the distal interphalangeal joints and Boucher's nodes if they involve the proximal joints.

When conservative treatment has failed, surgery may be contemplated, the aims being to provide pain relief and adequate stability, together with the maximum range of movement possible. The options for surgery range from soft tissue reconstruction to total arthrodesis.

Nursing actions

Therapeutic restriction and increasing physical mobility. Rest, support and movement play their part in the treatment of patients with rheumatoid or osteoarthritic changes to the hand. Splints to help prevent painful movements are useful, especially at night, and postoperatively they may be necessary to maintain the hand or wrist in an acceptable position whilst healing takes place. Orthopaedic nurses should understand how these splints work and be able to remove or apply them safely.

Altered body image.   Both types of arthritis cause disfigurement of the wrist and hands, which can have a profound effect on a patient's body image. Surgery may be corrective but the rehabilitation may consist of several months of splinting and dressings, which also impact on body image. For example, after distal interphalangeal joint silicone interpositional arthroplasty of the hand for osteoarthritis, the rehabilitation consists of external splinting of the distal joint in full extension, in addition to a K wire, for 4 weeks, followed by wire removal and a further 4 weeks with a mallet finger type splint worn continually. Night splinting is continued for the third and fourth postoperative months (Wilgis 1997).

Ineffective role performance.   The wrist and hands are used in most activities related to work or leisure so the effects of arthritis can therefore be wide-ranging. Referral to an occupational therapist may result in the provision of aids to help role performance.

Self-care deficit.   Similarly the ability to wash and dress may be impaired in both chronic conditions and postoperatively; help may need to be provided.

DE QUERVAIN'S TENOSYNOVITIS

The tendons of the extensor pollicis brevis and abductor pollicis longus pass under a tight fibrous bridge, proximal to the radial styloid process. This makes them prone to any localised swelling, the main cause of swelling being repeated twisting movements (Fig. 21.15). This causes pain on movement, which is reproduced by asking the patient to grasp the thumb with the other fingers and then pushing the hand into flexion and ulnar deviation.

Knowledge deficit. Patients need advice on eliminating the activities that cause the pain. If this is unsuccessful in reducing the pain, a steroid injection into the tendon is attempted. If the problem continues, the fibrous bridge can be divided surgically.

TRIGGER FINGER

The flexor profundus longus tendon is prone to friction where it enters its tendon sheath. This causes a 'pop' sound and sensation where the damaged tendon enters the sheath (see Fig. 15.10). Eventually the tendon becomes stuck in the flexed position. Symptoms usually occur following unaccustomed repetitive activity; rest and elimination of the cause are often successful management strategies. Local steroid injection or surgery to open the tendon sheath may be necessary.

Knowledge deficit. As with de Quervain's disease, the patient needs to understand the causes and strategies to help alleviate the situation.

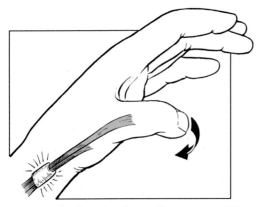

Figure 21.15 De Quervain's disease. The extensor pollicis brevis and abductor pollicis longus tendons are irritated as they pass beneath a fibrous bridge proximal to the radial styloid. (From Dandy & Edwards 2003.)

HAND INFECTIONS

The structures of the hand are prone to infection because many of them are superficial and the hand is often damaged during activities. Infections can be classified as follows (Dandy & Edwards 2003):

- nailfold infections; paronychia
- pulp space infections
- infections of the tendon sheaths
- web space infections
- infections of the deep spaces.

All of these are very painful because, with the exception of web space and deep space infections, there is little room for the infection to spread without causing pressure. The treatment and nursing care are similar for each type of infection.

Therapeutic restriction. High elevation of the arm is necessary (see Figs 21.4, 21.6) to reduce the pressure and prevent pooling of the infection. Antibiotic therapy is commenced.

Impaired skin integrity. If rest, elevation and antibiotics are not successful, incision and drainage are necessary, particularly for tendon sheath infections as adhesions may form if the infection is not treated rapidly. Following drainage of the area, pain relief is good but care should be taken with the wound as any wound infection can lead to extensive scarring.

FRACTURES OF THE UPPER LIMB

Fractures of the upper limb are relatively common, often related to falling on an outstretched hand. Many of these fractures are managed on an outpatient basis, requiring A & E and outpatient clinic nurses to have an understanding of the potential complications and patient problems, particularly the risk of peripheral neurovascular dysfunction and knowledge deficits. There are a variety of upper limb fractures, the most common of which are discussed here. Readers are referred to Chapter 6 for discussion of the nursing care issues relating to patients with a cast, traction care and for internal or external fixation of fractures.

CLAVICLE FRACTURES

These are among the most common fractures (Dandy & Edwards 2003). Fractures of the midshaft of the clavicle usually occur from a violent upwards and backwards thrust typically from falling with the arm outstretched.

Therapeutic restriction.   The arm is supported in a broad arm sling for up to 10 days. If there is malunion or non-union, internal fixation is normally successful.

Risk of peripheral neurovascular dysfunction.   There is a risk of damage to the great blood vessels near to the clavicle, the subclavian vessels and the lung (Dandy & Edwards 2003).

Fractures of the outer end of the clavicle involve the acromioclavicular joint, with the distal fragment often remaining attached to the acromion. Treatment depends on the degree of displacement. Simple fractures require a broad arm sling for a short period before mobilising. Other fractures require closed manipulation, then use of the sling. More seriously displaced fractures, involving the articular surfaces, need open reduction and internal fixation.

HUMERAL FRACTURES

Humeral neck fractures are generally seen in the elderly. These fractures are often impacted, requiring very little treatment other than a broad arm sling for 4–6 weeks while the pain settles. A more complicated comminuted fracture may require a shoulder hemiarthroplasty and rehabilitation similar to a shoulder arthroplasty. However, the Cochrane Review by Gibson et al (2002) concluded that the evidence does not confirm that an operative intervention will produce consistently better long-term outcomes.

Humeral shaft fractures are generally caused by a direct blow or fall onto the arm. The radial nerve is at risk of being trapped between the bone ends, therefore careful neurovascular observations are important. Depending on the position of the fracture, treatment is by:

• internal fixation used for displaced and pathological factures
• U-slab or hanging cast for undisplaced fractures. The weight of the cast applies traction to the fracture site and maintains correct alignment. A collar and cuff, not a broad arm sling, ensures the weight of the cast applies traction to the fracture site. Such a treatment is not always successful and requires careful monitoring on an outpatient basis to ensure the fracture is healing. There are also implications in terms of the patient's ability for self-care

and the potential for ineffective role performance, particularly as the patient is often elderly.

Supracondylar fractures are frequently seen in children. Particular problems arising from these are the high risk of damage to the brachial artery and median nerve, and compartment syndrome. Undisplaced fractures are normally treated in a backslab with the elbow in flexion for 2 weeks, while displaced fractures need either open or closed reduction with pin stabilisation prior to application of the backslab. Occasionally Dunlop traction is used if the position cannot be maintained (Fig. 21.16).

FRACTURES OF THE FOREARM AND WRIST

Many of these fractures are managed on an outpatient basis, whilst others are seen as inpatients especially if there are difficulties in treating the fracture or the social circumstances of the patient or the patient has other multi-trauma.

Both the proximal and distal radius and ulna are prone to several types of injury; the most common are discussed below. As these fractures are occasionally associated with more extensive injuries of the elbow and wrist joints, these joints must be carefully examined as well.

Head of radius

A fall on to the hand may produce a crack in the head of the radius. If undisplaced, it is left to unite, with reasonable results. If badly displaced and interfering

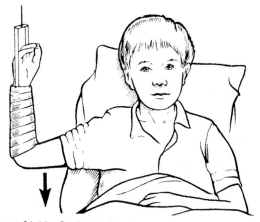

Figure 21.16   Dunlop traction for supracondylar fracture of the humerus.

with movements of the elbow, the treatment is usually excision of the radial head.

Olecranon fractures

The olecranon is easily fractured in direct falls on the elbow and the fracture is usually displaced. Internal fixation is required with either a screw or tension band wiring to hold the position. If the fragments cannot be reassembled, excision of the olecranon may be needed.

Proximal radius and ulna

It is rare to fracture the radius and ulna separately. When single fractures do occur they can be slow to unite. When both are fractured the muscles attached to the opposite ends of the bone can produce displacement of the fragments. Therefore fractures involving both the proximal radius and ulna are normally fixed internally to maintain the alignment.

Therapeutic restriction and increasing physical mobility. For conservative treatment of radial head fractures, a supporting bandage can be used, while a cast is occasionally used for proximal radius and ulna fractures if there is little displacement. The patient needs to understand the importance of maintaining mobility in the adjacent joints.

Risk of peripheral neurovascular dysfunction. As radial and ulna fractures can result in vascular damage and compartment syndrome, neurovascular observations are very important.

Knowledge deficit. As patients are likely to be in hospital for only a short period, if at all, it is important they understand the treatment and the complications to observe for.

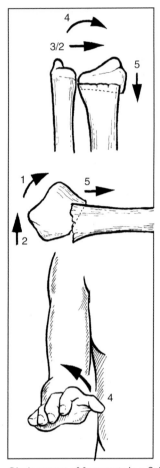

Figure 21.17   Displacement of fragments in a Colles' fracture. Five separate elements: (1) backward angulation; (2) backward displacement; (3) radial deviation; (4) supination; (5) proximal impaction. (From Dandy & Edwards 2003.)

Colles' fracture

This is the commonest fracture, with a classic dinner fork displacement of the distal radius (Fig. 21.17). It is normally seen in women over 50 years and is often the first indicator that a patient has osteoporosis.

Usually closed manipulation and the application of a cast for 4–6 weeks will provide adequate positioning and stability for normal healing. Manipulation can be performed with different types of anaesthesia, such as a haematoma block, but there is insufficient evidence to establish their relative effectiveness (Handoll et al 2002a). A plaster backslab is initially applied until the swelling has subsided, followed by a complete cast. Younger et al (1990) suggest that a full cast split to the skin, rather than a backslab, provides better accommodation for postreduction swelling and reduces the risk of neurological impairment.

Surgical interventions such as external or internal fixation are used when there is a displacement that cannot be corrected by manipulation. Handoll & Madhok (2002a, b) point out the need for further good-quality evidence for the outcomes of both surgical and conservative approaches.

Some units carry out check X-rays during the healing period to review the position of the fracture as these injuries have frequent complications, including median nerve injury, malunion, Sudeck's atrophy (reflex sympathetic dystrophy caused by a disturbance of the sensory and autonomic supply of bone and blood vessels) and rupture of the extensor pollicis longus tendon.

Knowledge deficit.   Patients need to be aware of the risks and to identify the early signs of potential complications. Patient education is particularly important to prevent Sudeck's atrophy, as regular finger and shoulder movements are vital in reducing the risk. Education must include care of the cast. Royal College of Physicians (1999) guidelines suggest that women under 50 with a low-impact distal radial fracture should be investigated for osteoporosis and given advice and information on how to reduce the risk of future fractures.

Risk of peripheral neurovascular dysfunction.   Neurovascular observations are needed to identify the early signs of Sudeck's atrophy and median nerve injury. Nurses undertake these observations while the patient is in hospital prior to discharge; the patients must be taught what to look for, especially during the acute phase when swelling is most likely.

Therapeutic restriction and increasing physical mobility.   Exercise and physiotherapy are beneficial for short-term and long-term recovery of function, although the evidence is inconclusive (Handoll et al 2002b). Initially the cast is supported with a broad arm sling, although this can be discarded after 10–14 days as there is a tendency for patients to keep the arm immobile while in a sling, increasing the risk of Sudeck's atrophy.

Self-care deficit.   As the majority of patients are elderly, consideration is needed of how they will manage with the cast or postoperative restrictions.

Smith's fracture

This is another fracture of the distal end of the radius, sometimes called a reverse Colles' fracture, as the displacement is anterior. It results from a backward fall, knocking the wrist forwards. The injury is commonest in middle-aged rather than elderly patients. The usual treatment is a forearm cast with the hand supinated and the wrist in full extension. Open reduction and internal fixation might be required as the fracture is often unstable. The nursing implications are similar to those of a patient with a Colles' fracture.

Scaphoid fractures

The scaphoid bone, situated on the thumb side of the proximal row of carpal bones (See Fig. 21.3), is injured by falls onto the hand or a blow to the wrist; usually these injuries are seen in young adults. The indicative symptoms are tenderness over the fracture site in the area known as the anatomical snuffbox, weakness of pinch position and power and pain on hyperextension. The fractures do not always show on initial X-rays so they should be repeated at 10 days to 2 weeks.

In the meantime if the history of the injury and symptoms are indicative, it is treated as a scaphoid fracture in a well-fitting cast that incorporates the thumb, holding the wrist in dorsiflexion and radial deviation. Stable fractures are treated in this cast for 6 weeks but an unstable fracture will require internal fixation.

However, stable fractures treated conservatively remain at risk, as the blood supply to the proximal fragment is poor and damaged by the fracture; internal fixation and grafting may be necessary after the 6 week cast immobilisation (Dandy & Edwards 2003). It has been argued that early fixation should be carried out on all scaphoid fractures, including stable fractures, as this injury is commonest in young working adults and the cast immobilisation may cause economic hardship (Dao & Shin 2001).

The period of splint immobilisation commonly causes wrist stiffness but this will clear up with exercise and use. The nursing implications are similar to those for patients with a Colles' fracture.

FRACTURES OF THE HAND

Fractures of the hand are either managed as outpatients or patients are admitted for only a short period if internal fixation is required. Thus the need for good patient education is paramount, particularly with regards to self-care deficit and ineffective role performance. There are many different types of fractures; only the most common are discussed here.

Metacarpal fractures and dislocations

Metacarpal injuries comprise 36% of hand and wrist fractures, with fractures of the fifth metacarpal neck accounting for around a third of these (Klein & Belsole 2000).

Bennett's fracture.   This is a fracture dislocation of the first carpometacarpal joint at the base of the thumb, caused by the thumb being knocked backwards in hyperextension. A Bennett's cast is used to hold the saddle joint in correct alignment after reduction. As maintaining the position can be difficult, open reduction and screw fixation may be required or percutaneous pin fixation for 3–6 weeks

(Klein & Belsole 2000). The joint can have a limited range of movement after this injury.

Metacarpal fractures. The commonest cause of metacarpal fractures is a punch with the fist clenched, the fifth metacarpal usually being angulated at the neck. If undisplaced, it can be supported by neighbour strapping the little finger to the ring finger (Dandy & Edwards 2003). If it is markedly displaced, reduction and straightening are needed prior to application of a dorsal plaster slab, percutaneous pin insertion or internal screw fixation (Klein & Belsole 2000).

Finger phalangeal fractures

These account for approximately 46% of fractures of the hand and wrist (Klein & Belsole 2000). These are generally treated by strapping to the neighbouring finger(s) if no angulation or rotational deformity is present (Lee & Jupiter 2000). The patient is encouraged to use the hand normally. Percutaneous wiring or internal fixation is required if the fracture is unstable, there is angulation or a deformity is present that cannot be corrected by conservative treatment.

Nursing considerations

Therapeutic restriction and increasing physical mobility. The majority of treatment for hand fractures involves some degree of therapeutic restriction such as neighbour strapping, a cast or bandaging after internal fixation. A splint is essential after percutaneous fixation, as this does not provide as rigid a fixation as internal fixation (Klein & Belsole 2000). The length of this restriction will vary from a few days, following internal fixation, to 5–6 weeks for neighbour strapping, a cast or splint. The nurse should ensure that the patient understands the importance of this restriction and the need for exercising the other fingers, wrist and arm joints when it is permitted.

Self-care deficit and ineffective role performance. Although the injury may be to one finger, it can have a major effect on a patient's ability to carry out everyday activities. Patients need advice on how to overcome problems, such as using a plastic bag to protect a cast or dressing whilst bathing. Some patients may not be able to work during the acute treatment stage, depending on the nature of their employment.

Risk of peripheral neurovascular dysfunction. Percutaneous wires may cause injuries to nerves and vessels; the incidence is reported as being 5–41% (Klein & Belsole 2000). Regular neurovascular observations of the hand are performed whilst the patient remains an inpatient, with the patient being taught to observe for any symptoms after discharge.

CONCLUSION

Upper limb conditions and injuries can lead patients to become dependent on others for many basic activities. With technological advances and the move towards shorter lengths of hospital stay, patients will spend less time, if any, in an acute patient area. Therefore, there is a need to communicate the essentials of care to the patient and to others who may care for them in clinic and primary care settings.

References

Balcombe K 1994 Using a nursing model: a model for orthopaedic nursing. In: Davis P (ed) Nursing the orthopaedic patient. Churchill Livingstone, Edinburgh

Constant CR, Murley AHG 1987 A clinical method of functional assessment of the shoulder. Clinical Orthopaedics and Related Research 214: 160–164

Damrel D 1998a Physiotherapy after unconstrained shoulder replacement. In: Wallace WA (ed) Joint replacement in the shoulder and elbow. Butterworth Heinemann, Oxford

Damrel D 1998b Rehabilitation after total elbow replacement. In: Wallace WA (ed) Joint replacement in the shoulder and elbow. Butterworth Heinemann, Oxford

Dandy DJ, Edwards DJ 2003 Essential orthopaedics and trauma, 4th edn. Churchill Livingstone, Edinburgh

Dao KM, Shin AY 2001 Scaphoid fractures: is early fixation the gold standard? Current Opinion in Orthopaedics 12(4): 280–285

Deuschle JA, Romeo AA 1998 Understanding shoulder arthroplasty. Orthopaedic Nursing 5: 7–15

Fealy S, Drakos MC, Answorth AA et al 2001 Arthroscopic Bankart repair. Clinical Orthopaedics and Related Research 390: 31–41

Fehringer EV, Kopjar B, Boorman RS et al 2002 Characterizing the functional improvement after total shoulder arthroplasty for osteoarthritis. Journal of Bone and Joint Surgery 84A(8): 1349–1353

Gartsman GM 2001 Arthroscopic rotator cuff repair. Clinical Orthopaedics and Related Research 390: 95–106

Gibson JNA, Handoll HHG, Madhok R 2002 Interventions for treating proximal humeral fractures in adults

(Cochrane Review). The Cochrane Library, Issue 4. Update Software, Oxford

Gill TJ, Lyle J, Michell MD et al 1997 Bankart repair for anterior instability of the shoulder. Journal of Bone and Joint Surgery 79A(6): 850–857

Green S, Buchbinder R, Glazier R et al 2002a Interventions for shoulder pain (Cochrane Review). Cochrane Library, Issue 3. Update Software, Oxford

Green S, Buchbinder R, Barnsley L et al 2002b Non-steroidal anti-inflammatory drugs for treating lateral elbow pain in adults (Cochrane Review). Cochrane Library, Issue 3. Update Software, Oxford

Gschwend N 2002 Present state-of-the-art in elbow arthoplasty. Acta Orthopaedica Belgica 68(2): 100–117

Gupta R, Bozentka DJ, Osterman AL 2001 Wrist arthroscopy: principles and clinical applications. Journal of the American Academy of Orthopedic Surgeons 9(3): 200–209

Handoll HHG, Madhok R 2002a Conservative interventions for treating distal radial fractures in adults (Cochrane Review). Cochrane Library, Issue 4. Update Software, Oxford

Handoll HHG, Madhok R 2002b Surgical interventions for treating distal radial fractures in adults (Cochrane Review). Cochrane Library, Issue 4. Update Software, Oxford

Handoll HHG, Madhok R, Dodds C 2002a Anaesthesia for treating distal radial fracture in adults (Cochrane Review). Cochrane Library, Issue 4. Update Software, Oxford

Handoll HHG, Madhok R, Howe TE 2002b Rehabilitation for distal radial fractures in adults (Cochrane Review). Cochrane Library, Issue 3. Update Software, Oxford

Klein DM, Belsole RJ 2000 Percutaneous treatment of carpal, metacarpal, and phalangeal injuries. Clinical Orthopaedics and Related Research 375: 116–125

Knowles M 1990 The adult learner: a neglected species, 4th edn. Gulf Publishing, London

Lee S-G, Jupiter JB 2000 Phalangeal and metacarpal fractures of the hand. Hand Clinics 16(3): 323–331

Lucas B 2002 Orthopaedic patient journeys: a UK perspective. Journal of Orthopaedic Nursing 6(2): 86–89

Lyons PM, Orwin JF 1998 Rotator cuff tendinopathy and subacromial impingement syndrome. Medicine and Science in Sports and Exercise 30(4): S12–S17

Metter EJ, Conwit R, Tobin J, Fozard JL 1997 Age-associated loss of power and strength in the upper extremities in women and men. Journal of Gerontology: Biological Sciences 52A(5): B267–276

Moro JK, King GJW 2000 Total elbow arthroplasty in the treatment of posttraumatic conditions of the elbow. Clinical Orthopaedics and Related Research 370: 102–114

North American Nursing Diagnosis Association (NANDA) 2001 Nursing diagnoses: definitions and classification 2001–2002. North American Nurses Diagnosis Association, Philadelphia

Owens RA 1997 Total shoulder arthroplasty. AORN Journal 65(5): 927–932

Park JY, Lee GW, Kim Y et al 2002 The efficacy of continuous intrabursal infusion with morphine and bupivacaine for postoperative analgesia after subacromial arthroscopy. Regional Anesthesia and Pain Medicine 27(2): 145–149

Price B 1990 A model for body-image care. Journal of Advanced Nursing 15: 585–593

Radford M, Carr A 2003 Total elbow replacement. Current Orthopaedics 16: 325–330

Rahman N, Thomas JJ, Rice MS 2002 The relationship between hand strength and the forces used to access containers by well elderly persons. American Journal of Occupational Therapy 56(1): 78–85

Redfern TR, Wallace WA 1998 History of shoulder replacement surgery. In: Wallace WA (ed) Joint replacement in the shoulder and elbow. Butterworth Heinemann, Oxford

Royal College of Physicians 1999 Osteoporosis – clinical guidelines for prevention and treatment. Royal College of Physicians, London

Santy J 2001 An investigation of the reality of nursing work with orthopaedic patients. Journal of Orthopaedic Nursing 5(1): 22–29

Shapiro JS 1996 The wrist in rheumatoid arthritis. Hand Clinics 12(3): 477–498

Smith JW, Murphy TR, Blair JSG et al 1983 Regional anatomy illustrated. Churchill Livingstone, Edinburgh

Stamm TA, Machold KP, Smolen JS et al 2002 Joint protection and home hand exercises improve hand function in patients with hand osteoarthritis: a randomised controlled trial. Arthritis Care and Research 47: 44–49

Wallace WA 1998a Revision shoulder replacement and rotator cuff problems. In: Wallace WA (ed) Joint replacement in the shoulder and elbow. Butterworth Heinemann, Oxford

Wallace WA 1998b Total elbow replacement. In: Wallace WA (ed) Joint replacement in the shoulder and elbow. Butterworth Heinemann, Oxford

Wallace WA (ed) 1998c Joint replacement in the shoulder and elbow. Butterworth Heinemann, Oxford

Wheeler D 1994 Shoulder and upper limb problems. In: Davis PS (ed) Nursing the orthopaedic patient. Churchill Livingstone, Edinburgh

Wilgis EFS 1997 Distal interphalangeal joint silicone interpositional arthroplasty of the hand. Clinical Orthopaedics and Related Research 342: 38–41

Yamaguchi K, Sethi N, Bauer GS 2002 Postoperative pain control following arthroscopic release of adhesive capsulitis: a short-term retrospective review study of the use of an intra-articular pain catheter. Arthroscopy 18(4): 359–365

Younger ASE, Curran P, McQueen MM 1990 Backslabs and plaster casts: which will best accommodate increasing intracompartmental pressures? Injury 21: 179–181

Zadeh HG, Calvert PT 1998 Recent advances in shoulder arthroplasty. Current Orthopaedics 12: 122–134

Chapter 22

Peripheral nerve injuries

Beverley Wellington

CHAPTER CONTENTS

INTRODUCTION

Nerve injuries are often viewed as complex injuries because of the physiological changes that occur, their medical management and the potential length and complexity of the patient's rehabilitation. Rehabilitation will at best facilitate the patient's complete recovery over a few weeks, months or years but can equally require a patient to adapt to permanent and severely disabling physical, psychological and social changes.

The nervous system is divided into the central nervous system and the peripheral nervous system. The central nervous system (CNS) consists of the brain, spinal cord and cranial nerves I and II; the care of patients with a spinal cord injury is addressed in Chapter 20. The peripheral nervous system (PNS) consists of cranial nerves III–XII, the spinal nerves and their branches.

This chapter focuses on the common peripheral nerve injuries seen in orthopaedic or trauma units. The more complex issues relating to the rehabilitation of severely disabled patients are not explored here in depth; readers interested in such areas are advised to refer to other relevant rehabilitation texts. Many patients with severe nerve injuries are referred to specialist neurological or orthopaedic units that are able to support the patient and their family in the immediate and long term through appropriate surgical and rehabilitation services. Developments in these centres have provided opportunities for orthopaedic nurses to expand specialist nursing roles and services that support patient care both in hospital and in the community.

INJURIES TO PERIPHERAL NERVES

Orthopaedic nurses need to understand the microanatomy and physiology of the PNS and the way injuries to the PNS occur, as these inform the management of such injuries and the related nursing actions.

MICROANATOMY

The microanatomy of nerve structures appears complex but can be thought of as a series of tubes with sheaths surrounding each one.

Each neuron is composed of a cell body, multiple dendrites and usually one axon. The cell body contains a nucleus surrounded by cytoplasm. The dendrites are the receiving portion of a neuron; they are usually short, tapered and branching. The axon must be connected to the cell body in order to be viable. This long, thin, cylindrical projection processes the nerve impulses, passing the impulse on at a synapse to another neuron, muscle fibre or gland cell.

All axons are surrounded by Schwann cells. These begin to form myelin sheaths around the axons during fetal growth. Each Schwann cell spirals around one axon to form the multilayered lipid and protein covering called the myelin sheath; the integrity of this sheath is vital for nerve conduction. When a single Schwann cell wraps around several axons, this forms an unmyelinated sheath (Tortora & Grabowski 2003).

Individual axons are wrapped in collagen, a fibrous tissue sheath called the endoneurium (Fig. 22.1). Clusters of axons are arranged in bundles or fascicles, surrounded by a larger fibrous sheath of connective tissue called the perineurium. The perineurial space is the area between the endoneurium and perineurium layers. A superficial collagen cover, known as the epineurium, then surrounds groups of fascicles and provides the strongest supporting structure of the nerve. The arrangement of the fascicles is more complex in the proximal area of peripheral nerves than at the distal end (Hems 2000).

NERVE RESPONSE TO INJURY

Generally, any part of a neuron detached from its nucleus will degenerate and be destroyed by phagocytes. However, myelinated axons are capable of repair if the cell body is intact and the Schwann cells are active.

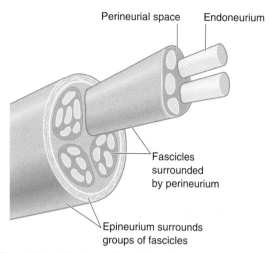

Perineurial space   Endoneurium

Fascicles surrounded by perineurium

Epineurium surrounds groups of fascicles

Figure 22.1   Structures of a peripheral nerve.

The degeneration of the distal part of the axon and myelin sheath is called Wallerian degeneration. This process occurs in stages.

- Two to three days after injury, the damaged distal portion of the nerve will break into fragments and the myelin sheath deteriorates.
- By day 7, the Schwann cells multiply by mitosis and phagocytose the myelin debris.
- By 25–30 days, the axonal debris is cleared and the Schwann cells remain present in the endoneurial tube. As they grow towards each other, they form a regenerated tube across the injured area; this directs any potential growth of a new axon from the proximal to the distal area. The regeneration progresses slowly as the axons are guided across the damaged area with a growth rate of 1–2 mm a day. In time, the Schwann cells form a new myelin sheath.

CLASSIFICATION OF NERVE INJURIES

Nerve injuries are classified according to the extent of the damage to the connective tissue layers. Most widely used is the Seddon classification, described by Sir Herbert John Seddon, Professor of Orthopaedic Surgery, Royal National Orthopaedic Hospital, in 1942. This classification divides nerve injuries into three types of increasing severity.

Neuropraxia: non–working nerve

This is a relatively mild injury, usually due to a compression mechanism. There is a local conduction block with localised demyelination of nerve fibres in the damaged area. The axons remain in continuity and the conduction distal to the injury site is normal. Removing the cause of the compression allows for complete recovery as the Schwann cells repair the demyelination, although it may take days, weeks or months to recover.

Axonotmesis: divided axons

These injuries are usually from a severe blow or, more commonly, from a traction or stretching injury to the nerve. The axons and their myelin sheaths are anatomically disrupted although the endoneurial tubes remain intact. Wallerian degeneration occurs distally to the site of injury, causing nerve conduction to be lost. Recovery is by axon regeneration along the same endoneurial tube at a rate of 1–2 mm a day. Prognosis is good, though sensory function is more completely restored than motor function.

Neurotmesis: whole nerve divided

This injury normally results from a penetrating wound from a high-energy traction injury or stabbing with a knife or glass. The nerve trunk is completely severed with disruption of the axons and connective tissue structures, resulting in distal Wallerian degeneration. There is no recovery unless surgical repair, if deemed appropriate, is undertaken. Following successful surgery, recovery may occur at the rate of 1–2 mm a day, although the quality of recovery is questionable. As the endoneurial tubes and other structures are disrupted, the regenerated nerve fibres often repair with a degree of 'miswiring', resulting in reduced or misconnected impulse transfer which consequently affects the innervation of muscles and organs (Hems 2000).

MECHANISM OF INJURY

Compression

The most frequently presenting nerve injuries are those caused by compression of one or more nerves. The areas commonly affected are the median nerve in the carpal tunnel and the ulnar nerve in the cubital tunnel.

Occasionally these injuries are caused in hospital. For example, the position of a patient on the operating table can lead to the following.

- The ulnar nerve may be damaged when the forearm is extended and pronated or when the elbow is in extreme flexion across the chest.

- The radial nerve can be compressed between the edge of the table and the humerus.
- The sciatic nerve can be damaged if the patient is thin and the table is not padded appropriately.
- The common peroneal nerve can be compressed either against the head of the fibula when the patient is in the lithotomy position or between the fibula and the table when the patient is in the lateral position.

Traction or stretch

These mechanisms are typified by brachial plexus injuries where there is violent displacement of the shoulder girdle and stretching of the sciatic nerve in operations requiring significant lengthening of the lower extremity (Sawyer et al 2000). These injuries are difficult to manage because the severity of the nerve injury may not be clear.

Open wounds

Clinical evidence of a nerve injury needs to be considered when a patient presents with a compound fracture, gunshot wound or penetrating injuries from a weapon such as glass or a knife.

DIAGNOSIS

An accurate diagnosis of the presence and extent of nerve injuries requires a thorough understanding of the anatomy and physiology of the PNS. The diagnosis is based on:

- the patient's presenting history, making it essential to establish the mechanism of injury
- a clinical examination that includes motor and sensory findings
- neurological investigations, for example nerve conduction studies and electromyography.

Nerve conduction studies are performed to evaluate the sensory and motor responses of the peripheral nerves anywhere along their course. Stimulation of a peripheral nerve should evoke a contraction in the muscle that it supplies. Electromyography is used to record motor activity at rest and on attempted contraction of a muscle.

The level of dysfunction is graded using the MRC classification (Box 22.1). Additional factors affecting the prognosis of nerve injury repair need to be taken into account at the time of diagnosis as they impact

Box 22.1 Assessing the return of muscle function after nerve injuries (Medical Research Council cited in Birch et al 1998)

Motor function

M0 =	no contraction
M1 =	return of perceptible contraction in proximal muscles
M2 =	return of perceptible contraction in proximal and distal muscles
M3 =	return of proximal and distal muscle power enough for all important major muscles to act against resistance
M4 =	return of function as stage 3 + synergic and independent movement possible
M5 =	complete recovery

Sensory function

S0 =	absence of sensibility in the autonomous area
S1 =	recovery of deep cutaneous pain within the autonomous area of the nerve
S2 =	return of some degree of superficial cutaneous pain and touch in the autonomous area
S3 =	return of some superficial cutaneous pain and touch in the autonomous area with disappearance of previous overreaction
S3+/S4=	as stage 3 with some recovery of 2-point discrimination in the autonomous area
S4/S5=	complete recovery

on the decisions made about the patient's management; these include the patient's age and the severity and level of the injury.

- **Patient's age**: the prognosis and results of nerve repair are less favourable with increasing age.
- **Severity of injury**: Seddon's classification relates the severity of injury to the expected outcomes. The condition of the nerve ends at the time of injury affects the prognosis; for example, a clean-cut nerve will repair better than a jagged cut nerve. Injuries associated with skin loss, vascular damage, soft tissue compromise and fractures are less likely to provide a satisfactory outcome. The risk of infection from compound injuries will also influence the outcome.
- **Level of injury**: generally, more proximal lesions have a lower success rate than distal lesions, principally because the proximal injury will affect a larger nerve bundle, nerve distribution and functional area.

FEATURES OF NERVE INJURIES

Horner's syndrome

This condition, first described in 1869 by Friedrich Horner, a Swiss ophthalmologist, occurs from a disorder of the sympathetic nerves in the brainstem or damage to the superior sympathetic trunk in the cervical region.

It is commonly associated with brachial plexus injuries, with patients presenting with (Hems 2000):

- **miosis/myosis**: a constricted pupil
- **ptosis**: a drooping upper eyelid
- **anhidrosis**: facial dryness because of a lack of sweating.

Tinel's sign

Described in 1917 by the French neurologist Jules Tinel, this sign indicates an injury to the nerve trunk from compression or percussion. The patient reports a tingling sensation in the cutaneous (sensory distribution) region of the nerve. This is often described as an 'electric shock' feeling or like 'ants crawling over the skin'. This descriptive sensation is known as formication. A progressive Tinel's sign, where the area of tingling sensation gradually increases, is encouraging as it indicates the course of nerve regeneration but does not always mean that complete recovery from the nerve injury will occur.

Autonomic function

When a peripheral nerve is disrupted, there is a vasomotor reaction and loss of sweating (anhidrosis). Initially, the area affected becomes pink from vasodilation, before becoming pale, cold and mottled in appearance. This can spread out from the area supplied by the nerve with atrophy of the fingers and nails occurring. If sweating is still present, the nerve damage is probably incomplete.

Nerve injury pain

The physiology and management of pain are discussed in full in Chapter 7. The issues raised here relate specifically to nerve pain.

The physiology of pain can be divided into two classifications: nociceptive and neuropathic. Nociceptive pain involves four basic principles (Wood 2003).

1 **Transduction of pain**: this process starts at the periphery of the site of cell damage. The cell

damage is caused by a mechanical, thermal or chemical noxious stimulus. The damaged cell releases excitatory neurotransmitters, which then activate the C-fibres and A-fibres. An action potential occurs and a pain impulse is transmitted.

2 **Transmission of pain**: this process occurs in three segments: along the nociceptor fibres to the spinal cord, from the spinal cord to the brainstem and through connections between the thalamus and cortex.

3 **Perception of pain**: this is when the pain becomes a conscious experience from activation of multiple cortical areas, including the reticular system, somatosensory cortex and the limbic system.

4 **Modulation of pain**: here the pain impulses are changed or inhibited. This process explains the wide variation of patient perceptions of pain.

Acute, normal, nociceptive pain results from a high-intensity stimulus at the nerve endings. The pain messages are carried via an intact nervous system, which relays pain messages from nociceptors through C-fibres to the spinal cord and brain. Inflammatory pain results from tissue damage at the peripheral nerve endings. Whilst the causes of inflammatory pain are different, the messages are carried in a similar way via the C-fibres to the spinal cord and brain (Pasero et al 1999).

The pathophysiology of neuropathic pain mechanisms is uncertain but includes changes to the nervous system resulting in the spontaneous generation of pain impulses along the C-fibres. Damage to the peripheral nervous system can also result in physiological changes, where pain signals in the nerve and central neurons are reorganised. A-fibres can be rewired so that normal, non-painful impulses such as pressure and touch result in the transmission of pain messages to the brain (Birch et al 1998, Wilson 2002, Wood 2003).

Neuropathic pain (Table 22.1) is a complex phenomenon, that causes distress for patients and can be difficult for the healthcare team to treat successfully.

Diagnosis of neuropathic pain. An accurate assessment and measurement of the patient's pain provides nurses with the information required to achieve appropriate pain relief. There are various pain measurement tools, including unidimensional visual analogue and verbal rating scales and the multidimensional McGill Pain Questionnaire, which provides qualitative and quantitative data.

Table 22.1 Neuropathic pain terms

Term	Definition
Allodynia	Hypersensitivity to usually non-painful stimuli of mechanical or thermal origin such as touch, cold or heat
Causalgia	Pain resulting from an injury to a major nerve, typically giving an intense burning pain. Often referred to as complex regional pain syndrome 2 (CRPS2)
Dysaesthesia	An unpleasant normal sensation
Hyperalgesia (hyperpathia)	An exaggerated pain response from painful stimuli
Hyperaesthesia	Excessive sensitivity, especially of the skin
Neuralgia	Pain in the nerve distribution area, described by patients as burning, aching, electric shock, tingling, shooting, jumping and paroxysmal where the pain is worsening or reoccurring
Reflex sympathetic dystrophy (algodystrophy)	Often known as complex regional pain syndrome 1 (CRPS1). This syndrome involves a cycle of pain and dysfunction, leading to a chronic state of sympathetic hyperactivity. It is important to recognise the condition early and to break the cycle

Fundamental to the pain assessment process is the need to take the patient's general medical history and their specific pain history, along with a thorough clinical examination. Defining and measuring the pain using the patient's terms and descriptions of their experiences gives a patient-centred assessment, increasing their involvement in their pain management and their confidence in the healthcare team. For some patients, especially those with chronic neuropathic pain, this can be the first time they feel their pain has been taken seriously by a team that is interested in helping them to adapt to and manage their life.

Consequences of neuropathic pain. The nature of this pain is multidimensional, affecting the patient in many different ways with degrees of physiological, psychosocial, economical and behavioural effects. These in turn affect the patient's quality of life including (Gureje et al 1998):

- changes to general health causing insomnia, fatigue, loss of appetite, weight loss and reduced mobility
- disruption of activities including self-care and all activities of daily living, housework and child-care, sports, hobbies and work, which can result in loss of employment with additional financial implications
- psychosocial function, which can be either decreased, from changes in concentration, memory, self-esteem, self-confidence, sense of control, auton-omy and libido, or an increased psychosocial func-tion that manifests as despair, depression, anxiety, frustration, anger, dependence on others and a focus on the pain.

Neuropathic pain management. Ashburn & Staats (1999) define the goal of therapy as the control of pain combined with rehabilitation, enabling the patient to function as well as possible. There are various modes of treatment, grouped here as phar-macological or non-pharmacological management (Wood 2003).

Pharmacological management involves the use of the principal drugs of pain management. Many patients find that a range or combination of medica-tions is needed for different circumstances.

- Simple analgesia, for instance paracetamol and co-proxamol, has a limited use in neuropathic pain.
- COX-1 and COX-2 NSAIDs, for example ibu-profen, diclofenac and rofecoxib, are rarely effective for neuropathic pain but can be used during the acute inflammatory phase.
- Opioids, for example morphine, tramadol and dihydrocodeine, are more useful for visceral and cancer pain, although an analgesic effect can be achieved with high doses.
- Tricyclic antidepressants such as amitriptyline, imipramine and lofepramine usually result in an improved sleep pattern, mood and anxiety but care-ful dosage monitoring is essential.
- Anticonvulsants, for instance carbamazepine, phenytoin and gabapentin, are not licensed in all countries for use with neuropathic pain but are use-ful for electric shock type pain.
- Local anaesthesia, principally with lidocaine (lignocaine), is useful for continuous dysaesthesia.
- Muscle relaxants such as baclofen and diazepam are commonly used for musculoskeletal pain.

- Topical treatments using EMLA cream and capsaicin can be useful for allodynia.
- Nerve blocks have a variable reputation with conflicting data suggesting that the analgesic effect is minimal. They are often ineffective in neuro-pathic pain but can be of use with complex regional pain syndrome (CRPS).

The non-pharmacological methods do not replace medications but are adjuncts that improve the patient's overall pain management. Many patients will try different therapies, accessing these either through their healthcare team or privately.

- Transcutaneous electrical nerve stimulation (TENS) is a patient-controlled non-invasive treatment.
- Cryoanalgesia provides pain relief through the application of cold. It needs to be used with caution if patients have thermal allodynia.
- Behavioural therapy is generally through pain management programmes involving physiother-apy, psychotherapy and education approaches. This often involves using stress management, relaxation and pain modulation techniques such as guided imagery.
- Alternative therapists using acupuncture, chiropractic, osteopathy, homeopathy, hypnotherapy and reflexology techniques aim to treat the patient holistically. These are valuable for some but not all patients.

Nurses need to ensure the patient's pain is man-aged appropriately, as it can make a real difference to the patient's quality of life. Continued and poorly treated pain has a human cost in terms of the activ-ities of daily living undertaken by the patient and a financial cost to the health service and society.

BRACHIAL PLEXUS INJURIES

A plexus is a network of nerves. The union of five spinal nerves from C5 to C8 and T1 forms the brachial plexus. Occasionally there is a significant contribution from the fourth cervical nerve root, when the plexus is described as 'prefixed', or the second thoracic root, when the plexus is described as 'postfixed'.

The brachial plexus is arranged into a series of roots, trunks, divisions and cords (Fig. 22.2). The brachial plexus descends into the posterior triangle of the neck, between the scalenus anterior and

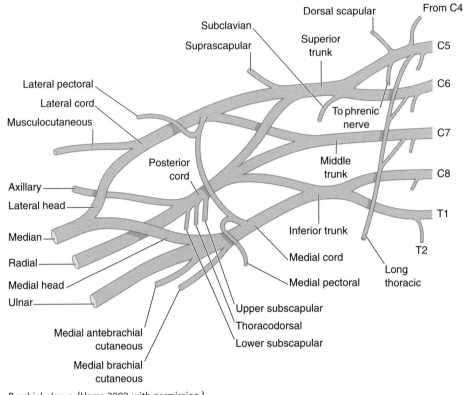

Figure 22.2   Brachial plexus. (Hems 2003 with permission.)

medius muscles. The roots are the ventral rami anterior branches of the spinal nerves; the ventral rami of C5 and C6 unite to form the upper trunk, C7 forms the middle trunk and the ventral rami of C8 and T1 unite to form the lower trunk. Each trunk divides into an anterior and a posterior division, which lie in the supraclavicular triangle.

The anterior divisions form the lateral and medial cords and the posterior divisions form the posterior cord. The cords are so named because of the position they occupy in relation to the axillary nerve.

- The posterior cord from C5 and C6 gives rise to the axillary nerve.
- The posterior cord from C5 to C8 and T1 gives rise to the radial nerve.
- The lateral cord from C5–7 gives rise to the musculocutaneous nerve.
- The lateral and medial cords, from C6–T1, give rise to the median nerve.

- The medial cord, from C8 and T1, gives rise to the ulnar nerve.

Each nerve has sensory and motor components (Tortora & Grabowski 2003); the cutaneous nerve supply of the arm is shown in Figure 22.3.

CAUSES OF INJURY

Injuries to the brachial plexus are of great importance because of the potentially devastating damage that can occur. There are various classifications of these injuries but commonly they are referred to as open or closed injuries. Open injuries are caused by penetrating wounds from a weapon or missile such as a knife, glass or gunshot. Closed injuries result from:

- a traction injury from a violent pulling or stretching force between the shoulder girdle and the clavicle

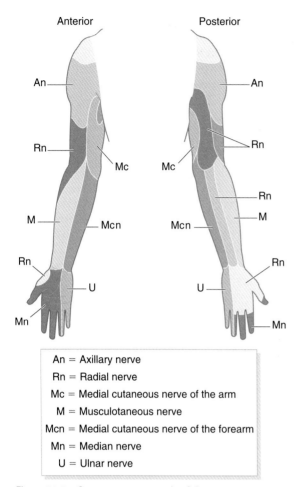

Anterior

Posterior

An

An

Rn

Rn

Mc

Mc

Rn

M

Mcn

Mcn

M

Rn

Rn

U

U

Mn

Mn

An = Axillary nerve

Rn = Radial nerve

Mc = Medial cutaneous nerve of the arm

M = Musculotaneous nerve

Mcn = Medial cutaneous nerve of the forearm

Mn = Median nerve

U = Ulnar nerve

Figure 22.3   Cutaneous nerve supply of the arm.

- compression of the plexus from adjacent injured tissues
- crushing of the plexus from blunt trauma to the neck and upper limb
- malignant infiltration at the base of the neck, with or without radiation-induced damage
- perinatal or obstetric palsys often referred to as Erb's or Klumpke's palsy.

LEVELS OF INJURY

Brachial plexus injuries occur at different levels, although many are at several levels.

A preganglionic lesion involves avulsion of the spinal nerve root from the spinal cord at a point proximal to the dorsal root ganglion. The thoraco-scapular muscles are supplied by the C5–7 nerve roots arising from the plexus close to the spine; paralysis of these muscles indicates proximal plexus damage. The clinical signs include:

- severe pain in an anaesthetic arm
- paralysis of the thoracoscapular muscles; normally the rhomboids retract the shoulder and serratus anterior stabilises the scapula to stop it 'winging'
- a positive Horner's syndrome
- swelling in the posterior triangle of the neck.

Preganglionic injuries are largely irreparable and have a poor prognosis. However, new innovative surgical techniques, where the ventral motor roots are repaired within the spinal canal, may offer hope for some patients in the future.

A postganglionic lesion involves rupture of the nerve root distal to the ganglion. If an assessment to determine the function of the thoracoscapular muscles elicits a positive action, the lesion is assumed to be postganglionic. There may be a neurotmesis where there is a complete nerve tear or division at the level of the plexus trunk, division or cord. Other clinical signs include an absence of pain, absent Horner's syndrome, sparing of the rhomboids and serratus anterior and a positive Tinel's sign. This injury will not recover spontaneously but has the potential to recover following surgical repair by suturing or grafting.

Plexus injuries are also described as supraclavicular or infraclavicular but there is a possibility of damage both above and below the clavicle.

Supraclavicular injuries to the upper brachial plexus involve the C5 and C6 nerve roots. Except for perinatal palsy, the most common mechanism of injury is a motorcycle accident. The bike rider hits the ground landing on their shoulder, the head is forced in the opposite direction creating a jerking, pulling or stretching force that separates the neck and shoulder, causing immense strain on the nerve roots. The main nerves affected in upper brachial plexus injuries are the axillary, musculocutaneous and suprascapular, resulting in a loss of shoulder abduction and external rotation, elbow flexion and forearm supination. Sensation is lost from the outer arm and hand. The degree of recovery depends on the extent of the damage.

Infraclavicular injuries to the lower brachial plexus involve the C8 and T1 nerve roots. These are less common injuries usually associated with an obstetric paralysis such as Klumpke's palsy. An injury here mainly affects the ulnar nerve, resulting in paralysis of the wrist and finger flexors, along with all the intrinsic muscles of the hand. There is also decreased sensation in the skin along the ulnar side of the forearm and hand.

If the entire plexus is damaged, there is flaccid paralysis of the entire arm with anaesthesia. It is important to determine the mechanism of injury as a high-velocity trauma may result in more complex injuries with damage potentially occurring at several levels. It is also vital to establish how far from the spinal cord the lesion is.

MANAGEMENT OF BRACHIAL PLEXUS INJURIES

For a confirmed diagnosis, it is vital to perform radiological tests to exclude other injuries to the head, neck and chest. A CT or MRI scan will show any avulsed dorsal spinal nerve sleeves. Neurophysiology tests are performed to study nerve conduction but they are not usually undertaken during the acute phase.

The medical management and nursing care will vary depending on the cause and type of injury. Closed injuries are often associated with a neuropraxia or axonotmesis; these should recover spontaneously as a surgical repair is only necessary after neurotmesis. If the injury is open, early surgical exploration is essential with early repair of the divided nerves if possible; simultaneous vascular repair may also be required. Patients treated conservatively must be followed up closely in the first few months and only if there is no clear evidence of recovery at this time is a surgical exploration considered.

Surgical options

With any neurosurgery, it is essential to have accurate restoration of the nerve ends within a healthy tissue bed and with no tension. There are a number of surgical options available to deal with brachial plexus injuries, depending on the particular nerve diagnosis.

Direct nerve suturing. The nerve ends must be placed in the correct pattern of alignment to minimise crossover or miswiring during the healing and recovery process. Guidance for the positioning of the nerves is provided by the nerve fascicles and surface blood vessels; the sutures are placed in the epineurium layer.

Nerve grafting. This is performed when direct nerve suturing is not possible. A length of nerve trunk considered expendable is harvested and cut up. This allows a number of strands to be used, building up a thickness similar to the nerve trunk being repaired. The nerves normally used for harvesting are the sural nerve in the leg and the medial cutaneous nerve in the forearm. The sural nerve is formed by the medial and lateral cutaneous sural branches from the common peroneal nerve. It provides sensation to the skin at the back and side of the lower leg, winding round the back of the lateral side of the ankle and lateral side of the foot. The medial cutaneous nerve originates from C8 and T1 roots and supplies the skin of the middle and posterior aspects of the forearm.

Nerve transfers. This allows a nerve to be transferred with its connection to the spinal cord and attached to the end of the nerve that has lost its spinal cord connection.

Following any of the above surgical procedures, the limb is immobilised to reduce tension on the suture line. The period of immobilisation depends on the severity of the injury and extent of the surgery. Following immobilisation, physiotherapy exercises are introduced to maintain a passive range of movements in all joints. Clinical monitoring will indicate if the nerve is recovering at the expected rate with a progressive Tinel's sign showing increased sensation that advances by approximately 1 mm per day, demonstrating the presence of axonal regeneration (Hems 2000).

The final outcome of brachial plexus reconstruction may take 2 or 3 years to become apparent. The main goal of treatment is to restore motor function to the M4 level of recovery (see Box 22.1). Of particular importance is promoting elbow flexion and to enable this, a variety of surgical interventions can be required.

Tendon transfer. Various muscles can be used to act as elbow flexors. The nerve supply to these muscles must stay intact but their original muscle function is sacrificed to replace or enhance another.

Free muscle transfer or transplantation. This is routinely performed for restoration of elbow flexors and wrist extensors. A variety of muscles are used including the latissimus dorsi, rectus femoris and gracilis. Two or three intercostal nerves are then used to innervate these muscles.

Shoulder arthrodesis. This is reserved for unstable or painful shoulders, the position being tailored to the individual patient.

Rehabilitation

The complex nature of these injuries creates a variety of challenges, both physical and psychological, that affect the patient's rehabilitation and long-term care. The aim of rehabilitation is to facilitate the patient's return to society, in a state of physical and psychological well-being.

The unaffected arm overperforms to compensate for the affected arm, making it more prone to stress-related injuries, resulting in bursitis, tendonitis, carpal tunnel syndrome and muscle strains.

Neuropathic pain can become protracted and as the cause is generally poorly understood it is difficult to treat. Care is focused on enabling the patient to adapt to their chronic pain so the involvement of the chronic pain team is essential to provide patient care and long-term support.

A brachial plexus injury can be life changing. It is important to provide as much information as possible for the patient but false expectations must be avoided. Many patients have difficulty understanding the nature of a brachial plexus injury and as every injury can be so different, they and their families find it hard to comprehend the diagnosis and treatment, especially as many of the expected outcomes following brachial plexus injuries are initially vague and rely on the passage of time to determine the prognosis.

Support and counselling must be offered from the outset and continue as patients face a long and slow period of treatment and rehabilitation with the ongoing nature of care often causing anxiety and depression. Recognition, treatment and monitoring of these conditions should be of the utmost importsance in the holistic care provided.

If the affected arm is noticeably disabled, the patient is likely to express concerns about their body image and how they appear to others. Having a flail arm with little or no motor function is most noticeable when attempting to perform basic activities of daily living. These limitations can lead to increased dependence on others and affect social and sexual relationships, which are placed under extreme pressure. Patients experience mood swings, frustration, anger and even guilt. Employment and financial problems need to be addressed soon after the injury with referral to the appropriate agencies.

If there is little or no recovery of limb function, an artificial brace or support for the limb is custom made. The orthosis works on biomechanical principles with the main function of maintaining the correct position of the upper arm and shoulder. These can be bulky and rather obtrusive when worn.

PERINATAL BRACHIAL PALSY

Perinatal or obstetric brachial palsy occurs when traction forces are applied to the fetus during birth causing any of the three classifications of injury: neuropraxia, axonotmesis and neurotmesis.

There are three groups of perinatal brachial plexus palsy described as upper, lower and total palsy.

Upper brachial plexus palsy

This is the most commonly affected area of the plexus. The injuries are also referred to as Erb–Duchenne palsy or simply Erb's palsy.

These injuries are due to traction on the shoulder girdle resulting in damage to the upper nerve roots of C5, C6 and possibly C7, the cause normally being:

- macrosomia: the excessive growth of the fetus, usually with enlarged organs
- forceps delivery
- shoulder dystocia: manoeuvres used to deliver the shoulder with downward traction.

The baby lies with the arm adducted, elbow flexed, forearm pronated, with the wrist and fingers flexed, typically known as the 'waiter's tip' position (Hems 2000).

Conservative management is advised as there is usually a good prognosis. However, if the baby has reached 3–6 months of age and has failed to regain elbow flexion or there is complete limb paralysis, then surgery is considered.

Lower brachial plexus palsy

Injuries to the lower plexus, known as Klumpke's paralysis or palsy, are the least common of this range of injuries.

It is generally associated with breech births where the baby's arm is pulled upwards and hyper-extended to be delivered with the head and not before it, leading to trauma of the lower nerve roots of C8 and T1. The baby has a 'claw hand' deformity with a poor hand grasp and loss of sensation due to the damage affecting the wrist and finger flexors and the intrinsic muscles of the hand.

A full evaluation of the arm function is needed during the baby's early months, followed by conservative management with an emphasis on exercises to promote any potential function.

Total brachial plexus palsy

A total palsy is the most devastating of all obstetric brachial palsies, leaving the baby with a flail and insensate arm (Dodds & Wolfe 2000, Pollack et al 2000) that cannot be treated.

UPPER LIMB NERVE INJURIES

RADIAL NERVE INJURIES

The radial nerve is the most frequently injured major nerve in the upper limb. The nerve exits the brachial plexus from the posterior cord, having contributions from the C5–8 and T1 spinal nerves. It supplies most of the posterior skin of the arm and the motor branches innervate the extensor muscles of the upper limb, producing elbow extension, supination of the forearm, extension of the wrist and fingers, plus abduction of the thumb (Tortora & Grabowski 2003).

The nerve travels along the shaft of humerus near the spiral groove and runs posterolaterally beneath the lateral head of the triceps (Lowe et al 2002a); any injury in these areas can affect the nerve function. Among the causes of radial nerve injury are the following.

- Fractures of the humerus shaft, for example a spiral fracture of the distal shaft with radial angulation resulting in a radial nerve paralysis.
- Dislocation of the radial head creates a traction injury; the resultant paralysis is usually temporary. Such dislocations are associated with a Monteggia fracture or a complex distal humeral fracture.
- Radial nerve compression occurs when the arm hangs from a trolley or over the back of a chair while the patient is asleep or inebriated. This is commonly referred to as Saturday night palsy (McRae & Kinninmonth 1997).
- Postoperative radial nerve palsy is also associated with the use of a tourniquet or blood pressure cuff.
- Other causes include direct nerve trauma from open wounds, triceps compression which can occur after strenuous activity, tumours and idiopathic neuritis (Lowe et al 2002a).

Typically, patients present with a decrease in their hand power grip and pinch, possibly with a sensory loss over the dorsum of the thumb and the first web space. Wrist drop occurs with severe injuries from paralysis of the wrist extensors, resulting in the hand being flexed at the wrist and flaccid.

As with all peripheral nerve injuries, a complete patient history and clinical examination are essential to establish the level of injury and the suspected cause. The Seddon classification system is used and the appropriate treatment option then considered.

All patients with true radial nerve palsy require a 'cock-up' wrist support and exercises to prevent joint stiffness or permanent loss of function.

An open injury is explored surgically and if the nerve is transected but retains its length with minimal soft tissue damage, a primary repair is performed. Closed injuries are more complex to manage, often requiring electrodiagnostic studies to determine the level and extent of the radial nerve injury before identifying a plan of care (Lowe et al 2002b). Tendon transfers are considered if nerve reconstruction fails or is not feasible; this can restore some wrist and finger extension function. Nerve transfers are performed as an alternative to tendon transfers when patients present late or with a high-level nerve injury causing radial nerve paralysis.

MEDIAN NERVE INJURIES

The median nerve exits the brachial plexus via two branches, the medial cord supplied by C8 and T1 and the lateral cord at C5–7. The nerve supplies the anterior forearm and most of the flexor muscles activating pronation of the forearm, wrist and finger flexion and opposition of the thumb. Sensory supply is to the lateral side of the palm, thumb, index, middle and lateral half of ring finger (Tortora & Grabowski 2003).

The median nerve is commonly injured at the forearm or wrist, for example from lacerations to the forearm and 'wrist slashing' suicide attempts. Other causes include associated distal radius fractures and compression in the carpal tunnel.

Patients present with paraesthesia along the distribution of the nerve with:

- loss of sensation in the lateral half of the palm
- paralysis of the forearm pronators, the wrist flexors and fingers
- loss of flexion at the index finger and thumb interphalangeal joints
- loss of opposition and abduction of the thumb.

Once the cause of injury has been determined, the appropriate management commences. For instance, an open wound should be explored or if carpal tunnel syndrome is suspected, a decompression is performed.

ULNAR NERVE INJURIES

The ulnar nerve arises from the medial cord of the brachial plexus with nerve fibres from C8 and T1 and in some patients from C7. It runs down the medial side of the arm and forearm supplying the skin on the medial aspect of the hand, the little finger and half of the ring finger. Its main action is in the hand where it supplies most of the small muscles, the two inner lumbricals and all interossei, to enable wrist, ring and little finger flexion and wrist adduction (Tortora & Grabowski 2003).

The nerve is commonly injured as it passes through the cubital tunnel at the elbow, often in association with fractures of the medial epicondyle of the humerus or from external pressure when the forearm is extended and pronated.

The patient will experience loss of sensation over the sensory pathway of the nerve distribution. The inability to spread out the fingers and flex the metacarpophalangeal joints or extend the interphalangeal joints results in a 'claw hand'. Hypothenar wasting and inability to flex the thumb also occur.

If cubital tunnel syndrome is diagnosed, a surgical decompression is advised. Otherwise, splinting of the hand to maintain a functional position is undertaken, along with exercises to prevent further joint stiffness (Birch et al 1998).

AXILLARY NERVE INJURIES

The axillary nerve originates from C5 and C6, branching off from the posterior cord of the plexus. It leaves the axilla and runs to the inferior aspect of the shoulder joint. It innervates the deltoid and teres minor muscles and provides sensation to the outer shoulder area over the lower half of the deltoid (Tortora & Grabowski 2003).

Injuries to the axillary nerve are commonly associated with dislocations of the shoulder joint; due to the proximity of the nerve to the surgical neck of the humerus, paralysis can occur following fractures in this area (Perlmutter 1999). Axillary nerve injuries result in a patch of anaesthesia over the outer aspect of the arm over the deltoid tuberosity, known as the 'sergeant's patch'. The deltoid function is affected, leading to a weakened shoulder function with loss of arm abduction.

It is essential to determine the underlying cause of injury and then treat accordingly. The patient must maintain their passive and active range of movement through regular exercises. A nerve transfer or graft is possible; if successful, deltoid renervation should show after 3–4 months.

MUSCULOCUTANEOUS NERVE INJURIES

The musculocutaneous nerve is the major end branch from the lateral cord of the brachial plexus arising from C5–7. It runs superficially within the anterior arm, supplying the skin of the anterior and lateral areas of the forearm, innervating the elbow flexors, the biceps brachii and brachioradialis. These areas and functions are therefore affected in any injury to the nerve.

THORACIC OUTLET SYNDROME

When the brachial plexus is compressed by a rib or band of fibrous tissue, it causes pain, numbness and tingling over the neck and shoulders along with weakness in the hands. Treatment is by improving the posture and strengthening the shoulders and neck with exercise. Operative measures may involve removal of the rib or fibrous tissue causing the problem.

LOWER LIMB NERVE INJURIES

SCIATIC NERVE INJURIES

The sciatic nerve is the largest branch of the sacral plexus, formed from the roots of L4, 5 and S1–3 spinal nerves. It divides into two nerves, the tibial and the common peroneal, that diverge proximal to the knee (Tortora & Grabowski 2003).

The nerve is occasionally injured by wounds but is commonly associated with acetabular fractures, especially posterior fracture dislocations of the hip joint when there is displacement through the greater sciatic notch. The three main nerves, the obturator, femoral and sciatic, are vulnerable during hip surgery, for example during hip arthroplasty surgery, but the sciatic nerve is the most frequently damaged. It can be 'nicked' or cut during the surgical exposure, stretched by traction during dislocation or after the prosthesis is inserted. Additional causes are damage from malpositioning of a retractor, by external compression from a haematoma or by the insertion of the circlage wire used to reattach the greater trochanter (Birch et al 1998, Russell et al 2001).

The patient typically presents with a loss of sensation below the knee, except at the medial border of the foot as the saphenous nerve supplys this area. Paralysis of the hamstrings causes an inability to flex the knee and weakness of ankle dorsiflexion results in plantar flexion or foot drop.

The prognosis is poor, particularly in proximal injuries. Management is mainly conservative, utilising orthosis and symptom control.

COMMON PERONEAL (LATERAL POPLITEAL) INJURIES

The common peroneal nerve originates from the sciatic nerve in the posterior aspect of the thigh and wraps around the head and neck of the fibula, just below the lateral side of the knee. It passes through the fibular tunnel before dividing into superficial and deep branches. These innervate the foot extensors (dorsiflexors) in the anterior compartment and the skin to the dorsum of the foot (Tortora & Grabowski 2003).

It is the most frequently damaged nerve in the lower limb. As it originates from the sciatic nerve, any sciatic nerve lesion proximal to this point will affect the common peroneal nerve as well.

The nerve is sensitive to injury from fracture dislocations around the knee (Sawyer et al 2000).

Pressure over the fibular head from restrictive casts or bandages can pose a problem but the symptoms are nearly always relieved when the pressure is removed. In the operating theatre, a patient in the lateral position is at particular risk from pressure of the fibular head against an operating table, causing compression of the nerve.

Patients often complain of difficulty in walking and dragging their foot on the ground when taking a step forward. This is from an inability to pull the foot and toes up in dorsiflexion and inability to evert the foot. There may also be paraesthesia or complete numbness on the top of the foot.

If the nerve injury is associated with compression by a tight-fitting cast, this must be removed. For any other suspected cause, a surgical exploration may be undertaken. An orthosis may be useful for the patient to regain an improved walking pattern.

CONCLUSION

Many nerve injuries occur with or as a result of musculoskeletal injuries and disorders. The changes that occur as a result can be short or long term, from mild alterations in sensation to severe chronic pain with no controlled movements. The changes in self-image can be equally varied depending on the person's ability to cope. The healthcare team need to enable the patient to adapt to these symptoms and changes in their physical, psychological, social and economic status, through appropriate support and rehabilitation care, the aim being to help them live as independently as possible.

Relevant websites

www.tbpiukgroup.homestead.com
This site is written by and for people who have a trauma brachial plexus injury, to provide them with support and information. Useful for healthcare professionals and provides a patient perspective.

www.orthoteers.co.uk
Originally developed for postgraduate orthopaedic trainees preparing for their FRCS exam, the Orthoteer orthopaedic education resource claims to be the largest orthopaedic e-textbook.

www.1uphealth.com
This provides comprehensive medical information on a range of topics, useful for health professionals and patients alike.

www.rad.washington.edu
This site contains online teaching material with radiographic displays and patient information links.

References

Ashburn MA, Staats PS 1999 Management of chronic pain. Lancet 353: 1865–1869

Birch R, Bonney G, Wynn Parry CB 1998 Surgical disorders of the peripheral nerves. Churchill Livingstone, Edinburgh

Dodds SD, Wolfe SW 2000 Perinatal brachial plexus palsy. Current Opinion in Orthopaedics 11(3): 202–209

Gureje O, von Korff M, Simon GE 1998 Persistent pain and well-being: a WHO study in primary care. Journal of the American Medical Association 280: 147–151

Hems TJ 2000 Nerves. In: Russell RCG, Williams NS, Bulstrode CJK (eds) Bailey and Love's short practice of surgery, 23rd edn. Arnold, London

Hems TJ 2003 Guidelines on the management and transfer of brachial plexus injury. Available online at: www.show.scot.nhs.uk/sguht/brachialplexus

Lowe JB III, Sen SK, Mackinnon SE 2002a Current approach to radial nerve paralysis. Plastic and Reconstructive Surgery 110(4): 1099–1113

Lowe JB III, Tung TR, Mackinnon SE 2002b New surgical option for radial nerve paralysis. Plastic and Reconstructive Surgery 110(3): 836–843

McRae R, Kinninmonth AWG 1997 Orthopaedics and trauma. Churchill Livingstone, Edinburgh

Pasero C, Paice JA, McCaffrey C 1999 Basic mechanisms underlying the causes and effects of pain. In: Wall PD, Melzack R (eds) Textbook of pain, 4th edn. Churchill Livingstone, Edinburgh

Perlmutter GS 1999 Axillary nerve injury. Clinical Orthopaedics and Related Research 368: 28–36

Pollack RN, Buchman AS, Yaffe H 2000 Obstetrical brachial palsy: pathogenesis, risk factors and prevention. Clinical Obstetrics and Gynaecology 43(2): 236–246

Russell GV Jr, Nork SE, Chip Routt ML Jr 2001 Perioperative complications associated with operative treatment of acetabular fractures. Journal of Trauma 51(6): 1098–1103

Sawyer RJ, Richmond MN, Hickey JD 2000 Peripheral nerve injuries associated with anaesthesia. Anaesthesia 55(10): 980–991

Tortora GJ, Grabowski SR 2003 Principles of anatomy and physiology. Wiley, New York

Wilson M 2002 Overcoming the challenge of neuropathic pain. Nursing Standard 16(33): 47–53

Wood S 2003 Pain management. Emap Healthcare, Thanet Press, London

Chapter 23

Care of patients with a pelvic injury

Julia D Kneale

CHAPTER CONTENTS

INTRODUCTION

The safe and effective management of patients with pelvic injuries creates a challenge for all clinical staff. According to Hakim et al (1996), pelvic fractures represent 3% of all skeletal injuries, with unstable injuries having the highest morbidity and mortality rate at 10–40% (Engle & Gruen 1993). Patients can present with complex problems, requiring a multi-faceted, multispecialty approach to their physical, psychological and social care. The orthopaedic nurse must be aware of the implications arising from the skeletal trauma, soft tissue trauma and associated major injuries. The nursing challenges include hypovolaemic shock, pain and coordination of the multidisciplinary team to ensure high-quality care.

This chapter reviews the nursing management through discussion of:

- the assessment of a patient presenting with a pelvic injury
- an overview of treatment options for pelvic, acetabular, sacral and coccyx injuries
- nursing management, including care of a patient with hypovolaemic shock
- the potential risks of pelvic soft tissue trauma.

The implications of injury during pregnancy and paediatric considerations are touched on but readers are encouraged to review these sections in line with critical care, maternity and paediatric texts for more specific information.

The classification of pelvic and acetabular fractures is not discussed in detail; readers are referred instead to relevant texts listed under References at the end of this chapter.

PELVIC ANATOMY

The pelvis is in two halves, each composed of three separate bones: the pubis anteriorly and inferiorly, the ischium posteriorly and inferiorly, and the ilium superiorly. They meet at the acetabulum, which encloses the femoral head, provides stability and allows a wide range of movements. Although the three bones are fused in adults to form each half of the pelvis, they are still referred to as three separate bones to distinguish the different sections (Fig. 23.1).

The two halves join anteriorly at the fibrocartilaginous symphysis pubis joint and posteriorly link to the sacrum at the sacroiliac joints. The bones are mainly cancellous tissue with a thin overlying cortex.

The pelvic ring is defined as being the pelvic bones, sacrum and coccyx, which together form a basin (Fig. 23.2). The greater or false pelvis is the upper portion bounded laterally by the iliac crests, posteriorly by the lumbar spine and anteriorly by the abdominal wall. This forms the abdominal cavity, protecting the bladder when full and the uterus in pregnancy.

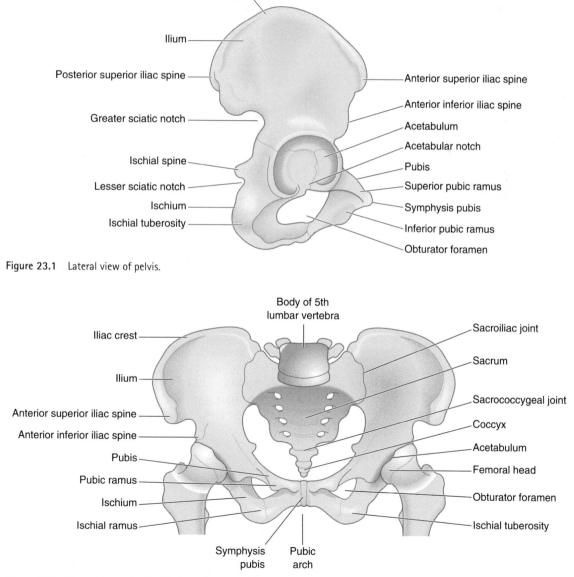

Figure 23.1   Lateral view of pelvis.

Figure 23.2   The pelvis: anatomical features (male pelvis).

Table 23.1   Gender differences in pelvic anatomy

Feature	Female	Male
False pelvis	Shallow	Deep
Pelvic inlet	Wide and oval	Narrow and heart shaped
Ilium	Wider and flatter	More vertical
Iliac fossa	Shallow	Deep
Iliac crest	Gentler curve	Pronounced curve
Acetabulum	Relatively small	Large
Obturator foramen	Oval	Round
Pubic symphysis	Relatively shallow	Deeper
Pubic arch	Greater than 90°	Less than 90°

Box 23.1   Functions of the pelvis

- To support the organs of digestion, excretion and reproduction.
- Protect the bladder, uterus, female reproductive organs, rectum and iliac blood vessels.
- Provide a strong, stable, mechanical support to carry the weight of the body while allowing ambulation.
- Act as a shock absorber through the ligaments and cancellous bone structures.

The lesser or true pelvis surrounds the pelvic organs, bounded laterally by the inferior ilium and ischium, posteriorly by the sacrum and coccyx, and anteriorly by the pubis. The differences between the male and female pelvis relate to musculature and accommodating pregnancy and childbirth (Table 23.1).

The principal functions of the pelvis (Box 23.1) are to provide stability and movement. The muscles attached to the pelvis allow flexion of the vertebral column, for instance by the iliacus, and movement of the thigh by, for example, the gluteus and adductor muscle groups. Pelvic stability depends on the integrity of the bones, joints and the sacroiliac ligaments: sacrospinous, sacrotuberous, anterior and posterior sacroiliac. Any disruption causing a change in pelvic stability can disrupt the structures within it, leading to soft tissue trauma and possibly a large blood loss.

PELVIC INJURIES

The majority of fractures are associated with the transfer of energy; the greater the energy transferred, the greater the resultant skeletal and soft tissue injury and the greater the risk of an unstable fracture occurring. Traumatic fractures are classified according to the resultant degree of pelvic stability (Table 23.2).

Table 23.2   Classification of pelvic fractures and potential management (McRae & Esser 2002, Tile 1988)

Classification	Options for medical management
Type A Stable and minimally displaced fractures A1 Fractures not involving the pelvic ring A2 Minimally displaced, stable fractures of the pelvic ring	Conservative symptomatic treatment involving: rest, observation, analgesia, graduated mobilising with crutches, partial then full weight bearing. Internal fixation if displaced 2 cm or more
Type B Rotationally unstable, vertically stable fractures B1 Anteroposterior compression fracture with disruption and widening of the symphysis pubis	C-clamp applied for initial stabilisation. Internal or external fixation if the anterior sacroiliac joint or symphysis pubis is widened by more than 2.5 cm. If surgery is contraindicated, then conservative treatment with pelvic traction is used with repeated X-rays to monitor the sacroiliac joint position
B2 (ipsilateral) and B3 (contralateral) compression injuries, unstable in internal rotation	C-clamp for initial stability. If stable then conservative treatment with pelvic traction is used. Internal and/or external fixation if there are multiple injuries, haemodynamic instability or pain control is difficult
Type C Rotationally and vertically unstable fractures C1 Unilateral C2 Bilateral C3 Associated with an acetabular fracture	C-clamp for initial stability, then internal fixation. Skeletal leg traction needed if acetabular involvement cannot be managed surgically

As the pelvis is a rigid ring, if broken in one place it is invariably disrupted or broken elsewhere. These double fractures, or double injuries, potentially cause instability and marked pelvic ring disruption. The potential medical management options for these injuries are summarised in Table 23.2.

Pelvic fractures are not solely trauma related. Henry et al (1996) define two types of stress fractures.

1 Fatigue fractures in normal bone occurring from bone metastases, bone malignancy or posttraumatic osteolysis. Generally these fractures cause pain but can be asymptomatic if no displacement occurs.

2 Insufficiency fractures in abnormal bone from conditions such as osteoporosis, long-term corticosteroid use, rheumatoid arthritis or local irradiation from radiation therapy treatment. These fractures can be misdiagnosed but typically patients present with severe hip or low back pain.

STABLE AND MINIMALLY DISPLACED FRACTURES

Here the integrity of the pelvic ring is maintained. If the fracture is minor, with minimal bruising and easily controlled pain, the patient may not require a hospital admission. Other bone and soft tissue injuries must be excluded.

Fractures to the wing of the ilium, generally from a direct blow, leave the weight-bearing mechanism unaffected. Some patients walk into the hospital although this can be painful, as is side-to-side compression of the ilium. The ilium protects the pelvic contents and is the point of attachment for muscles; consequently, the bruising can be extensive. Careful observation of the area is essential to monitor for severe blood loss, in which case admission is essential for fluid replacement, analgesia, bedrest and possibly surgical intervention. The nurse can encourage the patient to be mobile when the pelvis is stable and their pain is controlled.

Avulsion fractures (Box 23.2) are sudden muscle contraction injuries, best treated by rest, reassurance and analgesia. Bruising, swelling and ecchymosis make some movements or sitting uncomfortable. Non or partial weight bearing is encouraged until the pain is controlled or subsides, then gradually mobility is increased to strengthen the affected muscles and prevent a further or repeated injury. Some patients experience tenderness or severe pain lasting several months and need reassurance that this is normal.

> **Box 23.2   Avulsion fracture sites (McRae & Esser 2002)**
>
> Sudden muscle contraction can avulse the:
>
> - anterior superior spine – sartorius muscle
> - anterior inferior spine – rectus femoris muscle
> - ischial tuberosity – hamstrings
> - posterior spine – erector spinae muscle
> - iliac crest – abdominal muscles
>
> Direct violence can fracture the crest and blade

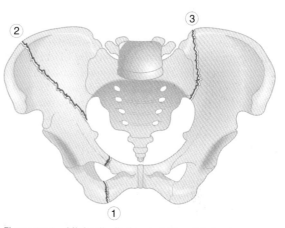

Figure 23.3 Minimally displaced, stable pelvic fractures. This group includes: (1), fractures of two rami on one side; (2), fracture of the ilium to the sciatic notch; (3), fracture of the ilium or sacrum involving the sacroiliac joint. (From McRae & Esser 2002.)

Single or unilateral fractures of the pubic and ischial rami are mostly seen in elderly patients following relatively minor trauma or stress to an abnormally weakened bone. These injuries are occasionally undiagnosed (Ryman 2001) but indicators such as difficulty in walking, tenderness over the superior rami, referred groin pain and pain on side-to-side compression should suggest the possibility of rami fractures. If the pain has a severe effect on the patient's mobility and ability to carry out activities of living, they are admitted for analgesia, rest and graduated mobility. A displacement of 2 cm or more increases the risk of non-union, chronic pain and disability; internal fixation reduces these risks.

Occasionally there is only one fracture across the pelvic ring, for instance fractures from the ilium to the sciatic notch or two fractured rami on one side (Fig. 23.3). Although there was another disruption of the pelvic ring, the secondary injury was either uncomplicated, it reduced immediately or there was a sprain injury to the symphysis pubis or sacroiliac joints. These injuries are more common in paediatrics as a child's symphysis pubis and sacroiliac joints allow movement and disruption without affecting the ring integrity. The patient is treated as if the pelvis were stable, with symptomatic pain management, possibly a short period of rest then gently increasing activity as the discomfort, referred pain and bruising allow.

In a straddle injury, where the legs fall either side of an object such as a wall, the anterior force fractures the four rami (butterfly fracture) or two rami on one side with a tear through the symphysis pubis. These are stable injuries if the posterior pelvis is unaffected and the displacement is slight because the separated bone segments remain attached to the bladder and urethra but not the pelvis. As unilateral rami fractures carry a 15% risk and bilateral fractures a 40% risk of urological trauma (Taffet 1997), these patients are admitted for urological observation with either symptomatic treatment or internal fixation as clinically required.

ROTATIONALLY UNSTABLE, VERTICALLY STABLE FRACTURES

These injuries involve incomplete disruption of the sacroiliac joint. They are associated with bladder, urethra and pelvic blood vessel trauma.

An anterior-posterior force injury, such as a crush injury from being run over, can result in an open book or sprung pelvis injury (Fig. 23.4) with damage to the symphysis pubis, pubic and ischial rami on one side, a fracture of the pelvic ring elsewhere or disruption of the sacroiliac joint. The disrupted symphysis pubis may not repair well, leaving a potentially weakened area.

A unilateral (ipsilateral) compression causes the rami on one side to fracture. With continued pressure the rami are forced to overlap, the anterior sacroiliac joint margin on the same side is crushed but the posterior sacroiliac ligament is intact. Due to the springing nature of the ligaments, spontaneous reduction from unilateral compression injuries can occur.

With a bilateral (contralateral) compression from a fall onto one side or crush compression, the ischial and pubic rami on one side fracture, with a second fracture through the sacrum or sacroiliac joint on the opposite side. The impact can then rotate the iliac wing inwards.

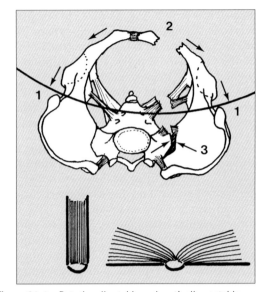

Figure 23.4 Rotationally stable and vertically unstable fractures. Example of an 'open book' fracture where the anterior superior iliac spines are forced outwards and backwards (1), the ring breaks anteriorly, e.g. at the symphysis pubis or rami (2), and posteriorly, e.g. at the sacroiliac joint (3). (From McRae & Esser 2002.)

The pelvis is unstable in a rotational plane but is vertically stable. These injuries can result in leg shortening (McRae & Esser 2002). Although these injuries can be treated conservatively, if the joints widen or the fractures are displaced, surgery is indicated.

ROTATIONALLY AND VERTICALLY UNSTABLE FRACTURES

Multiple fractures of the pelvic ring (Fig. 23.5) are normally due to deceleration, where the body suddenly stops after moving at speed, as with a fall from a height. The force results in a vertical and rotational movement of one half of the pelvis in relation to the other, plus disruption of the sacroiliac, sacrospinous and sacrotuberous ligaments, causing rotation and vertical instability. A combination of the following injuries can occur.

- Disruption of the anterior pelvis at the symphysis pubis or the rami on one side.
- Posterior loss of sacroiliac continuity from disruption of the joint.
- Fractures of the posterior iliac spine, the ilium, sacrum or acetabulum.
- A fracture of the L5 transverse process leading to bilateral vertical instability.

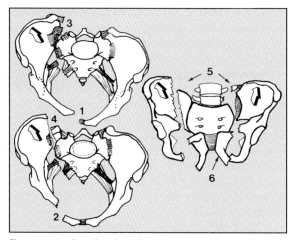

Figure 23.5 Rotationally and vertically unstable fractures. Complete pelvic ring disruption with injuries evident at, for example, the symphysis pubis (1), rami (2), sacroiliac joint (3) or posterior iliac spines (4). Bilateral injuries involve separation of both sides of the pelvis posteriorly (5) and often involve a butterfly fracture anteriorly (6). (From McRae & Esser 2002.)

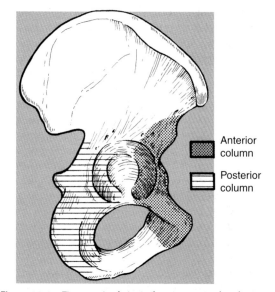

Figure 23.6 The anterior (stippled) and posterior (bars) columns of the pelvis. (From Dandy & Edwards 2003.)

Severe haemorrhage from muscle and abdominal trauma raises the intraabdominal pressure and restricts diaphragm movement. Sacral nerve root trauma causes sensory and motor changes such as saddle anaesthesia and incontinence. These neurological changes can be transitory but if they persist can cause severe lifestyle disruption. Diligent nursing care is essential as sacral pressure ulcers can develop without the patient being aware of the damage.

These life-threatening injuries require urgent external stabilisation to control pelvic movement, haemorrhage and hypovolaemia prior to definitive pelvic fracture management.

ACETABULAR INJURIES

Acetabular fractures are caused by high-energy impact trauma such as a dashboard injury or from a fall from a height. The force exerted up the femoral shaft or a lateral compression force results in damage to the hip and pelvic weight-bearing mechanism, driving the femoral head through the acetabular floor or dislocating the joint. If the injury is missed or the patient mobilised too early, the femoral head can push through the acetabulum, causing a fracture displacement or stove-in pelvis. Severe soft tissue trauma can result in the loss of 1.5 litres or more of blood.

Acetabular fractures are located in the anterior and posterior column (Fig. 23.6, Box 23.3). Anterior

---

Box 23.3   AO classification of acetabular fractures (McRae & Esser 2002)

Type A One column only involved
A1 Posterior column fracture with or without posterior dislocation of hip
A2 Posterior column fracture with no dislocation of hip
A3 Anterior column fracture

Type B Transverse fractures with part of the acetabular roof remaining attached to the ilium
B1 Transverse fracture with or without involvement of the posterior acetabular wall
B2 Transverse and vertical fracture form a T-fracture
B3 Transverse and vertical fracture involving the anterior column

Type C Anterior and posterior columns affected, with a fracture line above the acetabulum and no continuity between the acetabulum and ilium
C1 Anterior column fracture extends up to the iliac crest
C2 Anterior column fracture extends to the anterior border of the ilium
C3 Fracture involving the sacroiliac joint

---

column fractures have a good prognosis, as the weight-bearing area is less affected.

An anterior dislocation occurs when the leg is extended and the spine flexed, resulting in an externally rotated, abducted and flexed leg position. The rectus femoris muscle, attached at the anterior inferior iliac spine, prevents upward femoral head movement and leg shortening. The femoral head is palpable anteriorly and active movement is impossible.

Fractures of the posterior column and posterior dislocations of the hip joint typically result from a head-on car accident; the passenger has their hips and knees flexed, making the patella the point of impact (Klinger 1995). The force exerted up the femur can result in a range of injuries: patellar fractures, posterior cruciate ligament injury, femoral shaft fractures or fractures from the obturator foramen to the sciatic notch which separates the posterior ischio-pubic column and breaks the weight-bearing part of the acetabulum.

In a posterior dislocation without a posterior column fracture, the backward movement of the femoral head results in a shearing force, fracturing the acetabular rim. The leg is internally rotated, adducted and flexed, with no further active movement of the joint. The femoral head is often palpable in the buttock and on X-ray is behind the pelvis in an internally rotated, shortened position.

Complex fractures of the anterior or posterior columns with transverse fractures of the acetabulum (types B and C in Box 23.3) separate parts of the ilium, pubis and ischium. When the acetabular roof is disrupted, a central dislocation occurs with the femoral head being forced through the floor of the acetabulum. The leg can retain a normal position, with tenderness over the greater trochanter and joint, but there is minimal active movement. Often the thigh is grazed and bruised, indicating a lateral impact or fall onto the side. If the articular surface is totally detached from the axial (spinal) column, joint reconstruction is much harder, requiring internal fixation or acetabular prosthetic replacement. Although functional active movement is achievable, all movements with the exception of flexion and extension can remain impaired and there is a high risk of osteoarthritis in the long term.

PATIENT ASSESSMENT

Early immobilisation at the scene of injury is vital in preserving the level of pelvic function, preventing further injury and minimising muscle spasm and pain. Any immobilisation device used prior to admission is left in place until a full patient assessment and X-ray examination are complete. This prevents further trauma from bone movement or dislodging of a haematoma.

Pneumatic antishock garment (PASG) or military antishock trouser (MAST) systems are thought to provide effective lower limb splintage (Cardona et al 2002). However, they increase the intrathoracic pressure, creating problems with the respiratory, cardiovascular and renal systems. Although various centres internationally use PASG and MAST systems, Pignataro (1997) does not recommend them because they also prevent full abdominal and peroneal examination.

A multispecialty assessment of the patient starts in the A & E department resuscitation room. The American College of Surgeons Advanced Trauma Life Support protocols are followed to ensure the best opportunity for a safe recovery (Henry et al 1997). This involves a complete physical examination and establishes the mechanism of injury and relevant past medical and tetanus history. The airway, respiratory ventilation and appropriate oxygen supply are the initial priorities. The circulation check assumes hypovolaemic shock is present until proven otherwise. Patients with a multiple or unstable pelvic fracture are likely to be hypotensive and tachycardic, due to internal or external haemorrhage. Hypothermia is a major risk, making it vital to monitor body temperature and minimise heat loss.

PHYSICAL ASSESSMENT

Understanding the physical assessment process is essential as continued monitoring and reassessment will identify or exclude musculoskeletal and soft tissues injuries.

An initial systematic assessment of the patient includes examination of the abdomen, pelvis, back, perineum and thighs. This identifies the presence of abrasions, lacerations, grazes, foreign bodies, entry and exit wounds, previous injuries and surgery scars, swelling or bruising.

The presence of Cullen's sign (bruising around the umbilicus) or Grey Turner's sign (bruising in the flank) indicates a pool of blood in the retroperitoneal cavity. Regular girth measurements are of little help as a 1 cm increase can equate to a large intraabdominal haemorrhage. Observing for changed abdominal contours is more appropriate along with observation for hypovolaemic shock.

Auscultation and percussion enable the detection of bowel sounds, bruits, fetal heart sounds, hyperresonance indicating a collection of air or dullness indicating a collection of fluid. A systematic abdominal and pelvic palpation and examination prevents omission of an injury by:

- identifying evidence of an abdominal mass, guarding, rigidity or rebound tenderness
- examination of the back and buttocks for signs of skin or underlying injury
- full musculoskeletal pain assessment
- examination of the urethral meatus, genitalia and perineum for oedema, haemorrhage or haematuria
- rectal examination to confirm an intact rectal wall or the presence of a haematoma and the position of the prostate
- vaginal examination to confirm an intact vaginal wall, inferior pubic rami fractures or symphysis pubis disruption
- lower extremities for neurological status and function
- identification of hip joint instability. Pressure on the iliac crest will cause pain if a posterior pelvic fracture is present. Pressure on the symphysis pubis causes pain from fractured pubic rami.

These examinations must be done by experienced staff as repeated assessments can cause pain or discomfort.

RADIOGRAPHIC ASSESSMENT

As technology improves, more accurate and faster diagnosis of pelvis fractures and soft tissue trauma is possible with a reduced risk of omitting injuries. As patients will experience two or more types of radiographic assessments, they and their relatives need support and reassurance before and during these procedures, in particular with regards to what to expect, why it is being done and appropriate pain management before, during and after the event (Box 23.4).

STABILISING PELVIC FRACTURES

There are two approaches to managing pelvic injuries: traction and fixation.

Box 23.4   Radiographic assessments

Plain X-rays: used for initial screening, shows joint spaces, the presence and size of erosions or osteophytes, presence of an abdominal mass, dislocations and fractures. Commonly used views include the following.

- Anteroposterior (A/P) views to show the sacral wings, iliac bones, ischium, pubis, femoral head and neck, and lumbar vertebrae.
- Inlet projections identify posterior displacement of the true pelvis and pelvic rotation.
- Outlet views show superior displacement of the posterior hemipelvis and the presence of a superior or inferior displacement of the anterior pelvis.

Computer tomography (CT) scans: identify bony abnormalities, erosions, joint space changes and soft tissue trauma, including a retroperitoneal haematoma. Due to time, a CT scan is reserved for confirming fixation positions, to monitor bone healing and to exclude soft tissue trauma such as bladder entrapment (Morey 2000). Increasingly used for diagnosing posterior sacrum and sacroiliac fractures as 35% of these fractures are not diagnosed from a plain X-ray (Engle & Gruen 1993).

Bone scans: identify increased mechanical joint stress, fractures, infections, metabolic changes and neoplasms. This can identify stress fractures before they are visible on plain X-rays but a negative bone scan in the first few hours after injury may not exclude such a fracture (Lapp 2000).

Magnetic resonance imaging (MRI): allows assessment of muscle, cartilage and ligament structures and is effective in identifying early pelvic inflammatory conditions and soft tissue tumours.

TRACTION

Pelvic traction stabilises and immobilises fractures of the pelvic ring, closing any anterior diastasis. A balanced vertical pull suspension traction system with a canvas pelvic sling (Fig. 23.7) is used for patients with minimally displaced fractures or where a lateral compression is required. The aim is to align

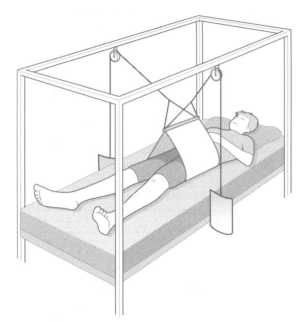

Figure 23.7 Pelvic traction using a canvas sling.

the bone ends to near normal, restore neurovascular function and reduce further soft tissue trauma.

The traction is maintained either as a temporary measure, prior to internal or external fixation, or for conservative fracture management.

The patient rests in the pelvic sling, which extends from the posterior iliac crests to the gluteal fold. The vertical pull of 4–8 kg should just elevate the buttocks off the bed. The countertraction is provided by the patient's body weight. The sides of the sling provide lateral compression; this can be increased to close a pubic diastasis by adjusting the traction pulleys so they are either closer together or crossed over the midline of the patient. This is avoided with compression injuries because additional lateral compression can distort the fracture position and override the bone ends. The patient is generally on traction for 6 weeks before mobilising non-weight bearing for 2–3 weeks prior to putting partial and then full weight through the affected leg. The degree of weight bearing depends on whether the fracture was through the weight-bearing area.

A patient with an acetabular or vertically displaced fracture may benefit from skeletal traction via a tibial tubercle pin for 4–6 weeks to reduce the pressure on the acetabulum.

For general nursing care of patients on traction, see Chapter 6. Specific nursing care implications for the patient with a pelvic injury on traction include the following.

- Remembering that the patient is supine. They may require additional pillows to support the head and a lumbar roll to support the lumbar spine but this must not cause an excessive lumbar arch.
- Communication, activities of daily living and independence are restricted, requiring additional support in most activities.
- Good assessment and management of discomfort and pain are essential.
- Moving and handling the patient requires planning before all procedures and ensuring adequate analgesic cover.
- Careful positioning of the bedpan and prompt peroneal hygiene after bedpan or urinal use is vital for patient comfort.
- Prevention of neurovascular injury from the traction, by frequent checks of neurovascular and motor function of the lower limbs and sacrum, and prevention of external rotation by allowing the patient slight hip and knee flexion if possible.

EXTERNAL AND INTERNAL FIXATION

Failure to ensure stability of the posterior pelvic ring causes long-term pain, reduced activity and a poor sitting balance. This is now a less common scenario due to the increased use of external fixation.

Using a pelvic stabiliser or C-clamp as a first-line measure is common practice in most units. This temporary external fixation device is applied under local anaesthetic and remains in situ until internal or external fixation can be carried out. The fixator enables any hypovolaemic shock to be stabilised by preventing fracture movement, disruption of blood clots and reduces the risk of haemorrhage. The pins are inserted into the pelvic bone either below the iliac crest or into the posterior superior iliac spine. Continued neurovascular monitoring is needed as damage to the sciatic nerve, gluteal nerve and blood vessels can occur during insertion.

A more permanent external fixation using a rigid frame with percutaneous pins attached to the anterior iliac crest (Fig. 23.8) or the anterior inferior iliac spine is applied once the patient is stable.

An unstable fracture cannot be reduced by closed manipulation; it is best treated by internal fixation. Hakim et al (1996) found open reduction and internal

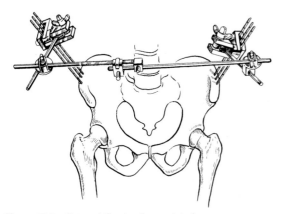

Figure 23.8   External fixation for a pelvic fracture.
(From Dandy & Edwards 2003.)

fixation of unstable fractures allowed a more accurate anatomical reduction, resulting in fewer long-term problems of back pain in comparison to bedrest and external fixation. Unstable fractures, especially if vertically displaced, have a higher incidence of long-term pain, pelvic and leg length discrepancy, sitting imbalance, mal- or non-union and post-trauma arthritis (Engle & Gruen 1993).

A combination of external fixation, reduction of displaced segments and internal fixation will hold fragmented fractures and ensures the pelvis is held rigid and stable, thus reducing the risk of mal- and non-union.

Once stability is assured, the patient can mobilise and bear weight, initially with physiotherapy and nursing assistance. They are discharged home once able to care for their pin sites. This requires patient support and education to enable acceptance of the fixator, ensure continued care of the fixator and pin sites and acceptance of the restrictions to normal activities and the change in body image.

ACETABULAR INJURY MANAGEMENT

There is a wide range of potential acetabular injuries; hence, an accurate patient assessment is essential before any treatment is commenced.

For a broad guide to the medical management options see Table 23.3. Internal fixation is essential to restore hip function and facilitate early mobilisation. Early intervention reduces the risk of early osteoarthritis changes especially if there is displacement of over 2 mm. Mears et al (2003) identify the presence of extensive femoral head impaction, damage to the

Table 23.3   Summary of acetabular fracture management options (McRae & Esser 2002)

Type of fracture	Management options
Minimally displaced fractures (less than 2 mm)	Conservative treatment on traction, followed by 3 weeks non-weight bearing then partial weight bearing
Severe fragmentation of acetabular floor	Conservative treatment on traction with or without skeletal leg traction, followed by 3 weeks non-weight bearing then partial weight bearing
Fracture with more than 2 mm displacement	Open reduction and internal fixation with acetabulum reconstruction or prosthetic replacement
Dislocation and fracture	Reduce under general anaesthetic, appropriate fracture management as above and potential period of traction
• Small, avulsed or minimally displaced fracture not affecting the acetabulum	• Period of bedrest or skin traction for 3–6 weeks to relieve pressure on the joint and allow bone and soft tissue healing
• Larger fractures	• May require internal fixation

articular surface and associated femoral head or neck fractures as indicators of potentially poor results from internal fixation. These patients may benefit from a total hip replacement or non-operative treatment (Mears et al 2003).

If the patient is treated conservatively using Hamilton Russell traction, active and passive hip movements are essential to reduce the risk of joint stiffness and assist later rehabilitation. The patient may experience a reduction in hip movement but the overall functional outcomes are good with conservative treatment.

Appropriate pain management is essential due to the potential for severe pain, especially when patients start to mobilise.

NURSING MANAGEMENT

Patients admitted with pelvic and acetabular fractures require diligent nursing care to prevent and preempt posttrauma complications. The nursing challenges increase if a stable fracture becomes unstable in the 24–48 hours following an injury as the muscles relax or hidden injuries become more evident. Constant reassessment, monitoring of vital signs and prompt action can preempt further complications.

Ideally the patient with multiple skeletal and organ trauma is admitted to a critical care unit but this need is not always identified or possible to meet. The orthopaedic nurse must therefore have the knowledge and skills to meet the patient's complex care needs.

Balcombe's orthopaedic model of nursing is used in Table 23.4 as a framework to illustrate nursing care issues. The orthopaedic nurse needs to relate these potential nursing diagnoses and care implications to individual patients' needs. The major trauma implications and potential for complex patient problems mean that this list is not exhaustive, but rather aims to be a starting point in the planning of patient care.

Hypovolaemic shock, soft tissue trauma and the potential complications of pelvic trauma are expanded on here to illustrate some of the nursing actions required and to highlight the issues a trauma nurse must be aware of. Good pain management is vital at all stages of the patient's care. This is not addressed further here but readers are advised to refer to Chapter 7.

HYPOVOLAEMIC SHOCK

The orthopaedic nurse should be able to differentiate between the types of shock (Table 23.5). Hypovolaemic shock is the most common form due to the extensive blood loss from femoral and pelvic fractures.

All patients presenting with a suspected or actual pelvic injury are assessed for their blood loss. A deceleration injury, for example, can separate the pelvic organs from their arterial blood supply, potentially resulting in bruising in the buttocks or scrotum, a retroperitoneal haematoma from an aortic rupture and leg ischaemia from a damaged iliac artery.

A patient can rapidly lose 3–4 litres of blood into the abdominal cavity, presenting with abdominal or back pain, a tender abdominal mass and the absence of bowel sounds. The resultant hypovolaemic shock requires emergency treatment to stabilise the patient prior to exploration and suturing of the affected blood vessels and organs.

Stages of shock

Hypovolaemic shock is an acute condition caused by inadequate tissue perfusion affecting the supply of oxygen and nutrients to cells. The cells and organs are then unable to function normally, leading to widespread hypoxia.

The main cause is reduced circulatory volume resulting in circulatory failure, a drop in blood pressure and cardiac output, leading to reduced oxygen perfusion of the brain, lungs, kidneys and other organs, creating a life-threatening situation. The causes of reduced volume are internal and external haemorrhage and extracellular fluid loss through severe vomiting, diarrhoea, thermal injuries or excessive diuresis.

Early detection prevents progression through the four identifiable stages of shock (Collins 2000, Kneale 2003).

1 Initial stage. The initial loss of 10–15% of circulatory volume deprives the tissue cells of oxygen, resulting in:

- the mitrochondria being unable to produce adenosine triphosphate (ATP), needed to create energy in cells
- cell membranes damaged increasing permeability
- cells using the less productive anaerobic rather than aerobic metabolism.

Anaerobic metabolism produces a build-up of lactic and pyruvic acid that is harmful to the cells. Normally, the circulatory system removes these toxins, which are broken down by the liver, but as this cannot occur metabolic acidosis develops.

2 Compensatory stage. The loss of 15–30% of the circulatory volume instigates the compensatory mechanisms and the first real symptoms occur.

- Hyperventilation to increase to the oxygen supply.
- A fall in blood pressure, detected by the aortic and carotid baroreceptors, stimulates the release of adrenaline (epinephrine) and noradrenaline (norepinephrine) leading to tachycardia.
- In response, peripheral vasoconstriction occurs, increasing the blood pressure and heart rate, resulting in a weak, thready pulse.
- Testing the rate of capillary refill of the nailbeds indicates vasoconstriction, the colour taking longer than 2 seconds to return. The skin, especially on the hands and feet, is cold from lack of circulating blood.
- The sweat glands are stimulated, increasing secretion and causing the skin to feel moist.

Table 23.4   Nursing diagnoses and nursing care implications in pelvic fractures

	Nursing diagnoses	Care implications
Breathing	• Hypovolaemic shock, reduced oxygen saturation or reduced tissue perfusion secondary to haemorrhage • Restricted respiratory intake and/or hyperventilation from abdominal or chest injuries	• Appropriate monitoring of cardiovascular and respiratory function • Observe for and treat continued blood loss
Pain	• Discomfort and pain from pelvic fracture, muscle spasms, soft tissue trauma • Swelling and bruising causing discomfort • Pain from constipation due to paralytic ileus or bedrest	• Appropriate pain assessment and management related to the cause and severity • Repositioning and support to relieve pain • Once pain decreases and the fracture is stable, mobilise partial weight bearing to generate fracture site stress so aiding bone healing • Avoid risk of further fractures by graduated, gentle, progressive weight bearing
Hygiene	• Unable to perform personal care due to pain, injuries, bedrest and position in traction • Altered urinary status indicating bladder or urethral trauma • Knowledge deficit related to personal care and need for independence at time of discharge • At risk of pin-site infection • Education needed on pin-site care	• Assistance needed to maintain personal hygiene due to restrictions imposed • Assistance and discretion in helping the patient with elimination needs • Preventive measures to protect the patient from healthcare-related infections • Support patient in acceptance of and management of traction, pin sites and external fixation frames • Patient education and support aiming towards self-care and maximising independence on discharge
Diet	• Fluid and nutrition deficit from trauma, haemorrhage and fracture • Unable to meet own dietary and fluid needs • Nausea and vomiting from paralytic ileus, abdominal or retroperitoneal haematoma	• Fluid replacement to correct hypovolaemic shock, dehydration and electrolyte imbalance • Nutritional assessment and monitoring • Provision of appropriate fluids and nutrition to maintain raised nutritional needs • Provision of nutritional supplements as required • Monitor, prevent and manage nausea and vomiting • Ensure bowel sounds present prior to giving oral fluids and diet • Positional problems for eating and drinking requiring appropriate aids and assistance
Movement	• Peripheral neurovascular deficit from fracture, limb positioning, traction or external fixator application • Altered sensory and motor function from sciatic or sacral nerve compression • Motor deficit from pelvic and gluteal muscle compression • Risk of compartment syndrome	• Ongoing assessment and observation for soft tissue trauma, vascular or neurological status changes • Provision of appropriate antibiotic regime, including tetanus cover • Support and assist patient when learning to mobilise • Ensure patient is safe transferring from, e.g. bed to wheelchair, to achieve a good sitting balance, and correct leg positioning if needed

(continued)

Table 23.4   (*Continued*)

	Nursing diagnoses	Care implications
		• Encourage appropriate graduated exercises: full range of movement, muscle strengthening to prevent contractures and muscle atrophy, gait training and cardiovascular exercises as appropriate • Ensure understanding of the need to continue exercises on discharge
Sleep	• Altered sleep pattern from trauma, pain, hospital regime and position in bed	• Develop and maintain a near natural sleep pattern for the patient
Mental state	• Anxiety from pain, trauma event and uncertainty of future • Knowledge deficit related to surgical and nursing management, rehabilitation and postdischarge care	• Ensure good communication between the patient and multidisciplinary team • Acknowledge and reduce limitations imposed by patient's position • Support patient education and reinforce multidisciplinary team teaching relating to the injuries, care and future needs
Behaviour	• Altered behavioural state following trauma event	• Acknowledge behavioural changes and encourage the patient to discuss fears
Self-concept	• Altered self-concept and body image from: sick role, altered physical self, external fixation mechanism, enforced bedrest or traction application	• Allow time, explanations, opportunity to discuss body image changes especially related to long-term issues raised by an external fixator and pin sites
Aspirations for health	• Altered life priorities and concepts of healthy self	• Allow opportunities for the patient to express concerns over health status, long and short term • Involve social care support as necessary
Home environment	• Knowledge deficit related to needs and ability to cope at home • Change of role in the family and work life • Change in interpersonal relationships	• Patient needs reassurance, explanations and support in adapting to, accepting and complying with lengthy or repeated surgery, prolonged bedrest, periods of non and partial weight bearing, limited activity and long periods away from home and work • Involve the patient and family in all aspects of care as appropriate

- Reduced renal circulation and release of antidiuretic hormone lead to reduced urine output.

3 Progressive stage.   Once 30–40% of the circulating volume is lost, the compensatory mechanisms begin to fail. There is:

- decreased cell perfusion; sodium collects in the cells and potassium leaks out
- increased anaerobic metabolism, resulting in systemic metabolic acidosis

- histamine release, causing fluid and protein leakage into the surrounding tissues, further increasing circulating fluid loss and blood viscosity
- sustained vasoconstriction, compromising vital organ function.

4 Refractory stage.   Once 40% or more of fluid volume is lost, the state of shock is irreversible. There is cell death leading to multiple organ failure and brain damage, death occurs within hours.

Table 23.5   Types of shock (Kneale 2003)

Type of shock	Main cause
Hypovolaemic	Reduced circulatory volume resulting in reduced cardiac output and low perfusion
Cardiogenic	Left ventricular failure, generally following a cardiac problem such as myocardial infarction or heart failure
Neurogenic	Caused by loss of sympathetic nerve activity due to disease, a drug, for example anaesthetic agents, or trauma such as spinal cord injury
Septic	Results from an overwhelming infection
Anaphylactic	Severe allergic reaction causing circulatory collapse. Damage to mast cells releases histamine and bradykinin, causing vasodilation

> **Box 23.5   Laboratory and diagnostic tests for hypovolaemic shock (Kneale 2003)**
>
> - Arterial blood gases
> - Serum electrolyes
> - Blood glucose concentration
> - Enzyme levels to indicate tissue damage: creatinine phosphokinase (CPK), serum glutamate oxaloacetate transaminase (SGOT), amylase
> - Renal and hepatic function tests: serum urea nitrogen, creatinine, bilirubin and ammonia
> - For covert bleeding: full blood count and coagulation studies

Prevention of hypovolaemic shock

To prevent and detect the early signs of hypovolaemic shock, the nurse must constantly reassess the patient's fluid balance by maintaining accurate records of fluid input and output to detect a negative balance. This includes estimating the fluid loss at the site of injury, through dressings, insensible loss, accurate intraoperative loss plus loss via chest and wound drains.

Nursing care of the patient in hypovolaemic shock

Regular physical observations, initially every 15 minutes, will give more immediate indicators of changes than other observations. Understanding the physiological changes enables early detection and treatment to manage or correct these.

Initially hypoxia from reduced circulatory volume stimulates the respiratory centre, increasing the respiratory rate and depth to twice the normal tidal volume in an attempt to improve circulating oxygen levels. As the stages of shock progress, the respiratory muscles tire and the patient begins to hyperventilate with rapid but shallow breaths. Ideally, the patient should be on 100% oxygen given via a non-rebreathe mask. Humidifying the oxygen increases expectoration of secretions and prevents damage to the bronchial mucosa and cilia. Monitoring of the respiratory rate, oxygen saturation level and blood gases is essential for indicators of oxygen circulation and perfusion (Box 23.5).

A tachycardia is present, with peripheral pulses being weak and thready from the reduced peripheral flow. Cardiac monitoring identifies any cardiac arrhythmias early.

The blood pressure is initially normal prior to the compensatory mechanisms starting. The fall in blood pressure relates to the drop in systolic pressure from the reduced cardiac stroke volume, while the diastolic pressure remains normal due to peripheral vasoconstriction giving a narrower systolic–diastolic range. As the circulatory volume decreases, the peripheral blood pressure readings become less accurate and invasive measurements such as central venous pressure are required.

Core and peripheral temperatures are measured as the loss of blood leads to a lower temperature from the lack of circulatory heat. Severe blood loss can therefore lead to hypothermia. Rapid rewarming is avoided as this leads to vasodilation and affects the physiological compensatory mechanism. Instead, gradual rewarming is essential, with warmed intravenous fluids being given if required.

In the early stages of shock, as the central nervous system is stimulated, there is increased blood supply to the main organs with less to the peripheral areas and the increased sweat gland activity makes the skin cool, pale and clammy. With sustained vasoconstriction, the oxygen supply to the peripheries is reduced further and the skin appears cyanotic, cold and mottled. As the skin is also dehydrated, there is poor skin turgor while the mucous membranes are dry and pale from the reduced blood supply.

Hourly monitoring of fluid balance is essential. Urine output via a catheter needs to be greater than 0.5 ml/kg/h or 20 ml/h; less than this indicates reduced renal perfusion. The specific gravity or osmolarity of the urine increases as urine concentration rises from the continued excretion of waste products and fluid retention. As the stages of shock progress, the kidneys excrete fewer waste products. As the volume is also low, the relative concentration remains stable or dilutes, as the kidneys are unable to concentrate the urine.

To prevent the progression of shock, measures are needed to treat the cause, prevent further blood loss and replace the circulating volume. Two large-bore cannulae are needed for the rapid infusion of large volumes of fluid. If insertion of peripheral lines is difficult due to vasoconstriction, a central line is required. A blood transfusion is ideal as this increases the circulatory volume and oxygen-carrying capacity to supply the tissues; hence 2–3 units of blood are crossmatched. In comparison colloid and crystalloid fluids increase the volume but not the oxygen capacity, further diluting the blood, as seen by haemoglobin (ideally 12.5–14 g/100 ml) and haematocrit (ideally above 30%) levels.

Most drugs are given intravenously to increase their rate of absorption, but adrenaline (epinephrine) is given intramuscularly if required.

The patient's level of consciousness decreases because of reduced cerebral blood flow leading to an inadequate oxygen supply to brain cells. Initially there are subtle changes generally presented as restlessness, agitation and irritability. As the cerebral ischaemia increases, confusion, personality changes, paranoia, poor judgement, loss of memory and altered sleep patterns occur. As the stages of shock progress, responses to verbal stimulation reduce. The nurse then needs to assess the patient's responses to pain which will likewise decrease until there is no response to any stimuli. Measuring these changes by using the Glasgow Coma Scale enables early detection of changes.

As the patient is nursed supine, there is a risk of fluid accumulation in their lungs and pressure ulcers occur from reduced tissue perfusion and increasing susceptibility to pressure area damage. Regular pressure area care with correct moving and handling to prevent fracture site movement is vital.

The patient will be nil-by-mouth in case they need surgery and to reduce their risk of aspiration. Regular mouth care increases patient comfort and counteracts oral discomfort from dehydration.

The patient and relatives need verbal and psychological support, through good communication skills and information on the effects and implications of the injury and nursing care.

PELVIC FRACTURE COMPLICATIONS

The complex nature of pelvic trauma puts the patient at risk of a wide range of complications. The nursing team needs to be alert to the potential risks, which are higher for those with open pelvic fractures due to the effects of large blood loss and increased infection risk.

The potential risks seen during the patient's admission can include the following.

- Altered bone continuity causing pain, angulation and possible overriding of the bone ends from poor stabilisation.
- Neurovascular injuries and fat embolisms are seen following the injury and during the subsequent medical and nursing management.
- A large blood loss, especially in the abdominal and peritoneal spaces, contributes to the risk of abdominal compartment syndrome or obstruction of the ureters, vena cava or aorta. Uncontrolled haemorrhaging can result in hypovolaemic shock, hypothermia, coagulopathy and, if untreated, death.
- A paralytic ileus can result from a retroperitoneal haematoma which, if treated by nasogastric suction and intravenous fluids, normally resolves in 2–3 days (McRae & Esser 2002).

Even well-managed pelvic injuries carry a risk of long-term complications that patients need to be aware of, for example:

- chronic pain, especially if the sacroiliac joint is affected
- secondary osteoarthritis
- myositis ossificans after surgical intervention or if there is an accompanying head injury
- impotence if there is urethral rupture, neurological damage or penile vascular insufficiency
- for women, a distortion of the true pelvis may rule out natural childbirth.

Acetabular fractures and hip joint dislocations can cause major complications at the time of injury and long term. For instance:

- any bone fragment in the joint requires removal before joint reduction is attempted
- femoral vein and artery compression from an anterior dislocation increases the risk of an embolism or thrombosis

- recurrent dislocations require repair of the acetabulum rim or acetabular replacement
- avascular necrosis of the femoral head from a disrupted blood supply
- nerve damage from the injury or during reduction of a dislocation. Sciatic nerve compression from a posterior dislocation causes drop foot, loss of dorsiflexion and lost sensation to the sole of the foot. Femoral nerve compression from an anterior dislocation causes difficulty in extending the leg and loss of sensation over the anteromedial aspect of the thigh.

MANAGING ASSOCIATED SOFT TISSUE TRAUMA

The pattern of the pelvic injury indicates potential soft tissue trauma. This varies depending on the mechanism of injury. The subsequent management of the patient can prevent or exacerbate such injuries. A broad outline of soft tissue trauma identification and management is discussed here because nursing care includes recognition of the relevant signs and symptoms, reporting these and instigating appropriate care.

Bladder trauma

An empty bladder is protected behind the symphysis pubis, but as the bladder fills, the dome rises, making it prone to injury. Vertical displacement of the hemipelvis or rami fractures stretches the bladder wall, causing trauma. Bladder trauma is associated with injuries to the urethra, rectum, vagina, uterus, vas deferens, peritoneum and the fourth sacral nerve that supplies the lower part and neck of the bladder.

Taffet's (1997) review suggests that 15% of patients with pelvic fractures have bladder trauma resulting in an:

- incomplete tear or contusion
- intraperitoneal rupture of the dome, causing urine seepage into the peritoneal cavity. The patient appears to develop ascites. If infected, peritonitis develops very quickly. This is a risk in ethanolic patients but may be missed if the alcohol masks the symptoms
- extraperitoneal ruptures which have an anterior tear near the base of the bladder, allowing urine to flow into the perivesical tissues but not beyond the urogenital diaphragm or into the peritoneal cavity.

All patients with unstable fractures need close monitoring of their fluid intake and output to enable early identification of bladder or urethral trauma. Depending on the position of the tear, patients present with:

- abdominal pain over the pelvic and suprapubic region
- perineal bruising or swelling of the scrotum, buttocks, vulva and perineum as urine seeps along the fascial plane
- blood at the tip of the urethra
- haematuria indicating a partial or extraperitoneal tear
- no urine output suggestive of an intraperitoneal rupture.

A urological referral is vital if a bladder or urethral injury is suspected because a small bladder or urethral tear can be extended by inappropriate urethral catheterisation. Suprapubic catheterisation is essential until the extent of the bladder or urethral damage is known. The catheter keeps the bladder empty for 7–10 days and is then removed after confirmation of healing.

Urethral trauma

Although partial and full urethral tears occur in women, the relatively longer male urethra is more prone to trauma. Urethral trauma is indicated by disruption of the symphysis pubis, bleeding at the urinary meatus, perineal bruising, a distended bladder, inability to pass urine, a penile haematoma or oedema.

Posterior urethral trauma involves the prostatic or membranous urethra, superior to the urogenital diaphragm. As the puboprostatic ligament attaches the prostate to the symphysis pubis, any disruption here causes a partial or full urethral tear. Blood and urine seepage into the pelvic cavity results in a haematoma around the prostate, giving a 'boggy feel' on rectal examination. Any superior displacement of the bladder and prostate makes them difficult to palpate on rectal examination.

Anterior urethral trauma involves the bulbar or penile urethra, inferior to the urogenital diaphragm. Straddle injuries and catheterisation trauma can result in partial or full tears. If the Buck's fascia is intact, blood and urine track down the penile sheath but if disrupted, a butterfly-shaped haematoma occurs from blood and urine loss into the scrotum and abdominal walls.

If the patient is able to pass urine, this is encouraged and prophylactic antibiotic cover provided. If unable to pass urine, suprapubic catheterisation is followed by urological assessments to diagnose the extent of the trauma and surgical repair is carried out as soon as possible.

If the patient is discharged with a catheter, they require support and education to understand the importance of their catheter care, how to prevent an infection and what to do should the catheter block. Suggested nursing diagnoses and nursing care points for the patient with urethral trauma are listed in Box 23.6. Long-term urological follow-up is required to prevent or exclude later stricture formation and impotence.

Genital trauma

Following a straddle injury, the genitalia require close examination as the labia, testicles, urethra and perineum are at risk of direct impact trauma. There is often severe pain in the area, with swelling and discoloration, especially of the scrotum. Nursing management includes analgesia and, if severe, bedrest to limit physical activity until the pain and swelling subside.

Bowel trauma

The body's reaction to stress and injury causes a reduction or absence of bowel sounds, abdominal pain and guarding. As these are seen with most pelvic injuries, trauma to the colon can be missed.

Rectal perforations occur from open fractures while crush injuries cause trauma to the small bowel. Faecal contamination of the pelvic and abdominal cavities increases the risk of peritonitis and septicaemia. Prophylactic broad-spectrum antibiotics are generally prescribed.

A sigmoidoscopy is done to assess for colon injuries (Engle & Gruen 1993). A diverting colostomy, if required for a colon tear, is positioned in the upper quadrant to avoid placement sites for a pelvic external fixator.

PELVIC TRAUMA IN PREGNANCY

The assessment and treatment of a pregnant woman with a pelvic fracture remains the same but requires consideration of the gestational stage, the physiological changes from pregnancy and potential

---

Box 23.6   Nursing diagnoses and care for patients with urethral trauma

Nursing diagnoses

- Urine output deficit secondary to urethral tract trauma
- Increased discomfort and pain from haemorrhage, oedema and trauma
- Increased risk of infection: from blood and urine loss into surrounding structures, disrupted lower urinary tract or an indwelling catheter
- Fear and anxiety related to loss of control over body function, embarrassment, loss of fertility or loss of penile erection

Nursing care actions

- Ensuring haemodynamic stability, including fluid and electrolyte balance, care of intravenous fluids and catheter management
- Monitor and record urine output
- Reduction of risk of complications such as urinary tract infection, urinary stricture and catheter blockage
- Management of the closed urinary drainage, initially by nursing staff then aiming for patient independence in catheter management on discharge
- Encourage a normal voiding pattern after removal of catheter
- Effective management of pain and discomfort
- Patient education relating to their injury, rationale for care interventions and treatment
- Give prescribed antibiotic therapy to preempt or treat identified urinary tract infection

complications of severe haemorrhage, uterine rupture or placental abruption.

By the end of the first trimester, the fundus is level with the symphysis pubis, the uterus occupies most of the pelvic cavity but remains protected by the pubic rami. At 20 weeks gestation, the fundus is level with the umbilicus and by 36 weeks, it occupies nearly all the abdominal cavity up to the costal margin, making the gravid uterus the most susceptible to pelvic trauma.

The mother's needs invariably override fetal protection when assessing the type and extent of a pelvic injury. For instance, the position of the uterus makes clear pelvic X-rays difficult to obtain while shielding the fetus from radiation. This creates ethical and moral dilemmas for the family and practitioners in terms of the rights of the unborn child.

Although there are two lives at risk, fetal resuscitation and survival is dependent on the prompt and accurate care of the mother (Manley & Santanello 1991, Pape et al 2000). Pape et al suggest that to protect the fetus, a modified version of the normal fracture treatment is used, providing this is in the best interests of the mother. A modified fracture management regime can increase the risk of long-term pain, discomfort, mobility or osteoarthritis for the mother.

All pregnant women require an obstetric referral no matter how minor their pelvic injury. Monitoring fetal movements and heart rate offers early signs of fetal distress while repeated assessment of the uterus contours and shape can indicate a concealed haemorrhage or uterine rupture.

Placental abruption, where the placenta shears away from the uterus, occurs in deceleration injuries. The uterus becomes tender, irritable or hardened, from vaginal blood or amniotic fluid loss. Restricted oxygen supply and carbon monoxide accumulation then cause fetal hypoxia, acidosis and bradycardia. Confirmation of placental abruption is by CT scan, but this procedure delays an emergency caesarean section that could save a viable fetus. In most cases of placental abruption and uterine rupture, fetal survival is rare.

The patient and family remain anxious for the health of the mother and baby throughout the initial assessment, treatment to stabilise the fracture and rehabilitation phases of care. Providing clear explanations about the care of both mother and baby, and listening to concerns expressed, can help the patient and family to cope. Equally, enabling grieving and offering appropriate support to those involved should the baby not survive are essential.

PAEDIATRIC CONSIDERATIONS IN PELVIC TRAUMA

Pelvic, sacrum and coccyx fractures in children are uncommon, even from severe falls and road traffic accidents. Children often have less extensive injuries compared to adults as their bones and joints absorb more of the impact energy. Equally, their pelvic joints are better able to compress and return to their normal position compared to those of adults (Glasgow & Graham 1997).

Stable fractures of the ilium, pubic rami or avulsion fractures usually respond well to rest and symptomatic treatment.

As the primary ossification centres meet at the acetabulum, trauma in this area can arrest further growth, causing acetabular dysplasia if the femoral head growth exceeds that of the acetabulum.

Unstable fractures of the pelvic ring are occasionally treated by fixation, depending on the extent of the damage, the stage of skeletal development and position of the injury. The majority of unstable fractures are treated with bedrest or pelvic sling traction to reduce and maintain stability of the fracture site.

These injuries carry the same potential risks of soft tissue trauma as for adults. Any alteration in respiration pattern, abdominal pain or bowel sounds can indicate pelvic or abdominal tissue trauma. The child's diaphragm is more horizontal, placing the spleen and liver anteriorly and at greater risk of injury. Abdominal breathing is affected sooner if the peritoneum, pelvic or abdominal cavities are affected by a haematoma, urine or bowel contents. A nasogastric tube is required to decompress the stomach as children have a tendency to swallow air. Any head and chest injuries, haemorrhage or soft tissue damage take precedence over the treatment of skeletal injuries.

THE SACROILIAC JOINT

The anatomical position of the sacroiliac joint (SIJ) makes it difficult to examine. Patients experience referred pain here from other lower spinal structures, making it the source of primary and secondary pain, accounting for up to 20% of patients presenting with low back pain (Schwarzer et al 1995).

Confusion over the sources of pain is seen in a straight leg raise of 60°, which normally generates some SIJ movement. If a patient experiences low back pain during this examination, the cause could be dural tension pain or an SIJ abnormality (Cole et al 1996).

SACROILIAC JOINT CHANGES

The SIJ evolves during the 10th to 12th week of gestation; it continues to develop through childhood to become the adult C-shape. The joint is mobile but the structural size, shape and contours vary between individuals and with age. After puberty, the articular surface of the ilium develops bony ridges that increase in size and number to enhance the stability of the joint, probably as adaptations to adult weight gain, but they do not cause pain.

The fibrous joint capsule is well developed anteriorly with the anterior sacroiliac ligament forming the anterior border, lying close to the obturator nerve and continuous with the anterior portion of the iliolumbar ligament. The posterior joint border is formed by the interosseous ligament, which is the strongest ligament supporting the joint but the posterior portion is more prone to trauma. The accessory muscles (iliolumbar, sacrotuberous and sacrospinous ligaments), gluteus maximus and medius muscles and the thoracodorsal fascia provide additional support to the joint.

Accessory articulations can develop behind the articular surface of the second sacral transverse process and the ilium, creating the saddle-shaped joint capsule. This occurs in 8–35.8% of the population but is rare before the age of 40 (Cole et al 1996). The joint spaces narrow with age; in Cole et al's (1996) estimation this can reduce to 0.1–0.2 cm by 50–70 years and is down to 0–0.1 cm by 70 years of age. These degenerative changes seen on X-ray are normally asymptomatic.

The SIJ is essentially a shock absorber, transmitting and dissipating weight from the trunk to the lower extremity, especially during walking and sitting. The accepted movements at this joint are:

- nutation: the backward rotation of the ilium on the sacrum
- counternutation: the forward rotation of the ilium on the sacrum.

These movements are not voluntary, but generated by movement such as changing weight or posture. In pregnancy the increased levels of relaxin cause the soft tissues to slacken, increasing the joint mobility and predisposing it to sprain injuries.

SACROILIAC JOINT INJURIES

Trauma to the joint occurs from falls onto the buttocks, tripping down steps, inappropriate lifting techniques or a repetitive rotation injury of the lumbar spine. These cause sharp, aching or dull pain at the joint or referred pain to the buttocks, groin, posterior thigh, knee or foot. Gait analysis often reveals an antalgic gait where the trunk shifts towards the normal side. When sitting, the patient leans away from the injury to relieve pressure on the joint.

Inflammation of the SIJ is due to metabolic changes, trauma, arthritis or an infection. Joint infections are usually unilateral, with a predisposing factor of pregnancy, trauma, endocarditis, intravenous drug abuse or immunosuppression. The infection causes distension of the joint capsule, potentially irritating the lumbar and sacral nerve roots.

The cause of the injury requires investigation followed by either conservative treatment or, if the symptoms are severe or there is joint instability, a joint fusion is required. Denervation at the fourth and fifth lumbar spinal nerve outlets can reduce protracted pain. Other patients prefer manipulation so consult a physiotherapist, osteopath or chiropractor in an effort to seek relief.

SACRUM AND COCCYX INJURIES

Sacral fractures (Fig. 23.9) are divided into fractures of the ala, from either side-to-side or anteroposterior compression of the pelvis, and transverse fractures resulting from a fall from a height. Patients experience pain and the area is tender to touch. Occasionally

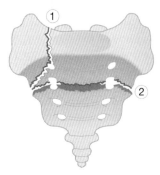

Figure 23.9 Fractures of the sacrum. These can be fractures of the ala (1) or transverse fractures that are either undisplaced (2) or laterally or anteriorly displaced. (From McRae & Esser 2002.)

neurological changes occur, for example changes of sensation over the sacral nerve root distribution area, causing symptoms such as leg weakness, saddle anaesthesia or incontinence.

The coccyx is injured from falls when the patient lands in a sitting position on a hard surface. Fractures of the coccyx, with or without subluxation, cause local pain; the area is tender to touch and on palpation, with pain on defaecation or when sitting on a hard surface. These injuries are detected by rectal examination. Coccyx dislocations are reduced by rectal manipulation.

Patients require appropriate advice to manage their pain, for example to use a cushion to sit on and not to become constipated during the healing process. If the pain becomes chronic, a local anaesthetic injection into the joint or excision of the coccyx is required.

References

Cardona VD, Hurn PD, Mason PJB et al 2002 Trauma nursing: from resuscitation through rehabilitation, 3rd edn. WB Saunders, London

Cole AJ, Dreyfuss P, Stratton SA 1996 The sacroiliac joint: a functional approach. Critical Reviews in Physical and Rehabilitation Medicine 8(1): 125–152

Collins T 2000 Understanding shock. Nursing Standard 14(49): 35–39

Dandy DJ, Edwards DJ 2003 Essential orthopaedics and trauma, 4th edn. Churchill Livingstone, Edinburgh

Engle C, Gruen GS 1993 Vertical shear fractures of the pelvis. Orthopaedic Nursing 12(5): 55–59

Glasgow JFT, Graham HK 1997 Management of injuries in children. BMJ Publishing Group, London

Hakim RM, Gruen GS, Delitto A 1996 Outcomes of patients with pelvic ring fractures managed by open reduction internal fixation. Physical Therapy 76(3): 286–295

Henry AP, Lachmann E, Tunkel RS, Nagler W 1996 Pelvic insufficiency fractures after irradiation: diagnosis, management and rehabilitation. Archives of Physical Medicine Rehabilitation 77(4): 414–416

Henry SM, Tornetta P, Scalea TM 1997 Damage control for devastating pelvic and extremity injuries. Surgical Clinics of North America 77(4): 879–895

Klinger DL 1995 Acetabular fractures. AORN Journal 61(1): 157–178

Kneale JD 2003 Understanding hypovolaemic shock. Journal of Orthopaedic Nursing 7(4): 207–213

Lapp JM 2000 Pelvic stress fracture: assessment and risk factors. Journal of Manipulative and Physiological Therapeutics 23(1): 52–55

Manley L, Santanello S 1991 Case review: trauma in pregnancy: uterine rupture. Journal of Emergency Nursing 17(5): 279–281

McRae R, Esser R 2002 Practical fracture treatment, 4th edn. Churchill Livingstone, Edinburgh

Mears DC, Velyvis JH, Chang CP 2003 Displaced acetabular fractures managed operatively: indicators of outcome. Clinical Orthopaedics and Related Research 407: 173–186

Morey AF 2000 Bladder entrapment after external fixation of traumatic pubic diastasis: importance of follow up computed tomography in establishing prompt diagnosis. Military Medicine 165: 492–493

Pape HC, Pohleman T, Gänsslen A, et al 2000 Pelvic fractures in pregnant multiple trauma patients. Journal of Orthopaedic Trauma 14(4): 238–244

Pignataro ED 1997 Use of pelvic stabilizers. International Journal of Trauma Nursing 3(2): 56–58

Ryman H 2001 Pelvic fractures in an elderly female. European Journal of Chiropractic 47: 15–20

Schwarzer AC, Aprill CN, Bogduk N 1995 The sacroiliac joint in chronic low back pain. Spine 20: 31–37

Taffet R 1997 Management of pelvic fractures with concomitant urological injuries. Orthopedic Clinics of North America 28(3): 389–396

Tile M 1988 Pelvic ring fractures: should they be fixed? Journal of Bone and Joint Surgery 70B(1): 1–12

Chapter 24

Care of patients with lower limb injuries and conditions

Julie Santy

INTRODUCTION

Lower limb injuries are the major cause of admissions to orthopaedic trauma units, the most common reason for adult orthopaedic surgery and, because of the human body's reliance on lower limb fitness for locomotion, a major cause of loss of independence and mobility during recovery and rehabilitation. The age of adult patients with lower limb conditions and injuries is rising in accordance with demographic trends. Lower limb injuries can lead to considerable disability and dependency in later life.

The lower limb provides support for standing upright and is instrumental in ambulation. A lower limb injury or problem has a severe effect on mobility, activities of living and self-care, requiring adaptation to a new or difficult situation. Understanding the anatomy and mechanics of the lower limb, including the skeletal structures, soft tissues, joints, nerve and blood supply, mechanisms and pathophysiology of injuries enables the orthopaedic nurse to give appropriate and sensitive care.

The management of lower limb conditions and injuries has moved forward considerably with expansion of surgical interventions and a notable decrease in the length of stay for hospitalised patients. However, orthopaedic nurses need to be aware that modern techniques do not always provide solutions to some of the more complex and difficult problems. Skeletal traction has become an uncommon method of treatment but there are occasions when surgery and other interventions cannot be used. On these occasions the nursing skills in traction care become essential. (see Chapter 6)

This chapter reviews the nursing diagnoses and management related to major injuries and conditions that affect the lower limb in adults. Due to the variety and complexity of these, only major and commonly met conditions are considered. Details related to other conditions can be found in the texts recommended for further reading at the end of the chapter.

An outline of the medical and surgical treatment and management is included to demonstrate the rationales for nursing care. A summary of the main nursing issues affecting patients can be found in Table 24.1. More detailed nursing management of patients with femoral neck fractures is discussed in the text as this constitutes a major client group on trauma wards.

HIP FRACTURES

The hip joint (Fig. 24.1) is normally very stable, the ball and socket arrangement allowing flexion, extension, abduction, adduction, rotation and circumduction. When hip fractures or fractures of the proximal femur occur, they are disabling injuries mostly affecting the elderly. The generic term 'fractured neck of femur' is inaccurate for describing this group of injuries as it applies to only a small number of fractures of this region.

As more people live into their ninth or even tenth decade, there is an increase in numbers of these injuries (Newman 1992) and nursing these patients has become an enormous issue for orthopaedic nurses. The report 'Caring for older people: a nursing priority' (SNMAC 2001) demonstrates that standards of fundamental care for older people in acute settings are in need of improvement. Nurses increasingly need the motivation, skills and appropriate philosophies for the effective care of older people. The challenges of caring for this vulnerable group are enormous because of their age, frailty and the pathophysiological and healthcare needs that affect recovery from a severe injury.

AETIOLOGY, EPIDEMIOLOGY AND RISK FACTORS

Fractures of the hip are normally caused by a fall on a biomechanically compromised proximal femur (Newman 1992). Patients often describe it as a minor fall, often with a twisting element as the mechanism of injury.

The incidence of hip fractures increases with age. Below the age of 60 they occur more frequently in men, generally from industrial trauma (McRae & Esser 2002). In later life they occur more in women, with postmenopausal osteoporosis being a contributing factor.

The major risk factors are seen in many vulnerable older adults: gender (female), previous falls, living alone or in institutional care, below normal body weight, smoking, excessive alcohol consumption, low weight-bearing activity levels, low bone density and deficiency of vitamin D. A great deal of credence is given to these risk factors in the literature with particular reference to prevention (Royal College of Physicians 1989).

As the incidence rate continues to rise it appears that to date, prevention strategies have largely been unsuccessful. The use of hip protector pads (Buckler et al 1997, Ekman et al 1997) has proven successful in preventing hip fractures in individuals who are prone to falls but the pads are difficult to put on, making compliance an issue for those who have no help. They are an ideal intervention in residential and nursing homes where the incidence of falls is high due to the frailty of those living in such settings.

Other strategies include prevention of osteoporosis through healthy lifestyles, although once old age is reached this is less effective and prevention of falls becomes the focus (DoH 2001). Musculoskeletal fitness in the elderly is of paramount importance if this major injury is to be avoided.

HIP FRACTURE MANAGEMENT

There are four main fracture sites (Figs 24.2, 24.3):

- subcapital and transcervical fractures occur within the capsule of the hip joint (intracapsular), while
- intertrochanteric or basal and pertrochanteric fractures occur outside the hip joint capsule (extracapsular).

Fractures of the proximal femur and femoral shaft are also classified according to the degree of displacement. Both the position and displacement of the fracture are important for the choice of management strategy.

It is vital orthopaedic nurses understand the rationale for surgical or other treatment interventions. The patient and relatives or carers must understand the implications of treatment before informed

Table 24.1 Nursing issues in lower limb conditions and injuries

Nursing diagnosis	Main associated conditions	Nursing interventions	Rationale
Pain and pain management deficit	All lower limb injuries and conditions	Pain assessment and evaluation Analgesic administration via all routes Alternative strategies, e.g. acupuncture, TENS, comfort strategies Management of swelling and bruising with elevation and ice	Pain assessment and evaluation allow sensitive use of analgesia and other pain management strategies Pain management must be responsive to individual needs
Impaired physical mobility	All lower limb injuries and conditions	Active and passive exercise Short- and long-term goal setting Gradual remobilisation Use of mobilisation aids	The need to prevent muscle wasting and joint stiffness. The need to gradually reintroduce mobility activities
Knowledge deficit of mobility skills	All lower limb injuries and conditions	Education and training	The need for information for the individual to be able to cooperate with rehabilitation programmes and treatment
Self-care deficit	All lower limb injuries and conditions	Assessment of nursing needs for intervention and level of intervention	Effective rehabilitation is brought about by appropriate nursing support Dignity is maintained by allowing individuals to self-care wherever possible
Activity intolerance	All lower limb injuries and conditions	Provision of balance between rest or sleep and activity Adequate nutritional intake	There is a fine balance between adequate rest and activity in recovery Remobilisation following lower limb injuries and conditions demands high energy levels
High risk for skin breakdown	Hip fractures Femoral shaft fracture Lower limb injuries and conditions in the elderly	Risk assessment and management Appropriate support surface Management of intrinsic and extrinsic factors Frequent evaluation	Intrinsic and extrinsic factors in pressure damage development must be managed in order to prevent skin breakdown
High risk of complications: DVT/PE	All lower limb injuries and conditions	Antiembolic measures	Prevention and early detection of complications are the two main nursing aims
Fat embolus syndrome Osteomyelitis	Femoral shaft fractures Compound fractures Associated infections	Stabilisation of fracture Aseptic management of wounds Wound assessment Vital sign observation	
Wound infection	Any lower limb injury or condition with a wound	Neurovascular observation Elevation of the limb	

(continued)

Table 24.1   (*Continued*)

Nursing diagnosis	Main associated conditions	Nursing interventions	Rationale
Chest infection	Any lower limb condition in the elderly which affects mobility or patients who smoke or have other respiratory problems	Early mobilisation where possible Deep breathing exercises	
Urinary/bowel complications	Any lower limb condition that restricts mobility and leads to the potential for urinary stasis or poor bowel motility	Provision of suitable toilet facilities with privacy. Oral fluids, high-fibre diet, cranberry juice	
High risk for ineffective coping	All lower limb conditions which cause any of the above effects	Provision of appropriate and understandable information Allowing fears and worries to be raised and discussed	The correct level of information delivered in an appropriate way enhances recovery. Fears and anxieties are tempered by discussion

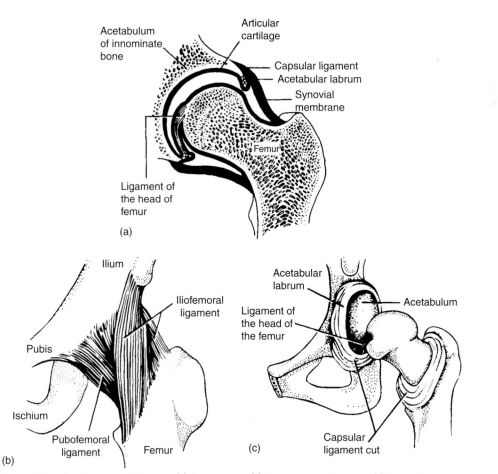

Figure 24.1   The hip joint, anterior view. (a) Cross-section. (b) The supporting ligaments. (c) Head of femur and acetabulum separated to show components. (From Wilson 1990 with permission.)

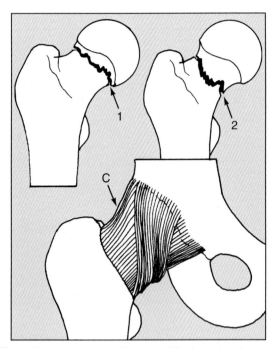

Figure 24.2   Intracapsular fractures of the femoral neck. Subcapital (1) and transcervical (2) fractures lie within the joint capsule (C). (From McRae & Esser 2002.)

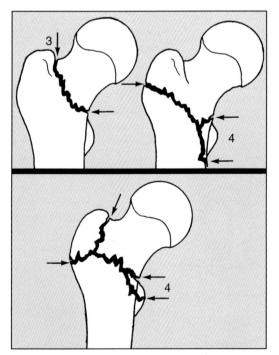

Figure 24.3   Extracapsular fractures of the femoral neck. Intratrochanteric or basal fractures (3) run between the trochanters. Pertrochanteric fracture lines (4) separate one or both trochanters from the femur. (From McRae & Esser 2002.)

consent can be obtained; this also assists in compliance with treatment and care interventions.

Conservative approaches take up to 12 weeks to heal a fracture for a fit healthy individual. However, for a frail older person with osteoporosis, it may take longer. In addition, long-term bedrest on skeletal or skin traction makes conservative management a high-risk approach for most patients. Therefore surgical management of these fractures is accepted as the treatment of choice.

Occasionally a decision is made to delay surgery or to treat the fracture conservatively if the patient is at greater risk from surgery, particularly if they are a high anaesthesia risk. For this reason spinal anaesthesia is increasingly common as the older person is at less risk than with a general anaesthetic.

The significance of the position of the fracture is vital when considering surgical management. If the fracture is below or around an existing prosthesis, this makes surgery difficult and the chances of a good outcome unlikely (Somers et al 1998).

Intracapsular fractures disturb the blood supply to the head of the femur (Fig. 24.4), leading to avascular

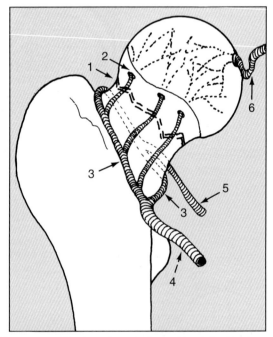

Figure 24.4   Blood supply to the femoral head. The blood supply is disrupted by intracapsular fractures (1), leading to avascular necrosis. The main supply penetrates the femoral head close to the cartilage margin (2) and arises from the arterial ring (3) fed from the lateral and medial femoral circumflex arteries (4,5), with a small portion of the head being supplied via the ligamentum teres (6). (From McRae & Esser 2002.)

necrosis and the consequent painful collapse of the femoral head. The femoral head comprises a shell of compact bone containing very fragile, sparsely woven cancellous bone that does not lend itself to firm internal fixation. For this reason intracapsular fractures are usually treated by hemiarthroplasty, except in adults under the age of 60–65 years. A total hip arthroplasty is considered when an otherwise fit patient has symptomatic arthritis. In patients less than 60 years of age, reduction and internal fixation is the treatment of choice. These patients may still require an arthroplasty if they remain fit and active for more than a decade following the initial surgery. A variety of internal fixation devices are available for the treatment of both intracapsular and extracapsular fractures, the most common being the dynamic hip screw and joint replacement.

SURGERY AND OLDER PEOPLE

Due to their age and the condition not being immediately life threatening, patients with a hip fracture are in danger of receiving a second-class service (Royal College of Physicians 1989). Research demonstrates clearly that patients should receive an operation by an experienced surgeon within 24 hours of admission (Parker & Pryor 1992) and many units are now striving to achieve this standard in the UK (Audit Commission 1995). Unfortunately all too often surgery is delayed, leading to the increased probability of complications and delayed recovery.

The National Confidential Enquiry into Perioperative Deaths (NCEPOD 1999) made a number of important recommendations applicable to older people undergoing surgery following orthopaedic trauma. These include:

- adequate fluid management
- a team approach, including surgeons, anaesthetists and physicians, to the management of older people with poor physical status or a high operative risk
- surgery performed by experienced surgeons
- provision of high-dependency or intensive care facilities where necessary
- older people should wait no longer than 24 hours once fit for surgery
- appropriate and specialised pain management provided by those with appropriate experience to ensure safe and effective pain relief.

PRINCIPAL NURSING CARE ISSUES

Preoperative traction

Historically preliminary skin traction (3–4 kg) has been used to relieve the initial pain and minimise further displacement of the fracture. The type of traction varied according to surgeon preference and unit protocol but was usually unilateral Pugh's or Hamilton Russell traction. This practice is now uncommon for a variety of reasons:

- the value and effect of the traction are questionable (Draper & Scott 1996)
- the patient should be transferred to the operating theatre soon after admission, making the application of traction pointless and likely to cause unnecessary distress
- traction adds to the risk of complications such as pressure damage and acute confusion, although research evidence has yet to demonstrate this
- research evidence (Draper & Scott 1997, Finsen et al 1992) throws doubt on the success of the traction in managing pain
- perhaps most significantly, if pain management is adequately considered and the limb supported by a pillow or other soft appliance, the effect is likely to be at least as good as when traction is applied (Draper & Scott 1997) and the traction is an additional cost.

Pain management

Fracture pain is not well described in the literature (Santy & Mackintosh 2001) and there is a tendency for pain management for these patients to be inadequately considered (Closs 1994).

Additionally postoperative pain is notoriously inadequate (Royal College of Surgeons and College of Anaesthetists 1990). The management of an elderly person with postoperative pain is often even more inadequate (Novy & Genge Jagmin 1997, Partridge 1994). This has grave implications for sleep, anxiety levels, recovery and rehabilitation (Closs et al 1997) – yet if these patients are to do well, their pain must be adequately managed.

Good pain management must begin with the use of a pain assessment that adequately fits the needs of older people (Hayes 1995, Novy & Genge Jagmin 1997). This includes taking into account the fact that older people tend to have been brought up in a culture of forbearance and are unlikely to request pain relief. Older people also have difficulty in communicating pain because of physical or cognitive impairment.

The use of analgesics in the elderly requires care and as a consequence there is a tendency to underprescribe and underadminister analgesia (Novy & Genge Jagmin 1997). This is demonstrated in Closs et al's (1993) study where older people having undergone hip surgery reported considerable postoperative pain but only a small proportion of the prescribed analgesia had been given.

During the early hours and days following surgery when mobilisation regimes begin and pain is most acute, small frequent doses of opiate analgesics are necessary. Patient-controlled analgesia is appropriate for patients with good cognitive function. However, the reduced function of the nervous system in the elderly means that opiate analgesia must be carefully administered and monitored for adverse effects such as drowsiness and respiratory depression. Bowel motility in the elderly also tends to be diminished and codeine-based analgesics are known to cause constipation. Careful assessment and management of bowel function are therefore important.

The efficacy of less potent analgesics such as paracetamol and aspirin-based products should not be underestimated once the severe pain subsides but neither should their effect be overestimated when the pain is severe.

Alternatives to pharmacological pain management such as transcutaneous electrical nerve stimulation (TENS), acupuncture and distraction techniques are being increasingly used.

One of the greatest difficulties in pain management is pain assessment of the cognitively impaired or confused older person. The nurse must learn to recognise non-verbal signs of discomfort such as changed breathing patterns, non-specific noise making and fidgeting (Miller et al 1996).

Cognitive state and psychological care

Patients with a hip fracture have undergone a major traumatic life event. Due to the common occurrence of this injury, healthcare staff can trivialise it and underestimate how the patient and relatives view it as a source of major concern and anxiety. Failure to deal with these fears can be detrimental to the rehabilitation process.

An acute confusion state is described by Brooking (1986, p242) as: 'an acute or subacute alteration in previously normal mental function which is often temporary and reversible, associated with impaired

Box 24.1	Causes of acute confusion (adapted from Matthiesen et al 1994)
Physiological	Dehydration and electrolyte imbalance
	Drug therapy (especially tranquillisers, antidepressants and analgesics)
	Pyrexial and apyrexial infections
	Metabolic disturbances, endocrine disease
	Nutritional deficits
	Hypothermia
	Constipation, cardiovascular and respiratory diseases
Psychological	Severe emotional distress
	Pain
	Anxiety
	Relocation
	Loss of control
	Bereavement
	Visual and/or hearing impairments
	Impaired communication
Environmental	Unfamiliar environment
	Sensory deprivation or overload
	Lack of environmental clues such as clocks and calendars
	Sleep deprivation
	Immobility
	Social isolation

brain function, usually secondary to a pathological process outside the nervous system' and tends to be characterised by disorientation, agitation and hyperactive behaviour (Schofield 1997). Unfortunately, acute confusional states are a common complication of hip fracture surgery.

Hip fracture is commonly associated with Alzheimer's disease and dementing illness. There is a danger that many nurses consider confusion to be inevitable and untreatable (Schofield 1997). The literature suggests the causes of acute confusion are likely to be any or a combination of physiological, psychological or environmental factors as seen in Box 24.1. It is important that orthopaedic nurses understand the causes and are able to assess and manage the reasons for this, especially factors within the hospital environment such as noise, of post-fall syndrome where the older person is reluctant to mobilise for fear of falling again. They have a tendency to clutch, grab and shuffle when asked to walk. This is a natural reaction and must be managed sensitively with clear explanations, realistic and achievable goal setting, followed by praise and encouragement when goals are achieved. Each patient will undertake the remobilisation process in a different way.

It is just as important to consider how the fall led to the injury, why the person fell and any measures that can be taken to prevent recurrence. The events surrounding the fall, underlying medical conditions, medication, social circumstances and the environment are among the factors that should be considered. It is inappropriate to discharge patients who have sustained an injury following a fall without adequately addressing the factors that led to it. The management of falls is a local and national problem. The orthopaedic team needs to liaise with the local falls service to ensure a team approach to the assessment, identification of risks and prevention of future incidents (DoH 2001).

Skin

These patients are automatically at high risk of a pressure ulcer (Lizi 2000) because of their age, the injury, consequent immobility and other underlying conditions and problems. Pressure ulcer prevention must be considered from the moment of admission. Sensitive and rapid handling in the A & E department must include the use of mattress overlays and the rapid transfer of patients to a specialised orthopaedic trauma ward within 1 hour (Audit Commission 1995).

On arrival on the ward, the patient must be placed on an appropriate support surface, minimally a mattress proven successful in preventing pressure ulcers in medium- or high-risk clients. For patients who are very frail or have a significant number of additional risk factors, an alternating pressure mattress or other more sophisticated support system should be employed. It is unacceptable to place patients on a standard-issue mattress that is known to be inadequate in these circumstances (Nuffield Institute/NHS CRD 1995).

Early mobilisation remains one of the most effective guards against pressure ulcers but it is vital to consider seating, cushions and frequent changes of position in the chair once this has commenced, as well as nutrition.

activity and changing the patient's bed position within the ward.

Nursing research in this area is scanty. Foreman (1986) suggested the lack of research was due to confused elderly patients not commanding academic attention as they are perceived as uninteresting, relatively unimportant, unworthy or beyond help. There is little to suggest this situation has changed.

The absence of physical harm and the maintenance of self-esteem during and after the period of acute confusion are priorities of nursing care (Schofield 1997). Schofield suggests a standard for managing acute confusional states and offers a detailed rationale for these (Box 24.2).

The fall

Most patients with a fracture of the hip have fallen. Downton (1993) describes the common phenomenon

Nutrition

Practices in preoperative fasting have been the source of much discussion in the literature. Current evidence suggests that food need only be withdrawn for 4–6 hours prior to surgery and clear fluids for only 2–3 hours preoperatively (Green et al 1996, Haines 1995, Hung 1992, Phillips et al 1993).

The difficulties arise because it is not always possible to predict the time of surgery due to competing priorities with other patients. In areas of good practice the surgery time can be predicted because operating lists are set aside daily for these patients (Audit Commission 1995, Parker & Pryor 1992), so food and drink can then be withdrawn at the appropriate time.

It is equally vital to assess the patient's hydration state. Intravenous rehydration or adequate oral fluids will prevent electrolyte imbalance and dehydration that may otherwise lead to acute confusion states, urinary problems and constipation. Nurses need to challenge systems in which excessive periods of fasting, dehydration and waiting for surgery remain an issue (NCEPOD 1999).

Many older people are nutritionally compromised from a combination of social, psychological and physical factors. The elderly frail person who has sustained a hip fracture has an increased demand for nutrition because of the trauma and its physiological effect. The correct nutritional intake, particularly increased calories, protein, calcium and fibre, allows healing of the fracture and surgical wound and provides additional energy for mobilisation and rehabilitation (D'Eramo et al 1994). Vitamin C has been identified as important in the healing process and there is evidence that supplements of this enhance recovery (Handel 1997).

There are many reasons for malnutrition while in hospital (Lennard Jones 1992, McWhirter & Pennington 1994). In most instances the normal hospital diet does not provide enough calories and other nutrients to meet physiological needs. The simplest way of providing nutritional support is to encourage the patient to eat more by ensuring food is available in the right form, in the right quantity, at the right time and that the patient is physically able to eat it (Bond 1998).

There is strong evidence to suggest that dietary supplementation with high-calorie, high-protein feeds significantly improves recovery outcomes and prevents complications such as wound healing problems, poor mobility and pressure ulcers as well as reducing the length of stay and preventing infection (Larsson et al 1990). Work by Bastow et al in 1983 showed that tube feeding at night following hip fracture is successful in improving recovery outcomes but the invasiveness and discomfort of a nasogastric tube make this unpleasant for the patient. Oral supplements, where they can be taken, are the product of choice.

Elimination

Urinary problems, particularly infections and urinary retention, are common due to immobility and stasis of urine.

An adequate fluid intake is essential to ensure effective renal function and to dilute urine. There is evidence to suggest that cranberry juice is effective in preventing urinary infection and would also increase the vitamin C intake (Winslow 1995).

Urinary retention is common after surgery. It can generally be resolved by assisting the patient to get out of bed and use a commode if their condition and treatment allow. Only in extreme circumstances should urinary catheterisation be considered as the procedure is associated with bacteraemia. If the catheter is left in situ it is likely to predispose the patient to infection around the orthopaedic implant (Levi et al 1997, Stickler & Zimakoff 1994).

Urinary incontinence is relatively common in patients with a hip fracture (Palmer et al 1997). It is easy but misguided to assume that incontinence is to be expected, is a chronic problem or cannot be treated. Urinary catheterisation is not the management option of choice for incontinence. Nurses need to become adept at assessing the reasons for incontinence, such as urinary tract infection, dehydration, poor bladder wall muscle and sphincter control or psychological problems (Pearson & Kelber 1996, Penn et al 1996), and identifying interventions which may solve the problem.

Mobility

Recovery in patients with a hip fracture is generally measured by the assistance required in activities of living, particularly mobility, in relation to the individual's prefracture abilities (Williams et al 1994). Remobilisation normally begins on the day following surgery providing fixation of the fracture is satisfactory. The reasons for early mobilisation must be fully explained to the patient and relatives, as they may view this as unreasonable at a time when postoperative pain is still expected.

Ambulation must be gradually introduced. In some cases partial weight bearing is recommended. The most rapid gain in mobility is in the first 8 weeks, with less rapid improvement following this (Williams et al 1994). It is important that rehabilitation measures are concentrated to match this period.

Mobilisation begins with standing for short periods, then progressing to walking gradually greater distances with decreasing levels of support. This is combined with active exercises to strengthen the quadriceps muscles as they are instrumental in standing from sitting in a chair. The quadriceps can become very weak in older people who do not exercise, leading to a greater likelihood of falling.

A full assessment of the patient's previous mobility is vital along with ascertaining their previous living arrangements, potential place of discharge and mobility requirements. Realistic goals and timescales are the key to successful rehabilitation and it is vital that these are negotiated with the patient. Most patients wish to return to their previous home circumstances and regaining independence gradually enables return to their physical and psychological normality (Gamroth 1991).

Mobilisation initially involves the use of a walking frame. When the patient has enough stability and confidence this is gradually replaced with crutches or a walking stick. A patient can make minor improvements compared to their prefracture mobility with the right rehabilitation strategies but generally it is wise to anticipate a return to previous mobility levels. It is unrealistic to expect the client to achieve this in a few weeks; they should be encouraged to gradually reintroduce and increase activities following discharge from hospital. Mobility in the home must be considered; for example, a walking frame may cause problems due to limited space and the need to negotiate steps or stairs.

REHABILITATION FOLLOWING HIP FRACTURE

Realistic, appropriate and achievable goals are keys to successful rehabilitation. The goals must be negotiated, with the patient taking an active part in decision making. A patient who has faced a lonely struggle at home and is poorly motivated to recover just to face the same circumstances on discharge requires sensitive and skilled psychological care and empowerment (Hawkey & Williams 2001).

It is vital that orthopaedic nurses avail themselves of the specialist skills required to effectively nurse older people with complex problems and needs. Studies have shown (Audit Commission 1995, Sluenwhite & Simpson 1998) that discharge planning and communication are points where care often fails, resulting in vulnerable older people returning to the community to face unacceptable risks.

A variety of models have developed, ranging from orthopaedic units including formalised input from a geriatrician on 'orthogeriatric' units to the development of specialist nursing roles (Coulson 1993, Shiell et al 1993), specialist rehabilitation units for elderly orthopaedic patients, early supported discharge and hospital at home schemes (Darlow et al 1998, Parker et al 1991, Pryor & Williams 1989, Renton & Brown 2001, Tudor 1998).

There is little doubt that early discharge provides the optimum environment for rehabilitation but continued support will be needed in the community. With the continued development of intermediate care services (DoH 2001) a number of new options for rehabilitation are likely to become available both in the home and in the hospital setting. Further community services are likely to develop to allow early discharge with outreach and community rehabilitation services. It is also possible that the private elderly care sector may become more deeply involved as the NHS begins to collaborate more often with commercial healthcare organisations.

OTHER INJURIES TO THE HIP AND FEMUR

Although hip fractures and osteoarthritis account for the majority of patients admitted for orthopaedic nursing care, there are other relevant conditions. Adults presenting with hip pain usually have an arthritic condition, avascular necrosis or a soft tissue or bony injury (Apley & Solomon 1994). Only bony injuries are addressed here: hip dislocation, femoral shaft and supracondylar fractures.

DISLOCATION OF THE HIP

The hip joint is relatively stable and not prone to dislocation unless the trauma is severe. The mechanism of injury involves transfer of a force up the lower limb. This typically occurs with a dashboard injury in a road traffic accident; this mechanism of injury is also linked to injuries of the knee and femur.

If the knee is flexed at the time of impact, there is a posterior dislocation. If the hip is widely abducted an anterior dislocation can occur. The patient will present with deformity and severe pain (McRae & Esser 2002).

Reduction is usually carried out as soon as possible under general anaesthetic or sedation. Following reduction, the hip must be kept at rest to allow healing of the soft tissues and prevent complications such as recurrent dislocation and secondary osteoarthritis. The time of this period of rest may vary from 1 to 6 weeks depending on the surgeon's preference. The use of fixed traction in a Thomas splint is debatable (McRae & Esser 2002). Other surgeons prefer to get patients up and mobilising in a removable brace to restrict adduction of the joint.

Following injury and reduction the nurse must closely observe the limb for signs of compromised circulation or neurological function as the sciatic nerve and the blood supply to the femoral head and lower leg are vulnerable to injury. This involves recording muscle power and the colour, warmth and sensation of the limb.

Once the dislocation is reduced the pain should be less but not absent due to the associated soft tissue trauma. In order to facilitate movement, pain assessment and analgesia must be carefully considered. During periods of bedrest, static quadriceps exercises along with hourly plantar and dorsiflexion of the foot ensure minimal muscle wastage and reduce the risk of deep vein thrombosis. A period of partial weight bearing with crutches can be necessary once mobilisation begins.

FRACTURES OF THE FEMORAL SHAFT

The femur is the largest and strongest bone in the human body, covered with the largest and longest muscles; it normally requires considerable force to fracture. This has implications for nursing management because of the amount of trauma sustained and the potential for other injuries.

The femoral shaft is defined as the area extending from the trochanters to the condyles (Fig. 24.5). Most fractures of the femoral shaft are the result of road traffic accidents (Taylor et al 1994) or industrial trauma, particularly those involving high velocity or great force.

Pathological fractures resulting from metabolic bone disease or malignancy do occur but require less force. Injuries range from simple transverse and oblique fractures to extremely complex compound injuries.

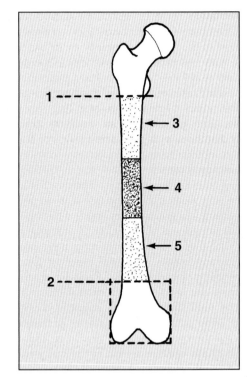

Figure 24.5   Classification of femoral shaft fractures. Under the AO classification of femoral fractures, the shaft extends from the inferior margin of the lesser trochanter (1) to the upper border of the distal femur (2). The shaft then divides into the proximal or subtrochanteric zone (3), middle (4) and distal (5) thirds. (From McRae & Esser 2002.)

Initial care

One of the greatest risks immediately following a femoral shaft fracture is hypovolaemic shock. Up to a litre of blood can be lost into the fracture site in a closed fracture (McRae & Esser 2002) and coupled with blood loss from the surrounding traumatised soft tissues, this can lead to rapid depletion in the circulating blood volume. It is vital to monitor the level and stability of the pulse and blood pressure, particularly during the first 12 hours following injury.

An intravenous infusion is vital for 24 hours or longer if eating and drinking are impaired or a blood transfusion is necessary. Blood loss can be replaced with isotonic intravenous fluids or plasma replacement products in most instances. However, where there is a drop in haemoglobin levels whole blood should be administered or later, if circulating volume is normal, packed cells. Postfracture anaemia is likely to be a major cause of lethargy and subsequently poor mobilisation and rehabilitation.

Fat embolisms are a rare but dangerous complication of femoral shaft fractures; they occur because of the size of the femoral fatty marrow-filled cavity. For the first 72 hours following injury the patient should be observed closely for petechial rash, pyrexia, confusion and anoxia. Similarly deep vein thrombus and pulmonary embolus development are potential complications and the risks should be managed according to the current best practice.

Multiple injuries

A considerable number of lower limb fractures are associated with multiple injuries, particularly in cases of fractures of the shaft of femur and tibia where high velocity and force have been involved in the mechanism of injury; compound fractures are common (Zavotsky & Banavage 1995). Although the femoral fracture is not likely to be viewed as life threatening in itself there is considerable evidence to demonstrate that early stabilisation and fixation of the fracture reduce morbidity and mortality.

Complications may be related to other multiple injuries to the spine, pelvis, abdominal and pelvic organs, pulmonary contusions or a head injury (Bone et al 1998). Consequently multiply injured patients receive initial interdisciplinary care in an intensive care or high-dependency unit. This highlights the importance of the availability of orthopaedic nursing skills in areas not designated as orthopaedic.

Equally the orthopaedic nurse receiving patients from an intensive care unit requires high-dependency nursing skills and sensitivity to the psychological problems experienced by the patient and family. Such patients present unrivalled challenges where complication rates are extremely high and place inordinate demands on nursing time and skills (Hefti 1995).

Management

Conservative treatment.   This is used when surgical intervention is contraindicated. Skeletal or skin traction is used to overcome the fracture displacement. It is important that the correct traction force, position and amount of padding beneath the fracture site are prescribed and maintained, with regular radiographic examination to check the alignment of the fracture. The patient should be taught static quadriceps exercises, encouraged to maintain their muscle tone and to plantar and dorsiflex the foot to improve venous return from the lower leg.

Once sufficient callus is evident any external splint can be discarded and the fracture site supported with a sling or cushion. Alternatively a Pearson knee flexion piece can be added to the traction apparatus. Flexion and extension exercises of the knee are now started.

After approximately 4 weeks, if sufficient callus is present, a femoral cast brace is applied to allow partial weight bearing through the limb to increase axial loading for correct bone healing. The femoral cast brace allows a controlled degree of flexion and extension but prevents rotation, maintaining the position of the fracture while the patient mobilises. The ankle may or may not be included in the cast. If the ankle is not incorporated, a plastic foot piece and ankle hinges are used and a good, firm shoe such as a trainer should be worn whilst mobilising. The upper half of the cast is shaped to lie just below the crease of the buttocks and up to the groin; both of these regions must be closely observed for signs of skin breakdown. If the fracture is in the upper third of the femur a hip hinge and waist strap are used to prevent rotation; the strap must always be fastened when the patient is mobilising.

Conservative treatment with skeletal traction is now rare unless surgical intervention is contraindicated.

Surgical management.   Surgery for femoral shaft fractures is the treatment of choice because it allows early mobilisation. The medical management has improved considerably since the advent of the interlocking nail. This allows firm internal fixation of the fracture without a surgical incision to the fracture site, placing the patient at less risk of infection. There are still considerable risks from the surgery, specifically fat emboli caused by reaming of the medullary cavity during surgery (Christie et al 1995) and thromboembolism.

If the fixation is considered to be sound the patient can mobilise bearing weight almost immediately. If the fixation is in doubt, weight bearing is allowed once callus is present at the fracture site. Occasionally external splintage is required if the fracture is highly contaminated, compound or complex.

External fixation is used for a fracture that is very complex or is compound (DeGeorge & Dunwoody 1995).

SUPRACONDYLAR FRACTURES

Supracondylar fractures of the femur are less common than fractures of the femoral shaft. However, the complexities of treating them, especially in the elderly, make them a challenge for the orthopaedic service. Fractures of the lower end of the femur around the condyles occur as a result of a high-velocity impact to the flexed knee when in a sitting position, a typical example being the driver of a car in a road traffic accident involving a frontal collision. Fractures of or around the femoral condyle provide specific challenges because the muscles and tendons cause displacement and the close proximity to the knee joint causes difficulty for internal fixation (Schatzker 1998).

INJURIES AND CONDITIONS AROUND THE KNEE JOINT

The knee is the most complex synovial joint in the human body. Under arthroscopic vision it appears as a series of blind alleys. Stability of the joint is provided by the complex arrangement of ligaments, tendons and cartilages within and exterior to the joint capsule. As one of the major weight-bearing joints of the body, it is placed under extreme stress in many activities, making it prone to injury.

FRACTURE OF THE PATELLA

The patella is suspended in the long tendon of the quadriceps muscles, giving it some protection from injury. Patellar fractures usually occur from a fall onto or a direct blow to the anterior aspect of the knee joint. The force required is considerable and often results in a comminuted, compound fracture with considerable damage to the surrounding soft tissues.

The primary nursing aims are to manage the pain and reduce swelling. Elevation and support of the limb and the application of ice to the anterior aspect of the knee can in part achieve both aims, although good pain assessment will indicate the need for additional pain management strategies. A haemarthrosis is likely (Maffulli et al 1993), requiring aspiration to reduce the pain and full joint assessment to rule out other soft tissue injuries such as ligament damage. Surgical management usually involves wiring of the patella if the fracture is displaced and occasionally a full or partial patellectomy if fragmentation is severe.

Alternatively a long leg cylinder cast is the conservative management option of choice (Braun et al 1993, Carpenter et al 1997). The knee is placed at approximately 15° of flexion in the cast, allowing an optimum resting position for the joint, preventing stiffness and making it easier for the patient to clear the floor with the foot when mobilising.

INTERNAL DERANGEMENT OF THE KNEE

Internal derangement of the knee comprises a group of soft tissue injuries of the knee joint. This group of injuries is usually, although not exclusively, the result of a sporting or leisure injury.

Meniscal injuries

The menisci are semilunar cartilages that help provide stability and lubrication for the knee joint. Injury to the menisci usually results from traction, compression, torque forces or a combination of all three. The meniscus becomes trapped between the femoral heads and the tibial plateau when the force exceeds the normal alignment of the joint (Cailliet 1992). This is a common turning or twisting injury in contact and field sports.

Meniscal injury or tear causes loss of continuity of the cartilage fibres. Such tears rarely heal because the outer area attached to the collateral ligaments is the only part with a blood supply. The patient with an acute injury will present with severe acute knee pain, loss of function, an effusion and, if severe, a haemarthrosis. The long-term signs are tenderness of the knee joint, locking, giving way, 'clicking' and wasting of the quadriceps from lack of use.

Diagnosis is made by examination of the knee and a variety of tests and signs described in the medical and physiotherapy literature. The value of X-rays is debatable. Diagnosis is confirmed by arthroscopic examination although many orthopaedic surgeons now prefer to use magnetic resonance imaging (MRI) as it is non-invasive and more cost effective.

With minor injuries when the patient's activity is not limited, conservative treatment is generally effective. This involves pain management, resolution of the effusion, 'unlocking' of the joint where necessary and restoration of quadriceps muscle function through active exercise, particularly straight leg raising.

Surgical treatment involves a full or preferably a partial meniscectomy which preserves the remaining normal meniscal tissue (Cailliet 1992). Removal of all or the majority of the meniscus predisposes the knee to secondary osteoarthritis.

Postoperative management includes a compressive bandage or dressing, keeping the leg elevated and isometric quadriceps exercises such as straight leg raising, within 24 hours of surgery. Gradual resistance, such as using weights on the foot or ankle, is encouraged once muscle strength begins to improve. Knee bending, flexion and extension exercises can be commenced once any restrictive bandaging is removed. It is vital that adequate pain relief is provided otherwise the rehabilitation programme is likely to be unsuccessful. The patient needs detailed information on the reasons for and the correct execution of these exercises.

Ligament injuries of the knee

A series of ligaments gives the knee some stability (Fig. 24.6). The main ligaments involved in knee injuries are the cruciate ligaments within the joint capsule and the external (medial and lateral) collateral ligaments attached to the outer aspect of the menisci. Excessive joint motion outside the normal physiological joint range leads to injury (strain, sprain or tear) of one or more of these structures. The knee is particularly vulnerable when fully extended, as both the cruciate ligaments and collateral ligaments are taut. At such a time any excessive rotation, as in twisting injuries or a blow to the lateral aspect of the knee, puts excessive pressure on the structures, making them prone to a tear or avulsion. The anterior cruciate ligament is particularly vulnerable during rotation as it stretches over the lateral femoral condyle at an angle (Cailliet 1992).

Medial collateral ligament (MCL). An injury here occurs from severe valgus forces exerted on the medial aspect of the knee, especially if the knee is slightly flexed at the time of impact. Such injuries are common in sporting activities and road traffic accidents. The patient complains of weakness of the knee but little initial pain, although there is marked tenderness over the medial aspect on palpation. Examination will reveal opening of the medial aspect of the knee joint under lateral pressure when compared to the normal knee. If there is effusion or haemarthrosis there may be other injuries.

Treatment of MCL injury involves immediate splinting of the knee at 30° of flexion with isometric quadriceps exercise and partial weight bearing.

From the second to sixth week flexion can be allowed from 30° to 90° in a hinged splint, which prevents lateral movement of the knee during flexion, along with isokinetic exercises and full weight-bearing ambulation. At 6 weeks the orthosis is removed and isokinetic exercises continued with increasing resistance. Full athletic activity is permitted once 80% of knee strength has been regained. This protocol may vary according to the surgeon's or physiotherapist's preference.

Lateral collateral ligament (LCL). Injuries to this ligament are less common. They are generally the result of a knee dislocation and are associated with nerve damage. Management tends to be similar to MCL injuries.

Anterior cruciate ligament (ACL). This is a major stabilising ligament. An ACL injury is a significant and common disabling condition of the knee responsible for disruption of sporting careers. The patient usually describes a twisting injury with the knee extended and in external rotation. An audible 'pop' is often reported at the time of the injury with immediate instability of the knee, disability and painful limited range of motion. There can be a noticeable haemarthrosis and associated effusion and spasm of the hamstring muscles.

Management of ACL damage varies. Conservative management is favoured if the tear is partial although there is an increasing tendency to treat ACL injuries surgically. Techniques vary by using a variety of graft materials and operative procedures. Allografts as well as autografts are increasingly being used (Harner et al 1996) and the patient needs to be fully informed, particularly in respect of having an allograft. There are a number of psychological issues for some patients related to the use of animal tissue grafts. The length of stay in hospital following surgery varies from an outpatient or day case visit to 3 days (Brown 1996).

Complete internal derangement. This may occur when there is a severe twisting force or a lateral blow to the knee. This places undue strain on the medial collateral ligament, which is likely to tear along with the medial meniscus as it is attached to the MCL, at the same time as a rupture of the anterior cruciate ligament, leaving the individual with an unstable knee that no longer functions (Fig. 24.7).

Orthopaedic nurses have yet to forge a clear role for themselves in the management of sports injuries, even though the patient often requires hospitalisation and lengthy outpatient management. There is no reason why in the future, the scope of

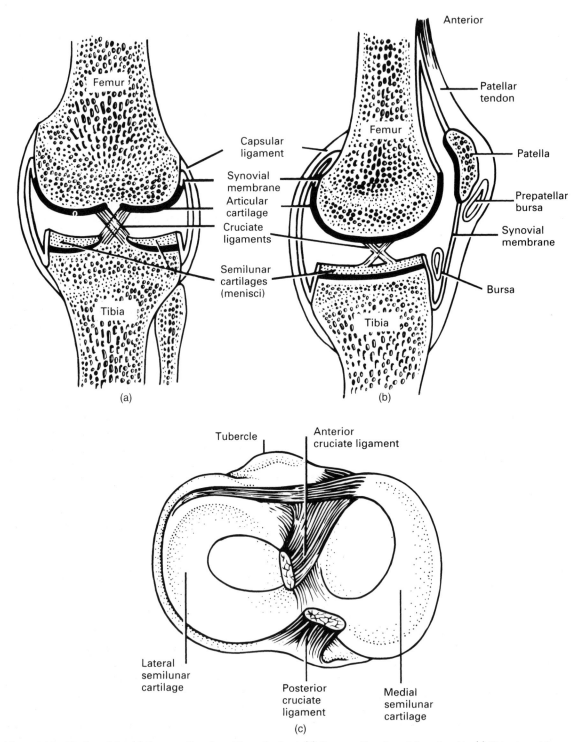

Figure 24.6 The knee joint. (a) Cross-section viewed from the front. (b) Cross-section viewed from the side. (c) Tibia viewed from the top. (From Wilson 1990 with permission.)

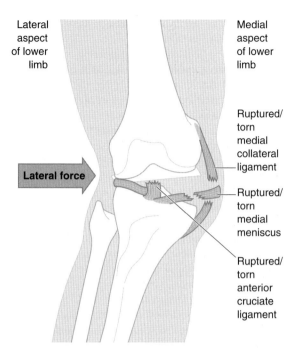

Lateral aspect of lower limb

Medial aspect of lower limb

Lateral force

Ruptured/ torn medial collateral ligament

Ruptured/ torn medial meniscus

Ruptured/ torn anterior cruciate ligament

Figure 24.7 Internal derangement of the knee.

practice should not be extended and expanded in this area (Santy 1999).

Arthroscopic knee surgery

Arthroscopic surgery allows the removal of most torn menisci and the repair or replacement of ruptured anterior or posterior cruciate ligaments. It is increasingly common for such surgery to take place in day surgery or outpatient units (Brown 1996, Neal 1996). Preadmission planning, assessment and discharge planning are essential if admission for such surgery is to be successful and a good experience for the patient (Dougherty 1996). During the preoperative phase the patient should have instruction on exercises and postoperative mobilisation techniques such as crutch walking.

This process should begin in the outpatients department followed by a specific appointment for preoperative nursing assessment (Brown 1996). Patients should arrive on the day of surgery having undergone all relevant diagnostic tests and be prepared both physically and psychologically. There is little doubt that a patient who is well informed about the procedure, its effects and the consequent rehabilitation programme will be more likely to achieve a successful recovery.

Wound closure is usually minimal, involving one suture or adhesive strip. The most feared complication is wound infection and subsequent failure of the surgical procedure. It is important to ensure that intra- and postoperative prophylactic antibiotics are administered correctly, that the wound and body temperature are monitored for signs of infection and, in particular, assessment for any undue pain is undertaken. In view of early discharge it is important that the patient understands the signs of infection and the potential complications.

It is easy to assume that pain is not a major feature of minimally invasive surgery. For this reason nurses involved in the recovery of patients undergoing arthroscopic knee surgery should be well acquainted with the procedure undertaken, which can be a source of considerable pain. The most important factor in determining the length of stay postoperatively is pain control. This needs to be individually provided to maintain sufficient pain relief to allow active use and exercise of the affected limb whilst avoiding side effects such as drowsiness and nausea. Local anaesthetics, narcotics and cryotherapy are increasingly common intra- and postoperative strategies (Brown 1996). Adequate analgesia should be provided for the patient to take home and they should be warned that the pain might increase once greater activity resumes.

Discharge is dependent on the ability to undertake static quadriceps exercises, to mobilise safely with crutches and the absence of significant pain and nausea.

Rehabilitation following arthroscopic knee surgery can last up to 1 year, the main aims of which are to (Brown 1996):

- protect any graft or repair
- restore the range of motion to the knee joint
- facilitate early weight bearing
- return to preinjury activities.

Many patients undergoing arthroscopic surgery are active sports enthusiasts with a positive attitude to their rehabilitation. Provided they have sufficient verbal and written information, they are likely to comply with the prescribed rehabilitation programme. However, the psychological effects of even temporary disability through injury to a competing athlete must be taken into account and the nurse should take the time to consider the likely effect on the rehabilitation performance to facilitate acceptance and motivation (Maher & Fout Rodts 1994).

ANTERIOR KNEE PAIN

Anterior knee pain is common, particularly in adolescents, and rarely requires treatment. Often this is treated in general practice or outpatients departments with the nurse being involved in health promotion and information giving. There are a variety of causes most of which resolve with conservative management and are not permanently disabling.

Chondromalacia patellae

One explanation for recurrent anterior knee pain is chondromalacia patellae, a common degenerative condition of the articular cartilage of the patella; it also occurs in other joints but less commonly. It usually arises in adolescents and young adults. The cause is unknown although injury is sometimes implicated (Cailliet 1992). The articular surface of the patella becomes soft, roughened, fibrillated and wears away. It causes pain, recurrent effusions and the knee sometimes 'gives way' unexpectedly. Pressure over the patella causes pain and there is often crepitus on moving the joint (Duckworth 1995).

The condition often resolves after some years but occasionally cases are persistent and difficult to treat. During this period the patient and family require support and good pain management. The surgical options include shaving off the rough surface of the patella and realignment of the patellar tendon. In severe cases a patellectomy is performed but other changes within the joint can make this unsuccessful in resolving pain. This condition often predisposes to osteoarthritis in later life.

The orthopaedic nurse must ensure the patient has sufficient information to make an informed choice about the treatment options and act as a health promoter, especially when obesity and overuse are placing additional pressure on the joint or advice on muscle strengthening may protect the knee.

FRACTURES OF THE TIBIA AND FIBULA

The lower leg is vulnerable to indirect violence from torsional stresses, violence transmitted through the feet and from direct blows, all causing tibia and fibula fractures. There are frequently additional injuries to the ankles or knees. For this reason it is vital that both legs are fully assessed to rule out injury to these joints even though they are away from the main site of pain.

The tibia is a main weight-bearing bone. Fractures occur from sporting injuries, falls from heights and motor vehicle accidents, generally, though not exclusively, in active children and younger adults.

Oblique and spiral fractures are particularly common. The medical management is dictated by the complexity of the fracture, the degrees of displacement and rotation and the integrity of the skin.

Undisplaced fractures of the tibia are treated with a long leg cast with the knee in approximately 15° of flexion, the optimum resting position for the knee joint. Children can mobilise non-weight bearing with crutches once any risk to the circulation is over; for adults this is after a few days. A walking heel is applied after approximately 4 weeks, allowing partial weight bearing and providing some degree of axial loading through the fracture. The fracture takes 4–5 weeks to unite in a young child and up to 12 weeks in an adult (McRae & Esser 2002), occasionally longer in the elderly.

Any patient in a lower limb cast requires appropriate information and advice on how to carry out activities of daily living (Pearson 1987). There is some evidence to suggest that functional cast bracing, which allows some movement at the fracture site and weight-bearing mobilisation of neighbouring joints, can stimulate healing and reduce the risk of non-union (Chapman et al 1996).

Compound fractures

As the anterior tibial crest lies just below the surface of the skin, compound injuries are extremely common (McRae & Esser 2002). There is a higher risk of osteomyelitis, making compound fractures a medical emergency (Brown et al 1996, Hersh & McGainty 1996).

They can be classed as incomplete amputations. The management priorities are firstly life preservation, then limb preservation, infection avoidance and lastly functional preservation (Zavotsky & Banavage 1995). For this reason any wound associated with the fracture is treated with extreme care, often by secondary intention. Suturing is not considered until the wound appears clean and free from any infection.

Minimal handling of the wound is vital, with a strict aseptic technique, dressings being left intact for as long as possible and the principles of moist wound healing utilised. An occlusive dressing provides visible observation of the wound, ensuring minimal contamination. Prophylactic antibiotics, initially intravenously, should be administered until wound healing is evident. The patient's temperature and the appearance of the wound should be monitored at least daily to detect signs of infection.

Internal fixation is avoided in compound fractures unless the fracture is not complex and the wound minor. External fixation is now commonly used when there is a complex fracture or extensive surrounding tissue damage (Checketts et al 1995). In some difficult cases skeletal traction via a calcaneal pin is used but the length of hospital stay with this option makes it uncommon.

The nurse must help the patient to understand the implications of these treatment options and to make informed choices that ensure optimum outcomes for maintaining quality of life (Brown et al 1996).

Potential complications

The major complications of lower leg fractures and surgery are compartment syndrome, deep vein thrombosis (Mosley-Koehler 1999) and Volkman's ischaemia.

The lower leg has three tightly packed compartments containing muscles, nerves and blood supply. Haemorrhage and swelling quickly lead to a build-up of pressure in these compartments (Tucker 1998), compromising the blood and nerve supply to the foot. The popliteal artery runs close to the posterior aspect of the upper tibia and if it is affected in upper tibial fractures (McRae & Esser 2002), this may lead to ischaemia of the calf muscles.

Until the swelling and inflammation subside, the limb is kept elevated to facilitate venous return. A Braun frame provides the ideal situation for this, facilitating a safe degree of flexion at the knee and sufficient elevation to ensure good perfusion. In the absence of such apparatus the foot of the bed is elevated and the lower leg supported on several firm pillows or a foam trough.

In some units, compartment catheterisation and pressure monitoring are performed in all cases of tibial fracture for the first 24–48 hours (McQueen et al 1996). Frequent observation of the patient and limb must be carried out for this period, especially for increasing and excessive pain, particularly on passive movement (Hersh & McGainty 1996). The affected and unaffected foot are compared to ensure

both are warm and pink, the pedal pulses are marked and felt, although an absent pulse is a late sign. The patient should be able to move their toes, with any splints or casts allowing movement and observation of this. Observations must be recorded to ensure continuity of care and to provide a record of actions taken, any discrepancies being reported immediately. If compartment syndrome or ischaemia is suspected, surgical intervention is always indicated. In the case of compartment syndrome a fasciotomy is performed to release the pressure. Ischaemia from displacement of the fracture requires internal fixation with careful isolation and examination of the popliteal artery.

INJURIES AND CONDITIONS AROUND THE ANKLE

The ankle is a vulnerable and complex joint, comprising articulation between the tibia, fibula and talus (Fig. 24.8). Plantarflexion and dorsiflexion of the ankle joint are the important movements in ambulation (Cailliet 1997). This combination provides great flexibility during ambulation and carries the body's weight on a relatively small surface area.

Stability is provided by a complex series of ligaments, the most important being the collateral ligament, which supports the lateral and medial aspects of the ankle (Cailliet 1997). The lateral malleolus of the fibula is firmly attached to the tibia by the strong anterior and posterior tibiofibular ligaments (McRae & Esser 2002). These ligaments are prone to injury when the ankle joint is placed under undue stresses, particularly during eversion and inversion.

Many ankle fractures are complex because of the close association of the bones and ligaments within the joint. In general these fractures tend to be classified as follows.

- First-degree fracture where one malleolus, either the lateral or medial, is fractured.
- Second-degree or bimalleolar fracture where both the lateral and medial malleoli are fractured.
- Third-degree, Potts or trimalleolar fracture where there is an additional fracture to the posterior part of the inferior articular surface of the tibia (Fig. 24.9).

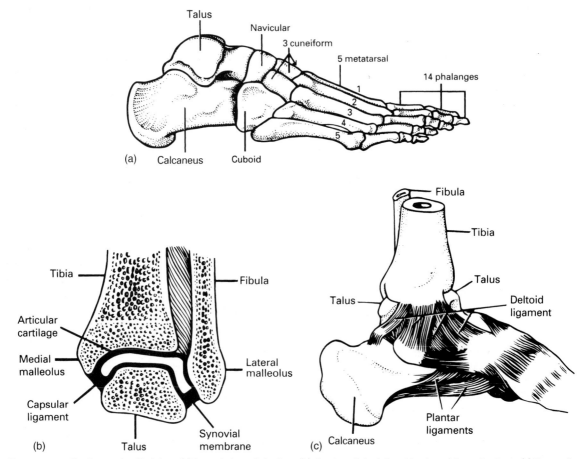

Figure 24.8   The foot and ankle joints. (a) Lateral view of the foot. (b) Section of the left ankle viewed from the front. (c) Supporting ligaments of the ankle, medial view. (From Wilson 1990 with permission.)

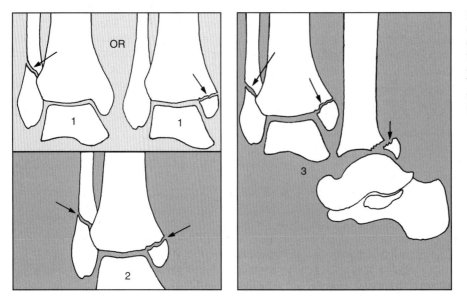

Figure 24.9   Classification of ankle fractures. (1) First-degree, single malleolus fracture. (2) Second-degree or bimalleolar fracture. (3) Third-degree or trimalleolar fracture. (From McRae & Esser 2002.)

The history and mechanisms of the injury, clinical examination and radiographs will give clues to the level of disruption of the joint. Rarely will the soft tissue and ligament structures remain intact if there is bony injury. In severe cases the ankle joint is completely unstable.

Ankle fracture management

The majority of ankle fractures are treated conservatively. The more complex and displaced the fracture, the greater the skill required to obtain accurate reduction and application of the cast. With severe disruption of the joint, adequate reduction and stabilisation require open reduction and internal fixation (McRae & Esser 2002).

The distal position of these fractures and soft tissue trauma mean ankle injuries are prone to severe swelling and bruising. Healing is quicker if the swelling and bruising are managed effectively by elevation and the use of ice as both improve the circulation to the surrounding tissues. Elevation, preferably with the ankle above the level of the pelvis on pillows or a Braun frame, is vital until swelling has subsided. This applies to fractures treated conservatively and surgically.

Ankle fractures are not encased in a full cast until the swelling has subsided but once any cast has been applied the risk of compromised circulation from swelling is high. The toes are observed for signs of impaired circulation and nerve supply, initially by the nurse who should teach the patient to observe for these signs as early discharge means complications are more likely to occur once home. If vascular compromise is suspected or considered likely, the cast is split and spread immediately (Younger et al 1990).

In most cases, during conservative management or following internal fixation, a below-knee cast is applied. Depending on the stability of the reduction, fixation and the surgeon's preference, mobilisation will begin with non-weight bearing using crutches until callus formation is evident. A walking heel is then applied, allowing partial or full weight bearing until union is considered sound at approximately 8 or 9 weeks following the injury. A supporting bandage may then be employed.

On discharge with a below-knee walking cast, the patient will require advice on how to cope with the activities of living. Classic work by Pearson (1987) noted that insufficient information was given to patients on discharge from hospital, severely restricting their activities. All verbal information given must be supported by written information to allow for gaps in the patient's memory.

In severe, complex and compression fractures external fixation or skeletal sliding traction through a calcaneal pin may be necessary.

Primary osteoarthritis of the ankle is rare, but secondary arthritis following an ankle injury that has disrupted the joint is very likely to lead to chronic pain and disability. In such cases ankle replacement is now becoming a more common option (Demetriades et al 1998).

SOFT TISSUE INJURIES TO THE ANKLE

The most common sports and leisure-related injuries are to the lateral ankle ligaments from eversion or inversion of the foot and ankle joints. If no bony injury is evident on X-ray examination, a soft tissue injury must be suspected. This can be ascertained by assessment of tenderness over the ligament, swelling and pain on movement of the ankle and, in severe cases, instability of the ankle.

In general sprains are often neglected and inadequately treated (Cailliet 1997). Treatment of acute ankle sprains involves (Cailliet 1997):

- local ice, elevation, compression bandaging and crutches for at least the first 24 hours to treat swelling
- early active movement of the ankle joint with a compression stocking plus dorsiflexion and plantarflexion exercises to prevent joint stiffness
- gradual toe raising and eversion–inversion exercises against increasing resistance
- a cast or elastic bandage worn for support. The length of time this should be required is controversial and varies according to medical preference.

Surgical treatment is considered where disruption or instability of the joint is severe.

RUPTURED ACHILLES TENDON

The Achilles tendon attaches the gastrocnemius muscle to the posterior calcaneum. Rupture of the tendo Achilles usually occurs from an overflexion injury of the ankle with excessive contraction of the calf muscle or a direct blow to the tendon. The patient describes sudden severe calf pain and a tangible 'snap' (Cailliet 1997).

If the tear is complete, early surgical intervention with approximation of the torn ends is indicated. Following surgery a cast is applied with the foot in plantarflexion to prevent stretching of the healing tendon. Mobilising with a cast in such a position can be more difficult. Once healing has occurred the tendon tends to be shortened and as a result may restrict some ankle dorsiflexion. However, this can be improved with exercise.

INJURIES AND CONDITIONS OF THE FOOT

SOFT TISSUE FOOT INJURIES

The foot is a very complex structure of bone and soft tissues. The structure and vulnerability of the foot make it prone to disorders related to its development and to short- or long-term injury.

Injury to the foot is due to sudden trauma or conditions that come about gradually through overuse or misuse, often related to inappropriate footwear. This can severely affect the person's life through chronic or acute pain and short- or long-term disability. Many patients are unaware of how to care for their feet properly and the orthopaedic nurse is in an ideal position to educate individuals regarding the importance of effective foot care (Fig. 24.10).

Unfortunately foot problems are particularly common in the elderly and may affect their ability to mobilise following injuries or conditions to any part of the lower limb. Where possible, podiatrists should be involved in the care and the teaching of appropriate foot care.

The 'normal' foot should be pain free and have appropriate muscle balance, absence of contracture, a central heel, straight and mobile toes and three sites of weight bearing while standing and during the stance phase of walking (Cailliet 1997).

SKELETAL INJURIES AND CHANGES TO THE FOOT

Tarsal fractures

Fractures of the calcaneum are associated with falls from a height and consequently tend to be crush fractures. This mechanism of injury can lead to associated injuries further up the leg, pelvis and spine.

Calcaneal fractures are often comminuted, extremely painful and associated with extensive swelling and bruising. Nursing management

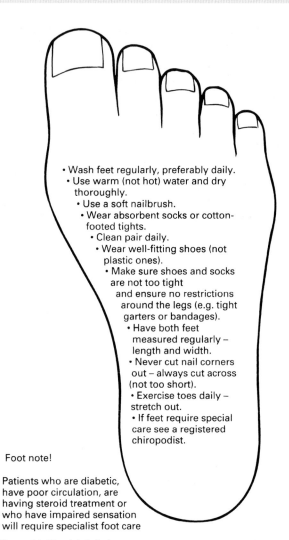

- Wash feet regularly, preferably daily.
- Use warm (not hot) water and dry thoroughly.
- Use a soft nailbrush.
- Wear absorbent socks or cotton-footed tights.
- Clean pair daily.
- Wear well-fitting shoes (not plastic ones).
- Make sure shoes and socks are not too tight and ensure no restrictions around the legs (e.g. tight garters or bandages).
- Have both feet measured regularly – length and width.
- Never cut nail corners out – always cut across (not too short).
- Exercise toes daily – stretch out.
- If feet require special care see a registered chiropodist.

Foot note!

Patients who are diabetic, have poor circulation, are having steroid treatment or who have impaired sensation will require specialist foot care

Figure 24.10   Adult foot care.

involves analgesia, high elevation with a Braun frame and ice therapy to control the pain and manage the swelling.

Medical options include closed reduction with a below-knee cast or open reduction and internal fixation with wires. During and following treatment ankle and toe exercises should be encouraged to prevent stiffness of the multiple joints of the foot and ankle (Apley & Solomon 1994).

Fractures of the other tarsal bones are unusual; they can require closed reduction and casting.

Metatarsal and phalanges injuries

The metatarsals are prone to injury through rotation, crush, traction or stress. Some displaced fractures

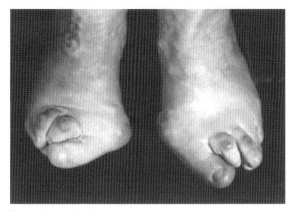

Figure 24.11   Hallux valgus.

require open reduction and internal fixation whilst the majority are managed by supporting the foot in a cast. Minimal casting of the foot is often used for a period of as little as 3 weeks. The effect of even minimal casts in foot injuries on the patient's activities of living must not be underestimated. In the case of compound fractures the usual wound management principles apply but there is even greater need for elevation to reduce swelling and for the wound to be protected from contamination from the floor once walking begins.

Fractured toes are usually the result of a heavy object falling on them. Phalangeal fractures are generally treated conservatively, often with 'neighbour' strapping to the adjacent toe. Any wound indicates a compound fracture requiring a sterile occlusive dressing and regular observation for signs of infection. Once again, the pain and the effects of swelling and bruising must not be underestimated.

Hallux valgus

A variety of other problems besides injuries may arise. However, there are two major conditions that orthopaedic nurses come into contact with regularly and these are hallux valgus and hammer toe.

Hallux valgus is a painful condition of the great toe (Fig. 24.11) commonly known as a bunion. This is a static subluxation of the first metatarsophalangeal (MTP) joint, in which there are three features.

1 The large toe angulates laterally towards the second toe.
2 The medial portion of the first metatarsal head enlarges.
3 The bursa over the medial aspect of the MTP joint becomes inflamed and thick walled (Cailliet 1997).

This combination leads to chronic pain and disability for some years if inappropriate footwear is worn but it may be asymptomatic.

In general this condition is managed with education and advice on good footwear and padding of the deformity. If there is severe deformity, pain and disability then surgery is considered. The most common surgery is a metatarsal osteotomy, where the bunion is removed, or an excision arthroplasty where the proximal part of the proximal phalanx is removed – a Keller's operation (Apley & Solomon 1994).

Hammer toe

A hammer toe is when the proximal joint is fixed in flexion whilst the distal and metatarsophalangeal joints are extended. The pressure of shoes over the deformity causes painful calluses. Operative correction involves excision arthrodesis (Apley & Solomon 1994).

FOOT SURGERY AND TRAUMA CARE

Foot surgery is often considered to be relatively minor. However, it has major implications for the patient as it is usually extremely painful and is likely to lead to considerable mobility problems in the short and medium term.

Patients having foot surgery need adequate information to allow them to take an active part in their recovery (Jackson 2001). In particular, they must be informed that they might experience considerable postoperative pain and how this will be managed. It is too easy to underestimate the amount of pain experienced following foot surgery. Individual pain assessment should ensure postoperative analgesia is sensitively prescribed and titrated. A combination of opiates and antiinflammatory drugs is often successful in the early stages. Patient-controlled analgesia is often valuable for these patients.

The patient is generally ambulant within hours of the procedure, if a day case, or on the following day. This causes patients much anxiety which is considerably abated if they are given the opportunity preoperatively to practise using crutches or sticks and to try walking strategies such as heel walking (Griffiths 1997).

Having fixation wires protruding from toes increases anxiety and poses an infection risk. Adequate padding, appropriate footwear and protection are needed to protect the foot from both trauma and infection. Pin sites are treated in the same manner as any other skeletal pin site.

Following foot injuries or surgery, footwear may be a problem for some time because of swelling and pain. Soft but supportive shoes such as a sports shoe, sandal or slipper are often required for some weeks after the injury.

AMPUTATION AND TRAUMATIC AMPUTATION

Many elective amputations of the lower limb or parts of the lower limb are carried out for vascular compromisation due to diabetic neuropathy or peripheral vascular disease. In many cases such surgery is carried out by the vascular surgeon. In some units the orthopaedic surgeon takes on this responsibility. In these situations the nurse has time to both physically and psychologically prepare the patient and relatives for the surgery and its aftermath.

Traumatic amputation of the lower limb is a feature of some crush injuries following entrapment, parasuicide or pedestrian traffic accidents. The very sudden, disabling and body image-changing nature of this injury presents unrivalled challenges for the orthopaedic nurse.

REHABILITATION

Young patients with lower limb injuries are usually also fit and healthy prior to the injury. The disability from the injury is usually temporary, but may be potentially long term if rehabilitation is not carried out effectively. Intensive rehabilitation can shorten the recovery period from the injury and significantly reduce the possibility of permanent disability (Hawkey & Williams 2001, Smith 1999).

Rehabilitation for the older age group is more complex when underlying medical conditions and social difficulties are considered and it is this aspect of care that poses the biggest challenge for the orthopaedic nurse and interdisciplinary team.

Further reading

Anders RL, Ornellas EM 1997 Acute management of patients with hip fracture: a research literature review. Orthopaedic Nursing 16(2): 31–46

Downton JH 1993 Falls in the elderly. Edward Arnold, London

Newman RJ (ed) 1992 Orthogeriatrics: comprehensive orthopaedic care for the elderly. Butterworth Heinemann, Oxford

Parker MJ, Pryor GA 1993 Hip fracture management. Blackwell, Oxford

Redfern S, Ross F (eds) 1999 Nursing older people, 3rd edn. Churchill Livingstone, Edinburgh

References

Apley GA, Solomon L 1994 Concise system of orthopaedics and fractures, 2nd edn. Butterworth Heinemann, Oxford

Audit Commission 1995 United they stand: co-ordinating care of elderly patients with hip fracture. HMSO, London

Bastow MD, Rawlings J, Allinson SP 1983 Benefits of supplementary tube feeding after fractured neck of femur: a randomised controlled trial. British Medical Journal 287: 1589–1592

Bond S 1998 Eating matters – improving dietary care in hospitals. Nursing Standard 12(17): 41–42

Bone LB, Anders MJ, Rohrbacher BJ 1998 Treatment of femoral fractures in the multiply injured patient with a thoracic injury. Clinical Orthopaedics and Related Research 347: 57–61

Braun W, Wiedemann M, Ruter A et al 1993 Indications and results of non-operative treatment of patellar fractures. Clinical Orthopaedics and Related Research 289: 197–201

Brooking J 1986 Dementia and confusion in the elderly. In: Redfern S (ed) Nursing elderly people. Churchill Livingstone, Edinburgh

Brown C, Henderson S, Moore S 1996 Surgical treatment of patients with open tibial fractures. AORN Journal 63(5): 873, 875, 877–878

Brown FM 1996 Anterior cruciate ligament reconstruction as an outpatient procedure. Orthopaedic Nursing 15(1): 15–20

Buckler JE, Dutton TL, MacLeod HL et al 1997 Use of hip protectors in a dementia unit. Physiotherapy Canada 49(4): 277–279, 310

Cailliet R 1992 Knee pain and disability, 3rd edn. FA Davis, Philadelphia

Cailliet R 1997 Foot and ankle pain, 3rd edn. FA Davis, Philadelphia

Carpenter JE, Kasman RA, Patel N et al 1997 Biomechanical evaluation of current patella fracture techniques. Journal of Orthopaedic Trauma 11(5): 351–363

Chapman H, MacDonald E, Smythe P 1996 Functional bracing of tibial shaft fractures. Nursing Times 92(23): 34–35

Checketts RG, Moran CG, Jennings AG 1995 134 tibial shaft fractures managed with the Dynamic Axial fixator. Acta Orthopaedica Scandinavica 66(3): 271–274

Christie J, Robinson CM, Pell AC et al 1995 Transcardiac echocardiography during invasive intramedullary procedures. Journal of Bone and Joint Surgery 77B: 450–455

Closs SJ 1994 Pain in elderly patients: a neglected phenomenon? Journal of Advanced Nursing 19: 1072–1081

Closs SJ, Fairclough HL, Tierney AJ et al 1993 Pain in elderly orthopaedic patients. Journal of Clinical Nursing 2: 41–45

Closs SJ, Briggs M, Everitt V 1997 Night time pain, sleep and anxiety in post operative orthopaedic patients. Journal of Orthopaedic Nursing 1(2): 59–66

Coulson I 1993 Co-ordinating an orthopaedic service. Nursing Standard 7(32): 37–40

Darlow M, Coast J, Richards SH et al 1998 Impact of a randomized controlled trial upon the development of a hospital-at-home service. Journal of Orthopaedic Nursing 2(3): 153–159

DeGeorge P, Dunwoody C 1995 Transfer techniques of the lower extremity with an external fixator. Orthopaedic Nursing 14(6): 17–21

Demetriades L, Strauss E, Gallina J 1998 Osteoarthritis of the ankle. Clinical Orthopaedics and Related Research 349: 28–42

Department of Health (DoH) 2001 The National Service Framework for Older People. Department of Health, London.

D'Eramo A, Sedlak C, Doheny M et al 1994 Nutritional aspects of the orthopaedic trauma patient. Orthopaedic Nursing 13(4): 13–20

Dougherty J 1996 Same day surgery: the nurse's role. Orthopaedic Nursing 15(4): 15–18

Downton JH 1993 Falls in the elderly. Edward Arnold, London

Draper J, Scott F 1996 An investigation into the application and maintenance of Hamilton Russell traction on three orthopaedic wards. Journal of Advanced Nursing 23(3): 536–541

Draper P, Scott F 1997 An evaluation of Hamilton-Russell traction in the preoperative management of patients with hip fracture. Clinical Effectiveness in Nursing 1: 179–188

Duckworth T 1995 Lecture notes on orthopaedics and fractures, 3rd edn. Blackwell, Oxford

Ekman A, Mallmin H, Michaelsson K et al 1997 External hip protectors to prevent osteoporotic hip fractures. Lancet 350(9077): 563–564

Finsen V, Borset M, Buvik GE et al 1992 Preoperative traction in patients with hip fractures. Injury 23(4): 242–244

Foreman M 1986 Acute confusional states in hospitalised elderly: a research dilemma. Nursing Research 35(91): 34–38

Gamroth LM 1991 Client valued outcomes for hip fracture clients in nursing homes. Unpublished PhD thesis, Oregon Health Sciences University

Green CR, Pandit SK, Schork MA 1996 Preoperative fasting time: is the traditional policy changing? Results of a national survey. Anaesthesia and Analgesia 83(1): 123–128

Griffiths H 1997 Pain assessment and relief in foot surgery. Journal of Orthopaedic Nursing 1(3): 131–135

Haines MM 1995 AANA journal course: update for nurse anaesthetists – pulmonary aspiration revisited: changing attitudes towards preoperative fasting. AANA Journal 63(5): 389–396

Handel C 1997 A review of the use and benefits of nutritional supplements in the wound healing of orthopaedic patients. Journal of Orthopaedic Nursing 1(4): 179–182

Harner CD, Olson E, Irrgang JJ et al 1996 Allograft versus autograft anterior cruciate ligament reconstruction: 3 to 5 year outcome. Clinical Orthopaedics and Related Research 324: 134–144

Hawkey B, Williams J 2001 Rehabilitation: the nurse's role. Journal of Orthopaedic Nursing 5(2): 81–88

Hayes R 1995 Pain assessment in the elderly. British Journal of Nursing 4(20): 1199–1204

Hefti D 1995 Complications of trauma: the nurse's role in prevention. Orthopaedic Nursing 14(6): 9–15

Hersh CK, McGainty P 1996 Meeting the challenge of common tibial fractures. Journal of Musculoskeletal Medicine 13(7): 45–50, 56–58

Hung P 1992 Preoperative fasting of patients undergoing elective surgery. British Journal of Nursing 1(6): 286–287

Jackson RJ 2001 An action research project introducing a leaflet for patients undergoing bunion surgery. Journal of Orthopaedic Nursing 5(2): 76–80

Larsson J, Unosson M, Ek A et al 1990 Effect of dietary supplement on nutritional status and clinical outcomes in 501 geriatric patients – a randomised study. Clinical Nutrition 9: 179–184

Lennard Jones JE 1992 A positive approach to nutrition as treatment. King's Fund, London

Levi N, Eiberg J, Skov Jensen J et al 1997 Mycoplasm in urine and blood following catheterisation of patients undergoing vascular surgery. Journal of Cardiovascular Surgery 38(4): 355–358

Lizi D 2000 Setting the standard for pressure sore prevention on a trauma orthopaedic ward. Journal of Orthopaedic Nursing 4(1): 22–25

Maffulli N, Binfield PM, King JB et al 1993 Acute haemarthrosis of the knee in athletes. A prospective study of 106 cases. Journal of Bone and Joint Surgery 75B(6): 945–949

Maher CA, Fout Rodts M 1994 Competitive athletes and injuries: a rehabilitation performance perspective. Orthopaedic Nursing 13(5): 31–37

McQueen MM, Christie J, Court-Brown C 1996 Acute compartment syndrome in tibial diaphyseal fractures. Journal of Bone and Joint Surgery 78B(1): 95–98

McRae R, Esser M 2002 Practical fracture treatment, 4th edn. Churchill Livingstone, Edinburgh

McWhirter JP, Pennington CR 1994 Incidence and recognition of malnutrition in hospital. British Medical Journal 308: 495–498

Miller J, Moore K, Schofield A et al 1996 A study of discomfort and confusion among elderly surgical patients. Orthopaedic Nursing 15(6): 27–34

Mosley-Koehler K 1999 Post-operative pain management in the patient with a tibial fracture. Journal of Orthopaedic Nursing 3(4): 197–202

NCEPOD 1999 Extremes of age. The report of the National Confidential Enquiry into Perioperative Deaths. Department of Health, London

Neal LJ 1996 Outpatient ACL surgery: the role of the home health nurse. Orthopaedic Nursing 15(4): 9–13

Newman RJ (ed) 1992 Orthogeriatrics: comprehensive orthopaedic care for the elderly. Butterworth Heinemann, Oxford

Novy CM, Genge Jagmin M 1997 Pain management in the elderly orthopaedic patient. Orthopaedic Nursing 16(1): 51–57

Nuffield Institute, NHS Centre for Reviews and Dissemination (CRD) 1995 Effective Health Care Bulletin 2 (1)

Palmer MH, Myers AH, Fedenko KM 1997 Urinary continence changes after hip fracture repair. Clinical Nursing Research 6(1): 8–24

Parker MJ, Pryor GA 1992 The timing of surgery for proximal femoral fractures. Journal of Bone and Joint Surgery 74B: 203–205

Parker MJ, Pryor GA, Myles JW 1991 Early discharge after hip fracture. Acta Orthopaedica Scandinavica 62(6): 563–566

Partridge C 1994 Pain in the confused patient. Elderly Care 6(5): 19–21

Pearson A 1987 Living in a plaster cast: how nursing can help. RCN research series. Royal College of Nursing, London

Pearson BD, Kelber S 1996 Urinary incontinence: treatments, interventions and outcomes. Clinical Nurse Specialist 10(4): 177–184

Penn C, Lekan-Rutledge D, Joers AM et al 1996 Assessment of urinary incontinence. Journal of Gerontological Nursing 22(1): 8–19

Phillips S, Hutchinson S, Davidson T 1993 Preoperative drinking does not affect gastric contents. British Journal of Anaesthesia 70(1): 6–9

Pryor GA, Williams DRR 1989 Rehabilitation after hip fractures. Journal of Bone and Joint Surgery 71B: 471–474

Renton S, Brown J 2001 An evaluation of an orthopaedic supported discharge service. Journal of Orthopaedic Nursing 5(3): 120–124

Royal College of Physicians 1989 Fractured neck of femur: prevention and management. Royal College of Physicians, London

Royal College of Surgeons and College of Anaesthetists Commission on the Provision of Surgical Services 1990 Report of the working party on pain after surgery. Royal College of Surgeons and College of Anaesthetists, London

Santy J 1999 Interprofessional boundaries between nursing and physiotherapy in the orthopaedic setting. Journal of Orthopaedic Nursing 3(2): 88–94

Santy J, Mackintosh C 2001 A phenomenological study of pain following fractured shaft of femur. Journal of Clinical Nursing 10: 521–527

Schatzker J 1998 Fractures of the distal femur revisited. Clinical Orthopaedics and Related Research 347: 43–56

Schofield I 1997 Patient-centred care in the management of postoperative orthopaedic patients with an acute confusional state. Journal of Orthopaedic Nursing 1(2): 71–75

Shiell A, Kenny P, Farnworth MG 1993 The role of the clinical nurse co-ordinator in the provision of cost-effective orthopaedic services for elderly people. Journal of Advanced Nursing 18: 1424–1428

Sluenwhite CA, Simpson P 1998 Patient and family perspectives on early discharge and care of the older adult undergoing fractured hip rehabilitation. Orthopaedic Nursing 17(1): 30–36

Smith M (ed) 1999 Rehabilitation in adult nursing practice. Churchill Livingstone, Edinburgh

SNMAC 2001 Caring for older people: a nursing priority. Report by the Standing Nursing and Midwifery Advisory Committee. Department of Health, London

Somers JF, Suy R, Stuyck J et al 1998 Conservative treatment of femoral shaft fractures in-patients with total hip arthroplasty. Journal of Arthroplasty 13(2): 162–171

Stickler DJ, Zimakoff J 1994 Complications of urinary tract infections associated with devices used for long-term bladder management. Journal of Hospital Infection 28(3): 117–194

Taylor MT, Banjerjee B, Alpar EK 1994 The epidemiology of fractured femurs and the effect of these factors on outcome. Injury 25(10): 641–644

Tucker R 1998 Compartment syndrome: the orthopaedic nurse's vital role. Journal of Orthopaedic Nursing 2(1): 33–36

Tudor M 1998 Case study of care provided by an orthopaedic early-discharge team for a patient with a fractured neck of femur. Journal of Orthopaedic Nursing 2(1): 37–41

Williams MA, Oberst MT, Bjorklyund BC 1994 Post hospital convalescence in older women with hip fracture. Orthopaedic Nursing 13(4): 55–64

Wilson K 1990 Ross and Wilson anatomy and physiology in health and illness, 7th edn. Churchill Livingstone, London

Winslow EH 1995 Research for practice. Support for folk wisdom on cranberry juice. American Journal of Nursing 95(5): 69

Younger AS, Curran P, McQueen MM 1990 Back-slabs and plaster casts: which will best accommodate increasing intracompartmental pressures? Injury 21(3): 179–181

Zavotsky KE, Banavage A 1995 Management of the patient with complex orthopaedic fractures. Orthopaedic Nursing 14(5): 53–57

Chapter 25

Sports injuries

Mike Smith

CHAPTER CONTENTS

INTRODUCTION

The major system affected by the clear majority of sporting injuries is the musculoskeletal system, namely the tendons, muscles, ligaments and bones. Injury to these will form the focus for this chapter. There are, however, other parts of the anatomy that may well be affected concurrently or individually and brief reference will be made to these as appropriate.

The prevention of sports injury is key to both sports management and healthcare promotion in sports. Nursing has a distinct and vital role to play in the management of sports injuries by:

- preventing injuries from occurring when possible
- the management of an injury
- prevention of repeated or future injuries.

A brief discussion of the epidemiology is essential in order to guide potential prevention strategies and reduce risk of recurrent injury. These should form part of patient education programmes within rehabilitation.

The principles of initial management of major trauma apply to any serious sports injury; however, many sports injuries are not classed as major trauma. The initial management of acute sports injury will be addressed and current practice subjected to critical analysis, including the essential RICE approach of rest, ice, compression and elevation.

As well as providing an outline of mechanisms contributing to regional sports injuries, both conservative and surgical management modalities are often possible, dependent on the eventual goals of the patient, as well as the severity and type of injury sustained, and these are discussed accordingly.

CLASSIFICATION OF SPORTS INJURIES

Sports injuries account for 12.5% of all injuries (Watson & Ozanne-Smith 2000) and historically sports injuries have been broadly classified into one of two categories: acute or traumatic injuries and chronic or overuse injuries.

There has been a gradual change in the pattern of sporting injuries. Acute injuries have traditionally been more common but there appears to be an increase in the frequency of overuse injuries. There may be many potential reasons for this; for instance, there are more people participating in sporting activities and this participation may often be for many years in a person's life rather than solely being restricted to younger years.

Patients with soft tissue injuries involving joints comprise the major cohort (Tall & DeVault 1993) but fractures too are common. Some of these may have life-threatening complications as with traumatic brain injury from fractures to the skull, spinal cord injury associated with vertebral fracture or hypovolaemic shock from major long bone and pelvic fractures. Sports injuries are also grouped together broadly into regional injuries, as with upper or lower limb injuries, or by the joint affected, for example knee injuries.

As a general rule overuse injuries occur when repeti-tive microtrauma overloads the capacity of the tissue to repair itself. The repeated acute inflammation, or in other words chronic inflammation, may often result in structural changes to the tissue. Such changes over time not only result in an inability to perform the desired sporting activity but also eventually impinge on the individual's functional capability in performing everyday tasks. Tendonitis, synovitis, chronic compartment syndrome, stress fractures and some medial collateral ligament damage may all be classed as overuse injuries. Readers are referred to Chapter 26 for a more detailed discussion of overuse injuries.

EPIDEMIOLOGY OF SPORTS INJURIES

Epidemiology is the study of distributions and determinants of injury rates with the aim of (Van Mechelen et al 1992):

- planning potential interventions
- setting up appropriate systems to guide diagnosis

- identifying benefits and implications of prevention strategies, for example rule changes, training regimes, health promotion campaigns
- establishing information regarding the degree of risk associated with particular activities.

Each sporting activity has specific common injuries associated with it; for example, knee, foot or ankle injuries are commonly associated with football while rugby can result in similar injuries and carries a higher risk of neck and shoulder injury. In the latter case epidemiological studies provided the impetus for changes to rules regarding the scrum.

Acute sports injuries are due to extrinsic and intrinsic factors (Box 25.1). Extrinsic factors pertain to the mechanism of injury such as a direct blow, contributory environmental conditions, for instance extremes of hot or cold, the state of any equipment used during the activity, adhering to safety rules or the pressure of competition.

Intrinsic factors pertain to the person's internal state and the condition of particular body parts put under stress during a sporting activity. To give a fairly obvious example, consider two athletes in a race who put the same amount of stress on a muscle group in the same environmental conditions. One is fully prepared through training so intrinsically his muscles are in a better condition to deal with those stresses and he is well prepared extrinsically by wearing appropriate footwear. Obviously an ill-prepared athlete with poor-quality footwear will be more likely to sustain an injury.

The complexity of risk factors is highlighted by the risks associated with having a previous injury (Fields et al 1992). These may be due to an inherent

Box 25.1 Intrinsic and extrinsic factors in sports injuries	
Intrinsic	*Extrinsic*
Fitness	Environment
Previous injury	Temperature
Risk taking	Equipment
Anxiety	Rules
BMI	Nature of sport, for
Previous medical history	example contact
Muscle flexibility/imbalance	Training
Warm–up	Surface
Gender	
Body shape	

weakness associated with the initial injury, inadequate rehabilitation or a disregard for, or failure to resolve, contributory extrinsic and intrinsic factors.

The psychological element of sports injury risk has been explored in a few studies. A recent review of such studies to date (Junge 2000) indicates a general consensus of the influence of 'life events', the competitive nature of the sports person and being more ready to take risks. There is a limit to the usefulness of some of the information gained from such studies. Apart from providing information on the potential risks, confirming the 2:1 male to female ratio of injuries and that women undertaking similar activities to men are far more likely to sustain anterior cruciate ligament injuries, data appear to be of minimal clinical use for nurses involved in sports injuries.

Epidemiological studies are useful if specific to particular populations. When a study is too broad in relation to age groups or gender or fails to take into account all the relevant factors, it will fail to deliver useful information for the sports injury practitioner. These aspects illustrate why it is essential to have standardised measures across healthcare research and data collation if meaningful epidemiological studies are to be undertaken.

A particularly good example of a useful study is the work undertaken by Stevenson et al (2000) focusing on injuries within Western Australia. This research is of good quality, covering variables that allow reviewing of the occurrence and potential for the planning of care related to sports injuries for a specific and defined population.

Finally, it is worth emphasising that sports injuries occur:

- across the lifespan
- to people from different backgrounds
- in those with chronic health problems or body changes due to ageing, including the elderly
- in those with previous unrelated injuries, for example those with a physical disability
- in children and adolescents, who comprise a major population group.

None of these should be viewed as a barrier to undertaking sports and indeed, the health benefits are substantial for all age groups and populations. Clearly, epidemiological studies must focus on these as specific populations along with treatment and rehabilitation programmes that allow and encourage return, if possible, to the desired sporting activity.

MAJOR SPORTS INJURIES

Clearly the potentially life-threatening injuries from sport also come under the acute injury umbrella. Such injuries are often the result of high-speed or force impacts. Spinal cord injuries (SCI), of which sporting injuries comprise between 10–20% as a mode of SCI (Grundy et al 1995), are generally seasonal in nature. In winter SCI would tend to result from sports such as skiing injuries, rugby and motor sport crashes. In the summer SCI may occur as a result of horse riding or diving in shallow water. The acute management of spinal cord injuries is addressed in Chapter 20.

Figures from some studies suggest that sports injury accounts for 10–13% of traumatic brain injury (Pickett et al 2001). Travelling at speed and falls without appropriate head protection account for a significant number of these.

Penetrating, blunt chest and abdominal injuries occur as a result of a crash in motor sports or any activity causing a fall from a height, such as mountain climbing. Often such incidents result in multitrauma to the individual concerned.

Scuba diving injuries, primarily due to a rapid ascent, are increasing as recreational diving becomes more popular. The two more common types of injury which may occur are decompression sickness or 'the bends' and damage to the respiratory system. The mechanism and management of these injuries are covered in Box 25.2.

PREVENTION OF SPORTS INJURY

Prevention is a key strategy within the sports injury field. The costs associated with the management of sports injuries, both nationally and internationally, are substantial due to healthcare costs and the costs to society from lost days at work. The costs to the individual can also be significant in loss of income and the 'suffering' element.

It has been concluded that generally recreational sports are safe (Stevenson et al 2000). It is worth reiterating that the health benefits and social enjoyment of sports participation undoubtedly outweigh the negative points outlined above.

Much has been spent on health promotion relating to playing sport in order to reduce both incidence and severity. Box 25.3 summarises some of the key principles. It is difficult to determine the efficacy of health promotion campaigns per se and

---

Box 25.2 Scuba diving injuries

Decompression sickness is a disorder resulting from the reduction of surrounding pressure, as in an ascent from a depth. It is attributed to the formation of bubbles from dissolved gas in the blood or tissues, usually characterised by pain and neurological manifestations.

When at depth a diver is under increased ambient pressure, so takes up additional quantities of oxygen (O_2) and nitrogen (N_2) in solution in the blood and tissues. O_2 is utilised continuously but the N_2 leaves the body only via the reverse of its entry through the lungs and circulation. The consequences of bubble formation from dissolved gas are known as decompression sickness, caisson disease or 'the bends'. Although 'the bends' refers strictly to painful manifestations, it is often used as a synonym for decompression sickness.

Repetitive dives are a major source of this condition. Some divers are unaware that an excess of inert gas remains in the body after every dive and this increases with each subsequent exposure.

Pain is present in a large proportion of cases of decompression sickness, often accompanied by neurological abnormalities. The pain is characteristically hard to describe and often poorly localised. At first the pain is mild or intermittent but it may increase steadily and can become very severe. Local inflammation and tenderness are often absent and the pain may not be affected by movement.

Neurological manifestations (occurring in over 50% of cases) may accompany pain or be present independently. The spinal cord is especially vulnerable and many divers are unaware of the dire significance of seemingly minor manifestations such as weakness or numbness in the extremities. They range from mild paraesthesia to major irreversible paralysis.

The condition known as the chokes, or respiratory decompression sickness, is rare but grave in significance. It arises from massive bubble embolisation of the pulmonary vascular tree. Some cases resolve spontaneously but rapid progression to circulatory collapse and death is not uncommon without prompt recompression. Substernal discomfort and coughing on deep inspiration or inhalation of tobacco smoke are often early manifestations of chokes.

Box 25.3 Prevention of sports injuries

Maintaining a healthy weight
Playing within the rules
Practising safety measures to help prevent falls
Wearing shoes that fit properly
Replacing sports shoes as soon as the tread wears out or the heel wears down on one side
Doing stretching exercises daily
Being in proper physical condition to play a sport
Warming up and stretching before participating in any sports or exercise
Wearing protective equipment when playing
Avoiding exercising or playing sports when tired, unwell or in pain
Not running on uneven surfaces

---

there are few good studies to indicate that a change in the behaviour of individuals is the result of health promotion. However, this should not detract from the principle that health promotion is a good philosophy.

Irrespective of health promotion, there will always be a cohort of individuals for whom the risk taking is part of the sporting 'buzz' and the competitive element in many sports by their nature will lead to sports injuries (Junge 2000, Kelley 1990). Of specific note on the prevention of injury, and perhaps personally for some readers, is a recent review of the clinical and science literature (Shrier 1999) suggesting that preexercise stretching does not reduce the incidence of injury. Nevertheless, it may be that stretching on a regular basis in between exercise and warming up through gentle jogging before activity is of benefit. Patients should be educated regarding this post injury in an attempt to avoid recurrence.

As well as rule changes and education, some prevention studies, particularly those related to ankle injuries, have focused on training methods for specific injuries and equipment such as footwear or bracing (Verhagen et al 2000). It is unfortunate that such studies seem rare as their benefit is undeniable.

MANAGEMENT PRINCIPLES

The initial management of major injuries, for instance a head or chest injury, follows the principles of primary and secondary surveys as with any major trauma, followed by early transfer to the relevant specialist unit for acute care and rehabilitation.

For the majority of injuries the objectives of initial management at the scene of the accident, during transfer to hospital and on admission are the:

- prevention of further injury
- protection of the injury
- reduction of pain
- prevention of secondary complications.

After this 'first aid' of injury management, the aims of medical and nursing treatment in the acute phase and long term will be to:

- restore optimal functional ability
- enable the patient to resume daily activities
- facilitate the patient's return to their desired sporting activities when possible, without recurrence of the injury.

SIGNS OF SOFT TISSUE INJURY

Pain

As with most injuries, the primary and most obvious symptom is the presence of pain. This is caused by damage caused by the trauma, cell hypoxia, chemical release (bradykinin, histamine, prostaglandin) or pressure on nerve endings resulting from the soft tissue swelling.

The traditional treatment with oral non-steroidal antiinflammatory drugs (NSAIDs) in acute soft tissue injuries is now the subject of debate. A review of the evidence (Almekinders 2000) suggested that although NSAIDs have proved efficacious in the treatment of pain, there is no strong evidence that they have any antiinflammatory benefit resulting in improvements in healing for such cases. Additionally the gastrointestinal upset associated with their use is obviously a concern, although the recent use of COX-2 inhibitors, for example celebrex, may have fewer side effects than the older NSAIDs. This review does not include their use within overuse or chronic injuries or with inflammatory conditions so any concerns regarding their use should therefore be restricted to acute injuries only.

Swelling

Tissue swelling is due to the chemical release of histamine, prostaglandin and serotonin, each contributing to an increase in cell membrane permeability and the consequent escape of proteins into the interstitial space. This creates an increase in the osmotic pressure gradient and draws in further fluid, so increasing oedema. The lymphatic system is unable to deal effectively with the increased demands put on it by this inflammatory exudate.

Redness and warmth

The release of histamine and substance P as a result of the injury causes a local vasodilation. This increases blood supply to the affected area so the area looks red and feels warm on clinical examination.

INITIAL TREATMENT OF SOFT TISSUE INJURIES

The most common approach to the initial treatment of sports injuries follows the acronym RICE (rest, ice, compression and elevation) and is used here to describe the initial treatment of soft tissue trauma. There are variations on this acronym seen in the sports injury literature but essentially they contain the same elements (Box 25.4).

Relative rest

Immobilisation that maintains the normal anatomical alignment of the traumatised structures is the initial aim until a full diagnosis has been made. This will assist in protecting the injured structures, minimising the likelihood of further injury and reducing the level of pain experienced.

Once a clear diagnosis is made a period of immobilisation, rest or a reduction in regular exercise or activities of daily living will be recommended. The patient may be advised to put no weight through the injured area for 48 hours. For an ankle or knee injury, crutches may help. If one crutch is used for an ankle injury, it should be used on the uninjured side to help the patient lean away from and relieve weight on the injured ankle.

For patients with a moderate or severe sprain, particularly of the ankle, a hard cast may be applied.

Box 25.4	Initial injury management acronyms	
RICE	*PRICE*	*RECIPE*
R Relative rest	**P** Protection	**R** Relative rest
I Ice	**R** Relative rest	**E** Elevation
C Compression	**I** Ice	**C** Compression
E Elevation	**C** Compression	**I** Ice
	E Elevation	**P** Pain limited
		E Exercise

Severe sprains and strains can require surgery to repair a torn ligament, muscle or tendons.

Complete rest for an extended period of time is not indicated in many injuries. Instead, the concept of 'pain-limited exercise' assists in a number of ways in the restoration of a preinjury state by:

- reducing the swelling through facilitation of lymphatic and venous drainage
- increasing the deep blood supply to assist regeneration through provision of micronutrients and oxygen to the damaged tissues
- facilitating appropriate restructuring of the collagen bundle by enabling the development of functional, rather than dysfunctional, scar tissue.

Returning to activity is influenced by these healing processes along with awareness that periods of immobilisation result in muscle atrophy. This atrophy in turn causes reduced muscle strength as a consequence of the decreased muscle weight and the size and number of muscle fibres (Appell 1990). Appell's review indicates two further issues of note:

1 the decrease is most dramatic during the first week of immobilisation
2 although complete recovery from atrophy is possible, the length of time recovery takes is substantially longer than the period of immobilisation.

Ice

The application of ice in the acute stage of sports injury serves four purposes:

1 reduction of inflammation
2 reduction of pain
3 reduction of muscle spasm
4 decrease in metabolism and therefore local requirement for oxygen, hence reducing the possibility of hypoxia.

Although ice or cold therapy is commonly used, and there is unanimous consensus in the literature of its benefit, there is substantial variation on the method, duration of application (5–40 minutes), frequency (1–6 hourly) and duration of treatment (6–72 hours). A systematic review by MacAuley (2001) indicates that the best evidence exists for:

- melting iced water through a wet towel
- application to the injured area for 10 minutes at a time, repeated as necessary to reduce the local skin temperature by 10–15°C, 4–8 times a day

- advising patients that they are more at risk of injury for 30 minutes after application due to locally impaired reflexes and motor function.

Repeated applications are preferable to allow the surface skin temperature to return to normal whilst the muscle temperature remains low; this reduces the possibility of compromising the skin. Readers should compare these standards against their local practice.

Compression

Compression is thought to increase the hydrostatic pressure of the interstitial fluid. This will counteract the osmolarity, so facilitating lymphatic and venous drainage. Consequently, this prevents the accumulation of, and improves the dispersal of, inflammatory exudate.

Care must be taken with the amount of compression applied to ensure it is not contributing to the patient's pain and the development of compartment syndrome. Examples of compression bandages are elastic wraps, special boots, air casts and splints. The method of compression will be dependent on the particular injury.

Although it is generally perceived as being of benefit in the sports medicine literature, in a Swedish study (Thorsson et al 1997) there was no apparent benefit from early compression in relation to the length of time taken to recover from an injury. This is strongly indicative of the need for further research within this standard intervention.

Elevation

Elevation of the affected part:

- decreases capillary pressure
- assists lymphatic drainage
- assists dispersal of inflammatory exudates
- reduces tissue pressure
- reduces pain by reducing tissue pressure.

Where possible, keeping the injured part elevated on a pillow, above the level of the heart, will help decrease the degree of swelling.

'Do no harm!'

Another acronym commonly quoted in the sports injury literature for initial management is that of 'do no HARM'. This useful approach provides patients with advice by referring to the need to avoid:

- **Heat** as it will increase vasodilation and the inflammation process, as well as increasing the oxygen demands of the tissue by raising metabolism

- **A**lcohol as it causes vasodilation
- **R**est; see previous points related to relative rest
- **M**assage as this may be painful and potentially increases the blood flow to the affected area, allowing the escape of fluid into the interstitial spaces thus increasing oedema.

GENERIC PRINCIPLES

The healing of sports injuries will be dependent on many factors both systemic and local (Box 25.5). Many of these are the same for healing any wound or injury. Although not specific to sports injuries alone, they are worth remembering when prescribing and implementing patient education, a rehabilitation programme or discharge plan.

Sprains and strains comprise the major group of soft tissue sports injuries. These are discussed prior to exploring specific regional injuries, as the general principles relate to many sports injuries.

Sprains

A sprain is an injury relating to a stretching or tearing of ligaments. It is not uncommon for a sprain to involve more than one ligament. The severity of the injury will be dependent on both the number of ligaments involved and the extent of the injury to each single ligament, namely whether it is a partial or complete tear.

A sprain can be caused by a fall, a sudden twist or a blow to the body that forces a joint out of its normal position. This results in an overstretch or tear of the ligament supporting that joint. Typically, sprains occur when people fall and land on an outstretched arm, slide, land on the side of their foot or

twist the knee with the foot planted firmly on the ground.

Although sprains can occur in both the upper and lower parts of the body, the most common site is the ankle (Wedmore & Charlette 2000).

A sprain may be classified as grade I, II or III.

- A grade I or mild sprain causes overstretching or slight tearing of the ligaments with no joint instability. A person with a mild sprain usually experiences minimal pain and swelling with little or no loss of functional ability. Bruising is absent or slight and the person is usually able to put weight on the affected joint.
- A grade II or moderate sprain results in a partial tearing of the ligament and is characterised by bruising, moderate pain and swelling. A person with a moderate sprain usually has some difficulty putting weight on the affected joint and experiences some loss of function.
- People who sustain a grade III or severe sprain completely tear or rupture a ligament. Pain, swelling and bruising are usually severe. Invariably the patient is unable to put weight on the joint.

Taking a thorough history of the injury is vital in the diagnosis of a sprain. This should include specific details of the forces and direction of the affected joint at the time of injury. Joint stability, movement and the ability to bear weight are also examined. An X-ray is usually taken to rule out a fracture to the affected part. Magnetic resonance imaging (MRI) may be used to differentiate between a significant partial injury and a complete tear in a ligament.

Strains

A strain is an injury caused by twisting or pulling a muscle or tendon. Severity of a strain ranges from a simple overstretching of the muscle or tendon to a partial or complete tear (Kannus & Natri 1997).

Strains can be acute or chronic. An acute strain is caused by trauma or an injury such as a blow to the body. Additionally strains are caused by lifting heavy objects awkwardly or overstressing the muscles, a particular issue in many jobs including nursing. Chronic strains are usually the result of overuse, for example prolonged, repetitive movements of muscles and tendons. Chronic injuries from overuse are addressed in more detail in Chapter 26.

Contact sports such as football, hockey, boxing and wrestling put people at risk of strains in many areas. Many sports have specific injuries common

Box 25.5	Factors in healing of sports injuries

Systemic factors	Local factors
Nutritional status (serum protein levels)	Degree of injury
	Infection
Vitamin levels (for example, vitamin C)	Local blood supply
	Synovial environment
Anaemia	Mediators of inflammation
Diabetes mellitus	Excessive scarring
Age	Mechanical stress

to that activity; for instance, gymnastics, tennis, rowing, golf and other sports that require extensive gripping can increase the risk of hand and forearm strains. Elbow strains occur from participation in racquet, throwing and contact sports.

Symptoms of a strain typically include pain, muscle spasm and muscle weakness. They can also have localised swelling, cramping or inflammation. A minor or moderate strain will usually cause some loss of muscle function. Patients typically have pain in the injured area and general weakness of the muscle when they attempt to move it. Severe strains that partially or completely tear the muscle or tendon are often very painful and disabling.

Treatment and rehabilitation for sprains and strains

The majority of sprains and strains will not require hospitalisation and will be managed conservatively (Jarvinen et al 2000) through the accident and emergency services initially, with subsequent follow-up as an outpatient for a variable period of time dependent on severity. Essentially, treatment for sprains and strains is similar and can be thought of as having two stages: acute treatment to reduce the swelling and pain, followed by rehabilitation.

In the acute treatment stage, doctors usually advise patients to follow the RICE formula for the first 24–48 hours after the injury. NSAIDs, such as ibuprofen, are often prescribed to help decrease pain although they may not actually reduce the antiinflammatory process (Almekinders 2000). Generally X-rays are taken to exclude the possibility of associated fractures. MRI and CT scans may also be utilised, particularly if surgical intervention is indicated or likely.

The goal of rehabilitation is to improve the condition of the injured part in order to restore functional ability. The healthcare provider, generally a physiotherapist, will prescribe an exercise programme designed to prevent stiffness, improve and maintain the normal range of movement and restore the joint's normal flexibility and strength. The range of movement or motion refers to the arc of movement of a joint from one extreme position to the other. Therefore, range of movement exercises help increase or maintain flexibility and mobility of muscles, tendons, ligaments and joints. If the patient remains in hospital during this stage, the nurse will be expected to assist in the continuation of the prescribed programme. It is essential therefore that

clear written guidelines are made available to assist all in this role.

The rehabilitation programme will often last for weeks, continuing past the patient's discharge date from hospital if they were admitted or beyond their outpatient physiotherapy period. It is therefore vital that the patient is familiar with all the prescribed exercises and can perform these without supervision.

The ultimate goal is for the patient to return to full daily activities, including sports when appropriate. Patients must work closely with their healthcare provider to determine their readiness to return to full activity. Sometimes people are tempted to resume full activity or play sports despite the pain or muscle soreness. Returning to full activity before regaining a normal range of movement, flexibility and strength increases the risk of reinjury and commonly results in a chronic problem.

Clearly the goal of returning to activity without recurrence of the injury must be foremost in the mind of the healthcare team and the patient. The principles of prevention and exploration of contributing extrinsic and intrinsic factors form part of a formal patient education programme. However, it is questionable how frequently this occurs in practice.

The amount of rehabilitation and the time needed for full recovery after a sprain or strain depend on the severity of the injury and individual rates of healing. For example, a moderate ankle sprain may require 3–6 weeks of rehabilitation before a person can return to full activity. With a severe sprain, it can take 8–12 months before the ligament is fully healed.

There are few studies that demonstrate the efficacy of various rehabilitation techniques so programmes have evolved and tend to be planned on a local basis rather than being based upon national or internationally proven standards of best practice. It is essential that this is addressed. Standardised measures of injury severity (Van Mechelen 1997), treatment modalities and patient outcomes are vital to undertake meaningful research which will impact positively on international sports injury practice.

It is also worth noting that the effect on the individual may be profound as it takes time to recover from a sports injury. Both work and financial status can be affected along with the person's social interaction, especially if it is some time before sporting activities can be resumed. An emotional response to the injury as a result of these factors would therefore not be uncommon (Crossman 1997, Smith et al 1990) and should be taken into account during rehabilitation. Not only may this be difficult for the individual to cope with at times, but it may encourage them to resume activities before the injured part is ready, with the obvious increased risk of recurrence.

Clearly, the feeling of loss may be severe for those whose injuries prevent them ever returning to their desired sport.

SPECIFIC SPORTS INJURIES

This section concentrates on the damage caused to the bone and soft tissues with a brief discussion of the medical management and rehabilitation of the patient, aiming towards recommencing the sport activity wherever possible.

There are many excellent reviews of specific regional sports injuries that outline aetiology and current management options in far more detail, beyond the scope of this chapter, on which the following sections are based. Readers are encouraged to obtain them for further information. A few examples include:

- shoulder: Doukas & Speer 2001, Gazielly 1989
- hand and wrist: Pitner 1990, Barton 1997
- hip and thigh: Mares 1998
- knee: Fadale & Noerdlinger 1999, Shelbourne & Klootwyk 2000
- Achilles tendon: DeMaio et al 1995
- ankle: Hockenbury & Sammarco 2001, Wedmore & Charlette 2000.

UPPER LIMB INJURIES

ROTATOR CUFF TENDONITIS AND TEARS

Rotator cuff tendonitis and tears are common disorders. They involve a series of four muscles whose function is to stabilise the shoulder and allow the arm to move through a full range of movement, with the subacromial bursa lubricating the muscle tendons. Rotator cuff tendonitis and tears are collectively known as impingement syndrome.

Impingement occurs when inflammation or bony spurs narrow the space available for the rotator cuff tendons. The syndrome is divided into three stages:

- stage I: swelling and mild pain
- stage II: inflammation and scarring
- stage III: partial or complete tears of the rotator cuff.

Rotator cuff tendonitis and tears occur from either a sudden violent movement of the shoulder or chronic overuse. Sports commonly associated with this diagnosis include tennis, swimming, baseball, softball and football.

A diagnosis of impingement syndrome is considered when patients complain of pain with overhead arm activities such as a tennis serve or pitching. A physical examination of the patient will reveal weakness of the rotator cuff muscles and commonly show a decreased range of movement of the shoulder: a painful arc. X-rays are taken to evaluate the bones of the shoulder. Occasionally, an MRI or shoulder arthroscopy is used to confirm the diagnosis.

Most cases of impingement syndrome respond to rest, antiinflammatory medication and a directed course of physiotherapy. Resolution of symptoms typically takes several weeks but return to full activity can take several months, depending on the severity of the problem. Occasionally, a steroid injection is used to help alleviate pain in older patients.

If non-operative measures fail to control the pain and restore full function, surgery is indicated to either remove the scarred and inflamed tissue (bursitis) or to open up the space available for the rotator cuff by shaving down bony spurs (subacromial decompression). Repair or reattachment of torn rotator cuff tendons can also be necessary. This is ideally performed using arthroscopic surgery, for patients with severe inflammation and partial rotator cuff tears. Open surgery is more often required for patients with complete rotator cuff tears.

See Chapter 21 for further discussion of the nursing issues relating to impingement syndrome and tears of the rotator cuff.

SHOULDER DISLOCATION

A shoulder dislocation occurs when the humeral head slips out of its socket, the glenoid cavity. Anterior dislocations are most common. When this occurs the anterior inferior labrum, the cartilage that stabilises the shoulder, is frequently torn; this is known as a Bankart lesion. A dent in the humerus bone known as a Hill-Sachs lesion may accompany the Bankart lesion in severe dislocations.

Shoulder dislocations can occur posteriorly and inferiorly. Repeated dislocations and multidirectional shoulder instability are also possible.

Falling is the most common cause of a new shoulder dislocation but it can occur when the arm is forcibly moved into an awkward position during a violent action such as tackling in rugby. If a dislocation or subluxation occurs with only minor force, a recurrent or multidirectional instability must be considered.

A shoulder dislocation is diagnosed when a patient presents with a history of a fall with subsequent pain around the shoulder, bruising, a visible deformity and an unwillingness to move the arm due to pain. X-rays confirm the dislocation and rule out any fracture around the shoulder.

For first-time dislocations, reduction under local anaesthesia, a sling and activity restriction for 3–4 weeks is the standard form of treatment. A supervised physiotherapy programme is also beneficial to regain the full range of movement and activity, preventing repeated dislocations by strengthening the muscles around the shoulder and upper back that help stabilise the shoulder joint.

For young patients, there is a high risk of recurrent dislocation. For these patients surgery may be indicated, involving repair and tightening of the structures within the shoulder damaged by the dislocations. Although the most common procedure is an open reconstruction, arthroscopic reconstruction techniques are evolving and may be utilised more frequently in the future.

ADHESIVE CAPSULITIS (FROZEN SHOULDER)

Adhesive capsulitis is defined as a loss of both active and passive motion, the common name being a frozen shoulder. The movement lost is due to tightening and thickening (fibrosis) of the ligaments and other supporting structures of the shoulder, resulting in restriction of movement that can severely limit function.

Most cases follow a three-stage specific pattern, the overall course being variable but can last 12–24 months.

1 Initial acute phase characterised by significant pain, difficulty sleeping and significant functional impairment.
2 Progressive stiffening phase when shoulder motion worsens.
3 The final resolution or 'thawing' phase identified by the gradual return of both movement and function.

A frozen shoulder can arise following a fracture or other arm injury. It is also related to a rotator cuff tear, degenerative arthritis or previous shoulder surgery. Many cases, however, have no known causes so are referred to as idiopathic or primary adhesive capsulitis. Despite this, primary adhesive capsulitis has been associated with systemic disorders such as diabetes and cardiovascular disease.

The loss of both active and passive movement on physical examination indicate a frozen shoulder. The patient will describe a pattern of pain that alternates between severe and mild, with the overall function of the shoulder in the acute phase being poor. X-rays are taken to rule out other shoulder disorders such as degenerative arthritis. An MRI scan is used to further evaluate the shoulder.

Antiinflammatory medications, stretching and physiotherapy are the primary conservative treatments along with cortisone injections if indicated. If these measures fail, manipulation under anaesthesia may be required.

ACROMIOCLAVICULAR SEPARATION (SHOULDER SEPARATION)

An acromioclavicular (AC) separation is an injury to the ligaments that connect the clavicle to the acromion. It is often classified by severity but more commonly is classified using the three grades of strain previously discussed.

The typical mechanism of injury is a fall on the point of the shoulder. A direct blow to the shoulder or a fall on an outstretched hand may also cause AC separation. Football and hockey are the common sports associated with this injury.

An AC separation is diagnosed by a history of pain, tenderness and swelling at the AC joint. If the injury is severe, significant deformity may occur. X-rays are taken for confirmation of the injury and to rule out fractures around the shoulder.

Most AC separations are treated with a sling and activity restriction followed by a physiotherapy programme. Recovery may take 6–8 weeks or more.

In injuries involving a complete tear, surgery is indicated.

Maintaining good strength and stability of the shoulder and upper back muscles may help prevent some AC separations.

FRACTURED CLAVICLE

The clavicle is one of the most commonly fractured bones. It is injured in a variety of ways, the most common being from a fall or from a direct blow to the bone. Almost any sport can be associated with clavicle fractures with football, rugby and hockey being typical activities.

A clavicle fracture is diagnosed from the history of the incident along with associated pain, deformity and swelling around the shoulder. X-rays are used to confirm the fracture. Rarely, further investigation by a CT scan is needed.

Most clavicle fractures are treated with a sling or a figure-of-eight splint. The typical time to healing is approximately 8 weeks with restriction of activity during that period.

The indicators for surgery include compound fractures, severely displaced fractures and some fractures of the outer part of the clavicle. Surgery normally involves a pin or a plate and screws.

PROXIMAL HUMERUS FRACTURE

Proximal humerus fractures are common in elderly women who fall and young adults with severe trauma to the shoulder. These fractures vary from very minor cracks to major injuries to the bone, nerves and blood vessels around the shoulder.

Falls or direct blows from collisions are the most common causes of proximal humerus fractures. Occasionally, there is an associated shoulder dislocation present.

Pain, swelling and deformity around the shoulder in association with a fall or collision are consistent with a proximal humerus fracture. X-rays are used to confirm the injury. Further testing by CT or MRI scan is rarely needed.

A simple sling or a functional brace can treat most proximal humerus fractures. Healing typically takes 6–8 weeks but varies considerably depending on the severity of the fracture.

Occasionally, surgery is needed to stabilise proximal humerus fractures using pins, plates and screws. In severe cases involving a fracture dislocation, a partial or total shoulder replacement is required.

Protective sports bracing or padding may prevent some proximal humerus fractures; however, the restrictions these impose on movements in high-risk activities may make this impractical or undesirable to use.

LATERAL EPICONDYLITIS (TENNIS ELBOW)

The muscles of the forearm that control the wrist and hand can become inflamed and partially tear if subjected to excess or repetitive stress. Pain from this inflammation can arise and progress suddenly or gradually.

Lateral epicondylitis arises from inappropriate or overuse of the tendons and muscles. Occasionally, it may begin after a sudden, traumatic movement of the elbow or wrist. Tennis, other racquet sports and weight training are commonly associated with this disorder, mainly due to incorrect technique or handle size in racquet sports.

Lateral epicondylitis is characterised by pain and tenderness on the outside of the elbow. This pain increases with any attempt to either play racquet sports or lift heavy objects with the wrist and hand.

Elbow X-rays are performed to evaluate the bone surrounding the muscles. Most cases will respond to rest, antiinflammatory medication and activity restriction. A compressive forearm band that reduces the tension at the elbow is frequently used. After controlling the inflammatory phase, physiotherapy designed to stretch and strengthen the forearm muscles may be added. A steroid injection can be tried if the above does not alleviate the symptoms.

Surgical intervention to excise the inflammation and scar tissue will be considered following failure of conservative measures. Repair or reattachment of the remaining tendon to its original bone at the elbow may also be required.

BICEPS TENDON TEAR

A biceps tendon tear is a rupture occurring at the point of insertion into the proximal radius. This is usually due to a sudden violent straightening force applied to an arm that is trying to bend. This can happen when a heavy object falls on the arm, for example when an attempt is made to catch an object with an open hand during contact sports or martial arts.

Biceps tendon tears are diagnosed by a history of an injury associated with immediate pain in the front of the elbow. A 'snap' or 'pop' may also be heard or felt. Typically, there is bruising and swelling in the elbow, difficulty in fully straightening the elbow or weakness with bending the elbow. Occasionally an MRI is needed to differentiate between a partial and complete tear.

Non-operative treatment consists of gentle range of motion exercises and antiinflammatory medication. This typically results in return of at least 60% of the normal strength of the biceps tendon.

Operative treatment is indicated for patients who wish to restore the original strength of the biceps tendon. The surgical reconstruction is complicated, involving an associated risk of damage to the nerves and blood vessels of the elbow and hand, so it should only be performed by an experienced surgeon. After the repair, a splint is used for a period of time prior to a structured rehabilitation programme under the direction of a physiotherapist.

MEDIAL EPICONDYLITIS (GOLFER'S ELBOW)

Medial epicondylitis is inflammation of the tendons and muscles of the forearm that control the wrist and hand. These muscles can become inflamed and may even partially tear if subjected to excess or repetitive stress. Although this is primarily an over-use injury, it may occur after a sudden, traumatic movement of the elbow or wrist. Golf and incorrect lifting techniques are commonly associated with this disorder.

The injury is characterised by pain and tenderness on the inside part of the elbow and may arise and progress suddenly or gradually. Direct pressure over the proximal portion of the muscles that control the wrist and hand reproduces the pain. Ruling out nerve injuries or other disorders around the elbow is essential. Elbow X-rays are needed to ensure integrity of the bones.

Most cases respond to rest, antiinflammatory medication and restriction of activity for a minimum of 3–4 weeks. A compressive forearm band that reduces the tension at the elbow is also frequently used. After controlling the inflammatory phase, physiotherapy to stretch and strengthen the forearm muscles may give added benefit. A steroid injection is used if this treatment plan does not alleviate the symptoms.

Occasionally, surgical intervention is needed if non-operative measures fail. A variety of procedures have been designed to excise the inflammation and scar tissue. Repair or reattachment of the remaining tendon to its origin on the bone at the elbow can be required.

DISTAL RADIUS AND/OR ULNA FRACTURE

Falling and landing on the hand or wrist, or direct force from a heavy object, are the most common ways to sustain this injury.

Pain associated with swelling and deformity of the wrist after a fall is consistent with a wrist fracture. X-rays are taken to confirm the diagnosis.

RICE initially is an important treatment for all wrist fractures. Fortunately, most of these fractures can be reduced under local or general anaesthetic followed by 4–6 weeks in a cast to maintain stability during healing. Following removal of the cast, stretching and strengthening exercises and physiotherapy are indicated to reduce joint stiffness.

Occasionally, surgery using internal or external fixation is needed to realign the bones.

LOWER LIMB INJURIES

ILIOPSOAS INJURY (HIP FLEXOR INJURY)

The iliopsoas is a large muscle that begins deep within the pelvis and inserts into the top of the femur, enabling flexion at the hip. Typically injury is a result of hyperextension of the leg at the hip joint so can occur with almost any sport, for example from tackling in rugby and collisions when a player is attempting to kick a football.

The patient will present with a sudden sharp pain in the groin area. On examination, bending or flexing the hip against resistance increases the pain. Often in severe injuries the patient cannot put weight on the affected leg.

Almost all of these injuries can be treated with rest and a progressive rehabilitation programme. This consists of 3–4 days of the RICE regime, then gentle stretching followed by strengthening exercises. Depending upon the severity of the injury, the patient may be able to resume light training within 4 weeks.

HAMSTRING STRAIN (PULLED HAMSTRING)

The hamstring muscles (semimembranosus, semitendinosus and biceps femoris) span the back of the leg and insert into points around the knee joint. These muscles work together to bend and control the knee. Hamstring strains are very common, especially from running or jumping. A lack of warm-up and stretching prior to activity is generally the cause amongst non-professional athletes.

Usually there is a history of a sudden onset of pain in the back of the leg above the knee. Patients present with pain while walking and tenderness around the area of the muscle strain. Additionally if the injury is severe, a balled-up portion of the muscle is felt or even seen down the posterior thigh.

Almost all hamstring strains can be treated without surgery. Immediate management is with RICE for the first 2 days with appropriate pain control, followed by gradual and gentle restoration of the range of movement over the first week. Flexibility can be increased over the following weeks through quadriceps and hamstring stretches. The return to various activities will be dependent on the individual patient.

QUADRICEPS INJURIES

Contusion of the quadriceps is the most common injury. It occurs from a direct blow, usually the result of collision. Patients will present with swelling, pain over the site of impact and reduced function. Very severe injuries with a major haematoma formation carry an increased risk of acute compartment syndrome. In rare cases surgery is performed to remove this major haematoma.

Quadriceps strains and ruptures are associated with major knee stresses. This also gives pain and reduced function along with point tenderness depending on the severity of injury. Most are treated conservatively, although complete rupture will necessitate surgical intervention.

Initial treatment for all quadriceps injuries follows the RICE steps and a programme to reduce the high risk of recurrence.

INJURIES TO THE KNEE

The four primary stabilisers of the knee are the anterior cruciate ligament (ACL), the posterior cruciate ligament (PCL), the medial collateral ligament (MCL) and the lateral collateral ligament (LCL). These ligaments function in collaboration with the muscles and menisci to help control movement of the knee. Proprioceptive fibres in these ligaments and the knee joint capsule augment this control via reflex feedback. Damage to these structures results in knee injuries being the most common of all joints injured in some sporting activities.

Developments in surgical techniques have lead to less invasive procedures through arthroscopic rather than open repairs (DeHaven & Bronstein 1997), which benefits patients because of the reduced recovery time and complications postoperatively.

Anterior cruciate ligament tear (ACL injury)

Located in the centre of the knee, the ACL is a strong band of tissue that limits hyperextension of the tibia.

An ACL injury may result from violent rotation of the knee often combined with sudden deceleration, as when a person plants their foot and then suddenly changes direction. The ACL can also tear if the knee is hyperextended. Therefore, almost any sport that involves jumping, cutting or twisting movements carries the risk of an ACL rupture. Basketball, skiing, football and rugby are among the most common sports associated with this injury.

Patients describe feeling a 'popping' in the knee at the time of injury. There is immediate swelling, a significant effusion and a reduced ability to fully straighten the knee immediately after the injury. ACL injuries often occur in association with fractures or a meniscus tear. The Lachman test (Fig. 25.1) is the best way to assess a knee for an acute ACL rupture. The test involves flexing the knee to approximately 20° and pulling the proximal tibia forward. Excessive anterior motion of the tibia is indicative of an ACL tear.

Non-operative treatment is indicated for patients with limited activity goals or with partial ACL tears. Initially RICE and antiinflammatory medication are recommended to control pain and swelling. Aspirating the effused knee may accelerate the recovery time. After the pain and swelling subside, a programme should be prescribed to increase the knee's range of movement and to strengthen the quadriceps and hamstring muscles. Sport-specific drills in the later treatment stages help restore balance and coordination. Using a knee brace when resuming sports is often advised.

Operative treatment is indicated for patients whose knee gives way during daily living activities, for patients who wish to return to cutting and twisting type sports or those sustaining severe injuries.

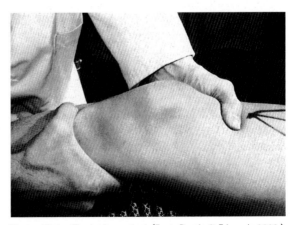

Figure 25.1   The Lachman test. (From Dandy & Edwards 2003.)

The combination of less invasive surgical techniques and more aggressive rehabilitation has improved the outcomes of ACL reconstruction surgery in the last few years.

The three most common ways to reconstruct the ligament are with a bone–patellar tendon–bone autograft, a hamstring autograft or with some form of allograft tissue, normally using either the patellar tendon or Achilles tendon. Screws or other devices are then used to secure the graft in position inside the knee.

After the surgery, rehabilitation begins within a few days. The initial goal is to restore the full range of movement of the knee which often involves the use of a supporting brace. Strength, endurance and coordination drills are added as the patient improves. Typically, the patient may return to activities of daily living in 1–3 weeks and progress to full sporting activity in 6 months, depending upon the surgeon's preference and the patient's recovery.

Medial collateral ligament tear (MCL sprain)

This ligament helps prevent outward movement of the leg at the knee. The two common modes of injury are a hard blow to the outside part of the lower thigh, causing the knee to buckle inwards, or any motion that forcefully moves the leg outwards at the knee as with football, rugby or skiing.

The patient presents with pain accompanied by mild to moderate swelling along the medial side of the knee. MCL injuries sometimes occur in combination with ACL, PCL or meniscus injuries: this should be borne in mind during examination.

Fortunately, most MCL injuries can be treated without surgery. Grade I and II and many grade III injuries are treated with rest, pain control and the use of a brace followed by a physiotherapy programme. MCL injuries that occur in combination with other ligament injuries may require surgical repair.

Posterior cruciate ligament tear (PCL injury)

The posterior cruciate ligament is located in the back of the knee and is responsible for limiting backward movement of the tibia. It is a relatively rare, isolated injury that occurs most often in rugby players, hockey players and skiers. A classic tear of the PCL is due to two mechanisms:

- falling on a bent knee, pushing the tibia backwards and tearing the PCL
- hyperextending the knee.

The PCL can be torn in conjunction with the ACL by a violent twisting of the knee. Obtaining a history of the injury is likely to reveal one of the above mechanisms diagnostic of a PCL injury. A physical examination will show moderate knee swelling and pain with motion.

Most PCL injuries can be treated by strengthening the quadriceps and hamstring muscles and bracing after initial RICE and pain control. Surgery is usually reserved for severe injuries that do not respond to conservative treatment and for those involved in professional sports. PCL tears that occur in combination with other ligament injuries may also require reconstructive surgery.

Meniscus tear

Meniscus tears result from a sudden traumatic injury such as a violent twisting of the knee. Tears also occur without significant trauma from repeated small injuries to the cartilage or meniscal degeneration in older patients. These cartilage injuries can occur during almost any sport or activity. They are also associated with ligament injuries such as a MCL sprain or an ACL tear.

Meniscus tears are typically associated with medial or lateral knee pain and mild to moderate swelling. The patient will often describe clicking or locking of the knee. X-rays are taken to rule out fractures and an MRI scan to confirm the tear.

Many meniscus tears respond well to RICE, anti-inflammatory medication and physiotherapy. If conservative treatment is unsuccessful, arthroscopic surgery is needed to remove the damaged tissue (meniscectomy) or repair the torn cartilage.

Iliotibial band friction syndrome

The iliotibial (IT) band is a long piece of muscle and tendon that starts around the hip and ends just below the knee. When the knee bends and straightens, this band can 'snap' across the outside part of the knee. Repetitive snapping of the IT band can cause friction and lead to inflammation in the area, scarring and subsequent tightening of the IT band. These are generally classified as overuse injuries commonly seen in long-distance runners and cyclists.

IT band friction syndrome typically causes pain on the lateral part of the knee during exercise and is often tender over the area when touched.

The initial treatment during an acute flare-up commences with the RICE approach and avoidance of any activity that makes the pain worse. A stretching programme and antiinflammatory medication are typically employed with steroid injections being used in severe or repeated injuries.

Patellar tendonitis (jumper's knee)

Patellar tendonitis is another overuse syndrome. Repetitive or power jumping as in basketball or volleyball contributes to swelling and inflammation in the patellar tendon. Small tears and the subsequent degeneration of the tendon may occur. Poor muscle flexibility is also responsible for causing patellar tendonitis.

This is diagnosed when an athlete complains of a sharp pain in the front of the knee on exercise, occasionally a dull ache at rest and tenderness when touched over the area between the patella and tibia. X-rays may show a high-riding patella.

In an acute flare-up RICE and pain control are indicated. A stretching and strengthening programme is prescribed and using strapping or bracing can be beneficial. The resumption of normal activities is dependent on the response to treatment. Rarely surgery is indicated to remove the inflamed tendon and stimulate healing, termed a patellar tendon debridement procedure.

Osteochondritis dissecans (articular cartilage injury)

Articular cartilage injuries are caused by a sudden acute knee injury or, less commonly, by a developmental disorder known as osteochondritis dissecans.

An articular cartilage injury is diagnosed by a history of an acute knee injury or a chronic dull ache inside the knee. Physical examination reveals isolated areas of tenderness around the outside of the knee. X-rays may reveal defects in the bone surface or advanced arthritis. An MRI should clearly demonstrate the extent of damage to the cartilage.

Management of the injuries occurs in three stages.

- Phase I: control of pain and inflammation through RICE, stretching and antiinflammatory medication.
- Phase II: restoration of strength and function.
- Phase III: return to work or sports-specific activities.

If this is unsuccessful, arthroscopic surgery may be required to smooth the cartilage or attempt to repair it. If the damage is severe more advanced techniques such as osteochondral transfer, osteotomy or even total knee replacement are considered.

Knee fracture

Falls from heights or a blow to the knee during almost any contact sport can result in a fracture. On physical examination, there will be moderate to severe swelling and usually an inability to bear weight on the affected leg. X-rays usually confirm the fracture but sometimes an MRI or CT scan is needed to further assess the damage. Both the quadriceps and patellar tendons can be injured if a knee fracture occurs.

Treatment for knee fractures is based on the severity of the fracture and the bone(s) involved. Usually fractures of the femur require some form of surgical stabilisation. Stable fractures of the patella are treated with immobilisation while displaced patellar fractures require surgery. Tibial fractures are highly variable and need individual assessment prior to developing a treatment plan.

ACHILLES TENDONITIS

Excessive running or jumping, especially without proper stretching and strengthening, are the most common causes of Achilles tendonitis (inflammation). Uphill running in particular causes this condition. Achilles tendonitis is diagnosed by a history of pain behind the ankle when running or jumping. It is confirmed by tenderness over the Achilles tendon and weakness when testing the calf muscles.

Most cases of Achilles tendonitis can be treated without surgery. Rest, antiinflammatory medications and stretching are the initial non-operative measures. Physiotherapy in combination with orthotics (shoe inserts) may also be needed.

Patients with severe tendonitis unresponsive to conservative treatment may need surgery. This consists of removing the degenerated portions of the tendon followed by an aggressive postoperative rehabilitation programme.

Warming up before exercising and proper stretching are essential to the prevention of Achilles tendonitis. This needs reinforcing otherwise repeat episodes will occur.

ACHILLES TENDON TEAR

Achilles tendon tears typically occur during cutting and jumping sports such as basketball, tennis or rugby although the injury does not usually involve contact with another player. These tears are the result of a violent contraction of the large calf muscles. In some cases, ruptures occur after a long history of Achilles tendonitis.

Achilles tendon tears are diagnosed by a history of a sudden injury followed by a 'pop' felt behind the ankle. The tear is confirmed by squeezing the calf muscles. If the foot does not move, the tendon is probably torn. Occasionally an MRI or ultrasound is needed to confirm that the tendon is ruptured.

The conservative treatment, used for example with inactive or less active patients, involves a cast for 4–6 weeks followed by rehabilitation. Non-operative approaches to care carry a higher risk of rerupture and possible loss of strength with pushing off activities as with walking, running and jumping.

For active patients, surgical reattachment of the torn tendon is recommended. This involves a 3–4 inch incision behind the ankle, suturing the torn tendon ends together and then splinting for 4–6 weeks. The risks inherent in the postoperative period include infection, scarring and poor wound healing. The benefits are a lower risk of rerupture and a better chance of restoring full power to the leg.

ANKLE SPRAIN

The talus bone and the distal tibia and fibula form the ankle joint. Several lateral and medial ligaments support this joint. Most ankle sprains occur when the foot turns inward (inversion injury) as when a person runs, turns, falls or lands on the ankle after a jump, often on an uneven surface. Equipment and surface conditions therefore play a role in causing and preventing ankle injuries.

Most sprains stretch or tear one or more of the lateral ligaments of the ankle. The anterior talofibular ligament is the commonest to be injured and the calcaneofibular ligament the second most frequently torn ligament. Occasionally the ligaments in between the bones of the ankle rupture. Rarely only the medial ligament will tear as a result of an eversion injury. Sports most commonly associated with ankle sprains include basketball, rugby and football.

An ankle sprain should be considered when a patient gives a history of turning their ankle accompanied by sudden pain and swelling. A physical examination will reveal bruising and point tenderness over the injured ligaments.

Most ankle sprains are treated with RICE. A short course of muscle strengthening and balance exercises is essential to prevent repeat sprain injuries. Occasionally surgery is needed to reestablish the stability of the ankle and to either repair or reconstruct the ligaments.

ANKLE FRACTURE

Ankle fractures result when the ankle is forced inwards or outwards past its normal range of motion. The modes and mechanisms of injury are the same as for sprains but with more severe forces at the time of injury.

The patient will complain of sudden pain at the time of injury, tenderness over the bones involved, deformity and severe swelling. Typically there are associated ligament and tendon injuries.

Less severe ankle fractures can be treated conservatively with immobilisation in a cast or splint for 6 weeks. A course of physiotherapy to strengthen the muscles around the ankle is then mandatory.

In more severe injuries surgery is needed to reduce and stabilise ankle fractures. A cast or splint is used for a variable period of time depending on the severity of the fracture. Weight bearing may be delayed until there is evidence of early fracture healing, which may take 4–8 weeks.

CONCLUSION

Health promotion incentives have increased participation in sports in many countries. Although recreational sports are generally safe, there has been a consequent increase in the incidence of sports injuries, from both acute trauma and overuse injuries.

The prevention of sports injuries through legislation and rule changes in some sports has been highly effective in reducing life-threatening injury but the efficacy of prevention strategies for other injuries is less well demonstrated. The recurrence of injury is common. Individual compliance with preventive measures, treatment regimes and instructions affects the outcome of rehabilitation programmes and the rate of recurrence.

Good-quality epidemiological studies and standardisation of severity and outcome measures will go some way to offering solutions to some of these problems. Such studies should take into account special problems associated with the elderly, people with disabilities and children and adolescents undertaking sports activities. None of these should be viewed as a barrier to returning to sports, therefore treatment and rehabilitation programmes that allow and encourage the return to desired sporting activities need to be devised.

The optimum management of sports injuries is unclear at every stage, from the time of injury through to completion of rehabilitation, due to the lack of available evidence. This is compounded by a lack of knowledge as regards the pathophysiology of soft tissue injuries and the recovery process not being entirely understood, although these areas have developed as a result of scientific study in recent years.

It is generally accepted that the acronym RICE comprises a good tool for immediate management although there are debates regarding actual implementation which have been addressed within this chapter.

The organisation of services to manage sports injuries may not contribute to optimum patient outcome and should be reviewed. The use of minor injury clinics is a positive step forward along with the benefits of the emergency nurse practitioner role. Expansion of this concept to nurse consultant or nurse-led sports injury clinics responsible for prevention and ongoing management programmes seems worth exploring in the future.

A sports injury has health, functional and social implications for the individual, some of which can be profound. These should all be borne in mind when planning and implementing sports injury rehabilitation programmes. Finally, a nursing knowledge of specific sports injuries as well as general principles will contribute positively to the optimum management, be it conservative or surgical, and to the rehabilitation of this patient group.

References

Almekinders LC 2000 Medscape Pharmacotherapy 2(2). Available online at: www.medscape.com/viewarticle/408954

Appell HJ 1990 Muscular atrophy following immobilisation: a review. Sports Medicine 10(1): 42–58

Barton N 1997 Sports injuries of the hand and wrist. British Journal of Sports Medicine 31(3): 191–196

Crossman J 1997 Psychological rehabilitation from sports injuries. Sports Medicine 23(5): 333–339

Dandy DJ, Edwards DJ 2003 Essential orthopaedics and trauma, 4th edn. Churchill Livingstone, Edinburgh

DeMaio M, Paine R, Drez DJ 1995 Achilles tendonitis. Orthopaedics 18(2): 195–204

DeHaven KE, Bronstein RD 1997 Arthroscopic medial meniscal repair in the athlete. Clinics in Sports Medicine 16(1): 69–86

Doukas WC, Speer KP 2001 Anatomy, pathophysiology and biomechanics of shoulder instability. Orthopaedic Clinics of North America 32(3): 381–391

Fadale PD, Noerdlinger MA 1999 Sports injuries of the knee. Current Opinion in Rheumatology 11(2): 144–150

Fields KB, Rasco T, Kramer JS et al 1992 Rehabilitation exercises for common sports injuries. American Family Physician 45(3): 1233–1243

Gazielly DF 1989 Sports injuries of the shoulder. Clinical Rheumatology 3(3): 627–649

Grundy D, Swain A, Russell J 1995 ABC of spinal cord injury. BMJ Publications, London

Hockenbury TR, Sammarco JG 2001 Evaluation and treatment of ankle sprains: clinical recommendations for a positive outcome. Physician and Sports Medicine 29(2). Available online at: www.physsportsmed.com/issues/2001/02_01/hockenbury.htm

Jarvinen TA, Kaariainen M, Jarvinen M et al 2000 Muscle strain injuries. Current Opinion in Rheumatology 12(2): 155–161

Junge A 2000 The influence of psychological factors on sports injuries: review of the literature. American Journal of Sports Medicine 28(5 suppl): S10–15

Kannus P, Natri A 1997 Etiology and pathophysiology of tendon ruptures in sports. Scandinavian Journal of Medicine and Science in Sports 7(2): 107–112

Kelley MJ 1990 Psychological risk factors and sports injuries. Journal of Sports Medicine and Physical Fitness 30(2): 202–221

MacAuley DC 2001 Ice therapy: how good is the evidence? International Journal of Sports Medicine 22(5): 379–384

Mares SC 1998 Hip, pelvic and thigh injuries and disorders in the adolescent athlete. Adolescent Medicine 9(3): 551–568

Pickett W, Ardern C, Brison RJ 2001 A population-based study of potential brain injuries requiring emergency care. Canadian Medical Association Journal 165(3): 288–292

Pitner MA 1990 Pathophysiology of overuse injuries in the hand and wrist. Hand Clinics 6(3): 355–364

Shelbourne KD, Klootwyk TE 2000 Low velocity knee dislocation with sports injuries: treatment principles. Clinics in Sports Medicine 19(3): 443–456

Shrier I 1999 Stretching before exercise does not reduce the risk of local muscle injury: a critical review of the clinical and basic science literature. Clinical Journal of Sports Medicine 9(4): 221–227

Smith AM, Scott SG, Wiese DM 1990 The psychological effects of sports injuries: coping. Sports Medicine 9(6): 352–369

Stevenson MR, Hamer P, Finch CF et al 2000 Sport, age, and sex specific incidence of sports injuries in Western Australia. British Journal of Sports Medicine 34(3): 188–194

Tall RL, DeVault W 1993 Spinal injury in sport: epidemiologic considerations. Clinics in Sports Medicine 12(3): 441–448

Thorsson O, Lilja B, Nilsson P et al 1997 Immediate external compression in the management of an acute muscle injury. Scandinavian Journal of Medicine and Science in Sports 7(3): 182–190

Van Mechelen W 1997 The severity of sports injury. Sports Medicine 24(3): 176–180

Van Mechelen W, Hlobil H, Kemper HC 1992 Incidence, severity, aetiology and prevention of sports injuries: a review of concepts. Sports Medicine 14(2): 82–99

Verhagen EALM, Van Mechelen W, De Vente W 2000 The effect of preventative measures on the incidence of ankle sprains. Clinical Journal of Sports Medicine 10: 291–296

Watson WL, Ozanne-Smith J 2000 Injury surveillance in Victoria, Australia: developing comprehensive injury incidence estimates. Accident Analysis and Prevention 32(2): 277–286

Wedmore IS, Charlette J 2000 Emergency department evaluation and treatment of ankle and foot injuries. Emergency Medicine Clinics of North America 18(1): 85–113

Chapter 26

Overuse injuries

Christine Love

INTRODUCTION

Overuse, repetitive strain or cumulative injuries are distinguished by virtue of their not arising from one specific identifiable event. They affect any of the musculoskeletal tissues.

This chapter addresses the causes and management of these injuries in relation to:

- injuries caused by tissue hypoxia
- the effect of overstretching tissues
- occupational and psychological implications.

The chapter provides generally applicable evidence with specific clinical examples being given to illustrate important aspects of cause, management or prevention.

OVERVIEW

Overuse injuries, according to Pitner (1990), arise from repeated submaximal loads causing trauma that exceeds the rate of repair or from compensatory maladaptive repair. In contrast, most other injuries result from a single supramaximal load.

The people affected include those engaged in repeated work actions over a long time, apparently unharmed, to those undertaking a new strenuous activity with symptoms developing within days. The cumulative nature of overuse injuries means they can develop over a few months or many years. However, if the right circumstances are present, then pain and disability can develop in 48–96 hours or in 1 week.

The progressive nature of these injuries means patients have no or few outward signs of injury. Pain and discomfort often precede obvious tissue damage, in comparison to acute injuries which are more overtly visible (Pitner 1990). Tissue damage is often insidious until a critical threshold is reached.

The absence of an obvious injury means it is not perceived in the same way as an acute injury. Patients can be reluctant to seek help, fear they will not be believed or economic and social pressures lead them to continue working despite an injury (Feuerstein 1996).

Prevention often relies on good risk assessments in the work or home situation and appropriate health promotion. When injury does occur, the available evidence indicates that tissue damage is often irreversible (Kalimo et al 1997, Woo & Hildebrand 1997). Consequently interventions are based on pain relief and protracted programmes of physiotherapy to enable the patient to adapt to the loss of function and consequent disablement (Netscher et al 1997). Complete restoration of function is not guaranteed.

CAUSES OF OVERUSE INJURY

Overuse injuries were initially identified in connection with different crafts and trades. Employment-related activities remain a significant factor, along with sports, as the main causes of these injuries.

Submaximal loads cause two broad categories of injury (Mense 1993):

1 through local tissue hypoxia
2 repeated bouts of overstretching with a hypoxic element.

Due to the prevalence of tissue hypoxia, more attention is given to these injuries.

MUSCLE INJURY FROM TISSUE HYPOXIA

Orthopaedic nurses are aware that tissue hypoxia occurs from tight bandaging and casts. The same effect can be caused by muscle tissue activity; this is the root cause of many overuse injuries (Elert et al 1992, Hagert & Christenson 1990, Larsson et al 1990).

MUSCLE TISSUE

To appreciate the tissue changes and the differences in muscle types, the differences in metabolism and contraction are discussed here with reference to the trapezius muscle as a classic example of an overuse injury.

Muscle types

Muscles are categorised according to their fibre type of which there are three: type 1, type 2 and type 3. Type 1 muscle fibres are found predominantly in postural muscles, such as the trapezius, and are the most at risk of an overuse injury. Protection from damage comes from the sequential use of the muscle fibres whilst others are resting and refuelling (Pheasant 1992). To maintain postural activity for long periods requires no more than 3% of type 1 muscle fibres to be active at one time (Bjorksten & Jonsson 1977).

Muscle metabolism

Type 1 muscle fibres require an immediate supply of oxygen to metabolise the nutrients they need. Their source of fuel and metabolic mechanism is entirely different from muscle types 2 and 3 which store glycogen in the muscle fibre. Glycogen provides a readily accessible source of energy for high-speed, high-intensity and short-lived movement.

Arm muscles are designed for quick bursts of activity so have a dominant number of type 3 fibres and fewer type 1 fibres (Powers & Howley 1994). Fatigue in type 3 muscle fibres relates to the speed, force and duration of activity as these govern the opportunity for refuelling. Marsh et al (1993) found that energy depletion from moderate activity occurred in 30 seconds, whilst refuelling took 2 minutes. If more than 30% of the muscle fibres are used, the fuel stores are depleted within 2 minutes and fatigue sets in, reducing the efficiency or function of the muscle to the point where it cannot be used (Marsh et al 1993). This explains why the arm muscles begin to ache when carrying loads over a distance in a fixed arm position.

Muscle contraction

Muscle tissue contracts in three ways:

1 isotonic contraction, where the length of the muscle shortens from a dynamic activity
2 eccentric contraction, where the muscle lengthens, as with resisting an applied force
3 isometric contraction, where the length does not change from its resting position; an isometric exercise is also called static exercise or work.

Eccentric and isometric activities are commonly implicated in overuse injury. These can occur together; for example, a postural muscle such as the trapezius uses isometric contraction but it needs eccentric contraction for working in an awkward position.

Eccentric contraction also controls the speed of motion or provides an opposing force; for example, when walking downhill the dorsiflexors control the speed of movement. This produces muscle tension but is efficient in its use of oxygen and glucose. However, if the contraction is increased, this efficiency of use is lost, causing ischaemia from loss of oxygen and glucose (Mense 1993). Sustained eccentric or isometric contraction, especially if the action is forced, causes tissue hypoxia or anoxia.

Prolonged static loading affects the blood supply and the muscles' ability to metabolise oxygen, replace nutrients and remove waste products. A slight or semicontracted position causes tension which reduces the blood supply and at full contraction the supply is shut off (Petrofsky & Phillips 1986). The blood pressure also rises with the force and duration of contraction. The resultant hypoxia and anoxia affect the muscle by:

- depriving it of oxygen and nutrients
- accumulation of toxic waste products causes a rise in osmotic pressure which further increases the intramuscular pressure.

Oedema. Oedema is an osmotic response where the direction of water exchange is always from low to high concentration. Accumulated waste products create a medium or high concentration; this attracts an inflow of fluid, causing intramuscular oedema. If the activity is continued, the oedematous changes compound and exacerbate anoxia. The tissue damage precipitates an inflammatory response characterised by the release of prostaglandins and bradykinin, increased membrane permeability and further oedema.

MUSCLE CHANGES

Prolonged submaximal loads, caused by, for example holding a muscle tense, will activate more than 3% of type 1 fibres at any one time. This affects the optimum function of the muscle especially if the position is held repetitively. To overcome this, the muscle tissue changes in two ways, both indicative of chronic muscle hypoxia.

1 A 'moth-eaten' appearance develops, indicative of a reactive hypertrophy. In the early stages the pain does not cause incapacity but the activity is

---

> ### Box 26.1   Changes in the trapezius muscle
>
> The trapezius is the main stabiliser of the shoulder girdle complex and is classified as a postural muscle with a predominance of type 1 muscle fibres. In women affected by trapezius myalgia, Larsson et al (1990) detected changes to the structure of the trapezius muscle. From biopsies Larsson et al found that changes were confined to the type 1 muscle fibres, specifically to the mitochondria of the muscle cell which process oxygen and glucose to produce energy and are reliant on a good blood supply.
>
> Larsson et al's study found both the moth-eaten appearance and ragged red fibres in the majority of patients. When the blood flow was assessed, it was reduced and linked to the degree of change and the level of reported pain. When muscle activity was examined, the trapezius was subjected to prolonged static use (loading). There was a direct link in that the more the muscle was held in a static position, the greater the level of tissue damage.

sufficient to reduce the blood flow. When this happens the moth-eaten appearance occurs even though the individual has not experienced discomfort (Bengtsson et al 1986).

2 A 'ragged red fibre' effect occurs, indicative of continual work in conditions of ischaemia.

See Box 26.1 for how this relates to changes in the trapezius muscle.

Muscle pain

Muscle ischaemia occurs when the activity is highly dependent on an isometric or eccentric type contraction. The risk is increased by a heavy load or by performing a task involving precision combined with strength and requiring the arm to be held in one position (Petrofsky & Phillips 1986). At first, the individual becomes aware of local discomfort and if the muscle is not rested, there is severe cramp followed by incapacity.

The free nerve endings in skeletal muscles have marked sensitivity to chemical stimuli, particularly disturbances of the local microcirculation. Type 1 muscle fibres are more sensitive to local blood supply disturbances because of their greater dependence on oxygen for contraction. As a result, they are more immediately sensitive to hypoxia and pain (Mense 1993). As all muscles contain a proportion of type 1 muscle fibres, this provides a protective effect from hypoxic conditions.

When ischaemic conditions cause muscle damage, endogenous E-type prostaglandins and the neuropeptide bradykinin are released as the normal inflammatory response ensues. If a muscle contracts when ischaemic, pain develops within 1 minute (Mense 1993) because the prostaglandin has an enhancing effect on the action of bradykinin which makes the nociceptors more sensitive. As a result the nerve endings cause pain, even during normal movements (Mense 1993).

Compartment pressure changes

Hagert & Christenson (1990) found raised intramuscular pressure in people with trapezius myalgia to a level associated with compartment syndrome even in a relaxed muscle. When contracted, the intramuscular pressure will rise to a level at which tissue death occurs. The intramuscular pressure values were:

- in a relaxed muscle: 27 mmHg ± 12 mmHg compared to a normal of 7.4 mmHg ± 3.8 mmHg
- in a contracted muscle: 49 mmHg ± 16 mmHg compared to a normal of 12 ± 4.9 mmHg.

Surgical intervention should begin when the intracompartmental pressure rises above 30 mmHg. Hagert & Christenson's (1990) findings explain the development of damage to type 1 muscle fibre from sustained muscle activity as they found this damage in all cases and on removal of the diseased tissue the pain was relieved.

PREDISPOSING OCCUPATIONAL CONDITIONS

Many work practices generate eccentric and isometric contractions. There is a positive correlation between the time spent with the head flexed forwards, the shoulders elevated and the upper arm in a position of flexion and abduction and the severity and incidence of neck and shoulder pain. In this posture, the trapezius muscle is actively resisting the gravitational pull of the arms for prolonged periods and is eccentrically loaded.

Eccentric contraction is observed in rotator cuff injuries. Repeatedly lifting a heavy box with both hands onto a shelf at waist height or above produces adduction and internal rotation of the shoulder. This requires eccentric contraction of the supraspinatus, infraspinatus and teres minor muscles to provide the necessary opposing forces of abduction and external rotation. The same situation would arise if supporting a load held away from the body, illustrating the need for correct moving and handling techniques.

Isometric or mild eccentric contraction can arise during small movements. The forearm muscles are at risk in hand-intensive activities such as using a computer keyboard, from fine finger or precision movements. Reactive inflammation leads to the onset of chronic compartment syndrome from the sustained tension, impeded blood flow, accumulated waste products, raised osmotic pressure and oedema.

In Veiersted et al's (1990) study to investigate the cause of neck and shoulder muscle pain, the single most important determinant, was prolonged muscular contraction. They found workers were unable to induce momentary spontaneous relaxation in their neck and shoulder muscles while working, causing the conditions in which muscle tissue hypoxia could arise. The onset of pain was unrelated to age or the period of employment but did show a prevalence amongst shorter people. Although the effect of a person's height in relation to the work surface was not investigated, shorter people would have to raise their arms more to do the same task, using more effort to achieve the same results. This exacerbates the conditions in which muscle hypoxia is already occurring.

Elert et al (1992) also noted that people suffering trapezius myalgia were unable to relax between repetitive work activities. The period of relaxation between activities is important for the health of muscle tissue as it prevents tissue anoxia from muscle contraction reducing the muscle microcirculation (Larsson et al 1990). Paradoxically, muscle hypoxia also causes the muscle to be unable to relax, compounding the situation.

In terms of prevention, Veiersted et al (1990) believed that increasing the time between repetitive work activities and optimum working conditions were more important than decreasing the length of the working day. This is important for prevention of overuse injury and for rehabilitation, as shortening the working day is not a solution if the work itself is not ergonomically correct.

NERVE INJURIES FROM HYPOXIA

Overuse injuries resulting from nerve tissue hypoxia occur mainly in the upper limb, affecting the peripheral nervous system. They are associated with the same activities as those causing muscle hypoxia and result in injuries such as carpal tunnel syndrome.

NERVE STRUCTURE

A peripheral nerve has its nerve cell located at the level of the spinal cord while the terminal structures are located in the target tissue some distance away. This elongated structure serves distant target tissues but is reliant on the centrally located segment for its oxygen, nutrients and removal of waste products (Szabo & Gelberman 1987). In some cases the distance can be over 1 metre (Carragee & Hentz 1988).

To reach their target tissues, these elongated structures or axons have to pass through tight anatomical spaces such as the carpal tunnel. These points make them vulnerable to entrapment or compression; it is here that overuse injuries occur.

Nerve coverings

The nerve cell is a strip of protoplasm surrounded by the neurilemma membrane and encased in protective coverings: the endo-, peri- and epineurium.

The endoneurium is a membranous tube covering the axon. It is highly vascular but contains no lymphatic channels. The axons together with their covering of endoneurium are arranged into bundles or fascicles.

The perineurium is a dense sheath of fibrous tissue covering each fasciculus separately. It is constructed from a multilayered network of collagen and elastic fibres arranged in concentric rings separated by perineural spaces. The elasticity of the perineurium protects individual fibres during stretching, for example when a joint is extended, and acts as a diffusion barrier to maintain intraneural pressure which prevents collapse (Szabo & Gelberman 1987).

Axonal transport

The nerve cell body produces all the substances needed for the survival and function of the nerve, including proteins, neurotransmitters, lipids, mitochondria and ribonucleic acid (RNA). These are transported to the peripheral or terminal areas of the nerve by antegrade transport. A return process, retrograde transport, transfers materials back to the cell body for recycling or excretion. The return process also transmits information to the cell body about the state of the peripheral nerve tissue, the

surrounding tissues and the presence of injury anywhere along the length of the axon.

Antegrade axonal transport occurs at two speeds:

1 up to 410 mm per day for substances serving the immediate energy demands of the target tissues
2 a slower rate of 3 mm per day for transporting materials for tissue repair; hence the healing process of nerve tissue injuries is very slow.

The speed of retrograde axonal transport is 300 mm per day. In a 1 metre peripheral nerve, any restriction to the retrograde flow of information could take up to 3 days to become acutely evident.

Axonal transport is impeded by compression, anoxia and the accumulation of waste products or the infiltration of toxic substances. Any compression along the length of the axon that prevents antegrade and retrograde flow can lead to nerve cell death. This has been found to occur from externally applied loads of more than 30 mmHg (Lundborg et al 1983).

COMPRESSION INJURIES

The underlying cause of nerve injury from overuse is compression, causing nerve damage in three ways.

1 Mechanical compression causes damage to the endoneurium from direct pressure, resulting in increased vascular permeability from direct injury to the capillary walls (Rydevik et al 1981).
2 Compression impeding blood flow in the epineurium causes hypoxia, the accumulation of venous fluid and blockage of retrograde axonal transport. The accumulation of waste products further exacerbates the development of oedema by creating a medium of high concentration which sucks fluid towards it by the effects of osmosis. As the endoneurium lacks lymphatic channels, any oedema is not easily removed. Moreover, when the damage occurs in a confined space, the effect of oedema becomes more marked as the local pressure rises.
3 Oedema causes changes in the electrolyte composition of endoneurial fluid, affecting its function (Lundborg et al 1983). As a consequence of both the direct tissue damage to the epineurium and raised osmotic pressure, intrafascicular pressure rises and further obstructs the microcirculation of the epineurium, leading to ischaemia (Lundborg et al 1983).

In an experimental study designed to assess the affect of compression on axonal transport, Dahlin &

McLean (1986) applied a pressure of 20 mmHg directly to nerve tissue for 8 hours. The results showed that fast and slow antegrade axonal transport were impeded. This level of compression has been found in patients with carpal tunnel syndrome (Dahlin et al 1987). See Box 26.2 for details of this condition.

In overuse peripheral nerve injury, the source of compression is the pattern of arm movements causing sustained isometric contraction at low submaximal loads. The static contraction causes a sequential rise in intramuscular pressure, further exacerbated by increasing hypoxia preventing the muscle from relaxing (Mense 1993).

Raised intramuscular pressure

Raised intramuscular pressure causes damage to the nerve by anoxia and acute compartment syndrome. This is shown by prolonged isometric contraction, especially in hand-intensive activities (Szabo & Gelberman 1987). Most nurses are familiar with compression from a sphygmomanometer cuff during blood pressure readings. The blood supply is temporarily interrupted at 30 mmHg above the systolic blood pressure before a reading can be made.

The normal endoneurial fluid pressure is 2 mmH$_2$O (Myers et al 1978). In experiments by Lundborg et al (1983), compressive forces of 30 and 80 mmHg were applied to a nerve. With the compressive force of 30 mmHg, there was no significant increase in endoneurial fluid pressure after 6 hours, but after 8 hours this had risen to 6 mmH$_2$O, three times the normal value. A compression of 80 mmHg for 3 hours produced a pressure of 6 mmH$_2$O, a threefold rise. When applied for 4 hours, this increased to 8.5 mmH$_2$O, four times the normal level.

In their experimental study, Szabo & Gelberman (1987) recruited volunteers with and without hypertension. Compressive forces of 40 and 50 mmHg were applied. No loss of sensation occurred with a compression of 40 mmHg. However, in the subjects with normal blood pressure, sensation was lost 10–60 minutes after application of the 50 mmHg pressure. At the time of sensation loss, motor function fell by 20–40% of the baseline values, reducing strength in the hand. In hypertensive subjects no changes were seen with 60 mmHg of compression but the above changes were present with a compression of 70 mmHg.

These findings show that contracted muscle tissue can impede blood flow to nerve tissue at levels lower than those to which a sphygmomanometer cuff is inflated when taking the diastolic blood pressure. According to the experimental findings of Marsh et al (1993) and Veiersted et al (1990), this could also arise if the working posture caused sustained or frequent contraction of a third or more of a muscle.

TISSUE DEFORMATION INJURIES

NORMAL REACTIONS

A force applied to a tissue causes it to undergo changes in size or shape. The strength of the tissue is judged by its ability to withstand this without injury.

Strain is the deformation of a tissue or a change in its length. There are three types of strain.

1 Tension causes the tissue to elongate.
2 Compression causes them to shorten.
3 Shear is a tension force that produces most deformation and is the most likely to cause injury.

Stress is the internal opposing force and refers to the elasticity of the tissue; this is the ability of the tissue to keep its shape when direct pressure is applied.

CHANGES ARISING FROM TISSUE STRETCHING

Each tissue has a finite stretch and buoyancy limit which is increased with use (Kalimo et al 1997, Woo & Hildebrand 1997) and reduced by disease and in older age (Pollock & Wilmore 1990). In normal circumstances the deforming force has no adverse effects and when removed, the tissue returns to its original shape and size. If overstretched, it either goes into a state of plastic deformation or snaps.

Plastic deformation refers to a situation in which a tissue is overstretched and does not spring back to its original shape when the tension force is removed. Strain is the clinical definition of deformation affecting contractile tissues such as muscle, while sprain injury affects non-contractile tissue such as ligaments.

Shearing injury

In normal usage, a pulling force is absorbed by muscle tissue. This requires the muscle to respond quickly and strongly enough to absorb and dissipate the applied load. The most vulnerable situations are when the muscle is:

- untrained, so is unable to contract strongly enough

Box 26.2   Carpal tunnel syndrome

This is the most common overuse injury. The incidence of carpal tunnel syndrome (CTS) is estimated at 1% of the population, with a further 10% experiencing symptoms on one or more occasions (Weirich & Gelberman 1993).

Epidemiological evidence reveals a population distribution split between young adults and people of retirement age. In younger people the prominent cause is either industrial or commercial activities resulting in repetitive, forceful movements with the wrist held in flexion, extension or oscillating rapidly between flexion and extension or is due to vibration (Weirich & Gelberman 1993). In older people, the cause can relate to previous hand usage, especially at work. Health and safety legislation and labour-saving devices in the workplace and at home have reduced the number of repetitive hand-intensive tasks. Any previous hand damage would become more obvious following a precipitating factor such as cervical spondylosis (Osterman 1988) or a Colles' fracture (Szabo & Gelberman 1987), both of which are known to trigger the onset of CTS symptoms.

Carpal tunnel anatomy.   The carpal tunnel is a concave arch created by the eight carpal bones situated on the dorsal surface and a transverse band of inelastic fibrous connective tissue on the palmar or volar surface (Fig. 26.1). This provides a fixed-sized passage for 10 structures supplying the fingers: four superficial and four deep flexor tendons, the flexor pollicis longus and the median nerve. Each tendon is enveloped in a synovial bursa providing protection from friction and compression.

The carpal tunnel is normally 5 mm in length and 10 mm wide. However, the size is not uniform in the population, being smaller in women than in men: it is up to 25% smaller in women with CTS (Dekel et al 1980).

The tunnel is narrower in the centre (Ham et al 1996) and the shape changes according to the angle at which the wrist is held. Flexion and extension reduce its size and increase the incidence of CTS. Extension stretches the soft tissues, enabling an increased angle to be achieved. Flexion reduces the space, bunching the contents.

Diagnosis of CTS.   Patients with CTS complain of loss of sensation from the median nerve. In severe cases, this extends to motor control. The tingling is worse at night and is relieved by shaking the hand; this is believed to be the most important clinical sign

(Weirich & Gelberman 1993). The condition is verified by provocative tests: the Phalen wrist flexion test (Weirich & Gelberman 1993) and the Tinel percussion test where tapping over the median nerve will reproduce the symptoms.

Treatment of CTS.   Treatment should start as early as possible. Prompt action can prevent the need for surgery to divide the carpal tunnel to achieve immediate nerve decompression.

Conservative treatment includes the use of diuretics or antiinflammatory agents. Depot steroid injections into the carpal space, for example 40 mg of methylprednisolone, followed by splinting in a neutral position are advocated (Weirich & Gelberman 1993) but their success relates to the severity of symptoms. Oral diuretics and NSAIDs are of unproven benefit. Prevention of further mechanical damage is achieved by using a removable wrist splint which limits flexion and extension and greatly relieves symptoms in mildly affected people. Patients should not wear the splint to overcome unergonomic work practices.

Surgery is used if the symptoms are not relieved and there is wasting of the thenar muscle. The aim of decompression surgery is to increase the volume of the carpal space which can be up to 25% (Weierich & Gelberman 1993). Division achieves decompression and permits forward displacement of the flexor tendons, causing continued and unresolved weakness of grip strength. Immediate relief is not always achieved from surgery with continued disability occurring for some patients.

Nursing issues.   Nurses need to be alert to the unique symptoms and highly characteristic patterns of onset of CTS. As it is a common complication of a Colles' fracture, this risk must be identified by staff in accident and emergency departments, fracture clinics and outpatient departments.

Postoperative health promotion involves avoidance of preventable complications (Tannahill 1985), including infection. Impaired dexterity occurs, especially if symptoms affect the dominant hand or both hands, so support in activities of daily living can be needed. Advice on the care of any splint is essential, including when and when not to wear it as some patients only need a splint for active provocative tasks. Advice on risks to the skin from pressure or friction from a splint and how to prevent these is essential. A well-fitting splint should not cause discomfort or skin damage.

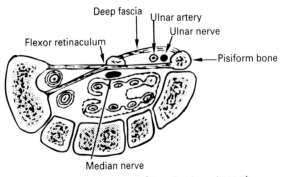

Figure 26.1   The carpal tunnel. (From Smith et al 1983.)

- unprepared, in which case it is not in a state of readiness
- contracted, in which case the force travels down the belly of the muscle to the myotendinous junction where distraction injury occurs as either a strain, sprain or in severe cases avulsion of bone.

Occasionally a pulling force occurs in opposing directions, leaving the muscle at risk of shearing (Kalimo et al 1997). This is potentially the most serious form of deformation, causing damage to the myofibrils and connective tissue framework. This results in an extensive haematoma and potentially extensive fibrous tissue development which reduces the muscle's function (Kalimo et al 1997).

MANAGING DEFORMATION INJURIES

Deformation injuries are part of the acute injury spectrum and include strain, sprain, tendon avulsion, ligament tears and stress fractures from supramaximal loads. Many are the consequence of overuse, where damage arises insidiously and cumulatively from tissue breakdown or microdamage exceeding the rate of adaptation or repair.

In the case of microdamage, healing that regains preinjury strength can take 6–12 months (Woo & Hildebrand 1997). The injury symptoms may be mild and short-lived, disguising the underlying damage and increasing the risk that the originating cause of injury will be repeated before full tissue strength is achieved.

When treating muscle tendon or ligament overuse injuries, attention should be given to the healing process which relies on a good blood supply to provide nutrients and to remove necrotic tissue.

Appropriate exercise of the tissue is essential. To prevent further damage, the patient needs to avoid the provoking action and then introduce it very gradually over the healing period of 6–12 months.

Three typical examples of overuse injury from repeated deformation which exceeds the rate of repair are rupture of the Achilles tendon, tears of the rotator cuff (see Chapter 21) and stress fractures (see Box 26.3).

PREVENTION OF INJURY

Prevention of overuse injuries is achieved by the gradual introduction of physical activity, allowing the muscle and bone to adapt to frequent repetitive cyclic loading. An ergonomically appropriate work or activity environment is essential, including the use of appropriate footwear, desk space and lifting aids.

Muscle fatigue must be regarded as an early warning sign. Any physical activity training programme should assume that most people have not been exposed to any endurance exercise. Endurance exercise is not required for most living activities; it is taken up as an extra and has to be maintained or fitness soon wanes.

Orthopaedic nurses need to be aware of the causes and potential indicators of overuse injuries to accurately assess and plan care and to offer appropriate advice for patients.

PSYCHOSOCIAL FACTORS IN OCCUPATIONAL INJURY

Occupational overuse injuries are the consequence of the manner in which a task is done (Feuerstein 1996). The way it is perceived and interpreted exerts a physiological influence in the development of symptoms.

Workstyle

Workstyle relates to why some people develop overuse injury while others do not, when apparently performing the same task (Feuerstein 1996). Workstyle consists of three components:

1 the method, which relates to the manner in which the task is performed
2 individual differences in anatomical, physiological and psychological variations and

Box 26.3   Stress fractures

Stress fractures occur from repeated submaximal loading. The normal cycle of adaptation and repair involves bone absorption before the formation of new bone. With repetitive cyclic loading, a time lag occurs during which the bone is structurally vulnerable.

Fracture cause.   In moderation and within the skeletal system strength and endurance, exercise is beneficial in the development of strong bones. Stress fractures occur when exercise exceeds the strength and endurance of a bone.

Unaccustomed and prolonged stress causes physical fatigue and microfractures occur which stimulate the repair process. Healing begins with osteoclast activity followed by osteoblasts developing new bone. Stress fractures do not occur if osteoblast activity keeps pace with osteoclast activity, especially if exercise is limited or stopped. As more exercise is undertaken, further microfractures occur which, if sufficiently extensive, can coalesce into a visible fracture.

Stress fractures normally develop over a few days but can occur from one episode. If the activity causes a significant number of microfractures of sufficient severity and in close proximity, this can break the bone. Commonly this arises from low bone density, inadequate dietary intake of bone-forming nutrients and exercise-induced oestrogen suppression (Haddad et al 1997).

Typical fractures.   The highest incidence of stress fracture is in the lower limb. Typical causes are exposure to endurance exercise when unfit and overly strenuous training programmes (Beck et al 1996, Hill et al 1996).

Muscle fatigue is a well-known feature of endurance exercise even in fit people. Sharkey et al (1995) showed that when fatigued, the weight-bearing force that should be absorbed by the plantarflexors contracting is directed to the metatarsals, subjecting them to increased loading and the risk of microfracture.

The most frequently reported incidence of stress fractures is in new recruits to the armed forces required to undergo strenuous training programmes (Beck et al 1996, Hill et al 1996). The onset arises within the first 10 weeks of recruitment, with a peak incidence during the first week of training (Jones et al 1989).

Hill et al (1996) reported 12 instances of pubic rami stress fractures in 11 military recruits in basic training. Eleven of the fractures were in women. The cause was attributed to mixed gender training that required female trainees to increase their stride length when marching. When the stride length was reduced, no further instances of pelvic stress were reported.

Professional and amateur athletes experience stress fractures from running (Jones et al 1989). The risk is increased by wearing inappropriate or worn-out footwear when walking or running and when the exercise is unaccustomed (Jones et al 1989).

Upper limb injuries are linked to racquet sports with fractures occurring in the proximal humerus (Boyd & Batt 1997) and the scaphoid.

Stress fractures have been reported following orthopaedic surgery. Fractures of the tibia following ankle arthrodesis occur as a late complication after full union of the arthrodesis site (Lidor et al 1997). Subcapital fractures have occurred following knee replacement surgery in patients affected by poor mobility preoperatively with a large varus or valgus deformity (Rawes et al 1995). Consequently any unexplained bone pain following surgery must be investigated for a possible stress fracture.

These fractures are more common in women because of their smaller bones and lower bone density. Caucasians have a higher risk than black people for the same reasons (Jones et al 1989). Risk also increases with age because of reduced bone density and a less active lifestyle (Jones et al 1989).

Diagnosis and treatment.   The most common feature is an obvious break in the bone but Jones et al (1989) have found evidence of four preceding stages which provide the diagnostic grading system shown in Table 26.1.

Treatment relates to the fracture type, site and severity. Delays in healing occur if the bone trauma has not been sufficiently severe to provoke osteogenesis. In this circumstance bone healing can be stimulated by capacitive coupling which involves passing an alternating sinusoidal wave electrical current through the fracture site (Benazzo et al 1995) or bone drilling (Orava et al 1995).

Table 26.1 Five grades of stress fracture (adapted from Jones et al 1989)

Grade	Bone response	Orthopaedic action
0	• Asymptomatic • Physiologic response to a change in the mechanical environment either from the amount of load (stress) or the frequency of repetition	• Detected only by bone scan • No detectable changes on X-ray • Structural integrity of bone still intact
1	• History of recently increased activity frequency or loading • Local pain exacerbated by the provoking activity but ceases when activity stops • Minimal local tenderness on palpation • No local swelling or mass	• Detected only by bone scan • No detectable changes on X-ray • Structural integrity of bone still intact • Scaling down of activity needed until physiological adaptation has occurred • Purchase of new footwear should be considered where appropriate if walking or running
2	• History of recently increased activity frequency or loading • Local pain exacerbated by the provoking activity but ceases when activity stops • More noticeable local tenderness on palpation • No local swelling or mass over site of pain	• Significant stress reactions seen on bone scan • Barely detectable damage on standard X-ray • Structural integrity of bone still intact • Scaling down of activity needed until physiological adaptation has occurred • Purchase of new footwear should be considered where appropriate if walking or running
3	• Pain more acute and persists after activity has stopped • Marked local tenderness • Palpable fullness or mass over site of pain	• Changes detectable on X-ray • Structure of bone in jeopardy • Activity stopped until symptoms and signs abate • Protected weight bearing with crutches during healing phase
4	• Pain very severe • Not able to bear weight	• Evidence of a fracture on X-ray • Treatment according to fracture type and location. Stable fractures generally require a cast, unstable fractures normally require internal or external fixation. Stimulation via capacitive coupling or drilling for delayed union

cognitions, which includes the person's attitude to the work and level of self-confidence

3 the nature of the work environment, its ergonomic status and the effect of internal and external pressures.

Individuals vary in the amount of force they apply to the same task. Veiersted et al (1990) found that symptomatic workers applied greater muscle activity compared to unaffected people and had fewer periods when the muscle was relaxed, predisposing the tissues to anoxia.

It is important that people only use the force needed to do a task. In some cases a lack of skill is the root cause whilst in others it is a lack of awareness, an inappropriate work environment or is due to motivational factors; for example, a highly goal-directed state of mind will increase the person's state of arousal and along with it muscular tension.

Prevention needs to look at the individual, their methods of working and the work environment to assess the risk of injury. This risk needs to be reassessed as working practices, resources or equipment change and when an employee returns from a period of absence or when someone is new to the job.

PERCEPTION AND INTERPRETATION OF INJURY

There is often a psychological component to occupational overuse injury (Feuerstein 1996).

Social cognitive theory

This theory explains how people develop somatic interpretations of physical symptoms; that is, how they make links between pain and situational experiences. It offers an explanation of the mechanism whereby people infer cause and effect links between a work process and their physical symptoms.

Social cognitive theory suggests that the associations between the symptoms and attributed cause provide the basis of illness schemata. An illness schema is the cognitive process that organises and represents understanding of an illness. In childhood, this mechanism equips people with a schema to link pain to actual or potential tissue damage and understanding that the tissue damage is harmful.

The basic premises are that the situation overwhelms the usual behaviour or performance and that learning is based on increments of situational experiences. It contends that people attempt to understand the context and situation to maintain a sense of control over events that affect them or could do so in the future. These cause and effect relationships describe and explain past, present and future events, including somatic experiences such as pain and discomfort. The process is referred to as somatic information processing.

When a physical sensation is noticed, so are associated situational and contextual features. The sensation is identified by the person; this is influenced by the experience of colleagues, prior knowledge, the media, in-service education and what has happened to family members or friends. This provides the basis for a naive explanation, or theory, of the presumed cause. For example, if a certain wrist position causes pain and is identified as being potentially harmful, it is then avoided if others similarly affected have had to give up work. If the pain is attributed to the previous evening's recreation, work is not an attributed cause and if the evening's activity was voluntary there is less or no perceived threat of harm. The pain is then memorised so it can be recalled if it recurs.

The impact of symptoms is therefore influenced by the context of the situation, possible causative links, the behaviour and beliefs of others, personal mood, feelings and interpretations, general personality traits and states and the individual's current position on the confident–diffident, success–failure, approved of–disapproved of continua. If workloads are high, autonomy and work satisfaction are often low; if there is a concurrent risk of disapproval, any pain may lead to a sense of not being in control, eliciting a stress response which overlays physical symptoms. However, if the person has control over their work, the initiating symptoms may be the same but they are not exacerbated by a sense of powerlessness and associated stress. Avoiding stress requires people to have a sense of autonomy and belief that they can meet the demands required of them. Workloads therefore need to be realistic for the individual's current capabilities and where possible should be worker, rather than machine, paced.

Effects of stress

High states of arousal cause muscle tension. Added to a stressful work situation, this exacerbates muscle contraction and the tension required to do the work task.

Arousal is caused by increased levels of noradrenaline (norepinephrine). The action of noradrenaline (norepinephrine) is to enhance prostaglandin and bradykinin; as these are already present due to tissue damage, the conditions exist for a self-sustaining cycle of pain even during normal levels of muscle contraction (Mense 1993).

In accordance with social cognitive theory, the reflex responses that release the neurochemicals can become part of a learned response. For example, as soon as a person sits at a computer keyboard, they immediately become tense in anticipation of pain or reprisals because their work is thought to be of substandard quality or their output not up to the required speed. As they work the muscle tension from using the keyboard causes physical pain and their sense of arousal is further increased.

Another source of stress is the perception that complaints of pain are not believed. The pain and disability which accompany severe physical trauma are easy for the onlooker to understand as they are related to a specific identifiable historical event and produce obvious outward clinical signs. This is not so with injuries which arise from seemingly normal activities, especially when others are doing the same kind of movement and the same level of work but are seemingly unaffected. It calls for absolute trust in the patient's complaint of pain and the need to believe the patient's experience of pain. The fact that only some people are affected requires understanding of the causes of overuse injury rather than disbelief of the effect.

Negligence

Individuals and groups, including employers, have a legal duty to act in a responsible way and not cause others physical or psychological harm. The legal duty is subsumed within the law of tort which exists to protect people from harm by others and to provide a mechanism whereby the injured party can be compensated.

Although there are a number of torts, the one most applicable to overuse injuries is negligence. Negligent acts occur as a result of an omission in which there is either a failure to appreciate an obvious risk or a failure to take appropriate preventive measures when a risk is identified (Pitchfork 1996).

In all cases, negligence is judged on the basis of what is reasonable and practicable in the circumstances and in accordance with the prevailing scientific evidence at the time of injury. In the case of overuse injuries, negligence could arise if a trainer failed to appreciate the risk of injury from a training programme or if a nurse failed to undertake a suitable and sufficient patient assessment resulting in, for example, a missed stress fracture.

In both sporting and occupational settings complaints of pain, cramp and muscular fatigue, with or without sickness absence, should be regarded as the early warning signs that control measures are failing and suggest the need for further risk assessment and work design.

CONCLUSION

There is now sufficient evidence to suggest that repetitive use which exceeds physiological function causes tissue damage and as yet, with the exception of bone, no studies have shown that the effects are reversible. It must therefore be concluded that when someone suffers an overuse injury the tissue damage is permanent. The two main effects are from tissue hypoxia and repeated tissue injury from submaximal loads that exceeds the rate of tissue repair. In respect of hypoxia, prolonged isometric or eccentric contraction creates greatest risk. Whilst it is recognised that stress can enhance the effect of isometric or eccentric muscular contraction, its contribution as a disease mediator must be kept in balance. Stress cannot, in itself, cause an overuse injury but will exacerbate any damage present which may result in an injury.

Prevention of overuse injury from physical activity requires that the level and duration are increased gradually to allow musculoskeletal tissue time to adapt to a changed mechanical environment. In all aspects of overuse injury, the key to prevention lies in the processes of risk assessment and health promotion and, above all, absolute trust in the complaints of the affected.

References

Beck TJ, Ruff CB, Mourtada FA et al 1996 Dual-energy X-ray absorptiometry derived structural geometry for stress prediction in male US Marine Corps recruits. Journal of Bone and Mineral Research 11(5): 645–653

Benazzo F, Mosconi M, Beccarisi G et al 1995 Use of capacitive coupled electric fields in stress fractures in athletes. Clinical Orthopaedics and Related Research 310:145–149

Bengtsson A, Henriksson KG, Larsson J 1986 Muscle biopsy in primary fibromyalgia: light miroscopical and histochemical findings. Scandinavian Journal of Rheumatology 15(1): 1–6

Bjorksten M, Jonsson B 1977 Endurance limit of force in long-term intermittent static contractions. Scandinavian Journal of Work, Environment and Health 3(1): 23–27

Boyd KT, Batt ME 1997 Stress fracture of the proximal humeral epiphysis in an elite junior badminton player. British Journal of Sports Medicine 31(3): 252–253

Carragee EJ, Hentz VR 1988 Repetitive trauma and nerve compression. Orthopedic Clinics of North America 19(1): 157–164

Dahlin LB, McLean WG 1986 Effects of graded experimental compression on slow and fast axonal transport in rabbit vagus nerve. Journal of the Neurological Sciences 72(1): 19–30

Dahlin LB, Nordborg C, Lundborg G 1987 Morphologic changes in nerve cell bodies induced by experimental graded nerve compression. Experimental Neurology 95(3): 611–621

Dekel S, Papaioannou T, Rushworth G et al 1980 Idiopathic carpal tunnel syndrome caused by carpal stenosis. British Medical Journal 280: 1297–1299

Elert JE, Rantapaa-Dahlqvist SB, Henricksson-Larson K et al 1992 Muscle performance, electromyography and fibre type composition in fibromyalgia and work related myalgia. Scandinavian Journal of Rheumatology 21(1): 28–34

Feuerstein M 1996 Workstyle: definition, empirical support and implications for prevention, evaluation and rehabilitation of occupational upper extremity disorders. In: Moon SD, Sauter SL (eds) Beyond biomechanics: psychosocial aspects of musculoskeletal disorders. Taylor and Francis, London

Haddad FS, Bann S, Hill RA et al 1997 Displaced stress fracture of the femoral neck in an active amenorrhoeic adolescent. British Journal of Sports Medicine 31(1): 70–72

Hagert CG, Christenson JT 1990 Hyperpressure in the trapezius muscle associated with fibrosis. Acta Orthopaedica Scandinavica 61(3): 263–265

Ham SJ, Kolkman WF, Heeres J et al 1996 Changes in the carpal tunnel due to action of the flexor tendons: visualisation with magnetic resonance imaging. Journal of Hand Surgery 21A(6): 997–1003

Hill PF, Chatterji S, Chambers D et al 1996 Stress fracture of the pubic ramus in female recruits. Journal of Bone and Joint Surgery 78B(3): 383–386

Jones BH, Harris JM, Vinh TN et al 1989 Exercise-induced stress fractures and stress reactions of bone: epidemiology, etiology and classification. Exercise and Sport Science Reviews 17: 379–422

Kalimo H, Rantanen J, Jarvinen M 1997 Muscle injuries in sports. Clinical Orthopaedics 2(1): 1–24

Larsson SE, Bodegard L, Henriksson KG et al 1990 Chronic trapezius myalgia: morphology and blood flow studied in 17 patients. Acta Orthopaedica Scandinavica 61(5): 394–398

Lidor C, Ferris LR, Hall R et al 1997 Stress fracture of the tibia after arthrodesis of the ankle or the hindfoot. Journal of Bone and Joint Surgery 79A(4): 558–564

Lundborg G, Myers R, Powell H 1983 Nerve compression injury and increased endoneurial fluid pressure: a 'miniature compartment syndrome'. Journal of Neurology, Neurosurgery and Psychiatry 46(12): 1119–1124

Marsh GD, Paterson DH, Potwarka JJ et al 1993 Transient changes in muscle high-energy phosphates during moderate exercise. Journal of Applied Physiology 75(2): 648–656

Mense S 1993 Peripheral mechanisms of muscle nociception and local muscle pain. Journal of Musculoskeletal Pain 1: 133–170

Myers RR, Powell HC, Costello MC et al 1978 Endoneurial fluid pressure: direct measurement with micropipettes. Brain Research 148: 510–515

Netscher D, Mosharrafa A, Lee M et al 1997 Transverse carpal ligament: its effect on flexor tendon excursion, morphologic changes of the carpal canal and on pinch and grip strengths after open carpal tunnel release. Plastic and Reconstructive Surgery 100(3): 636–642

Orava S, Karpakka J, Taimela S et al 1995 Stress fracture of the medial malleolus. Journal of Bone and Joint Surgery 77A(3): 362–365

Osterman AL 1988 The double crush syndrome. Orthopedic Clinics of North America 19(1): 147–155

Petrofsky JS, Phillips CA 1986 The physiology of static exercise. Exercise and Sport Science Reviews 14: 1–44

Pheasant S 1992 Ergonomics, work and health. Macmillan, London

Pitchfork ED 1996 Law of tort, 10th edn. HLT Publications, London

Pitner MA 1990 Pathophysiology of overuse injuries in the hand and wrist. Hand Clinics 6(3): 355–364

Pollock ML, Wilmore JH 1990 Exercise in health and disease: evaluation and prescription for prevention and rehabilitation. WB Saunders, Philadelphia

Powers SK, Howley ET 1994 Exercise physiology: theory and applications to fitness and performance, 2nd edn. Brown and Benchmark, New York

Rawes ML, Patsalis T, Gregg PJ 1995 Subcapital stress fractures of the hip complicating total knee replacement. Injury 26(6): 421–423

Rydevik B, Lundborg G, Bagge U 1981 Effects of graded compression on intraneural blood flow. Journal of Hand Surgery 6A(1): 3–12

Sharkey NA, Ferris L, Smith TS et al 1995 Strain loading of the second metatarsal during heel lift. Journal of Bone and Joint Surgery 77A(7): 1050–1057

Smith JW, Murphy TR, Blair JSG et al 1983 Regional anatomy illustrated. Churchill Livingstone, Edinburgh

Szabo RM, Gelberman RH 1987 The pathophysiology of nerve entrapment syndromes. Journal of Hand Surgery 12A(5 part 2): 880–884

Tannahill A 1985 What is health promotion? Health Education Journal 44(4): 167–168

Veiersted KB, Westgaard RH, Anderson P 1990 Patterns of muscle activity during stereotyped work and its relation to muscle pain. International Archives of Occupational Health 62(1): 31–41

Weirich SD, Gelberman RH 1993 Changing concepts in the diagnosis and treatment of carpal tunnel syndrome. Current Orthopaedics 7: 218–225

Woo SLY, Hildebrand KA 1997 Healing of ligament injuries: from basic science to clinical practice. Clinical Orthopaedics 2(1): 63–79

Index

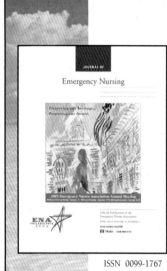